Principles of

Dear Epi,

May this gift from me becomes a stimulus for you to write better textbooks on Molecular Rheumatology. May it inspire you to improve and advance this field of Medicine.

If we, women-doctors, don't do it, who else will?

Olga
4-12-12

current
MOLECULAR MEDICINE

series editor:
J. Larry Jameson, MD, PhD

Principles of Molecular Rheumatology, edited by
George C. Tsokos, MD, 2000

Current Molecular Medicine

Principles of Molecular Rheumatology

Edited by

George C. Tsokos, MD

Walter Reed Army Institute of Research, Silver Spring, MD
Uniformed Services University of the Health Sciences, Bethesda, MD

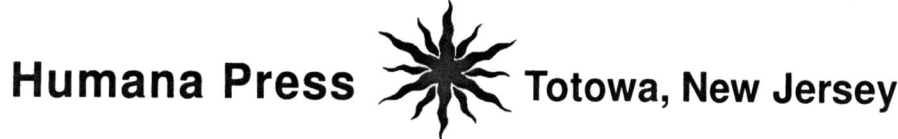

Humana Press   Totowa, New Jersey

To Sophia and Christos
To Maria

© 2010 Humana Press Inc.
999 Riverview Drive, Suite 208
Totowa, New Jersey 07512
All rights reserved.

No part of this book may be reproduced, stored in a retrieval system, or transmitted in any form or by any means, electronic, mechanical, photocopying, microfilming, recording, or otherwise without written permission from the Publisher.

All authored papers, comments, opinions, conclusions, or recommendations are those of the author(s), and do not necessarily reflect the views of the publisher.

For additional copies, pricing for bulk purchases, and/or information about other Humana titles, contact Humana at the above address or at any of the following numbers: Tel.: 973-256-1699; Fax: 973-256-8341; E-mail: humana@humanapr.com

This publication is printed on acid-free paper. ∞
ANSI Z39.48-1984 (American Standards Institute) Permanence of Paper for Printed Library Materials.

Due diligence has been taken by the publishers, editors, and authors of this book to assure the accuracy of the information published and to describe generally accepted practices. The contributors herein have carefully checked to ensure that the drug selections and dosages set forth in this text are accurate and in accord with the standards accepted at the time of publication. Notwithstanding, as new research, changes in government regulations, and knowledge from clinical experience relating to drug therapy and drug reactions constantly occurs, the reader is advised to check the product information provided by the manufacturer of each drug for any change in dosages or for additional warnings and contraindications. This is of utmost importance when the recommended drug herein is a new or infrequently used drug. It is the responsibility of the treating physician to determine dosages and treatment strategies for individual patients. Further it is the responsibility of the health care provider to ascertain the Food and Drug Administration status of each drug or device used in their clinical practice. The publisher, editors, and authors are not responsible for errors or omissions or for any consequences from the application of the information presented in this book and make no warranty, express or implied, with respect to the contents in this publication.

Cover design by Patricia F. Cleary.
Cover art from:

Photocopy Authorization Policy:
Authorization to photocopy items for internal or personal use, or the internal or personal use of specific clients, is granted by Humana Press Inc., provided that the base fee of US $10.00 per copy, plus US $00.25 per page, is paid directly to the Copyright Clearance Center at 222 Rosewood Drive, Danvers, MA 01923. For those organizations that have been granted a photocopy license from the CCC, a separate system of payment has been arranged and is acceptable to Humana Press Inc.

Printed in the United States of America. 10 9 8 7 6 5 4 3 2 1

Library of Congress Cataloging-in-Publication Data
Principles of molecular rheumatology / edited by George C. Tsokos.
    p. ; cm. -- (Current molecular medicine)
  Includes bibliographical references and index.
  ISBN 978-1-61737-182-0   e-ISBN 978-1-59259-018-6
  1. Rheumatism--Molecular aspects. 2. Arthritis--Molecular aspects. 3. Rheumatism--Pathophysiology. 4. Arthritis--Pathophysiology. I. Tsokos, George C. II. Series.
    [DNLM: 1. Rheumatic Diseases--genetics. 2. Rheumatic diseases--physiopathology. 3. Rheumatic Diseases--therapy. WE 544 P9567 2000]
RC927 .P676 2000
616.7'23'07--dc21
                              00-24930

Preface

"...we simply do not know enough, we are still a largely ignorant profession, faced by an array of illnesses which we do not really understand, unable to do much beyond trying to make the right diagnosis, shoring things up whenever we can by one halfway technology or another..."

Lewis Thomas,
The Fragile Species, TOUCHSTONE, *New York, 1992*

Principles of Molecular Rheumatology has been organized to help Rheumatology Fellows, House Officers, and Rheumatologists better understand the molecular and cellular aspects of Rheumatic Diseases. The ambition of the editor and the authors is to present and discuss the pathogenesis of rheumatic diseases in a concise manner. We hope that *Principles of Molecular Rheumatology* will facilitate the introduction of clinical trainees to the science of Rheumatology and will serve as a helpful accessory in reviewing basic and clinical articles with reference to basic science issues. Furthermore, it is our intention to help those students of human disease who do not have a formal medical training gain an informed perspective on rheumatic diseases.

The first section of *Principles of Molecular Rheumatology* discusses the molecular mechanisms that are central to many rheumatic diseases. Established authors present the biochemical mechanisms by which apoptosis, cell signaling, complement, lipids, and viruses contribute to disease expression. The second section reviews immune and nonimmune cell function as it relates to rheumatic diseases. The function of lymphocytes, monocytes, neutrophils, synoviocytes, chondrocytes, and bone cells is discussed. The third section takes a synthetic approach to disease. The authors present integrated discussions of the cellular, biochemical, and molecular biological mechanisms that are directly important to disease pathogenesis. Major diseases are reviewed and concepts are formulated. In the final section, the molecular aspects of those therapeutics that are routinely used in rheumatic diseases are discussed. The emphasis on mechanisms rather than clinical pharmacology aims at familiarizing the reader with what is being accomplished at the molecular and cellular levels following the administration of each medication.

Principles of Molecular Rheumatology does not replace any of the classic textbooks in Rheumatology. Rather, it adopts a fresh perspective designed to enhance the understanding of Rheumatology by emphasizing the importance of knowledge of molecular and cellular pathophysiology to the mastery of rheumatic diseases.

I am grateful to the authors for many exciting discussions on the format and content of the book and for their enthusiasm and support, which provided me with the stamina to see the project to its completion. I learned so much from my interactions with my esteemed colleagues, authors of *Principles of Molecular Rheumatology*, that I do not seek reward. My only hope is that *Principles of Molecular Rheumatology* will help our fellow Rheumatologists better serve the patients who suffer from rheumatic diseases. The unwavering support of Paul Dolgert is once more appreciated. Craig Adams and Elyse O'Grady are responsible for all the good things in this book, whereas I am responsible for its shortcomings

George C. Tsokos, MD

Contents

Preface v
Contributors xi

PART I. MOLECULAR MECHANISMS IN RHEUMATIC DISEASES

1 Genetics
  Peter K. Gregersen 3

2 Viruses
  Andras Perl 15

3 Apoptosis
  John D. Mountz, Hui-Chen Hsu, Huang-Ge Zhang, and Tong Zhou 35

4 Humoral Response
  Gary S. Gilkeson 59

5 T-Cell Signaling
  Gary A. Koretzky and Erik J. Peterson 75

6 Adhesion and Costimulatory Molecules
  Vassiliki A. Boussiotis, Gordon J. Freeman, and Lee M. Nadler 87

7 Transcription Factors
  Henry K. Wong 109

8 Immune Complexes
  Mark H. Wener 127

9 Complement
  V. Michael Holers 145

10 Eicosanoids and Other Bioactive Lipids
  Leslie J. Crofford 161

11 Collagens
   Sergio A. Jiménez *175*

PART II. CELLULAR MECHANISMS IN RHEUMATIC DISEASES

12 T-Lymphocytes
   Nilamadhab Mishra and Gary M. Kammer *199*

13 B-Lymphocytes
   Robert F. Ashman *213*

14 Monocytes and Macrophages
   James M. K. Chan and Sharon M. Wahl *225*

15 Polymorphonuclear Cells
   Michael H. Pillinger, Pamela B. Rosenthal, and Bruce N. Cronstein *243*

16 Synoviocytes
   David E. Yocum *259*

17 Chondrocytes
   Tariq M. Haqqi, Donald D. Anthony, and Charles J. Malemud *267*

18 Osteoblasts and Osteoclasts
   Stavros C. Manolagas *279*

19 Animal Models
   Thomas J. Lang and Charles S. Via *293*

PART III. PATHOGENESIS OF RHEUMATIC DISEASES

20 Systemic Lupus Erythematosus
   Stamatis-Nick C. Liossis and George C. Tsokos *311*

21 Rheumatoid Arthritis
   Richard M. Pope and Harris Perlman *325*

22 Inflammatory Myopathies
   Norbert Goebels and Reinhard Hohlfeld *363*

23 Systemic Sclerosis
   Timothy M. Wright *375*

24 Vasculitis
   Jörg J. Goronzy and Cornelia M. Weyand *385*

25 Osteoarthritis
   A. Robin Poole and Ginette Webb *401*

26 Osteoporosis
   Stavros C. Manolagas *413*

27 Heritable Disorders of Connective Tissue
   Petros Tsipouras *423*

PART IV. MOLECULAR ASPECTS OF TREATMENT OF RHEUMATIC DISEASES

28 Corticosteroids
   Henry K. Wong and George C. Tsokos *439*

29 Cytotoxic Drugs
   David A. Fox and W. Joseph McCune *451*

30 Complement Inhibitors
   Savvas C. Makrides *465*

31 Cytokine Response Modifiers
   Richard E. Jones and Larry W. Moreland *477*

32 Restoration of Immune Tolerance
   Woodruff Emlen *487*

33 Metalloproteases and Their Modulation as Treatment in Osteoarthritis
   *Johanne Martel-Pelletier, Ginette Tardif, Julio Fernandes,
   and Jean-Pierre Pelletier* *499*

34 Gene Therapy
   Robert P. Kimberly *515*

Index *525*

Contributors

DONALD D. ANTHONY, MD, PhD • *Division of Rheumatic Diseases, Department of Medicine, Case Western Reserve University, Cleveland, OH*

ROBERT F. ASHMAN, MD • *Division of Rheumatology, Department of Medicine, University of Iowa College of Medicine and Department of Veterans Affairs Medical Center, Iowa City, IA*

VASSILIKI A. BOUSSIOTIS, MD • *Department of Adult Oncology, Dana Farber Cancer Institute and Department of Medicine, Harvard Medical School, Boston, MA*

JAMES M. K. CHAN, PhD • *Oral Infection and Immunity Branch, National Institute of Dental and Craniofacial Research, National Institute of Health, Bethesda, MD*

LESLIE J. CROFFORD, MD • *Division of Rheumatology Internal Medicine, University of Michigan, Ann Arbor, MI*

BRUCE N. CRONSTEIN, MD • *Bellevue Hospital Center, and Division of Rheumatology, Departments of Medicine and Pathology, New York University School of Medicine, New York, NY*

WOODRUFF EMLEN, MD • *Exploratory Medicine, Connetics Corporation, Palo Alto, CA*

JULIO C. FERNANDES, MD, MSc • *Osteoarthritis Research Unit, Centre Hospitalier de l'Université de Montréal, Hôpital Notre-Dame, Montréal, Canada*

DAVID A. FOX, MD • *Division of Rheumatology, University of Michigan Multipurpose Arthritis and Musculoskeletal Diseases Center, University of Michigan Medical Center, Ann Arbor, MI*

GORDON J. FREEMAN • *Department of Adult Oncology, Dana Farber Cancer Institute and Department of Medicine, Harvard Medical School, Boston, MA*

GARY S. GILKESON, MD • *Division of Rheumatology, Medical University of South Carolina, Charleston, SC*

NORBERT GOEBELS, MD • *Department of Neurology and Institute for Clinical Neuroimmunology, Klinikum Grosshadern, Ludwig Maximilians-University of Munich, Munich, Germany*

JÖRG J. GORONZY, MD • *Division of Rheumatology, Department of Medicine, Mayo Clinic and Foundation, Rochester, MN*

PETER K. GREGERSEN, MD • *Departments of Medicine and Pathology, New York University School of Medicine and Chief, Division of Biology and Human Genetics, North Shore University Hospital, Manhasset, NY*

TARIQ M. HAQQI, PhD • *Division of Rheumatic Diseases, Department of Medicine, Case Western Reserve University, Cleveland, OH*

REINHARD HOHLFELD, MD • *Department of Neurology and Institute for Clinical Neuroimmunology, Klinikum Grosshadern, Ludwig Maximilians-University of Munich, Munich, Germany*

V. MICHAEL HOLERS, MD • *Divison of Rheumatology, Departments of Medicine and Immunology, University of Colorado Health Sciences Center, Denver, CO*

HUI-CHEN HSU, PhD • *Division of Clinical Immunology and Rheumatology, Department of Medicine, University of Alabama at Birmingham, and the Birmingham Veterans Administration Medical Center, Birmingham, AL*
SERGIO A. JIMÉNEZ, MD • *Division of Rheumatology, Department of Medicine, Jefferson Medical College, Thomas Jefferson University, Philadelphia, PA*
RICHARD E. JONES, MD, PhD • *Division of Clinical Immunology and Rheumatology, Department of Medicine, University of Alabama at Birmingham, Birmingham, AL*
GARY M. KAMMER, MD • *Section on Rheumatology and Clinical Immunology, Department of Internal Medicine, Wake Forest University School of Medicine, Winston-Salem, NC*
ROBERT P. KIMBERLY, MD • *Division of Clinical Immunology and Rheumatology, and University of Alabama at Birmingham Arthritis and Musculoskeletal Center, Birmingham, AL*
GARY A. KORETZKY, MD, PhD • *Leonard and Madlyn Abramson Family Cancer Research Institute, Department of Pathology and Laboratory Medicine, University of Pennsylvania School of Medicine, Philadelphia, PA*
THOMAS J. LANG, MD, PhD • *Division of Rheumatology, Department of Medicine, University of Maryland School of Medicine, Baltimore Veterans Affairs Medical Center, Baltimore, MD*
STAMATIS-NICK C. LIOSSIS, MD • *Division of Rheumatology and Immunology, Department of Medicine, Uniformed Services University of the Health Sciences, Bethesda, MD*
SAVVAS C. MAKRIDES, PhD • *EIC Laboratories Inc, Norwood, MA*
CHARLES J. MALEMUD, PhD • *Division of Rheumatic Diseases, Department of Medicine, Case Western Reserve University, Cleveland, OH*
STAVROS C. MANOLAGAS, MD, PhD • *Center for Osteoporosis and Metabolic Bone Diseases, Division of Endocrinology and Metabolism, University of Arkansas for Medical Sciences, and the Central Arkansas Veterans Healthcare System, Little Rock, AR*
JOHANNE MARTEL-PELLETIER, PhD • *Osteoarthritis Research Unit, Centre Hospitalier de l'Université de Montréal, Hôpital Notre-Dame, Montréal, Canada*
W. JOSEPH MCCUNE, MD • *Division of Rheumatology, Department of Internal Medicine, University of Michigan Medical Center, Ann Arbor, MI*
NILAMADHAB MISHRA, MD • *Section on Rheumatology and Clinical Immunology, Department of Internal Medicine, Wake Forest University School of Medicine, Winston-Salem, NC*
LARRY W. MORELAND, MD • *Division of Clinical Immunology and Rheumatology, Department of Medicine, University of Alabama at Birmingham, Birmingham, AL*
JOHN D. MOUNTZ, MD, PhD • *Division of Clinical Immunology and Rheumatology, Department of Medicine, University of Alabama at Birmingham and the Birmingham Veterans Administration Medical Center, Birmingham, AL*
LEE M. NADLER • *Department of Adult Oncology, Dana Farber Cancer Institute and Department of Medicine, Harvard Medical School, Boston, MA*
JEAN-PIERRE PELLETIER, MD • *Rheumatic Disease Unit, Université de Montréal, and Osteoarthritis Research Unit, Centre Hospitalier de l'Université de Montréal, Hôpital Notre-Dame, Montréal, Canada*
ANDRAS PERL, MD, PhD • *Section of Rheumatology, Department of Medicine, State University of New York Health Science Center, College of Medicine, Syracuse, NY*

Contributors

HARRIS PERLMAN • *Division of Rheumatology, Northwestern University Medical School, Chicago, IL*

ERIK J. PETERSON, MD • *Division of Rheumatology, Department of Medicine, University of Pennsylvania and the Abramson Family Cancer Research Institute, Philadelphia, PA*

MICHAEL H. PILLINGER, MD • *Division of Rheumatology, Department of Medicine, New York University School of Medicine, Department of Rheumatology, The Hospital for Joint Diseases, and Department of Rheumatology, Manhattan VA Hospital, New York, NY*

RICHARD M. POPE, MD • *Division of Rheumatology, Northwestern Multipurpose Arthritis and Musculoskeletal Diseases Center, Northwestern University Medical School, Chicago, IL*

A. ROBIN POOLE, PHD, DSC • *Departments of Surgery and Medicine, McGill University and Shriners Hospitals for Children, Montreal, Canada*

PAMELA B. ROSENTHAL, MD • *Divison of Rheumatology, Department of Medicine, New York University School of Medicine, and Department of Rheumatology, The Hospital for Joint Diseases, New York, NY*

GINETTE TARDIF, PHD • *Osteoarthritis Research Unit, Centre Hospitalier de l'Université de Montréal, Hôpital Notre-Dame, Montréal, Canada*

PETROS TSIPOURAS, MD • *Department of Pediatrics, University of Connecticut Health Center, Farmington, CT*

GEORGE C. TSOKOS, MD• *Department of Cellular Injury, Walter Reed Army Institute of Research, Silver Spring, and Division of Rheumatology and Immunology, Department of Medicine, Uniformed Services University of the Health Sciences, Bethesda, MD*

CHARLES S. VIA, MD • *Division of Rheumatology, Department of Medicine, University of Maryland School of Medicine, and Baltimore Veterans Affairs Medical Center, Baltimore, MD*

SHARON M. WAHL, PHD • *Oral Infection and Immunity Branch, National Institute of Dental and Craniofacial Research, National Institute of Health, Bethesda, MD*

GINETTE WEBB, PHD • *Joint Diseases Laboratory, Shriners Hospitals for Children and Department of Surgery, McGill University, Montreal, Canada*

MARK H. WENER, MD • *Immunology Division, Department of Laboratory Medicine, and Rheumatology Division, Department of Medicine, University of Washington, Seattle, WA*

CORNELIA M. WEYAND, MD • *Division of Rheumatology, Department of Medicine, Mayo Clinic and Foundation, Rochester, MN*

HENRY K. WONG, MD • *Department of Dermatology, and Division of Rheumatology and Immunology, Department of Medicine, Uniformed Services University for the Health Sciences, Bethesda, MD, and Department of Cellular Injury, Walter Reed Army Institute of Research, Washington, DC*

TIMOTHY M. WRIGHT, MD • *Division of Rheumatology and Clinical Immunology, Department of Medicine, University of Pittsburgh Arthritis Institute, University of Pittsburgh, Pittsburgh, PA*

DAVID E. YOCUM, MD • *Arizona Arthritis Center, University of Arizona, Tucson, AZ*

HUANG-GE ZHANG, PHD, DVM • *Division of Clinical Immunology and Rheumatology, Department of Medicine, University of Alabama at Birmingham, Birmingham, AL*

TONG ZHOU, MD • *Division of Clinical Immunology and Rheumatology, Department of Medicine, University of Alabama at Birmingham, Birmingham, AL*

I

MOLECULAR MECHANISMS IN RHEUMATIC DISEASES

1
Genetics

Peter K. Gregersen

1. Introduction

With a few exceptions, rheumatic diseases are similar to many other common medical conditions in that they are genetically complex, with a multifactorial etiology. Simple Mendelian disorders (autosomal dominant, recessive, or sex linked) are encountered relatively infrequently in rheumatologic practice, although some exciting successes in this area (notably the cloning of the gene for familial Mediterranean fever; *see* ref. *1*) may ultimately lead to new approaches to the general problem of inflammation. It is clearly important for the rheumatologist to be aware of the Mendelian diseases that can rarely underlie common rheumatologic conditions such as gout (e.g., PP-ribose-P synthetase overactivity or hypoxanthine guanine phosphoribosyltransferase (HGPRT) deficiency). Beyond this, the problem of genetics in rheumatic disease may strike the newcomer as dauntingly complicated and of limited utility. The purpose of this chapter is to provide the tools to approach this topic with confidence. It will be necessary for the educated rheumatologist to have some ability to interpret the wealth of genetic information that is likely to emerge over the next few years because of the completion of the Human Genome Project *(2)* and the application of genetic mapping techniques to the major rheumatic diseases.

2. Multifactorial Diseases and the Concept of Genetic Risk

It is useful to consider many of the rheumatic diseases, such as systemic lupus and rheumatoid arthritis, as the result of an interaction among genetic and nongenetic factors. Over time, this process may lead to the clinical expression of disease. The nongenetic factors may include specific environmental exposures (such as infection, blood transfusion or smoking; *see* refs. *3–5*), as well as a variety of stochastic factors (i.e., random events that may occur from early fetal life on into adulthood; discussed in ref. *6*). These etiological factors combine to produce disease, as well as the variable manifestations and degree of severity that is observed in patient populations with rheumatic diseases. Given the complexity of these interactions, it is not surprising that a simple one-to-one correlation between genes and disease is not observed.

Nevertheless, it is possible to assign a weight to the role of particular factors in susceptibility to, or risk for, a specific disease or clinical manifestation. In the case of

---

From: *Current Molecular Medicine: Principles of Molecular Rheumatology*
Edited by: G. C. Tsokos © Humana Press Inc., Totowa, NJ

genetic factors, we wish to identify particular genetic variants (alleles; see Subheading 12. for an explanation of genetic terms used in this chapter) that confer risk for disease. In the simplest formulation, an allele confers increased risk when the conditional probability of disease, D, in a population of individuals (over a lifetime) is greater in the presence of particular allele, A, than in its absence. This can be formally expressed as:

$$P(D \mid A) > P(D \mid \text{not } A)$$

An estimate of the ratio of these two probabilities can be assessed in various ways, as discussed later. The important point here is that modern approaches to genetics and epidemiology allow us to quantify these effects and ultimately identify genes that confer disease risk, even when many other factors may contribute "noise" and obscure the underlying genetic component.

3. Estimating the Strength of the Overall Genetic Component in Rheumatic Disease

We know for a fact that genetic background contributes to the risk for almost all autoimmune diseases; it is well established that genes within the major histocompatibility complex (MHC) confer risk for these disorders in both humans and animals [7–9]. However, it is also apparent that MHC genes are not the only genes involved in susceptibility, and it is therefore useful to have some idea of size of the overall genetic component. In the absence of knowledge about specific alleles, the only way to obtain this information is by comparing the prevalence of disease among populations with different degrees of genetic relatedness.

The most useful types of populations for these comparison are (1) genetically identical individuals (MZ twins), (2) individuals who have approximately 50% of their genes in common (DZ twins and siblings), and (3) unrelated individuals in the population. For the latter group of unrelated individuals, the overall degree of genetic similarity (at polymorphic loci) is relatively low, with approximately a 0.1% difference over the entire genome [2]. (Note that a 0.1% difference over the entire human genome of 3.2×10^9 base pairs implies approximately 3 million base pair differences between any two unrelated individuals, assuming that single nucleotide polymorphisms account for the majority of these differences.)

For identical (MZ) twins, the concordance rates for most autoimmune diseases are between 15% and 30% [10,11]. Put another way, if one takes 100 probands with autoimmunity who are members of MZ twin pairs, then between 15 and 30 of their genetically identical co-twins also will have the disease. As discussed, the fact that these concordance rates are substantially below 100% clearly indicates that nongenetic factors play a role. However, if one compares this MZ twin concordance rate with the concordance rate among DZ twins or siblings (who only have half their alleles in common), the rate drops considerably to around 2–5%. This fact alone indicates that complete sharing of genetic background with an affected individual substantially increases one's risk for disease. (In this case, we are assuming that shared environmental factors are approximately equivalent among MZ and DZ twin pairs).

In order to get a sense of the overall genetic risk, we need to compare these rates to the prevalence of disease in a genetically unrelated population (i.e., the background population prevalence). Depending on the autoimmune disease, background popula-

Table 1
Estimates of $\lambda_s{}^a$ and λ_{MZ} for Some Common Autoimmune Disorders

Disease	λ_s	λ_{MZ}
Systemic Lupus	20	250
Rheumatoid arthritis	3–10	20–60
Multiple sclerosis	20	250
Type I diabetes	15	60
Ankylosing spondylitis	54	500

^{a}See ref. 12.

tion prevalence ranges from 0.1% to 1%. These values can then be used to calculate two ratios, termed the relative risk to siblings (λ_s) and the relative risk to MZ twins (λ_{MZ}):

$$\lambda_s = \frac{\text{Disease prevalence in siblings of affected individuals}}{\text{Disease prevalence in general population}}$$

$$\lambda_{MZ} = \frac{\text{Disease prevalence in monzygotic co-twins of affected individuals}}{\text{Disease prevalence in general population}}$$

The values of these two ratios for various autoimmune disorders is given in Table 1. Clearly, if you have a sibling (or an identical twin) with one of these disorders, you are at substantially increased risk for the disease, compared with the general population. It is likely that genetic factors are largely responsible for this increased risk, although, of course, these risk ratios also take into account environmental factors that may be preferentially shared among family members. It has been estimated that MHC genes account for 50% or less of this risk in most cases *(12)*.

4. Measuring the Risk Associated with Particular Genes

The above calculations establish that genetic background contributes to risk for rheumatic disorders, but they do not provide us with insight into the role of particular genes. There are a variety of approaches to this problem. The most widely used method is the case control study design, and it is important to thoroughly understand the rationale, terminology, and conventions used to report the results from such studies.

In an ideal world, in order to determine whether there is an association between a particular allelic polymorphism and a disease, one would identify subjects with and without the allele of interest and follow them from birth until death to see if disease is more common in the group carrying the test allele. This is known as a cohort study and it is the most direct approach to comparing the probabilities referred to earlier. The data from such a study can be tabulated as shown in Table 2, and used to calculate the relative risk (RR):

$$RR = a/(a+b) \div c/(c+d)$$

The relative risk is a measure how much more (or less) likely you are to get the disease (over a lifetime) if you inherit the allele of interest. If the disease is uncommon

Table 2
Contingency Table for Cohort Study

	Disease	No disease
Exposed	a	b
Not exposed	c	d

Table 3
Contingency Table for Case Control Study

	Exposed	Not exposed
Disease	a	b
No disease	c	d

(a and c are small), then the relative risk can be estimated from the quantity $(a \times d)/(c \times b)$, also known as the cross-product of Table 2.

In reality, cohort studies are either impractical or very expensive because they require extended periods of follow up of the two populations. Therefore, rather than select the initial populations on the basis of genotype, the test and control populations are selected on the basis of whether they have disease, and the frequency of the allele is measured in each group. This is a case control design and the results are tabulated as shown in Table 3. If the disease is rare (as is the case for the major rheumatic diseases), an estimate of the relative risk, also known as the odds ratio, can be calculated as before using the cross product $(a \times d)/(c \times b)$ from Table 3.

The vast majority of data showing the association between human leukocyte antigen (HLA) alleles and autoimmune disease have been generated using a case control study design *(7–9)*. In general, the estimated relative risks are less than 10, with the exception of HLA-B27 and the spondyloarthropathies, where the RR values approach 100 for ankylosing spondylitis. Even when HLA analysis is done on the basis of particular amino acid sequences, such as the association of the "shared epitope" on HLA DR4 with rheumatoid arthritis, the overall risk calculations are still rather modest *(7)*.

5. Interpreting Case Control Genetic Association Studies: The Concept of Linkage Disequilibrium

When a positive association (RR > 1) is found between an allelic polymorphism and a disease, one is tempted to assume that the allele being investigated has something directly to do with the pathogenesis of the illness with which it associates. Although this may be the case, other explanations are more likely, at least initially. First, one must establish whether the association is statistically significant. This usually involves the calculation of a χ^2 and determination of a *p*-value and confidence interval using standard approaches *(13)*. Beyond the statistical considerations however, there are several issues that are specific to genetic association studies and are critical for their interpretation.

First, genetic polymorphisms occur at particular locations on chromosomes and are surrounded by many other polymorphisms nearby in the genome. These "neighborhoods" of particular alleles tend to cluster together on haplotypes in human populations, a phenomenon in population genetics known as linkage disequilibrium. This means that alleles that are located very near to one another (say, less than 500,000 base pairs apart) are often found together in the same individual, that is, more often than you would expect by chance.

To take an example, hemochromatosis is a disease of iron absorption (which, incidentally, can cause a distinct form of arthritis). This disease is autosomal recessive and is expressed in approximately 0.2–0.3% of Caucasian populations. It is caused by mutations in the *HFE* gene on chromosome 6 *(14)*, quite near the major histocompatibility complex (MHC). A typical class I allele within the MHC, HLA-A3, is present in approximately 25% of the Caucasian population. Because HLA-A3 has nothing to do with causing hemochromatosis, one might also expect that only 25% of patients with this disease would carry HLA-A3. However, what has been frequently observed in Caucasian populations is that upward of 70% of hemochromatosis patients carry HLA-A3. This is because HLA-A3 is in linkage disequilibrium with common mutations in the *HFE* gene. Indeed, it was the early observation of an association between particular HLA alleles and hemochromatosis that led to the initial localization of the *HFE* gene. Although *HFE* shares some homology with MHC class I genes, it does not have the classical functions of HLA molecules in antigen presentation, but rather interacts with transferrin, a key regulator of iron transport *(14)*. The estimated RR for HLA-A3 and hemochromatosis is in the range of 10, yet HLA-A3 has nothing whatsoever to do with the pathogenesis of hemochromatosis. This emphasizes that many, indeed most, genetic associations are likely the result of linkage disequilibrium between the test allele and the disease alleles; the actual genes responsible for the association are somewhere else in the genetic neighborhood. Using case control methods, it is nearly impossible to definitively prove that a particular allele is the "cause" of the association without resorting to other experimental methods that show the mechanism underlying the association.

6. The Problem of "Population Stratification" in Studies of Genetic Association

The second major issue that needs to be considered in genetic case control studies is the problem of "population stratification." This refers to the fact that, in order for the results to be valid, the control group must be matched to the disease group for every parameter except the disease under study. One obvious parameter is ethnicity, because it is well known that genetic polymorphisms differ in their prevalence in different ethnic groups; it is clearly not appropriate to study the association of lupus with blue eyes in Sweden if the control group is taken from Italy! However, there may be other hidden differences between the disease and control groups that are not immediately apparent. This is especially true in the United States, where the population is very heterogeneous and where local controls drawn from laboratory or hospital personnel may actually differ in genetic background despite belonging to the same general racial group as the disease population.

In order to get around the problem of population stratification, the use of family-based controls has become very popular in recent years. One such method is to calculate the "haplotype relative risk" *(15)*. Consider the nuclear family shown in Fig. 1,

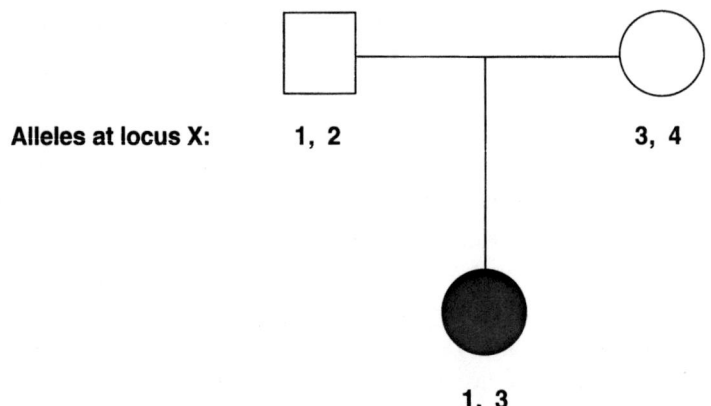

Fig. 1. A nuclear family with an affected child and both parents heterozygous at an autosomal marker locus, X. Alleles are indicated by the numbers. This family is useful for family based association studies, such at transmission disequilibrium testing (TDT).

with an affected individual carrying alleles 1 and 3 at a candidate locus, X. Both parents are heterozygous at this locus, with 1,2 and 3,4 carried by the father and mother, respectively. The parental haplotypes carrying the 2 and 4 alleles are not inherited by the affected child. These two noninherited haplotypes therefore can be used to construct a genotype for a control "individual." Although the generation of this control genotype requires typing two people instead of one, it has a major advantage: The test alleles (those transmitted to the child) are derived from exactly the same population (the parents) as the control alleles. There can be no question of population stratification here, because, in effect, the same individuals are used as a source for the two groups of alleles (those found in affecteds and those found in controls). These data can be used to construct a contingency table, just like the one shown in Table 3.

A variant of this approach is termed "transmission disequilibrium testing" or TDT *(16,17)*. Again, consider the family shown in Fig. 1. For a heterozygous parent (such as 1,2 in the father), there is a probability of 0.5 that any given allele, say allele 1, will be transmitted to a child. Thus, if this allele has no bearing on disease risk, the probability of transmission (T) to an affected child is equal to the probability of nontransmission (NT). This is stated simply as $P(T|D) = P(NT|D)$, where D indicates the presence of disease in the child. However, if the allele being examined is associated with disease risk, then $P(T|D) > P(NT|D)$. By examining large numbers of heterozygous parents with affected offspring, transmission disequilibrium testing can establish differences in disease association between test alleles and control alleles, both derived from the same individuals (the parents). Like the haplotype relative risk method, the problem of population stratification is avoided.

7. Why Is It Important to Understand Genetic Association Data?

From the perspective of the clinical rheumatologist, the preceding discussion of genetic association studies is probably the most important aspect of genetics to understand, because it is likely that most of the new knowledge about the genetic basis of rheumatic disease will derive from such studies. In addition, these association data

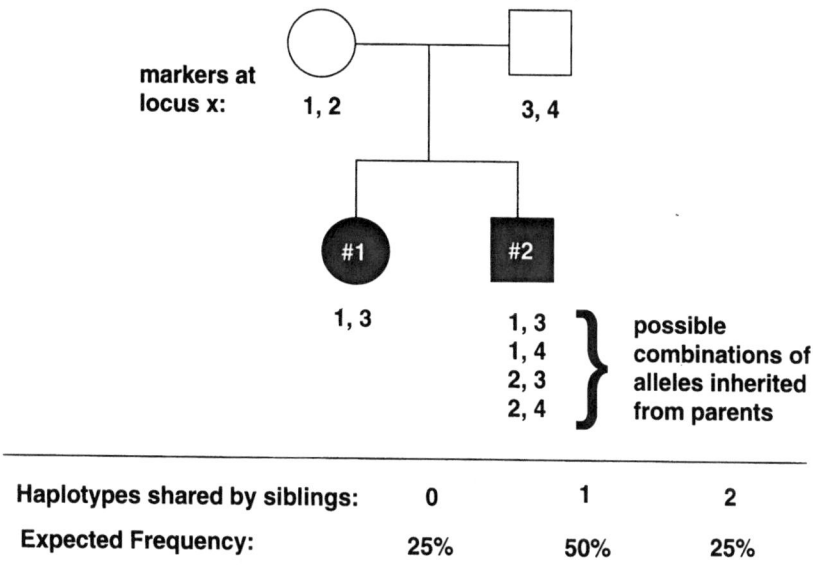

Fig. 2. A nuclear family with two affected children (affected sibling pair). The possible distribution of alleles at an autosomal locus, X is shown for sib 2, along with the predicted frequency of shared haplotypes among the sibs.

may well inform clinical decision making in the future. It is important to point out that most case control studies so far have simply examined the genetic influence on the presence or absence of a particular disease. However, it is likely that future studies will reveal associations between allelic polymorphisms and disease prognosis or response to therapy. Indeed, in the case of rheumatoid arthritis, it appears that genes in the MHC also influence disease outcome *(18,19)*, as well as risk for disease *per se*. In addition, hardly any data has been gathered on the role of particular *combinations* of alleles *(20)*. Because multiple genes probably contribute to the major rheumatic disorders, addressing this issue will become increasingly important over the coming decade. An understanding of the relative risk calculation will be essential in making intelligent use of these genetic data in the context of patient care.

8. The Concept of Genetic Linkage and Affected Sibling Pair Analysis

Despite the fact that association studies are likely to dominate the field in the future, it is nevertheless important to have some understanding of other approaches to finding disease genes. This involves the concept of linkage. A thorough discussion of this topic is beyond the scope of this chapter and can be found elsewhere *(21)*. However, genetic linkage underlies some of the most important current studies of genetics in rheumatic diseases, many of which utilize an analytic method known as affected sibling pair (ASP) analysis.

Briefly, linkage methods seek to find a relationship between a phenotype or disease and particular *genetic locations, within families*. This is in contrast to association methods, which are designed to look for relationships between a disease and particular *alleles, in populations*. Consider the family shown in Fig. 2, in which there are two siblings, each affected with a disease or phenotype. In these cases, the affected siblings *within each family* are highly likely (although not certain) to be carriers of the same disease gene(s). This assumption is based on the fact that the λ_s calculation is high enough to indicate a substantial genetic component to the disease (as discussed earlier) and that the genes involved are not so heterogeneous and so common in the population that affected sib pairs within a family are likely to have the disease on the basis of inheriting different susceptibility genes.

In the family shown in Fig. 2, both siblings are affected; given the fact that the first born sibling (sib #1) is 1,3, sibling #2 could have inherited one of four genotypes (1,3; 2,3; 1,4; or 2,4) with equal probability. There is a 25% chance that sib #2 inherited the identical alleles found in sib #1. By a similar reasoning, there is a 50% probability that these two siblings will share only one allele, and a 25% chance that they will share nothing in common at all at this locus. If, however, the marker locus X is located very near to a disease gene, one would expect that such affected siblings would tend to share alleles more frequently than predicted by these Mendelian segregation ratios. By examining large numbers of affected sibling pairs, one can develop statistical evidence that this is the case for a given test marker locus, using a straightforward χ^2 analysis, with the null hypothesis being that there is no increased sharing of alleles at the marker locus. This is the essence of ASP analysis; a discussion of some additional aspects of the method can be found in ref. *20*.

The ASP method has been used to search for genes involved in a number of autoimmune diseases including systemic lupus and rheumatoid arthritis *(22–25)*. Although the results are still preliminary, overall they suggest that there are a number of different regions outside the MHC that are involved in disease susceptibility. Confirmation of these findings will ultimately require detailed association studies in large populations.

9. The Nature of Genetic Markers

Genetic variability among individuals underlies all forms of genetic analysis, whether it be association- or linkage-based methods. However, different types of genetic markers may be used, depending on the specific question being addressed.

Until recently, most genetic studies of rheumatic disease have involved the study of allelic variation with the major histocompatibility complex. Early on, these studies utilized detection methods based on variation in the HLA proteins themselves, either by alloantisera or T-cell reactivity. Although these methods do not directly assess DNA sequence variation, they, nevertheless, constitute "genetic" markers and these detection methods serve to emphasize the fact that these genetic variations are relevant to immune recognition. Currently, HLA alleles are detected by searching directly for differences in DNA sequence at precisely defined locations within each HLA gene. This is usually done after amplification of these genes using polymerase chain reaction (PCR), followed by oligonucleotide hybridization or direct DNA sequencing; large databases of the different HLA alleles are available for comparison on the Web (http://www.ebi.ac.uk/imgt/hla/). In the case of HLA, particular polymorphisms are assessed because they are candidates for being directly involved in disease susceptibility *(7–9)*. Many other candidate genes have been proposed for study in a similar manner *(26)*. Thus, some genetic markers are selected because of their intrinsic biological interest, regardless of their "informativeness" at a genetic level (*see* Subheading 10.).

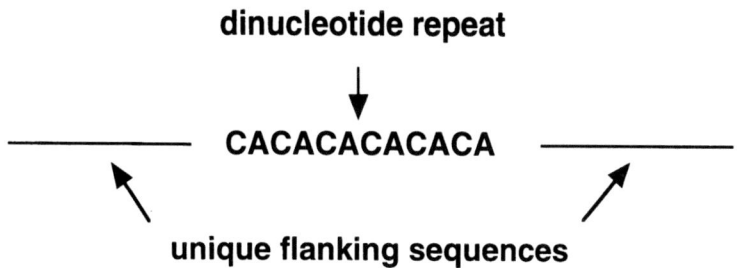

Fig. 3. Essential features of a microsatellite marker locus. A highly variable tandem repeated sequence (in this case a dinucleotide repeat) is flanked by a unique DNA sequence, which can be used to make primers for PCR amplification.

In the absence of a specific hypothesis about a particular allele, genetic analysis can also be done using genetic markers that do not themselves have biological relevance. Commonly used markers of this type are so-called "microsatellites" *(27)*, which contain variable numbers of tandem repeats (VNTRs). These tandem repeated elements most often consist of di-, tri-, or tetranucleotide sequences. Most importantly, as outlined in Fig. 3, these repeated elements are flanked by regions of unique sequences that occur only once in the genome. Thus, one can design PCR primers that specifically amplify a particular VNTR, at a particular location in the genome. The different alleles are easily distinguished on the basis of size, because this is a function of the number of repeats. Many thousands of microsatellites have been identified in the human genome, and semiautomated methods for their analysis are standard in genetic research laboratories.

10. How Useful Is a Genetic Marker? Calculation of Heterozygosity

Because microsatellites have a well-defined location in the genome, they are clearly useful for ASP analysis or other approaches based on linkage. This is because, as discussed earlier, linkage methods seek to find a relationship between a genetic location and a disease. Microsatellites can also be used for association studies if there is linkage disequilibrium between the microsatellite locus and a disease locus. However, some microsatellites are more useful, or "informative," than others. This depends on a quantity called heterozygosity.

Heterozygosity *(H)*, or the overall degree of polymorphism at a particular locus in a population, can be assessed in two ways: empirically and by calculation from allele frequencies. The empirical method involves genotyping a large number of subjects and recording the frequency of individuals who are heterozygous at the particular locus. This kind of information is generally not available for a large number of markers in different populations.

Heterozygosity is more frequently calculated from knowledge about the frequency of the various alleles at the marker locus:

$$H = 1 - \sum p_i^2$$

where p_i is the frequency of the ith allele at the marker locus. For example, if there are three alleles at the locus with a frequency of 0.1, 0.4, and 0.5, then the heterozygosity would be 1 − (0.01 + 0.16 + 0.25) = 0.68; that is, 68% of the population will be heterozygous and 42% will be homozygous for one of these three alleles. Note that the probability of being homozygous for a particular allele is simply the square of the population frequency of that allele. It is apparent that the level of heterozygosity is primarily dependent on two factors: (1) the number of different alleles and (2) their pattern of distribution. The higher the number of alleles and the more evenly distributed they are, the higher the level of heterozygosity. Thus, for a locus with five alleles, equally frequent, $H = 1 − 5(0.2^2) = 0.8$. Many microsatellite loci have H values of 0.8 or better, and these highly informative markers are preferred for genetic mapping studies.

11. Summary and Conclusions

This chapter has attempted to cover the major concepts underlying modern genetic approaches to the common rheumatic disorders. HLA-linked genes clearly play a major role in susceptibility to autoimmune disease, yet the exact identity of the predisposing alleles remains in dispute, as does the precise mechanism responsible for these associations *(7–9)*. In addition, the HLA associations are not of themselves sufficiently predictive of disease to warrant routine incorporation of this information into clinical practice. It is likely that further advances in this area will depend in part on identifying other genes involved in susceptibility to rheumatic diseases, as well as basic research into disease mechanisms. Therefore, genetic information will be important at many levels, from basic research to population screening and clinical evaluation of specific patients. Both the basic and clinical researcher, as well as the practicing rheumatologist will need to have an understanding of these genetic concepts in the coming decade.

12. Glossary

Alleles: Alternative forms, or variants, of a gene at a particular locus.

Haplotype: A group of alleles at adjacent or closely linked loci on the same chromosome, which are usually inherited together as a unit.

Heterozygosity: A measure, at a particular locus, of the frequency with which heterozygotes occur in the population (see text for details).

Heterozygote: An individual who inherits two different alleles at a given locus on two homologous chromosomes.

Linkage: The coinheritance, within a family, of two (nonallelic) genes that lie near one another on the genome.

Linkage disequilibrium: The preferential association, in a population, of two alleles or mutations, more frequently than predicted by chance. Linkage disequilibrium is detected statistically and, except in unusual circumstances, generally implies that the two alleles lie near one another on the genome.

Polymorphism: The degree of allelic variation at a locus, within a population. Specific criteria differ, but a locus is said to be polymorphic if the most frequent allele does not occur in more than 98% of the population. Occasionally, the term "polymorphism" can be used in the same way as "allele" to refer to a particular genetic variant.

References

1. Samuels, J., Aksentijevich, I., Torosyan, Y., Centola, M., Deng, Z., Sood, R., et al. (1998) Familial Mediterranean fever at the millennium. Clinical spectrum, ancient mutations, and a survey of 100 American referrals to the National Institutes of Health. *Medicine (Baltimore)* **77**, 268–297.

2. Collins, F. S., Patrinos, A., Jordan, E., Chakravarti, A., Gesteland, R., Walters, L., et al. (1998) New goals for the U.S. Human Genome Project: 1998–2003. *Science* **282,** 682–689.
3. Conrad, K., Mehlhorn, J., Luthke, K., Dorner, T., and Frank, K. H. (1996) Systemic lupus erythematosus after heavy exposure to quartz dust in uranium mines: clinical and serological characteristics. *Lupus* **5,** 62–69.
4. Symmons, D. P., Bankhead, C. R., Harrison, B. J., Brennan, P., Barrett, E. M., Scott, D. G., et al. (1997) Blood transfusion, smoking, and obesity as risk factors for the development of rheumatoid arthritis: results from a primary care-based incident case-control study in Norfolk, England. *Arthritis Rheum.* **40,** 1955–1961.
5. Cooper, G. S., Dooley, M. A., Treadwell, E. L., St. Clair, E. W., Parks, C. G., and Gilkeson, G. S. (1998) Hormonal, environmental, and infectious risk factors for developing systemic lupus erythematosus. *Arthritis Rheum.* **41,** 1714–1724.
6. Gregersen, P. K. (1993) Discordance for autoimmunity in monozygotic twins. Are "identical" twins really identical? *Arthritis Rheum.* **36,** 1185–1192.
7. Nepom, G. T. (1998) Major histocompatibility complex-directed susceptibility to rheumatoid arthritis. *Adv Immunol.* **68,** 315–332.
8. Zamani, M. and Cassiman, J. J. (1998) Reevaluation of the importance of polymorphic HLA class II alleles and amino acids in the susceptibility of individuals of different populations to type I diabetes. *Am. J. Med. Genet.* **76,** 183–194.
9. Reveille, J. D. (1992) The molecular genetics of systemic lupus erythematosus and Sjogren's syndrome. *Curr. Opin. Rheumatol.* **4,** 644–656.
10. Silman, A. J., MacGregor, A. J., Thomson, W., et al. (1993) Twin concordance rates for rheumatoid arthritis: results from a nationwide study. *Br. J. Rheumatol.* **32,** 903–907.
11. Jarvinen, P. and Aho, K. (1994) Twin studies in rheumatic diseases. *Semin. Arthritis Rheum.* **24,** 19–28.
12. Vyse, T. J. and Todd, J. A. (1996) Genetic analysis of autoimmune disease. *Cell* **85,** 311–318.
13. Elston, R. C. and Johnson, W. D. (1994) *Essentials of Biostatistics*, F. A. Davis & Co., Philadelphia.
14. Feder, J. N., Penny, D. M., Irrinki, A., Lee, V. K., Lebron, J. A., Watson, N., et al. (1998) The hemochromatosis gene product complexes with the transferrin receptor and lowers its affinity for ligand binding. *Proc. Natl. Acad. Sci. USA* **95,** 1472–1477.
15. Falk, C. R. and Rubinstein, P. (1987) Haplotype relative risks: an easy reliable way to construct a proper control sample for risk calculations. *Ann. Hum. Genet.* **51,** 227.
16. Spielman, R. S., McGinnis, R. E., and Ewens, W. J. (1993) Transmission test for linkage disequilibrium: the insulin gene region and insulin-dependent diabetes mellitus (IDDM). *Am. J. Hum. Genet.* **52,** 506–516.
17. Schaid, D. J. (1998) Transmission disequilibrium, family controls, and great expectations. *Am. J. Hum. Genet.* **63,** 935–941.
18. Weyand, C. M., Hicok, K. C., Conn, D. L., et al. (1992) The influence of HLA-DRB1 genes on disease severity in rheumatoid arthritis. *Ann. Intern. Med.* **117,** 801–806.
19. Criswell, L. A., Mu, H., Such, C. L., and King, M. C. (1998) Inheritance of the shared epitope and long-term outcomes of rheumatoid arthritis among community-based Caucasian females. *Genet. Epidemiol.* **15,** 61–72.
20. Seldin, M. F., Amos, C. I., Ward, R., and Gregersen, P. K. (1999) The genetics revolution and the assault on rheumatoid arthritis. *Arthritis Rheum.* **42,** 1071–1079.
21. Ott, J. (1992) *Analysis of Human Genetic Linkage*, Johns Hopkins University Press, Baltimore.
22. Cornelis, F., Faure, S., Martinez, M., Prud'homme, J. F., Fritz, P., Dib, C., et al. (1998) New susceptibility locus for rheumatoid arthritis suggested by a genome-wide linkage study. *Proc. Natl. Acad. Sci. USA* **95,** 10,746–10,750.

23. Tsao, B. P., Cantor, R. M., Kalunian, K. C., Chen, C. J., Badsha, H., Singh, R., et al. (1997) Evidence for linkage of a candidate chromosome 1 region to human systemic lupus erythematosus. *J. Clin. Invest.* **199,** 725–731.
24. Gaffney, P. M., Kearns, G. M., Shark, K. B., Ortmann, W. A., Selby, S. A., Malmgren, M. L., et al. (1998) A genome-wide search for susceptibility genes in human systemic lupus erythematosus sib-pair families. *Proc. Natl. Acad. Sci. USA* **95,** 14,875–14,879.
25. Moser, K. L., Neas, B. R., Salmon, J. E., Yu, H., Gray-McGuire, C., Asundi, N., et al. (1998) Genome scan of human systemic lupus erythematosus: evidence for linkage on chromosome 1q in African-American pedigrees. *Proc. Natl. Acad. Sci. USA* **95,** 14,869–14,874.
26. John, S., Hajeer, A., Marlow, A., Myerscough, A., Silman, A. J., Ollier, W. E., et al. (1997) Investigation of candidate disease susceptibility genes in rheumatoid arthritis: principles and strategies. *Rheumatology* **24,** 199–201.
27. Todd, J. A. (1992) La carte des microsatellites est arrivee! *Hum. Mol. Genet.* **1,** 663–666.

2
Viruses

Andras Perl

1. Introduction

Viruses are considered as key environmental factors that may cause inflammatory arthritis and autoimmune diseases in genetically susceptible hosts. Viruses can elicit acute or subacute and, less often, chronic forms of arthritis. These viral arthritis syndromes can be diagnosed by recognition of well-defined clinical signs and detection of viral antibodies and nucleic acids. Moreover, viral elements may also play a role in the pathogenesis of idiopathic autoimmune rheumatic diseases. The concordance rate of the most common autoimmune disease, such as rheumatoid arthritis (RA) or systemic lupus erythematosus (SLE), in monozygotic twins is about 25% *(1)*. Although these data show that genetic factors influence susceptibility to autoimmune diseases, alternatively, a 70% discordance rate emphasizes the importance of environmental factors. Forensic studies of archeological sites revealed the presence of RA-like erosive bony changes in pre-Columbian New World populations dating back 6500 yr and the absence of RA in the Old World before the 18th century *(2)*. This geographic distribution suggest that RA may have spread from the Americas through environmental factors, possibly by a virus, another microorganism, or an antigen. The potential etiological role of viruses in chronic rheumatic diseases have been recently reviewed *(3)*. This chapter will focus on known viruses capable of causing rheumatic diseases, review molecular techniques suitable to identify viruses, describe the latest experimental evidence implicating known and unidentified viruses in the causation of idiopathic autoimmune rheumatic diseases, and review mechanisms of viral pathogenesis, molecular mimicry, and altered apoptosis that can result in autoimmunity.

2. Virus-Induced Arthritis Syndromes

Viral infections are often associated with arthralgias, whereas arthritis occurs less commonly. Most cases of virus-induced arthritis are short-lived and self-limited as a result of an efficient elimination of the organism by the immune system. Examples of these viral syndromes include rubella and parvovirus B19-induced arthritis. Chronic joint diseases have been associated with persistent or latent viral infections, largely the result of an inability of the immune system to eliminate the pathogen, virus-induced autoimmunity, characterized by molecular mimicry, polyclonal B-cell activation, and immunodeficiency resulting in opportunistic infections. This latter group of pathogens include human immunodeficiency virus 1 (HIV-1), human T-cell lymphotropic virus type I (HTLV-I), and hepatitis C virus (HCV).

2.1. Virus-Induced Transient Arthritis Syndromes

2.1.1. Parvovirus B19

This small single-stranded DNA virus is one of the most frequent causes of viral arthritis in humans *(4)*. The majority of parvovirus B19 infections occur in children 5–15 yr of age. The virus spreads through respiratory or oral secretions. After a 1- to 4-wk incubation period, most children present with erythema infectiosum with a typical facial rash (slapped cheeks), headache, low-grade fever, coryza, cough, conjunctivitis, and/or mild gastrointestinal symptoms. Whereas arthritis occurs in 5% of childhood infections, 50% of adults freshly infected by the virus develop joint pain and swelling (Table 1). Joint pain develops with equal frequency in boys and girls. In the adults, arthritis is more frequent in females, and skin eruptions are far less conspicuous. The virus can infect bone marrow cells, preferentially erythroid progenitors, thus causing anemia, neutropenia, and thrombocytopenia with transient aplastic crises. Vasculitic peripheral neuropathies and liver disease with elevated transaminases have been also reported. Parvovirus B19 arthritis usually presents with acute, moderately severe, symmetric polyarthritis first affecting the hands and knees, then rapidly spreading to the feet, elbows, and shoulders. Joint manifestations are temporally associated with production of anti-B19 IgM antibodies. These antibodies clear the viremia, thus rendering the patient noninfectious. IgM antibodies are present for up to 3 mo after infection. Whereas IgM antibodies are diagnostic for a recent B19 infection, IgG antibodies are long-lived and not useful for diagnosis. Seroprevalence of IgG antibodies may be as high as 80% in the adult population. Joint pain and synovitis usually lasts for 2–8 wk and rarely persists for more than 3 mo. Patients have morning stiffness that can last for more than 1 h, symmetrical swelling of the wrist and metacarpophalangeal and proximal interphalangeal joints. Patients may have low-titer rheumatoid factors. Failure to recognize sometimes minimal skin eruptions and obtain B19 IgM antibody titers may lead to a diagnosis of early RA. However, erosions and joint destructions have not been described in B19 arthropathy. Whereas involvement of B19 has been repeatedly raised in classic RA *(5)*, large surveys failed to demonstrate an association between erosive RA and parvovirus B19 *(4)*. B19-Specific DNA can be detected in synovium and synovial fluid of patients with chronic B19 arthropathy. B19 DNA was also detected in normal noninflammatory synovium as well *(6)*. It is presently unclear whether intraarticular viral infection is prerequisite of B19 arthropathy.

2.1.2. Rubella Virus

Rubella virus has a single-stranded RNA genome. Viral infection is a mild and self-limited disease characterized by skin rash, lymphadenopathy, and low-grade fever. Infection may also lead to subclinical illness. Infection during pregnancy can result in fetal malformations. Rubella is known to cause arthralgias and acute arthritis in one-third of patients after both natural infection and vaccination *(7)*. Similar to parvovirus B19, joint symptoms are more common in women than in men or children. Rubella arthritis affects the small joints of the hands, wrist, elbows, or knees and rarely lasts more than 1 wk. Chronic arthropathy was reported in 1–4% of postpartum female

Table 1
Arthritis in Viral Infections

Virus	Genome	Arthritis frequency	Arthritis type	Duration	Erosion	Diagnosis	Ref.
HCV	RNA	10–50%	Polyarticular, symmetrical	Chronic	No	ELISA, WB[a], PCR	20,21
HBV	DNA	10–25%	Symmetrical, migratory	1–3 wk	No	ELISA, WB	3
Parvovirus B19	DNA	Children: 5–10% Adults: 50–70% Female : male = 2 : 1	Polyarticular, small and large joints, symmetrical	2–8 wk	No	ELISA	4
Rubella	RNA	10–30%	Multiple small joints	5–10 d	No	ELISA, WB, PCR	3,7
VZV	DNA	<1%	Monoarthritis	1–7 d	No	ELISA, WB	18
EBV	DNA	1–5%	Poly- or monoarthritis	1–12 wk	No	ELISA, WB	110
HSV-1	DNA	Case reports	Monoarthritis	1–10 d	No	ELISA	111,112
HTLV-I	Retrovirus	<1%	Oligoarthritis, large joints	Chronic	Yes	ELISA, WB, PCR	30,113
HIV-1	Retrovirus	10–50%	Painful joint syndrome	1–2 d	No	ELISA, WB, PCR	13
			Reiter's syndrome	Chronic	Yes		
			Psoriatic arthritis	Chronic	Yes		

[a]WB = Western Blot analysis.

recipients of the RA27/3 vaccine strain *(8)*. Other studies found no increase of chronic arthritis in women receiving the RA27/3 rubella vaccine *(9)*. No rubella virus can be recovered from peripheral blood lymphocytes of persons with chronic arthropathy following rubella infection or vaccination *(10)*. Neuropathic syndromes, such as carpal tunnel syndrome, does not appear to have an increased rate among recipients of the RA27/3 vaccine *(9)*. These data support the continued vaccination of rubella-susceptible females to reduce the risk of congenital malformations.

The rubella vaccine is part of a combined measles–mumps–rubella preparation. Arthritis is not uncommon in natural mumps infection, especially in adult man. Arthritis occurs 1–3 wk after the onset of parotitis and may be associated with low-grade fever. Mumps can cause migrating polyarthritis, monoarthritis of the knee, hip, or ankle, or arthralgias alone. Mumps arthritis is self-limited, rarely lasting more than 4 wk *(11)*. Measles have not been associated with joint symptoms. A recent survey failed to show evidence for involvement of measles, mumps, or rubella virus in chronic arthritis *(12)*.

2.1.3. Herpesviruses

Members of the Herpesviridae family have a large (> 100 kb) double-stranded DNA genome. After initial infection, herpesviruses persist in the host with lifelong latency. Therefore, several of these viruses have been considered as etiologic agents in autoimmune diseases, such as SLE, RA, or Sjogren's syndrome (*see* Subheading 4.).

The cytomegalovirus (CMV) infects most individuals during their life. Major syndromes associated with CMV include inclusion disease in neonates, heterophile antibody-negative mononucleosis in healthy individuals, and pneumonitis, arthritis, vasculitis, and chorioretinitis in immunocompromised individuals *(13)*.

The Epstein–Barr virus (EBV) commonly causes subclinical infections of heterophil antibody-positive mononucleosis in young adults. Arthralgias lasting for up to 4 mo occur in 2% of patients with mononucleosis. Recently, EBV-positive lymphomas were described in methotrexate-treated RA patients *(14–17)*. Interestingly, remission of lymphomas was noted after discontinuation of methotrexate *(14,15)*.

Herpes simplex virus 1 (HSV-1) can cause monoarthritis few days after the onset of oral or genital lesions. HSV-1 arthritis rarely last longer than 2 wk. Varicella–zoster virus (VZV) can cause monarthritis, mostly in the knee, as a rare complication of chickenpox *(18)*. HZV causes shingles in the elderly or immunosuppressed host after reactivation from dorsal root ganglia.

2.1.4. Hepatitis B Virus

Arthralgias and arthritis occur early after hepatitis B virus (HBV) infection. Arthritis is characterized by a sudden onset, symmetrical polyarticular synovitis of the small joints of the hands and knees, erythematous and pruritic rash, anorexia, malaise, and fever. Arthritis resolves in 2–6 wk with the onset of jaundice. Hepatitis B virus has been also associated with polyarteritis nodosa and cryoglobulinemia. Erythema nodosum, uveitis, and polyarthritis were rarely reported following immunization with recombinant HBV vaccine.

2.2. Virus-Induced Chronic Arthritis

2.2.1. Hepatitis C Virus

Hepatitis C virus (HCV) is a single-stranded RNA virus. Based on genomic variability, at least six subtypes have been identified. The virus is transmitted parenterally, primarily through the exchange of body fluids. Viral infection can be detected by PCR within 2 wk of exposure. Serum transaminases and antibody titers become elevated after 4–8 wk. Despite high-titer antibody levels, >80% of infected individuals become chronic virus carriers. HCV has a wide pathogenic potential that is not limited to diseases of the liver, chronic active hepatitis, cirrhosis, and hepatocellular carcinoma *(19)*. Identification of HCV as the cause of most cases (>90%) of type II or essential mixed cryoglobulinemia (EMC) is a major breakthrough in rheumatology *(20)*. Type II cryoglobulins are immune complexes comprised of a monoclonal IgM/kappa rheumatoid factor and polyclonal IgG. HCV-RNA is concentrated 1000-fold in the cryoprecipitate in comparison to the serum *(21)*. The clinical syndrome of EMC is an immune-complex vasculitis characterized by purpura, arthralgias, inflammatory arthritis, peripheral neuropathy, and glomerulonephritis *(22)*. IgM/kappa-bearing B cells are clonally expanded in the peripheral blood of EMC patients *(23)*. Infection by HCV may be directly responsible for the clonal expansion of B cells *(24)*. This process may lead to development of B-cell non-Hodgkin's lymphomas *(19)*.

The HCV infection is associated with production of autoantibodies. Up to 75% of the patients have high-titer rheumatoid factors, presumably produced by HCV-infected and thus clonally expanded B-lymphocytes. Half or more of the patients have anti-smooth-muscle antibodies. Low-titer antinuclear antibodies and anticardiolipin antibodies were noted in 10–30% of HCV-infected patients. Five percent of patients may develop Sjogren's syndrome. SLE, autoimmune thyroiditis, erosive/rheumatoid arthritis, and polymyositis/dermatomyositis were rarely documented *(19)*.

Cryoglobulinemia is detectable in 40–50% of HCV-infected patients *(19,25)*. Treatment with interferon-α and ribavirin appears to be effective in reducing viral RNA and cryoglobulin levels. Unfortunately, only 20% or less of the patients will have a sustained remission after discontinuation of antiviral therapies.

2.2.2. Human T-Cell Lymphotropic Virus I (HTLV-I)

Infection by human T-cell lymphotropic virus I (HTLV-I) has been associated with adult T-cell leukemia (ATL), mycosis fungoides/Sézary syndrome, HTLV-I-associated myelopathy/tropic spastic paraparesis (HAM/TSP), HTLV-I associated arthritis (HAA), polymyositis, and Sjögren's syndrome *(26)*. HTLV-I infection occurs in endemic areas of southwest Japan, the Caribbean basin, the southeastern United States, and parts of Africa. Despite very high rates of infection in endemic areas where 30% or more of the population may be infected, relative few (<1%) infected individuals show disease manifestations attributable to HTLV-I. The lifetime risk of developing a HTLV-I-associated disorder is less than 5%. The vast majority of virus carriers remain disease-free and serve as a huge reservoir for further transmission of the virus. The virus spreads through three major routes: from mother to child via breast-feeding, sexual intercourse, and contaminated blood products via transfusion or intravenous drug use. ATL usually presents in middle-aged adults in the forms of acute high-grade leukemia with widespread systemic involvement resulting from infiltration of the skin, liver, spleen, lungs, lymph nodes, bone marrow, salivary glands, and/or synovium. A chronic cutaneous involvement is characterized by leukemic cell infiltration of the dermis and subcutaneous tissue. Polymyositis, Sjögren's syndrome, and inflammatory arthritis may occur in the absence of leukemia. These latter conditions clinically are indistinguishable from the idiopathic autoimmune syndromes. They are characterized by infiltration of the skeletal muscle, salivary glands, or synovium with HTLV-I infected T-lymphocytes. T-cells infiltrating the joint have indented cerebriform nuclei similar to those seen in ATL. HAA patients develop chronic oligoarthritis, primarily affecting the larger joints (knees and shoulders). Patients may have rheumatoid factors and X-ray films show joint-space narrowing with erosions. HTLV-I infection can be diagnosed with enzyme-linked immunosorbent assay (ELISA) and confirmed by Western blot. PCR techniques are more sensitive that serological assays and allow the differentiation between HTLV-I and a less common virus, HTLV-II. Clinical significance of HTLV-II infection, most often found among intravenous drug abusers in the United States, is presently unknown. Transgenic mice carrying the *tax* transactivator gene of HTLV-I develop Sjögren's syndrome and rheumatoid-like arthritis *(26)*. These studies provided experimental evidence for a pathogenic role of the HTLV-I p40/tax protein. Prevalence of RA is increased in the HTLV-I-infected population (0.56%) with respect to the uninfected population of Japan (0.31%) *(26)*. Thus, the relatively low disease frequency in virus-infected individuals strongly advocates for the role of factors other than HTLV-I in the development of RA.

2.2.3. Human Immunodeficiency Virus 1

In the United States, more than 1 million individuals are infected by human immunodeficiency virus 1 (HIV-1). HIV-1 enters cells by fusion at the cell surface, triggered by binding of the gp120 envelop protein to the CD4 molecule of the host cell. A second receptor for HIV was recently identified as the receptor for β-chemokines *(27)*. Interestingly, homozygous defects in the β-chemokine/HIV-1 coreceptors CCR2 and CCR5 appear to be responsible for resistance of some individuals (<10%) to HIV-1 infection. These new findings may provide new means in preventing or slowing HIV disease. During the course of HIV-1 infection, three major phases can be distinguished. Within a few weeks after infection, extensive viremia occurs, giving rise to an acute mononucleosis-like syndrome. This period is characterized by flu-like symptoms, arthralgias, and lymphadenopathy, accompanied by a robust activation of the immune system. When humoral and cellular immune responses to HIV become established, a subclinical phase of disease with relatively minor changes in CD4 T-cell counts ensues. Recently, however, it became clear that this second or latent period represents an ongoing fierce battle between virus replication and replenishing of the CD4 T-cell reservoir. On the average, 10 yr following infection, virus-infected cells and viral RNA levels drastically increase with a sharp decline of CD4 T-cell counts in the peripheral blood. Both direct infection of various cell types and tissues and secondary changes in the lymphokine milieu are important for the pathogenesis of HIV disease. Disease progression has been attributed to a shift from Th1-type to Th2-type helper-T-cell predominance resulting in polyclonal B-cell activation, hypergammaglobulinemia, and production of autoantibodies. Rapid decline of CD4 T-cell counts is mediated by increased apoptosis sensitivity of HIV-infected cells. Diminished CD4 T-cell function gives rise to opportunistic infections, lymphomagenesis, and autoimmune phenomena at the final stages of disease. Autoimmune rheumatic diseases most commonly noted in patients with autoimmunodeficiency syndrome (AIDS) include Reiters syndrome, psoriatic arthritis, spondylarthropathies, and diffuse infiltrative lymphocytosis syndrome (DILS). Interestingly, all of these syndromes have been associated with relative expansion of CD8 T-cells, thus suggesting that HIV-1 infection accelerates HLA class I-restricted CD8 T-cell-mediated autoreactivity (28). In turn, SLE, RA, and polymyositis, which are thought to be mediated by CD4 T-cells, remit in some patients following infection by HIV-1 (13).

3. Molecular Techniques for Detection of Viruses

Diagnosis of viral infections can be made by serologic testing of virus-specific antibodies or detection of viral nucleic acids. ELISA or radioimmunoassays are best suited for rapid screening of antibody reactivities (29). Immunoreactivities to viral proteins generally require confirmation by Western blot. In comparison to ELISA, Western blot allows detection of antibodies to virion proteins of distinct molecular weight. As an example, specific immunoreactivity to HTLV-I requires detection of antibodies to a core protein, gag p19 or p24, *and* an envelop protein, gp41 (30). Along the same line, seroreactivity to HIV-1 is first tested by ELISA and confirmed by Western blot reactivity to a gag antigen, p24, and an envelope protein, gp41 or gp120. In response to antigenic stimulation, formation of IgM antibodies requires at least 2 wk, whereas high-titer IgG antibodies are generally detectable after 6–8 wk.

Polymerase-chain-reaction (PCR)-based detection of nucleic acids has been used for early diagnosis of viral infections, between viral exposure and production of detectable antibodies. Theoretically, a single viral RNA or DNA molecule may be sufficient for amplication by PCR. Viral DNA can be amplified with a set of sense and antisense primers. Viral RNA requires reverse transcription into complementary cDNA, prior to PCR. Reliable detection of viral sequences usually requires Southern blot hybridization with a probe internal to the location of oligonucleotide primers utilized for PCR. Gene amplification by PCR is currently the most sensitive diagnostic assay to detect any viral infection; nevertheless, it is not problem-free. Whereas DNA is fairly stable, RNA is prone to degradation by ubiquitous ribonucleases. Ironically, extreme sensitivity also represent an Achilles' heel of PCR-based methods. DNA contamination of clinical specimen can come form several sources: (1) another clinical specimen containing an abundant supply of target molecules for amplification by PCR, (2) contamination of reagents with PCR products, and (3) introduction of contaminants from skin, body fluids, or clothing of laboratory workers (31). DNA products of PCR amplification should be handled separately from unprocessed clinical samples. Multiplex PCR allows detection of different viral nucleic acids in a single specimen. This technique is the diagnostic method of choice for testing of organs prior to transplantation. Quantitative PCR is useful for monitoring viral load in HIV-1 or HCV-infected patients in correlation with clinical course and responses to medications.

4. Viral Pathogenesis in Common/Idiopathic Autoimmune Diseases

Independent lines of evidence have implicated environmental and genetic factors in the development of autoimmune rheumatic diseases. A discordance of approximately 70% for SLE and RA in monozygotic twins argues for a significant role for exogenous agents. The possibility of a viral etiology was raised by findings of virionlike tubuloreticular structures in endothelial cells and lymphocytes as well as demonstration of elevated serum levels of type I interferon (IFN) in lupus patients (32). Viruslike particles were also noted in RA synovium *(33)*. Retroviruses were implicated by detection of retroviral p30 gag protein in renal glomeruli and serum reactivities towards p30 gag antigen in patients with SLE *(34)*. Many viral infections are accompanied by production of autoantibodies and viral proteins have profound effects on both antigen presentation and effector functions of the immune system. Dysregulation of programmed cell death has been documented in HIV-infected *(35)* and lupus patients as well *(36)*. Similar to SLE, anemia *(37)*, leukopenia *(38)*, thrombocytopenia *(39)*, polymyositis *(40)*, and vasculitis have been widely reported in patients with AIDS *(41)*. Direct virus isolation and transmission attempts from tissues of autoimmune patients have not been successful *(42)*. Nevertheless, it is possible that a (retro)virus, responsible for provoking an immune response cross-reactive with self-antigens, has been cleared from the host, so the absence of viral particles is not conclusive. An alternative retroviral etiology (i.e., activation of endogenous retroviral sequences [ERS]) was initially proposed by a study of the New Zealand mouse model of SLE *(43)*. Endogenous retroviral envelope glycoprotein, gp 70, was found in immune-complex deposits of autoimmune lupus-prone NZB/NZW mice *(43)*. Abnormal expression of an ERS was noted in the thymus of lupus-prone mouse strains *(44,45)*. More recently, expression and autoantigenicity of human ERS has been demonstrated in patients with SLE *(46–50)*.

Below, two lines of evidence for possible viral pathogenesis of autoimmunity will be reviewed. The first scenario involves molecular mimicry causing abnormal self-reactivity. Naturally, viral infections elicit potent antiviral immunity that may lead to crossreactivity against self-antigens. Analysis of molecular mimicries that is a delineation of autoantigenic epitopes of self-antigens may provide clues to the identity of viral antigens responsible for triggering the cross-reactive immune responses. Second, infection of genetically susceptible hosts by a potentially large number of commonly occurring viruses may lead to T- and B-cell dysfunction and autoimmunity. Immunoregulatory aberrations triggered by well-defined viral proteins at the level of antigen presentation, modulation of cytokine activities, and disruption of cell-death pathways, will be discussed.

4.1. Molecular Mimicry Between Viral Antigens and Self-Proteins

Molecular mimicry between self antigens and viral proteins has long been considered a trigger of autoimmunity *(51)*. Under normal conditions, the immune system of the host is able to develop a potent virus-specific immune response that rapidly eliminates the virus with only minimal tissue injury. Thus, only minimal amounts of self-antigens are released, which are insufficient to induce autoreactive B- and T-lymphocytes and autoimmune disease will not ensue. However, in the event that the host and the virus share antigenic determinants, virus infection may result in autoimmunity because virus-specific T-cells and antibodies are cross-reactive with self-antigens. This scenario does not preclude the possibility that the infecting virus is eliminated by the crossreactive immune response. Similarities between proteins of the major histocompatibility complex (MHC) and microbial antigens, especially viral antigens, may allow the host to regard an infectious agent as self and, thus, forego an immune response. Molecular mimicry (i.e., immunological crossreactivity between autoantigens and viral proteins) has been documented in human autoimmune disorders.

Table 2
Molecular Mimicry Between Viral Proteins and Autoantigens

Autoantigen	Prevalence[a]	Viral protein	Virus	Ref.
70k/U1 snRNP	30%	gag	MoMLV[b], HRES-1[c]	47,55
La	15%	gag	FSV	66
Sm B/B'	30%	gagp24	HIV-1	58
HRES-1	21–52%	gagp24	HTLV-I	46–49
C/U1 snRNP	30%	ICP4	HHV-1	64
Sm D	36%	EBNA-1	EBV	59
Sm B/B'	25–40%	EBNA-1	EBV	63
p542	10–50%	EBNA-1	EBV	60,61
ERV-3	32%	env	MoMLV	50

[a]Prevalence of antibodies in patients with SLE.
[b]MoMLV = Moloney murine leukemia virus.
[c]HRES-1 = human T-cell leukemia virus-related endogenous sequence 1.

The presence of the unique amino acid sequence QTDRED in the nitrogenase protein of Klebsiella and HLA B27 is thought to be a pathogenetic factor in seronegative spondylarthropathies *(52)*. Along the same line, the "shared epitope" QKRAA sequence from the third hypervariable region of HLA DRB1*0401, which has been found in numerous human pathogens, is associated with susceptibility to RA *(53)*.

A hallmark of the self-destructive autoimmune process in patients with SLE is the production of circulating antinuclear autoantibodies (ANAs). ANAs are important markers for diagnosis and classification and are possibly related causally or consequentially to the pathology of SLE. Targets of these antibodies include naked DNA and nuclear proteins involved in transcription and RNA processing. Autoantibodies to uridine-rich small nuclear ribonucleoproteins (UsnRNPs) frequently occur in patients with SLE and in overlap syndromes of SLE, scleroderma, and polymyositis (OLS) *(54)*. Sm (Smith) - type antibodies are directed to U1, U2, U5, and U4/U6 snRNPs, whereas RNP antibodies mainly react with different components of U1 snRNP *(54)*. The 70K protein of U1snRNP was the first lupus autoantigen shown to contain a region of homology and immunological crossreactivity with a conserved p30 gag protein of most mammalian-type C retroviruses (Table 2). Based on this observation, Query and Keene proposed that autoimmunity to U1RNP may be triggered by expression by an endogenous retroviral gag protein *(55)*. Anti-gag antibodies elicited by the ERS could crossreact with the 70K protein and, subsequently, recognition could expand to additional 70K epitopes.

The ERS capable of triggering antibodies crossreactive with the 70K protein may correspond to *HRES-1*, a human T-cell lymphotropic virus-related endogenous sequence *(47,56)*. In different laboratories, prevalence of HRES-1 antibodies may be as high as 52% *(47)* or as low as 21% *(49)* in patients with SLE. Fifty-nine percent (10/15) of scleroderma, 44% (8/18) of primary SJS, and 19% (3/16) of polymyositis/dermatomyositis patients also had HRES-1 antibodies. By contrast, 3.6% (4/111) of normal donors and none of 42 patients with AIDS or 50 asymptomatic HIV-infected patients had HRES-1 antibodies *(47)*. Thus, HRES-1 antibodies are detectable in a significant subset of autoimmune patients, whereas they are conspicuously absent in states of nonspecific polyclonal B-cell hyperactivity such as AIDS. The retroviral gag-related region of the 70K protein shares three consecutive highly charged amino acids, Arg-Arg-Glu (RRE), an additional Arg, and functionally similar Arg/Lys residues with HRES-1/p28, which represent crossreactive epitopes between the two proteins *(46,47,55)*. Interestingly, the RRE triplet is repeated three times in the 70K protein at residues 248–250, 418–420, and 477–479, respectively (GenEmbl accession number X04654). This suggests that recognition of the retroviral domain may lead to epitope spreading through binding to RRE triplets within the 70K protein. It is well known that highly charged polypeptides can elicit high-titer antibodies *(57)*. Therefore, the presence of charged amino acids in the mimicking epitopes may have important implications in triggering crossreactive antibodies of high affinity.

A mimicking epitope between another lupus autoantigen, Sm, and HIV-1 p24 gag was defined based on crossreactivity with monoclonal antibody 4B4 *(58)*. A proline-rich domain present in both the B/B' subunit of Sm and HIV p24 gag was suggested to be the core of crossreactive epitopes. Antibodies binding to HIV-1 p24 gag were found in 22/61 patients with SLE *(58)*. A region of considerable homology, comprised of 11 highly charged residues (GRGRGRGRGRG), was identified as a site of crossreactivity between the D component of Sm and the Epstein–Barr virus nuclear antigen 1 (EBNA-1) *(59)*. Mimicry between EBNA-1 and another self-protein, the 71 kD p542, has been revealed in patients with SLE and other autoimmune diseases *(60,61)*. The mimicking epitope, a 28-mer glycine-rich sequence, was selectively recognized by sera from autoimmune patients, whereas it was uncommonly targeted by sera from normal donors. Autoimmune sera recognized two additional epitopes of p542 in addition to its mimicking 28-mer. The concept that EBV can trigger IgG antibodies that crossreact with autoantigens is an attractive one. EBV is a ubiquitous human DNA virus which infects B cells and causes their polyclonal activation and thus polyclonal antibody production. Such polyclonal B-cell activation may be an early step in pathogenesis of SLE *(62)*. Interestingly, prevalence of EBV infection was reported to be as high as 99% in young SLE patients in comparison to a 70% prevalence in controls *(63)*. Therefore, EBV has the potential to trigger lupus by two mechanisms: polyclonal B-cell activation and molecular mimicry. The ICP4 protein of another ubiquitous human DNA virus, human herpesvirus type I (HHV-1), shows crossreactivity with the C component of U1 snRNP *(64)*.

Antibodies to p24 gag of HTLV-I were also noted in patients with SLE *(65)*, possibly secondary to crossreactivity with HRES-1 *(46)*. A region with limited sequence homology to the feline sarcoma virus (FSV) gag protein was noted in the La antigen *(66)*. Antibodies to the env protein of an ERS, ERV-3, were reported in patients with SLE with the highest prevalence in mothers of babies with complete heart block (CHB) *(50)*. A limited sequence similarity was revealed between the env of ERV-3 and MoMLV. Relationship between CHB-associated Ro/La and ERV-3 reactivities has not yet been directly addressed *(50)*.

Endogenous retroviral sequences, in addition to serving as crossreactive targets of antiviral immunity, may also have a direct role in regulating immune responses. ERS and other retrotransposable elements possess a relatively high mobility and thus represent a major factor in the shaping and reorganization of the eukaryotic genome *(67)*. The ERS HERV-K10 was found to have an integration site in the human complement C2 gene *(68)*. Variable repeats of this element may have a role in polymorphism and differential expression of C2 loci. Integration of a 5.3-kb ETn retrotransposon in the FasR gene locus resulted in disruption of this apoptosis pathway in lupus prone MRL/lpr mice *(69,70)*. A synthetic heptadecapeptide corresponding to the transmembrane domain of the env protein conserved among many exogenous and endogenous retroviruses has been shown to have potent immunosuppressive properties *(71,72)*.

4.2. Viral Proteins Mimic Immunoregulatory Abnormalities of Autoimmune Patients

Tissue injury in rheumatic disease patients is often mediated by autoantibody-containing immune complexes. In turn, production of autoantibodies appear to be antigen-driven, polyclonal, and T-cell dependent *(73)*. A lack of tolerance to a variety of nuclear autoantigen is correlated with a profound dysfunction of both T- and B-cells. T-cell abnormalities include deficiencies of early activation events, proliferative responses to mitogens and antigens, T-helper, T-suppressor, and cell-mediated cytotoxic activities and decreased cell counts in the active stages of disease *(74,75)*. Functional abnormalities of T- and B-cells have been correlated with an altered cytokine production profile in patients with active SLE *(75)*. Secretion of T-helper type 1 (Th1) cytokines, interleukin-2 (IL-2), interferon-γ (IFNγ), and IL-12, necessary for maintenance of a classical T-cell-mediated immunity, is diminished *(75)*, whereas production of Th2 cytokines, in particular, IL-4, IL-5, IL-6 and IL-10, promoting B-cell function, is increased in patients with SLE *(76)*. This marked shift in cytokine production may be related to a fundamental biochemical defect manifested in deficiencies of protein kinase A activity, increased phosphatidylinositol turnover, and diminished protein kinase C activities in lupus T-cells *(74)*.

Changes in production of cytokines similar to those in patients with SLE have been described as a result of infection by HIV-1 *(77)*. Immune dysregulation in HIV-infected individuals observed during progression toward AIDS has been accounted for by a shift from a Th1-type to a Th2-type cytokine profile *(77)*. CD4 T-cell decline is mediated by an increased rate of apoptosis or programmed cell death (PCD) *(35)*. Interestingly, Th1-type cytokines protect against apoptosis, whereas Th2 cytokines increase PCD *(77)*. Accelerated apoptosis has also been described in SLE *(36)*. Moreover, apoptosis has been associated with a compartmentalized release of autoantigens in patients with SLE *(78)*. These observations raise the possibility that increased apoptosis and autoantibody production may be mediated by somewhat similar mechanisms both in AIDS and SLE.

Apoptosis or PCD represents a physiological mechanism for elimination of autoreactive lymphocytes during development *(79)*. Viral infections may have a role in dysregulation of apoptosis in autoimmune patients. Many viruses have evolved genes that can selectively inhibit or stimulate PCD. The suicide of an infected cell by internal activation of apoptosis or the killing of an infected cell by a cytotoxic T-lymphocyte or natural killer (NK) cell may be viewed as a defense mechanism of the host to prevent viral propagation. In the early stages of infection, viral inhibitors of apoptosis allow for more extensive production of progeny. At later stages, viral inducers of apoptosis facilitate spread of progeny to uninfected cells.

E1A of adenovirus *(80,81)* and E7 protein of human papilloma virus (HPV) activate p53-dependent apoptosis, which leads to elimination of virus-infected cells *(82)*. HIV

Table 3
Viral Proteins Stimulating Apoptosis

Protein	Virus	Pathway	Ref.
E1A	Adenovirus	Activates p53	80,81
E7	HPV	Activates p53	82
tat	HIV-1	Fas, oxidative stress	83,85
Protease	HIV-1	bcl-2 cleavage	86
tax	HTLV-I	bcl-2	100
ND[a]	Parvovirus B19	ND[a]	87
NS-1	Influenza	Fas, bcl-2	89

[a]ND = not determined.

may employ several mechanism to deplete CD4+ T-cells at the later stages of disease (Table 3). The tat protein induces oxidative stress *(83,84)* and enhances surface expression of the Fas ligand resulting in accelerated signaling through the Fas pathway *(83,85)*. In addition, cleavage of bcl-2 by HIV protease may expose the cell to a variety of apoptotic signals *(86)*. Parvovirus B19 depletes erythroid progenitor cells by apoptosis *(87)*, which raises the possibility of a similar mechanism in triggering arthritis in parvovirus-infected adults *(88)*. Cells infected by influenza virus undergo PCD that can be inhibited by bcl-2 and facilitated through the Fas pathway *(89)*. It is intriguing to consider the possibility that viruses causing common cold may stimulate antinuclear autoantibody production through periodic release of nucleosomes from apoptotic cells.

Inhibition of apoptosis by viral proteins help infected cells to evade inflammatory responses, such as killing by cytotoxic T-cells through the Fas and TNF pathways (Table 4). Moreover, blocking of cell-cycle-linked apoptotic mechanisms, mainly though interaction with the p53 tumor suppressor, can lead to increased viral replication and tumorigenesis. SV40 large T antigen binds directly to the p53 DNA binding region and blocks interactions with p53-specific promoter elements *(90)*. E6 of HPV promotes rapid degradation of p53 *(91)*. The pX protein of hepatitis B virus (HBV) inhibits binding of p53 to DNA by an unknown mechanism *(92)*. The *vpr* gene of HIV-1 causes cells to arrest in the G2 phase of the cell cycle when virus expression is highest *(93,94)*. *vpr* arrests cells in G2 by preventing activation/dephosphorylation of the p34cdc2/cyclin B complex that is required for entry into the M-phase. Therefore, *vpr*, by preventing p34cdc2 activation, may prevent apoptosis and, thus, increase viral replication in HIV-infected cells *(95)*. Viral homologs of bcl-2 can functionally substitute for bcl-2 in binding to the apoptosis-accelerating proteins, bax, bad, and bag *(96–98)*. Persistence of herpes simplex virus (HSV) in neurons has been linked to its apoptosis-inhibitory protein $\gamma_1 34.5$ *(99)*. The p40/tax protein of HTLV-I appears to possess both apoptosis-inducing *(100)* and apoptosis-inhibiting capabilities *(101,102)*. A proposed role of p40/tax in blocking Fas-dependent cell death may be involved in autoimmune arthropathy *(103)* and Sjögren's syndrome documented in HTLV-I/tax-transgenic mice *(104)*. Upregulation of thioredoxin, a NADPH-dependent antioxidant *(101)*, and inhibition of Fas-dependent signaling have been implicated in the antiapoptotic effect of HTLV-I tax protein *(102)*. These two mechanisms are not

Table 4
Viral Proteins Inhibing Apoptosis

Protein	Virus	Pathway	Ref.
Large T	SV40	Inactivates p53	90
E1B 19K	Adenovirus	bcl-2 homolog	96
$\gamma_1 34.5$	HSV	ND[a]	99
BHRF1	EBV	bcl-2 homolog	97
HMW5-HL	ASFV	bcl-2 homolog	98
pX	HBV	p53 antagonist	92
E6	HPV	p53 antagonist	91
p35, Iap	Baculovirus	Protease inhibitor	114
CrmaA	Cowpox	Protease inhibitor	106
vpr	HIV-1	Mitotic arrest	93,94
tax	HTLV-I	Fas, oxidative stress	101,102
23K E8-FLIP	EHV-2	Fas, vFLIP	107,108
ORF159L-FLIP	MCV	Fas, vFLIP	107,108
ORF71-FLIP	HVS	Fas, vFLIP	107,108
ORF189-FLIP	HHV-8	Fas, vFLIP	107,108

[a]ND = not determined.

mutually exclusive because Fas-induced cell death is accompanied by the formation of reactive oxygen intermediates (ROI) and is subject to regulation by enzymes of the pentose phosphate pathway, providing NADPH as a source of reducing equivalent for intracellular antioxidants *(105)*. The CrmA protein of the coxpoxvirus effectively blocks Fas- and TNF-induced cell death through inhibition of the family of IL1β-converting enzyme (ICE)-like cysteine proteases *(106)*. A new family of viral inhibitors, designated as vFLIPs (viral FLICE-inhibitory proteins), has recently been discovered *(107,108)*. vFLIPs are produced by several γ-herpesviruses, including the Kaposi-sarcoma-associated human herpesvirus 8 (HHV-8), the tumorigenic human molluscipoxvirus (MCV), herpesvirus saimiri (HVS), and equine herpesvirus 2 (EHV-2). vFLIPs block the early signaling events triggered through the death receptors Fas, TRAMP, TRAIL-R, and TNFR1. Thus, herpesviruses evolved a series of genes allowing selective blocking of the Fas- and TNFR-dependent signaling pathways.

5. Conclusions

The experimental evidence presented above reveals immunological crossreactivities between autoantigens and viruses. The concept that autoimmunity is triggered in genetically susceptible hosts by trivial environmental factors, possibly different from patient to patient, is consistent with the general epidemiology (i.e., a relatively sporadic occurrence) of the disease *(109)*. Moreover, proteins of commonly occurring viruses have profound effects on immune responses. Thus, molecular mimicry and immunomodulation by viral proteins may potentially account for both crossreactivity with autoantigens and abnormal T- and B-cell functions in autoimmune disorders. Therefore, continued research on viral pathogenesis is likely to provide new clues for understanding the causation of rheumatic diseases.

Acknowledgments

This work was supported in part by grant RO1 DK 49221 from the National Institutes of Health and grant RG 2466A1/3 from the National Multiple Sclerosis Society, the Arthritis Foundation, and the Central New York Community Foundation.

References

1. Arnett, F. C. and Reveille, J. D. (1992) Genetics of systemic lupus erythematosus. *Rheum. Dis. Clin. North Am.* **18,** 865–892.
2. Rothschild, B. M., Woods, R. J., Rothschild, C., and Sebes, J. I. (1992) Geographic distribution of rheumatoid arthritis in ancient North America: implications for pathogenesis. *Semin. Arthritis Rheum.* **22,** 181–187.
3. Inman, R. D., Perl, A., and Phillips, P. E. (1997) Infectious agents in chronic rheumatic diseases, in *Arthritis and Allied Conditions. A Textbook of Rheumatology.* (Koopman, W. J., ed.), Lea & Febiger, Philadelphia, p. 585.
4. Naides, S. J. (1998) Rheumatic manifestations of parvovirus B19 infection [Review]. *Rheum. Dis. Clin. North Am.* **24,** 375–401.
5. Takahashi, Y., Murai, C., Shibata, S., Munakata, Y., Ishii, T., Ishii, K., et al. (1998) Human parvovirus B19 as a causative agent for rheumatoid arthritis. *Proc. Natl. Acad. Sci. USA* **95,** 8227–8232.
6. Soderlund, M., von Essen, R., Haapasaari, J., Kiistala, U., Kiviluoto, O., and Hedman, K. (1997) Persistence of parvovirus B19 DNA in synovial membranes of young patients with and without chronic arthropathy [see comments]. *Lancet* **349,** 1063–1065.
7. Phillips, P. E. (1997) Viral arthritis. *Curr. Opin. Rheumatol.* **9,** 337–344.
8. Tingle, A. J., Mitchell, L. A., Grace, M., Middleton, P., Mathias, R., and MacWilliam, L. (1997) Randomised double-blind placebo-controlled study on adverse effects of rubella immunisation in seronegative women. *Lancet* **349,** 1277–1281.
9. Ray, P., Black, S., Shinefield, H., Dillon, A., Schwalbe, J., Holmes, S., et al. (1997) Risk of chronic arthropathy among women after rubella vaccination. Vaccine Safety Datalink Team [see comments]. *JAMA* **278,** 551–556.
10. Frenkel, L. M., Nielsen, K., Garakian, A., Jin, R., Wolinsky, J. S., and Cherry, J. D. (1996) A search for persistent rubella virus infection in persons with chronic symptoms after rubella and rubella immunization and in patients with juvenile rheumatoid arthritis. *Clin. Infect. Dis.* **22,** 287–294.
11. Gordon, S. C. and Lauter, C. B. (1984) Mumps arthritis: a review of the literature. *Rev. Infect. Dis.* **6,** 338–344.
12. Zhang, D., Nikkari, S., Vainionpaa, R., Luukkainen, R., Yli-Kerttula, U., and Toivanen, P. (1997) Detection of rubella, mumps, and measles virus genomic RNA in cells from synovial fluid and peripheral blood in early rheumatoid arthritis. *J. Rheumatol.* **24,** 1260–1265.
13. Espinoza, L. R. and Cuellar, M. L. (1998) Retrovirus-associated rheumatic syndromes, in *Arthritis and Allied Conditions.* (Koopman, W. J., ed.), Williams & Wilkins, Baltimore, p. 2361.
14. Le Goff, P., Chicault, P., Saraux, A., Baron, D., Valls-Bellec, I., and Leroy, J. P. (1998) Lymphoma with regression after methotrexate withdrawal in a patient with rheumatoid arthritis. Role for the Epstein-Barr virus. *Rev. D Rhumatisme, Eng. Ed.* **65,** 283–286.
15. Vassilopoulos, D., Waltuck, J., Clarke, G., Farhi, D. C., Williams, J., and Fanucchi, M. P. (1998) Reversible Epstein-Barr virus associated T cell non-Hodgkin's lymphoma in a patient with rheumatoid arthritis undergoing chronic immunosuppressive therapy. *J. Rheumatol.* **25,** 389–391 (letter).
16. Natkunam, Y., Elenitoba-Johnson, K. S., Kingma, D. W., and Kamel, O. W. (1997) Epstein-Barr virus strain type and latent membrane protein 1 gene deletions in lymphomas in patients with rheumatic diseases. *Arthritis Rheum.* **40,** 1152–1156.

17. Paul, C., Le Tourneau, A., Cayuela, J. M., Devidas, A., Robert, C., and Molinie, V. (1997) Epstein–Barr virus-associated lymphoproliferative disease during methotrexate therapy for psoriasis. *Arch. Dermatol.* **133,** 867–871.
18. Stebbings, S., Highton, J., Croxson, M. C., Powell, K., McKay, J., and Rietveld, J. (1998) Chickenpox monoarthritis: demonstration of varicella-zoster virus in joint fluid by polymerase chain reaction. *Br. J. Rheumatol.* **37,** 311–313.
19. Ferri, C., La Civita, L., Longombardo, G., Zignego, A. L., and Pasero, G. (1998) Mixed cryoglobulinaemia: a cross-road between autoimmune and lymphoproliferative disorders. *Lupus* **7,** 275–279.
20. Ferri, C., Greco, F., Longombardo, G., Palla, P., Moretti, A., Marzo, E., et al. (1991) Association between hepatitis C virus and mixed cryoglobulinemia. *Clin. Exp. Rheumatol.* **9,** 621–624.
21. Agnello, V., Chung, R. T., and Kaplan, L. M. (1992) A role for hepatitis C virus infection in type II cryoglobulinemia. *N. Engl. J. Med.* **327,** 1490–1495.
22. Gorevic, P. D., Kassab, H. J., Levo, Y., Kohn, R., Meltzer, M., Prose, P., et al. (1980) Mixed cryoglobulinemia: clinical aspects and long-term follow-up of 40 patients. *Am. J. Med.* **69,** 287–308.
23. Perl, A., Gorevic, P. D., Ryan, D. H., Condemi, J. J., Ruszkowski, R. J., and Abraham, G. N. (1989) Clonal B cell expansions in patients with essential mixed cryoglobulinaemia. *Clin. Exp. Immunol.* **76,** 54–60.
24. Ferri, C., Monti, M., La Civita, L., Longombardo, G., Greco, F., Pasero, G., et al. (1993) Infection of peripheral blood mononuclear cells by hepatitis C virus in mixed cryoglobulinemia. *Blood* **82,** 3701–3704.
25. Akriviadis, E. A., Xanthakis, I., Navrozidou, C., and Papadopoulos, A. (1997) Prevalence of cryoglobulinemia in chronic hepatitis C virus infection and response to treatment with interferon-alpha. *J. Clin. Gastroenterol.* **25,** 612–618.
26. Nishioka, K. (1996) HTLV-I arthropathy and Sjogren syndrome. *J. Acquired Immune Deficiency Syndromes Hum. Retrovirol.* **13(Suppl. 1),** S57–S62.
27. Paxton, W. A., Dragic, T., Koup, R. A., and Moore, J. P. (1996) The β-chemokines, HIV type 1 second receptors, and exposed uninfected persons. *AIDS Res. Hum. Retrovirus* **12,** 1203–1207.
28. Weitzul, S., and Duvic, M. (1997) HIV-related psoriasis and Reiter's syndrome [Review]. *Semin. Cutan. Med. Surg.* **16,** 213–218.
29. Carpenter, A. B. (1997) Enzyme-linked Immunoassays, in *Manual of Clinical and Laboratory Immunology*, 5th ed., (Rosc, N. R., Conway de macario, E., Folds, J. D., Lane, H. C., and Nakamura, R. N., eds.), ASM, Washington, DC, pp. 22–29.
30. McCallum, R. M., Patel, D. D., Moore, J. O., and Haynes, B. F. (1997) Arthritis syndromes associated with human T cell lymphotropic virus type I infection [Review]. *Med. Clin. North Am.* **81,** 261–276.
31. Podzorski, R. P., Kukuruga, D. L., and Long, P. M. (1997) Introduction to molecular methodology, in *Manual of Clinical Laboratory Immunology* (Rose, N. R., Conway de macario, E., Folds, J. D., Lane, H. C., and Nakamura, R. N., eds.), ASM, Washington, pp. 77–107.
32. Rich, S. A. (1981) Human lupus inclusions and interferon. *Science* **213,** 772–775.
33. Stransky, G., Vernon, J., Aicher, W. K., Moreland, L. W., and Gay, R. E. (1993) Virus-like particles in synovial fluids from patients with rheumatoid arthritis. *Br. J. Rheumatol.* **32,** 1044–1048.
34. Mellors, R. C. and Mellors, J. W. (1978) Type C RNA virus-specific antibody in human SLE demonstrated by enzymoimmunoassay. *Proc. Natl. Acad. Sci. USA* **75,** 2463–2467.
35. Meyaard, L., Otto, S. A., Jonker, R. R., Mijnster, M. J., Keet, R. P. M., and Miedema, F. (1992) Programmed death of T cells in HIV infection. *Science* **257,** 217–219.
36. Emlen, W., Niebur, J. A., and Kadera, R. (1994) Accelerated in vitro apoptosis of lymphocytes from patients with systemic lupus erythematosus. *J. Immunol.* **152,** 3685–3692.

37. McGuinnis, M. H., Macher, A. H., and Rook, A. H. (1996) Red cell autoantibodies in patients with AIDS. *Transfusion* **26**, 405–409.
38. Geissler, R. G., Rossol, R., Mentzel, U., Ottmann, O. G., Klein, A. S., Gute, P., et al. (1996) Gamma delta-T cell-receptor positive lymphocytes inhibit human hematopoietic progenitor cell growth in HIV type I-infected patients. *AIDS Res. Hum. Retrovirus* **12**, 577–584.
39. Karpatkin, S. (1990) HIV-1-related thrombocytopenia. *Hematol. Oncol. Clin. North Am.* **4**, 193–218.
40. Dalakas, M. C., Pezeshkpour, G. H., Gravell, M., and Sever, J. L. (1986) Polymyositis associated with AIDS retrovirus. *JAMA* **256**, 2381–2383.
41. Calabrese, L. (1989) The rheumatic manifestations of infection with the HIV. *Semin. Arthritis Rheum.* **18**, 225–239.
42. Hicks, J. T., Aulakh, G. S., McGrath, P. P., Washington, G. C., Kim, E., and Alepa, F. P. (1979) Search for Epstein–Barr and type C oncornaviruses in systemic lupus erythematosus. *Arthritis Rheum.* **22**, 845–857.
43. Yoshiki, T., Mellors, R. C., Strand, M., and August, J. T. (1974) The viral envelope glycoprotein of murine leukemia virus and the pathoegenesis of immune complex glomerulonephritis of New Zealand mice. *J. Exp. Med.* **140**, 1011–1025.
44. Krieg, A. M. and Steinberg, A. D. (1990) Analysis of thymic endogenous retroviral expression in murine lupus. *J. Clin. Invest.* **86**, 809–816.
45. Krieg, A. M., Gourley, M. F., and Perl, A. (1992) Endogenous retroviruses: potential etiologic agents in autoimmunity. *FASEB J.* **6**, 2537–2544.
46. Banki, K., Maceda, J., Hurley, E., Ablonczy, E., Mattson, D. H., Szegedy, L., et al. (1992) Human T-cell lymphotropic virus (HTLV)-related endogenous sequence, HRES-1, encodes a 28-kDa protein: a possible autoantigen for HTLV-I gag-reactive autoantibodies. *Proc. Natl. Acad. Sci. USA* **89**, 1939–1943.
47. Perl, A., Colombo, E., Dai, H., Agarwal, R. K., Mark, K. A., Banki, K., et al. (1995) Antibody reactivity to the HRES-1 endogenous retroviral element identifies a subset of patients with systemic lupus erythematosus and overlap syndromes: correlation with antinuclear antibodies and HLA class II alleles. *Arthritis Rheum.* **38**, 1660–1671.
48. Brookes, S. M., Pandolfino, Y. A., Mitchell, T. J., Venables, T. J. W., Shattles, W. G., Clark, D. A., et al. (1992) The immune response to and expression of cross-reactive retroviral gag sequences in autoimmune disease. *Br. J. Rheumatol.* **31**, 735–742.
49. Bengtsson, A., Blomberg, J., Nived, O., Pipkorn, R., Toth, L., and Sturfelt, G. (1996) Selective antibody reactivity with peptides from human endogenous retroviruses and nonviral poly(amino acids) in patients with systemic lupus erythematosus. *Arthritis Rheum.* **39**, 1654–1663.
50. Li, J., Fan, W. S., Horsfall, A. C., Anderson, A. C., Rigby, S., Larsson, E., et al. The expression of human endogenous retrovirus-3 in fetal cardiac tissue and antibodies in congenital heart block. *Clin. Exp. Immunol.* **104**, 388–393.
51. Oldstone, M. B. A. (1987) Molecular mimicry and autoimmune disease. *Cell* **50**, 819–820.
52. Baum, H., Davies, H., and Peakman, M. (1996) Molecular mimicry in the MHC: hidden clues to autoimmunity? *Immunol. Today* **17**, 64–70.
53. Albani, S. and Carson, D. A. (1996) A multistep molecular mimicry hypothesis for the pathogenesis of rheumatoid arthritis. *Immunol. Today* **17**, 466–470.
54. Reichlin, M. (1994) Antibodies to ribonuclear proteins. *Rheum. Dis. Clin. North Am.* **20**, 29–43.
55. Query, C. C. and Keene, J. D. (1987) A human autoimmune protein associated with U1 RNA contains a region of homology that is cross-reactive with retroviral p30^{gag} antigen. *Cell* **51**, 211–220.
56. Perl, A., Rosenblatt, J. D., Chen, I. S., DiVincenzo, J. P., Bever, R., Poiesz, B. J., et al. (1989) Detection and cloning of new HTLV-related endogenous sequences in man. *Nucleic Acids Res.* **17**, 6841–6854.

57. Sela, M. (1969) Antigenicity: some molecular aspects. *Science* **166**, 1365–1374.
58. Talal, N., Garry, R. F., Schur, P. H., Alexander, S., Dauphinee, M. J., Livas, I. H., et al. (1990) A conserved idiotype and antibodies to retroviral proteins in systemic lupus erythematosus. *J. Clin. Invest.* **85**, 1866–1871.
59. Sabbatini, A., Bombardieri, S., and Migliorini, P. (1993) Autoantibodies form patients with systemic lupus erythematosus bind a shared sequence of SmD and Epstein–Barr virus-encoded nuclear antigen EBNA I. *Eur. J. Immunol.* **23**, 1146–1152.
60. Vaughan, J. H., Valbracht, J. R., Nguyen, M., Handley, H. H., Smith, R. S., Patrick, K., et al. (1995) Epstein–Barr virus-induced autoimmune responses I. Immunoglobulin M autoantibodies to mimicking and nonmimicking Epstein–Barr virus nuclear antigen-1. *J. Clin. Invest.* **95**, 1306–1315.
61. Vaughan, J. H., Nguyen, M., Valbracht, J. R., Patrick, K., and Rhodes, G. H. (1995) Epstein–Barr virus-induced autoimmune responses II. Immunoglobulin G autoantibodies to mimicking and nonmimicking epitopes. Presence in autoimmune disease. *J. Clin. Invest.* **95**, 1316–1327.
62. Steinberg, A. D., Gourley, M. F., Klinman, D. M., Tsokos, G. C., Scott, D. E., and Krieg, A. M. (1991) Systemic lupus erythematosus. *Ann. Intern. Med.* **115**, 548–559.
63. James, J. J., Kaufman, K. M., Farris, A. D., Taylor-Albert, E., Lehman, T. J. A., and Harley, J. B. (1997) An increased prevalence of Epstein-Barr virus infection in young patients suggests a possible etiology for systemic lupus erythematosus. *J. Clin. Invest.* **100**, 3019–3026.
64. Misaki, Y., Yamamoto, K., Yanagi, K., Miura, H., Ichijo, H., Kato, T., et al. (1993) B cell epitope on the U1 snRNP-C autoantigen contains a sequence similar to that of the herpes simplex virus protein. *Eur. J. Immunol.* **23**, 1064–1071.
65. Phillips, P. E., Johnston, S. L., Runge, L. A., Moore, J. L., and Poiesz, B. J. (1986) High IgM antibody to human T-cell leukemia virus type I in systemic lupus erythematosus. *J. Clin. Immunol.* **6**, 234–241.
66. Kohsaka, H., Yamamoto, K., Fujii, H., Miura, H., Miyasaka, N., Nishioka, K., et al. (1990) Fine epitope mapping of the human SS-B/La protein. Identification of a distinct autoepitope homologous to a viral gag polyprotein. *J. Clin. Invest.* **85**, 1566–1574.
67. Perl, A. and Banki, K. (1993) Human endogenous retroviral elements and autoimmunity: data and concepts. *Trends Microbiol.* **1**, 153–156.
68. Zhu, Z. B., Hsieh, S., Bentley, D. R., Campbell, D., and Volanakis, J. E. (1992) A variable number of tandem repeat locus within the human complement C2 gene is associated with a retroposon derived from a human endogenous retrovirus. *J. Exp. Med.* **175**, 1783–1787.
69. Watanabe-Fukunaga, R., Brannan, C. L., Copeland, N. G., Jenkins, N. A., and Nagata, S. (1992) Lymphoproliferation disorder in mice explained by defects in Fas antigen that mediates apoptosis. *Nature* **356**, 314–317.
70. Nagata, S. and Golstein, P. (1995) The Fas death factor. *Science* **267**, 1449–1456.
71. Cianciolo, G. J., Copeland, T. D., Oroszlan, S., and Snyderman, R. (1985) Inhibition of lymphocyte proliferation by a synthetic peptide homologous to retroviral envelope proteins. *Science* **230**, 453–455.
72. Haraguchi, S., Good, R. A., and Day, N. K. (1995) Immunosuppressive retroviral peptides: cAMP and cytokine patterns. *Immunol. Today* **16**, 595–603.
73. Harley, J. B. and Gaither, K. K. (1988) Autoantibodies in systemic lupus erythematosus. *Rheum. Dis. Clin. North Am.* **14**, 43–56.
74. Dayal, A. K. and Kammer, G. M. (1996) The T cell enigma in lupus. *Arthritis Rheum.* **39**, 23–33.
75. Tsokos, G. C. (1992) Overview of cellular immune function in systemic lupus erythematosus, in *Systemic Lupus Erythematosus* (Lahita, R. G., ed.), Churchill Livingstone, New York, p. 15.
76. Klinman, D. M. and Steinberg, A. D. (1995) Inquiry into murine and human lupus. *Immunol. Rev.* **144**, 157–193.

77. Clerici, M. and Shearer, G. M. (1994) The Th1–Th2 hypothesis of HIV infection: new insights. *Immunol. Today* **15**, 575–581.
78. Casciola-Rosen, L. A., Anhalt, G., and Rosen, A. (1994) Autoantigens targeted in systemic lupus erythematosus are clustered in two populations of surface structures on apoptotic keratinocytes. *J. Exp. Med.* **179**, 1317–1330.
79. Cohen, J. J., Duke, R. C., Fadok, V. A., and Sellins, K. S. (1992) Apoptosis and programmed cell death in immunity. *Ann. Rev. Immunol.* **10**, 267–293.
80. White, E., Cipriani, R., Sabbatini, P., and Denton, A. (1991) The adenovirus E1B 19-kilodalton protein overcomes the cytotoxicity of E1A proteins. *J. Virol.* **65**, 2968–2978.
81. Whyte, P., Buchkovich, K., Horowitz, J. M., Friend, S. H., Raybuck, M., Weinberg, R. A., et al. (1988) Association between and oncogene and an anti-oncogene: the adenovirus E1A proteins bind to the retinoblastoma gene product. *Nature* **334**, 124–129.
82. Pan, H. and Griep, A. E. (1995) Temporally distinct patterns of p53-dependent and p53-independent apoptosis during mouse lens development. *Genes Dev.* **9**, 2157–2169.
83. Ehret, A., Westendorp, M. O., Herr, I., Debatin, K., Heeney, J. L., Frank, R., et al. (1996) Resistance of chimpanzee T cells to human immunodeficiency virus type I tat-enhanced oxidative stress and apoptosis. *J. Virol.* **70**, 6502–6507.
84. Banki, K., Hutter, E., Gonchoroff, N. J., and Perl, A. (1998) Molecular ordering in HIV-induced apoptosis: oxidative stress, activation of caspases, and cell survival are regulated by transaldolase. *J. Biol. Chem.* **273**, 11,944–11,953.
85. Westendorp, M. O., Frank, R., Ochsenbauer, C., Stricker, K., Dhein, J., Walczak, H., et al. (1995) Sensitization of T cells to CD95-mediated apoptosis by HIV-1 tat and gp120. *Nature* **375**, 497–500.
86. Strack, P. R., Frey, M. W., Rizzo, C. J., Cordova, B., George, H. J., Meade, R., et al. (1996) Apoptosis mediated by HIV protease is proceeded by cleavage of bcl-2. *Proc. Natl. Acad. Sci. USA* **93**, 9571–9576.
87. Morey, A. L., Ferguson, D. J, and Fleming, K. A. (1993) Ultrastructural features of fetal erythroid precursors infected with parvovirus B19 in vitro: evidence for cell death by apoptosis. *J. Pathol.* **169**, 213–220.
88. Naides, S. J., Scharosch, L. L., Foto, F., and Howard, E. J. (1990) Rheumatologic manifestations of human parvovirus B19 infection in adults. Initial two-year clinical experience. *Arthritis Rheum.* **33**, 1297–1309.
89. Hinshaw, V. S., Olsen, C. W., Dybdahl-Sissoko, N., and Evans, D. (1994) Apoptosis: a mechanism of cell killing by influenza A and B viruses. *J. Virol.* **68**, 3667–3673.
90. Bargonetti, J., Reynisdottir, I., Friedman, P. N., and Prives, C. (1992) Site-specific binding of wild-type p53 to cellular DNA is inhibited by SV40 T antigen and mutant p53. *Genes Dev.* **6**, 1886–1898.
91. Scheffner, M., Werness, B. A., Huibregtse, J. M., Levine, A. J., and Howley, P. M. (1990) The E6 oncoprotein encoded by human papillomavirus types 16 and 18 promotes the degradation of p53. *Cell* **63**, 1129–1136.
92. Wang, X. W., Gibson, M. K., Vermeulen, W., Yeh, H., Forrester, K., Sturzbecher, H. W., et al. (1995) Abrogation of p53-induced apoptosis by the hepatitis B virus X gene. *Cancer Res.* **55**, 6012–6016.
93. Bartz, S. R., Rogel, M. E., and Emerman, M. (1996) Human immunodeficiency virus type 1 cell cycle control: vpr is cytostatic and mediates G_2 accumulation by a mechanism which differs from DNA damage checkpoint control. *J. Virol.* **70**, 2324–2331.
94. Planelles, V., Jowett, J. B. M., Li, Q., Xie, Y., Hahn, B., and Chen, I. S. Y. (1996) Vpr-induced cell cycle arrest is conserved among primate lentiviruses. *J. Virol.* **70**, 2516–2524.
95. He, J., Choe, S., Walker, R., Di Marzio, P., Morgan, D. O., and Landau, N. R. (1995) Human immunodeficiency virus type 1 viral protein R (vpr) arrests cells in the G2 phase of the cell cycle by inhibiting p34cdc2 activity. *J. Virol.* **69**, 6705–6711.

96. Rao, L., Debbas, M., Sabbatini, P., Hockenberry, D., Korsmeyer, S., and White, E. (1992) The adenovirus E1A proteins induce apoptosis which is inhibited by the E1B 19K and bcl-2 proteins. *Proc. Natl. Acad. Sci. USA* **89,** 7742–7746.
97. Henderson, S., Huen, D., Rowe, M., Dawson, C., Johnson, G., and Rickinson, A. (1993) Epstein–Barr virus-coded BHRF1 protein, a viral homologue of bcl-2, protects human B cells from programmed cell death. *Proc. Natl. Acad. Sci. USA* **90,** 8479–8483.
98. Neilan, J. G., Lu, Z., Afonzo, C. L., Kutish, G. F., Sussman, M. D., and Rock, D. L. (1993) An African swine fever virus gene with similarity to the proto-oncogene bcl-2 and the Epstein-Barr virus gene BHRF1. *J. Virol.* **67,** 4391–4394.
99. Chou, J. and Roizman, B. (1992) The gamma$_1$34.5 gene of herpes simplex virus 1 precludes neuroblastoma cells from triggering total shutoff of protein synthesis characteristic of programmed cell death in neuronal cells. *Proc. Natl. Acad. Sci. USA* **89,** 3266–3270.
100. Yamada, T., Yamaoka, S., Goto, T., Nakai, M., Tsujimoto, Y., and Hatanaka, M. (1994) The human T-cell leukemia virus type I tax protein induces apoptosis which is blocked by the bcl-2 protein. *J. Virol.* **68,** 3374–3379.
101. Masutani, H., Hirota, K., Sasada, T., Ueda-Taniguchi, Y., Taniguchi, Y., Sono, H., et al. (1996) Transactivation of an inducible anti-oxidative stress protein, human thioredoxin by HTLV-I tax. *Immunol. Lett.* **54,** 67–71.
102. Kishi, S., Saijyo, S., Arai, M., Karasawa, S., Ueda, S., Kannagi, M., et al. (1997) Resistance to Fas-mediated apoptosis of peripheral T cells in human T lymphocyte virus type I (HTLV-I) transgenic mice with autoimmune arthropathy. *J. Exp. Med.* **186,** 57–64.
103. Iwakura, Y., Tosu, M., Yoshida, E., Takiguchi, M., Sato, K., Kitajima, I., et al. (1991) Induction of inflammatory arthropathy resembling rheumatoid arthritis in mice transgenic for HTLV-I. *Science* **253,** 1026–1028.
104. Green, J. E., Hinrichs, S. H., Vogel, J., and Jay, G. (1989) Exocrinopathy resembling Sjögren's syndrome in HTLV-I tax transgenic mice. *Nature* **341,** 72–74.
105. Banki, K., Hutter, E., Colombo, E., Gonchoroff, N. J., and Perl, A. (1996) Glutathione levels and sensitivity to apoptosis are regulated by changes in transaldolase expression. *J. Biol. Chem.* **271,** 32,994–33,001.
106. Ray, C. A., Black, R. A., Kronheim, S. R., Greenstreet, T. A., Sleath, P. R., Salvesen, G. S., et al. (1992) Viral inhibition of inflammation; cowpox virus encodes an inhibitor of the interleukein-1β converting enzyme. *Cell* **69,** 597–604.
107. Thome, M., Schneider, P., Hofman, K., Fickenscher, H., Meinl, E., Neipel, F., et al. (1997) Viral FLICE-inhibitory proteins (FLIPs) prevent apoptosis induced by death receptors. *Nature* **386,** 517–521.
108. Bertin, J. (1997) Death effector domain-containing herpesvirus and poxvirus proteins inhibit Fas- and TNFR1-induced apoptosis. *Proc. Natl. Acad. Sci. USA* **94,** 1172–1176.
109. Hochberg, M. C. (1990) Systemic lupus erythematosus. *Rheum. Dis. Clin. North Am.* **16,** 617–639.
110. Ray, C. G., Gall, E. P., Minnich, L. L., Roediger, J., De Benedetti, C., and Corrigan, J. J. (1982) Acute polyarthritis associated with active Epstein-Barr virus infection. *JAMA* **248,** 2990–2993.
111. Friedman, H. M., Pincus, T., Gibilisco, P., Baker, D., Glazer, J. P., and Plotkin, S. A. (1980) Acute monoarticular arthritis caused by herpes simplex virus and cytomegalovirus. *Am. J. Med.* **69,** 241–247.
112. Remafedi, G. and Muldoon, R. L. (1983) Acute monarticular arthritis caused by herpes simplex virus type. *Pediatrics* **72,** 882,883.
113. Sato, K., Maruyama, I., Maruyama, Y., Kitajima, I., Nakajima, Y., Higaki, M., et al. (1991) Arthritis in patients infected with human T lymphotropic virus type I. Clinical and immunopathologic features. *Arthritis Rheum.* **34,** 714–721.
114. Clem, R. J. and Miller, L. K. (1994) Control of programmed cell death by the baculovirus genes p35 and iap. *Mol. Cell. Biol.* **14,** 5212–5222.

3
Apoptosis

John D. Mountz, Hui-Chen Hsu, Huang-Ge Zhang, and Tong Zhou

1. Introduction

Apoptosis is a physiologic process that mediates the death of selected cells. In contrast to necrosis, which results from a strong nonspecific or toxic cell injury, apoptosis is initiated by ligand–receptor interactions that are highly regulated and tightly coupled to the phagocytosis of cells undergoing apoptosis. Several molecules that mediate or inhibit apoptosis of immune cells have now been identified, including Fas, tumor necrosis factor-receptor (TNF-R), and death domain related (DR) DR3, DR4, and DR5 *(1–7)* (*see* Fig. 1).

Apoptosis initiated by ligand–receptor interactions usually requires energy and results in distinctive changes in cell morphology. Early stages of apoptosis are indicated by loss of cell and nuclear volume *(8–10)*. Membrane changes are visible using light microscopy and include blebbing of the membrane. One of the distinctive features of apoptotic cell death is endonuclease degradation of chromosomal DNA into oligomers consisting of multiples of 180 base pairs. This pattern of degradation results in the "ladder" of DNA on gel analysis that is often used as an assay for apoptosis. Nuclear condensation and fragmentation is visible microscopically (Fig. 2). Although in vitro apoptosis leads to cell fragmentation, apoptosis in vivo is associated with uptake of these cells by macrophages; thus, apoptotic cells are usually observed only within macrophages. This is important because engulfment of apoptotic cells may be defective in systemic lupus erythematosis (SLE). Several macrophage receptors, including the scavenger receptor (SR-A) for phosphatidylserine, the thrombospondin receptor (including CD36 and the $\alpha_v\beta_3$ vitronectin receptor), and glycoproteins that have lost terminal sialic acid residues *(11)*. In lymphocytes, an asymmetric distribution of phospholipids across the plasma membrane is maintained by an ATP-dependent translocase, which specifically transports aminophospholipids from the outer to the inner leaflet of the bilayer. During apoptosis, this enzyme is downregulated and a lipid 'floppase' and the scramblase, are activated. Together, these events lead to the appearance of phosphatidylserine (PS) on the cell surface *(12,13)*.

2. Function of Apoptosis in the Immune System

Apoptosis is responsible for efficient removal of thymocytes and B-cells that express inappropriate receptors including thymocytes that either do not rearrange the T-cell

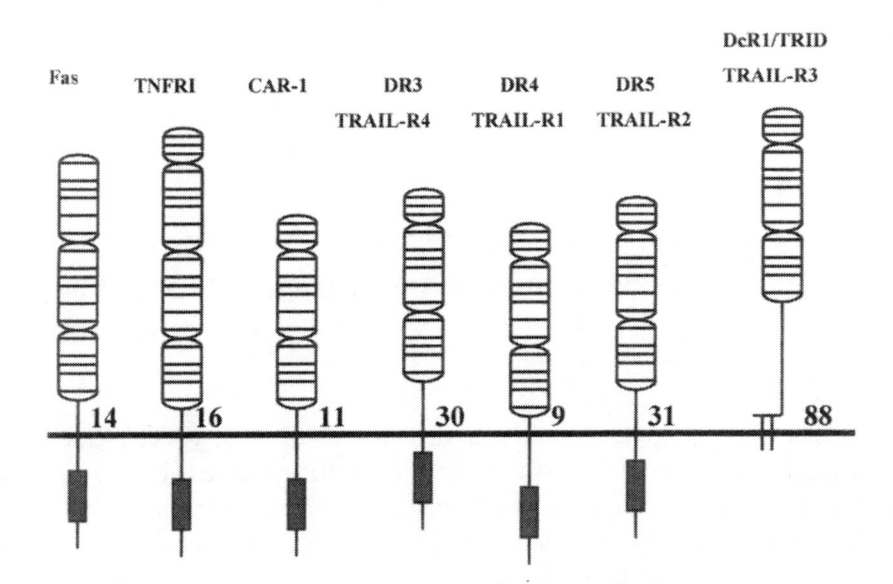

Fig. 1. Death domain family of receptors. The death domain family receptors include Fas, TNFR1, CAR-1, DR3, DR4, and DR5. The decoy receptor (DCR1/TRID) does not have a death domain but binds to the TNF receptor apoptosis-inducing ligand (TRAIL). Cystine repeat domains are shown in the extracellular (upper) part of the figure. Fas has three cystine-rich repeats and TNFR1 has four. The number of amino acids between the cystine-rich domain and the membrane are shown to the right of the molecule. The intracytoplasmic death domain is shown by the rectangular box.

receptor or fail to undergo appropriate positive or negative selection and B-cells that do not rearrange immunoglobulin genes normally. Thus, apoptosis plays a key role in shaping the T- and B-cell repertoire *(14)*. In young individuals, approximately 2% of progenitor T- cells or B-cells develop fully; the other 98% are eliminated by apoptosis during development. Thus, apoptosis is responsible for removing 5×10^7 thymocytes per day together with an equivalent number of B-cells. Although 98% of thymocytes undergo apoptosis, thymocytes are susceptible to apoptosis only during a 3-d time span, which takes place early in T-cell development. Moreover, the process of apoptosis occurs rapidly, taking only 1 h to complete. On analysis of the thymus, therefore, only 1% of thymocytes are undergoing visible apoptosis and these reside within macrophages *(15)*.

Apoptosis also is involved in the removal of immune cells after they have undergone activation and proliferation during a normal immune response, called activation-induced cell death (AICD) *(16–20)* (Fig. 3). This process efficiently removes inflammatory cells producing proinflammatory cytokines and likely plays a key role in downregulating the immune response. Thus, defects in AICD, even if minor, may contribute to chronic autoimmune rheumatic diseases. Activation-induced cell death is a highly regulated event that involves several apoptosis signaling molecules, including Fas and TNF-R, which are expressed on different cell types, including B-cells, T-cells, and macrophages.

Apoptosis also plays an important role in the removal of damaged or senescent immune cells *(21–23)*. Selective deletion of senescent T-cells throughout life is neces-

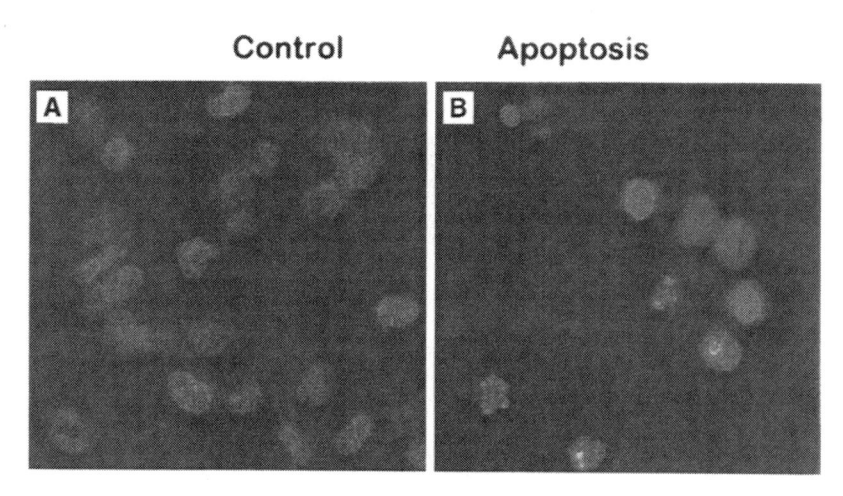

Fig. 2. Nuclear condensation and apoptosis. Jurkat T-cells were either untreated (control) or treated (apoptosis) with anti-Fas antibody. Apoptosis is characterized by nuclear condensation and cell shrinkage.

sary to prevent accumulation of these T-cells. It is, therefore, of interest that some aspects of apoptosis, including the expression and function of Fas, are decreased in T-cells obtained from aged mice *(21)*. Defective apoptosis and resulting accumulation of senescent T-cells and B-cells may contribute to late-age onset autoimmune disease and autoantibody production.

In summary, apoptosis is critical for the proper removal of immune cells at all stages of development. The complexity of apoptosis signaling pathways underlying removal of inflammatory cells during these events provides many potential points at which defects in apoptosis could give rise to a prolonged or autoimmune inflammatory reaction resulting in a chronic rheumatic disease.

3. Fas-Mediated Apoptosis

3.1. Regulation of the Fas Apoptosis Signaling Pathway

Fas/APO-1 (CD95) triggers apoptosis through a 90-amino-acid death domain (amino acids 201–292) of Fas, which is required to signal apoptosis *(24,25)*. Upon trimerization by the Fas ligand (FasL), the cytoplasmic death domain forms a death-inducing signaling complex (DISC) *(26)*. This DISC acts to dock adapter and signaling molecules that signal apoptosis, including Fas-associated protein with death domain (FADD or MORT1) *(27–31)*, which then recruits FADD-like interleukin-1β converting enzyme (ICE) (FLICE), now referred to as caspase 8 *(32–37)* (Fig. 4A).

T-cell apoptosis is associated with sequential caspase activation. Caspases are expressed constitutively in most cells, residing in the cytosol as a single-chain proenzyme. These are activated to fully functional proteases by proteolytic cleavage that first divides the chain into large and small caspase subunits and a second cleavage to remove the N-terminal domain (prodomain). The subunits assemble into a tetramer with two active sites *(38)*. Inefficient activation of caspase 8 results in direct activation of Bid, a pro-apoptotic member of the Bcl-2 family, and the C-terminal fragment acts on mitochondria triggering cytochrome-*c* release *(39,40)* (Fig. 4B). The released cyto-

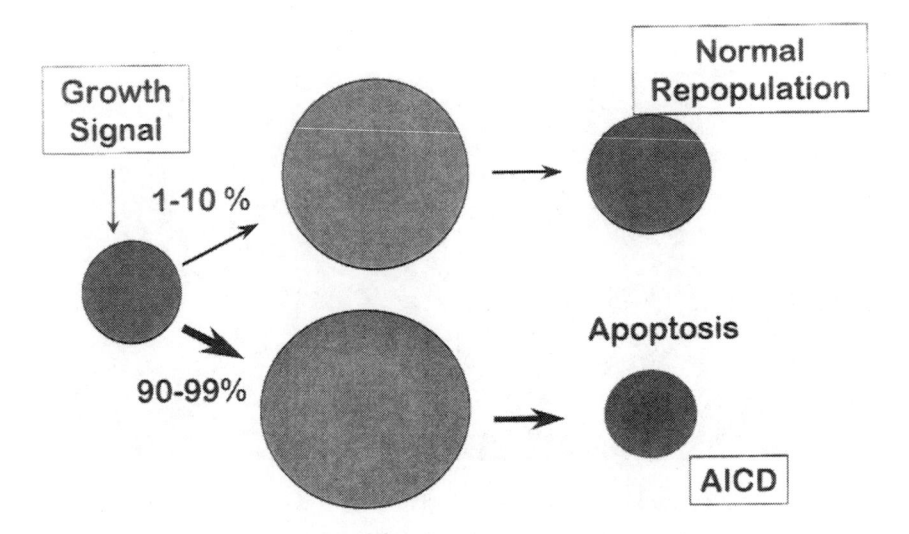

Fig. 3. Activation-induced cell death. Cells receiving an activation or growth signal enter into cell cycle and enlarge in size and proliferate. One to ten percent of the cells survive and eventually enter G_o or the resting cell phase. Most of the cells, 90–99%, do not survive and undergo AICD. AICD can result from an excessive activation signal, such as excessive amounts of IL-2 and PMA in the case of T-cells. Also, it can result from cells receiving a growth signal in the absence of supportive growth and differentiation factors or media.

chrome-*c* binds to Apaf-1, which self-associates and binds to caspase 9 *(41)*. This is associated with a drop in inner mitochondria membrane potential corresponding to the opening of the inner membrane permeability transition (PT) pore complex and loss of the ability to take up certain dyes *(42)*. In cells in which this mitochondria amplification loop is important, antiapoptotic Bcl-2 family members can suppress Fas-induced apoptosis *(43)*. Bcl-2 and Bcl-X act to prevent cytochrome-*c* release and thus interfere with this pathway. Caspases 9 and 8 then act on terminal caspases 3, 6, and 7 associated with apoptosis *(44)*. Alternatively, strong signaling through Fas leads to high levels of caspase 8 activity and direct activation of terminal caspases 3, 6, and 7, and apoptosis *(45–49)*.

The inhibitor of apoptosis (IAP) gene products play an evolutionarily conserved role in regulating programmed cell death in diverse species ranging from insects to humans. Human XIAP, cIAP1, and cIAP2 directly inhibit caspase 3, 6, and 7 *(50–53)*. The IAPs also can block cytochrome-*c*-induced activation of pro-caspase 9 and inhibit Fas-mediated apoptosis *(49)*. The murine homolog of the human X-linked IAP, called $_m$IAP, has been mapped to the X chromosome *(50–54)*.

3.2. TNF-Related-Apoptosis-Inducing-Ligand, a New Member of the FasL/TNFα Family

The tumor-necrosis-factor (TNF)-Related apoptosis-inducing ligand (TRAIL) was found as a new member of the TNF family, which mediates cell death in a wide variety of malignant cell lines and primary tumor cells *(55)*. There are currently five receptors that interact with TRAIL, including DR3, DR4, DR5, DR6, and a decoy receptor. TRAIL induces two different signals, cell death mediated by caspases, and gene induction mediated by nuclear factor κb (NF-κB). Inhibition of TRAIL-induced activation

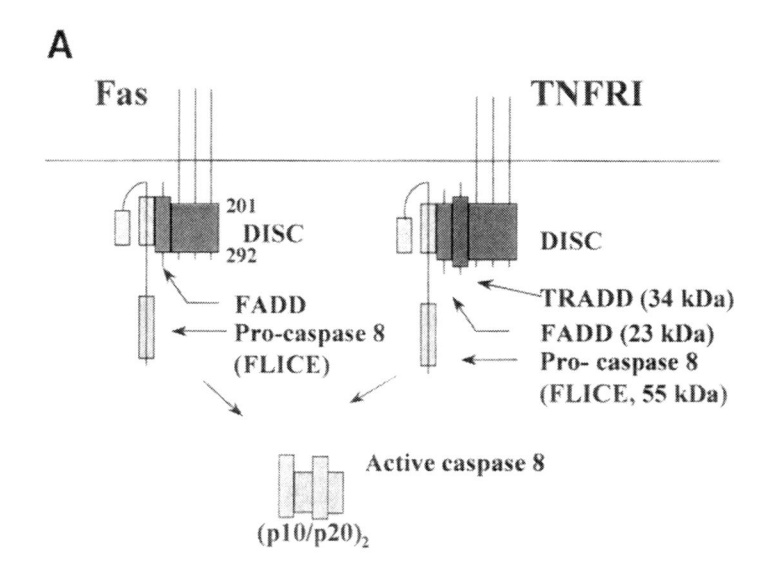

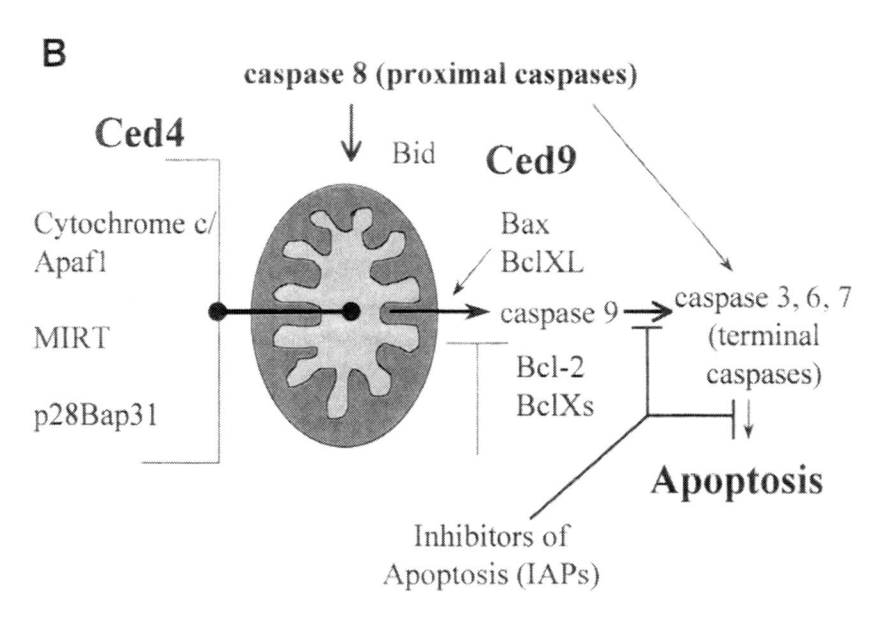

Fig. 4. Apoptosis signaling pathway. (A) Apoptosis signaling by a death-inducing signaling complex (DISC) were mediated by binding of Fas-associated death domain (FADD) and Fas-like ICE (FLICE, otherwise known as caspase 8) to Fas. The formatting of the DISC depends on crosslinking of the Fas molecule. This leads to the production of active caspase 8. In the case of TNFR1, the first molecule to bind to DISC is the TNF receptor apoptosis death domain (TRADD), followed by assembly of the same molecules as described for Fas. (B) The activated caspase 8 is regulated by Bcl-2 family members and mitochondrial signaling. Active caspase 8 directly activates Bid. In combination with other pro-apoptosis Bcl-2 family members (Bax, BclXL) or antiapoptosis Bcl-2 family members (Bcl-2, BclXS), this regulates the release of cytochrome C/Apaf-1 from mitochondria. This, in turn, acts on caspase 9 and terminal caspases 3, 6, and 7. Inhibitors of apoptosis (IAPs) act to prevent inversion of the procaspase to the caspase in the case of caspase 9 or prevent active caspase 3, 6, and 7 induction apoptosis.

of NF-κB augments apoptosis induction by TRAIL and attenuates apoptosis resistance. Currently, these molecules are of major interest due to their potential roles and application in cancer therapy.

3.3. Defective Apoptosis and Tolerance Loss in Mice and Humans

The role of apoptosis in the induction and maintenance of tolerance was first indicated by the identification of mutations of *Fas*L and *Fas* in the C3H-*gld/gld* and MRL-*lpr/lpr* autoimmune strains of mice *(56–62)*. CBA-*lpr/lpr* mice were first discovered to have a point mutation in the cytoplasmic death-domain-signaling region for Fas *(57)*. We and others have described that the genetic defect in MRL-*lpr/lpr* mice was an insertion of a 5kB retrotransposon in the second intron leading to abnormal splicing and premature termination of transcription *(63,64)*. In *gld/gld* mice, a point mutation at the carboxy terminus leads to a single amino acid change. This amino acid is located on the interface of the functional Fas ligand trimer resulting in an unstable trimer which is incapable of inducing trimerization of Fas *(62)*.

In order to study apoptosis of autoreactive T cells, we have analyzed autoreactive T-cell populations in the D^b/HY T-cell receptor (TCR) transgenic mice crossed to B6-*lpr/lpr* mice. In these mice, there was a minimal difference in expression of either CD8 or the D^b/HY T-cell receptor identified by the M33 clonotypic antibody *(65,66)*. However, there was a greatly increased and specific proliferative response of T-cells from the D^b/HY TCR male *lpr/lpr* mice to D^b male antigen-presenting cells (APCs) compared to the same population of autoreactive T-cells from D^b/HY TCR transgenic B6++ male mice. Similar results were obtained using Staphylococcal enterotoxin B (SEB) *(66–71)* for neonatally tolerized Vβ8 TCR transgenic MRL-*lpr/lpr* and MRL+/+ mice. Although the phenotype of the cells were different after neonatal tolerization, there was a greatly increased proliferative response of the autoreactive Vβ8-positive T-cells in MRL-*lpr/lpr* mice but not MRL+/+ mice. Of interest, this autoreactivity required new T-cells from the thymus because thymectomy after induction of tolerance eliminated the increased response of autoreactive T-cells in the MRL-*lpr/lpr* mice. These results demonstrate that (1) there is no detectable apoptosis defect of autoreactive T-cells in Fas-deficient *lpr/lpr* mice and (2) the primary tolerance defect in *lpr/lpr* mice is a failure to downregulate proliferation of autoreactive T-cells after stimulation with self-antigen.

These types of experiments have not been analyzed in humans with SLE. First, in contrast to experiments using T-cell-receptor (TCR) transgenic mice, self-reactive T-cells in humans cannot be identified. Autoreactive T-cells are only a small fraction of the activated T-cell population and have only been made visible for the first time by using TCR transgenic mice. Second, tolerance experiments such as introduction of a self-reactive T-cell or neonatal tolerance as described cannot be carried out in humans. Experiments using human peripheral blood mononuclear cells (PBMCs) must resort to the total population of T-cells that express multiple specificities. Therefore, it has not been possible to determine if there is a defect in activation-induced cell death of a minor population of T-cells with autoreactive specificities. The future direction and challenge in this area is to obtain T-cells from autoimmune diseases where the autoreactive specificity may be known, such as myelin basic protein autoreactive T-cells in patients with multiple sclerosis. Analysis of defective or normal AICD of these T-cells should help clarify if there is or is not an AICD defect of autoreactive T-cells in humans with autoimmune disease.

4. Regulation of Apoptosis in SLE and SLE-like Syndromes

4.1. Is There Defective Apoptosis in Patients With SLE?

The pathogenesis of SLE is multifactorial and multigenetic. Chronic inflammation associated with lupus is thought to result from loss of self-tolerance resulting from molecular mimicry, environment triggers, hormonal factors, or apoptosis defects. Defects in apoptosis can lead to abnormal clonal deletion of autoreactive cells or failure to down modulate an inflammatory response. Although the Fas death domain family of molecules are the primary pathway for elimination of inflammatory cells, defects in these death domain molecules are rarely observed in patients with SLE. Other death domain family molecules such as DR3, DR4, DR5, and DR6 have not been studied in SLE. Also, there are signaling pathways for apoptosis, including FADD, TNRFI-associated death domain (TRADD), and FADD-like ICE (FLICE) which are important in apoptosis signaling. The Bcl-2 family modulates apoptosis and has been reported to be abnormal in human autoimmune disease.

4.2. Fas Mutations and Autoimmunity in Patients With Autoimmune Lymphoproliferative Syndrome (ALPS)

In humans, Fas mutations have been identified in some individuals from families with autoimmune lymphoproliferative syndrome (ALPS) *(72–74)* (Fig. 5A). Heterozygous expression of the Fas mutations in these individuals results in a decrease in Fas-mediated apoptosis function. The Canale–Smith syndrome exhibits mutation of Fas and lymphoproliferative disease and is now considered to be identical with ALPS syndrome *(75)*. We have identified one patient with a mutation of the Fas ligand, and lymphoproliferative disease also exhibits AICD defect of PBMCs *(76)* (Fig. 5B). Interestingly, although these patients and one of their parents exhibit a heterozygous mutation of Fas, the parents do not develop ALPS. Also, heterozygous mutations in mouse Fas (*lpr/+*) or Fas ligand (*gld/+*) do not develop lymphoproliferative disease. Heterozygous mutations of Fas lead to production of mutant Fas molecules, which act as dominant negatives and prevent functional trimer formation *(73)*.

4.3. Evidence that there is Increased Apoptosis in Human SLE

Based on experiments in *lpr/lpr* and *gld/gld* mice that develop systemic autoimmune disease, we first propose that humans with autoimmune disease may exhibit apoptosis and/or AICD defects *(77)*. In contrast to ALPS syndrome, most studies of lupus patients report increased apoptosis and increased AICD of PBMCs. Accelerated in vitro apoptosis of PBMCs from patients with SLE was first analyzed by Emlen et al. *(78)*. There was a 2–3-fold increase in spontaneous apoptosis of lymphocytes from patients with SLE compared to normal controls. Several investigators then reported that PBMC from patients with SLE exhibited increased apoptosis after AICD *(79–81)*. In contrast, short-term established cell lines from patients with SLE exhibit a decrease in anti-CD3-mediated AICD, and this could be blocked in both control and SLE T-cells by an IgG anti-Fas antibody *(82)*. The analysis of activation pathways in lupus needs to take into account not only the differences between the in vitro and in vivo environments but

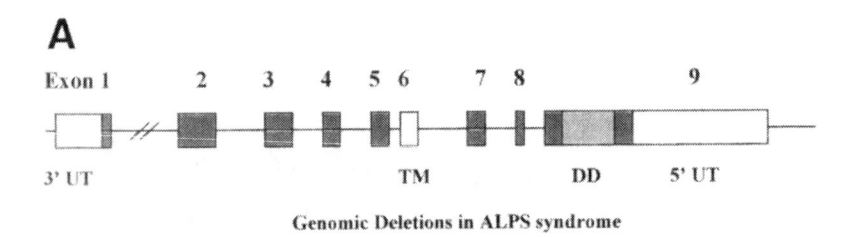

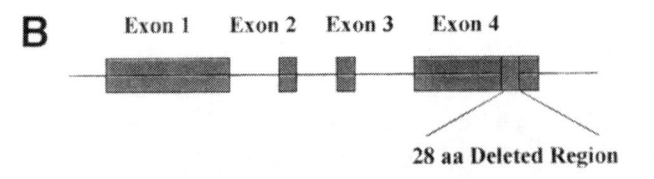

Fig. 5. Fas and Fas ligand mutations in patients with ALPS and SLE. **(A)** There are several Fas mutations that have been identified in ALPS patients that involve both the extracellular domain as well as the death domain. Shown is the genomic organization of Fas with nine exons including a transmembrane exon (exon 6) and a death domain which is entirely encoded within exon 9. **(B)** Fas ligand mutation identified in the patient with SLE. This consists of a 28 amino acid deletion within exon 4.

also the mechanisms of activation of T-cells. Different subpopulations of T-cells may be more or less susceptible to AICD. There was increased anti-CD3-induced apoptosis of CD28 positive T-cells in patients with SLE compared to controls, consistent with the downregulation of CD28 on peripheral T-cells in patients with SLE *(83)*.

T-cells from patients with SLE express increased levels of functional Fas ligand after anti-CD3 signaling *(84–86)*. These types of experiments are normally carried out using TCR signaling of T-cells from patients with SLE and normal controls, and testing these T-cells on a ^{51}Cr-labeled Fas-expressing target cell. The distinction between the membrane Fas ligand, as determined by functional assays described earlier, and the soluble Fas ligand as can be measured in sera is important because the soluble Fas ligand is reported to be an inhibitor of Fas apoptosis *(87)*.

4.4. Evidence for Dysregulation of Bcl-2 and IL-10 in Patients with SLE

Many *(88–91)* but not all *(92)* investigators reported high levels of BcL-2 protein in circulating T-cells or PBMC from patients with SLE. IL-10 has been shown to promote AICD of SLE patients and that increased spontaneous cell death in vitro results from in vitro T-cell activation and induction of IL-10 and Fas ligand *(93)*. A genetic linkage has been established between IL-10 and Bcl-2 genotypes, which determines susceptibility to SLE *(94)*. Short tandem repeat sequences (microsatellites) within the noncoding region of these genes were identified and used as genetic markers. This was used to examine a large Mexican-American SLE cohort of 128 patients and 223 ethnically matched controls. The DNA was analyzed using florescent-labeled primers and semiautomatic genotyping. The results revealed a synergistic effect between susceptible alleles of Bcl-2 and IL-10 in the determination of disease susceptibility, and two alleles together increased the odds of developing SLE by more than 40-fold. This is

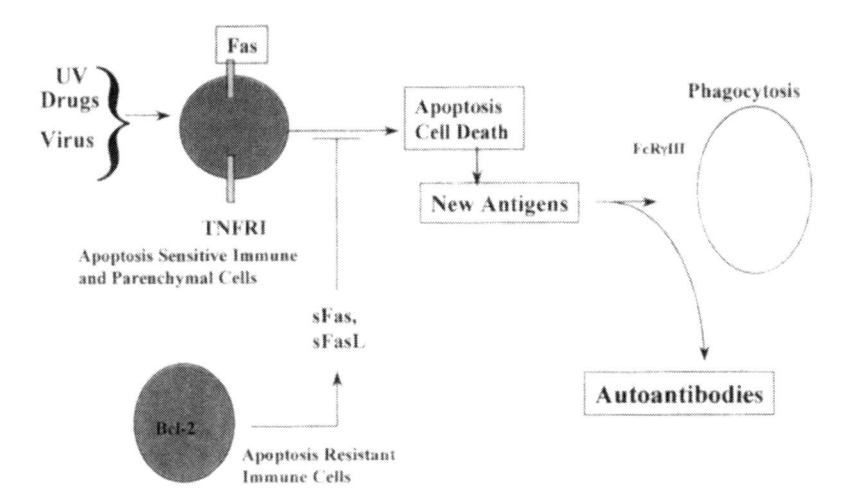

Fig. 6. Decreased Clearance of Antigen-Antibody Complex in SLE. Different environmental stimuli or toxins including UV light, drugs, or viruses can induce apoptosis of cells and release of new antigens including nucleoli or novel phosphorylated proteins, that occur during apoptosis. This may be influenced by regulatory mechanisms such as Bcl-2 or soluble Fas (sFas) or sFas ligand. Failure to clear new antigens in an efficient manner leads to autoimmunization and production of autoantibodies.

first time a specific combination of two distinct genes that regulate apoptosis have been found to predispose humans to an autoimmune disease.

These results suggest a model of dysregulated apoptosis in patients with SLE *(95)*. Increased in vivo apoptosis resulting from activation, ultraviolet (UV) light, and IL-10 leads to the release of intracellular antigens such as phosphorylated apoptosis signaling pathway molecules and also certain inhibitors of apoptosis such as soluble Fas, soluble Fas ligand, and upregulation of Bcl-2 by bystander cells (Fig. 6). A secondary immune dysfunction may occur because of defective apoptosis or the presence of antiapoptosis molecules and bystander immune cells. This effect of increased apoptosis may be potentiated by dysregulation of apoptosis signaling leading to production of new antigens or the failure of rapid clearance of cells that would normally occur if the apoptosis process was normal. Taken together, these results suggest that dysfunctional apoptosis in patients with SLE may underlie disease pathogenesis. This may be the result of increased apoptosis through pathways and, at the same time, decreased apoptosis through other pathways.

4.5. Decreased Clearance of Apoptotic Cell Residue may Result in Production of Autoantibodies in SLE

One possible mechanism for the decrease in clearance is an increase in SLE disease activity if there is increased binding of the Fc receptor by certain FcγRIII alleles. More severe SLE disease is associated with a polymorphism of FcγRIII (CD16) *(96)*, which alters the function of this receptor and predisposes to autoimmune disease. Patients with this polymorphism have more severe disease, as well as a greater level of NK cell activation and more rapid induction of AICD associated with the higher binding of the allele of FcγRIII. There is a strong association with the low-binding phenotype with lupus nephritis. These results suggest that increased apoptosis signaling through the FcγRIII receptor is beneficial for patients with lupus.

Increased apoptotic cells or fragments in patients with SLE could be the result of increased apoptosis and/or decreased clearance of these fragments *(97)*. High levels of circulating apoptotic PBMCs nuclear cells have been observed by many investigators in patients with SLE *(98)*. These cells were analyzed by annexin-V- FITC staining in flow cytometry of PBMCs from patients with SLE compared to normal controls. There is no correlation between percentage of apoptotic cells and the Systemic Lupus Activity Measure (SLAM)-SCORE or to therapy. Defective phagocyte function and not defective apoptosis was observed in PBMCs of patients with SLE *(99)*. In vitro phagotosis of autologous apoptotic cells in culture with PBMCs was examined microscopically and found to be defective in patients with SLE. These results suggest the persistently circulating apoptotic waste due to defective removal pathways and serve as an immunogen for the induction of autoreactive lymphocytes and as an antigen for immune complex formation.

Apoptosis in PBMC from patients with SLE is associated with generation of novel autoantigens and decreased clearance. In vivo nucleosomes are generated during apoptosis and may lead to the production of antinucleosomal antibodies *(100)*. One mechanism of protein fragments during apoptosis is the activation of caspases. Surface blebs of apoptotic cells constitute an important immunologic and potentially autoantigenic particle in SLE *(101)*. Apoptosis is associated with translocation of the phosphatidyl serine (PS) from the inner membrane leaflet to the outer membrane leaflet. Phosphatidyl serine is a potent pro-coagulant and can also lead to generation of antiphospholipid antibodies *(101–103)*. Different apoptotic stimuli, including Fas ligation, γ-radiation, and UV irradiation, but not anti-CD3 ligation leads to generation of several distinct serine phosphorylated proteins *(104)*. This protein phosphorylation precedes or is coincident with the induction of DNA fragmentation related to apoptosis. Over 75% of patients with SLE that produced antinuclear antibodies also product antibodies to these novel phosphorylated proteins *(105)*. A 72-KD signal recognition particle (SRP) protein is cleaved to a 66-KD immunoterminal fragment by caspase 3 and is an autoantigen in some patients with SLE. Therefore, new proteins phosphorylated during apoptosis may be preferred targets for autoantibodies in patients with SLE.

4.6. sFas Is Elevated in SLE and Is Correlated with Organ Damage

We have isolated chromosomal DNA for the human *Fas* gene and characterized the intron/exon organization as well as the promoter region *(106)*. We have also identified a naturally occurring soluble, alternatively spliced form of human *Fas* capable of binding to the Fas ligand and inhibiting apoptosis *(107,108)*. Soluble Fas is normally present at serum levels of 0.2–2.0 ng/mL, and despite original controversy *(109,110)*, it is now known to be increased in patients with SLE *(111–116)* (Fig. 7). We initially hypothesized that sFas may play a role in both immune regulation and regulation of Fas ligand-mediated tissue damage in SLE *(117)*. Levels of sFas were measured over a period of 4 yr (277 visits) in 39 patients with varying degrees of disease activity and disease severity. Healthy age- and sex-matched volunteers served as controls. SLE Disease Activity Index (SLEDAI) scores for disease activity were registered, as were SLICC/ACR

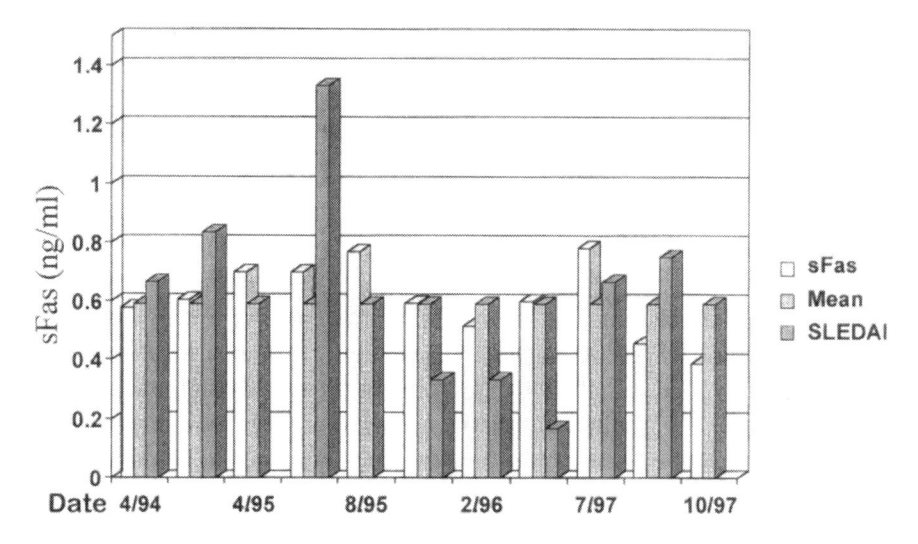

Fig. 7. Elevated sFas in SLE does not correlate with SLEDAI. Shown is a graph of a typical patient with SLE. Soluble Fas (sFas) and systemic lupus erythematosis disease activity index (SLEDAI) was determined that different times ranging from 1994 to 1997, over a 4-yr period. The level of soluble Fas does not vary much from the mean value as shown in this stippled bar. However, SLEDAI varies greatly. These results are typical and indicate that sFas is elevated in patients with SLE and does not vary over time for a given patient. Also, sFas does not correlate with SLEDAI.

scores for accumulative organ damage. Autoantibodies, liver and kidney function tests, as well as serum complement were determined. sFas levels were elevated in patients with SLE (0.60 ng/mL) compared to controls (0.26 ng/mL). sFas was found to correlate with the SLICC/ACR damage index but did not correlate with the SLEDAI. sFas was strongly correlated with liver and renal function tests measured by serum albumin, AST, serum creatinine, and creatinine clearance but did not correlate with inflammatory activity measured by erythrocyte sedimentation rate (ESR) and acute-phase reactants. These result further confirmed that sFas is elevated in patients with SLE. Because sFas correlates with indices of organ damage and not with disease activity, we suggest that sFas might be a marker of organ damage in SLE. We propose that in patients with SLE, sFas is primarily produced at sites of organ damage to inhibit the Fas ligand. These results are consistent with previous reports of increased sFas associated with liver disease.

4.7. Mapping of Genes Associated with Human SLE

There is a strong genetic predisposition for SLE among monozygotic twins (57%) and a relatively low concordance rate in dizygotic twins (5%) and first-degree relatives (5–12%). This strongly supports the hypothesis that SLE susceptibility is inherited as a multiple factorial genetic disease. Because of the complex and heterogeneous nature SLE, it has been difficult to collect sufficient patient samples for genetic analysis. However, certain genetic loci related to lupus are just now being identified, but can be mapped to regions on chromosome 1q41, 6p11–21 (near the HLA), 16q13, 14q21–23, and 2op12.3 *(118–121)*. These loci do not yet have specific apoptosis genes associated with them in general and could include genes such as FcγRII, MHC genes, TGFβ, as well as other genes.

4.8. Mapping of Genes Associated with Mouse Models of SLE

Several investigators have analyzed mouse models of lupus to identify the location of genes that confer disease susceptibility in several murine SLE models *(122–129)*. The mouse models studied include the MRL strain, NZB, NZW, and NZB/W. The strongest susceptibility genes that are common to all these mouse models are in the telemetric region of chromosome 1, the middle of chromosome 4, and the centromeric region of chromosome 7. Splenomegaly is associated with the susceptibility locus on chromosomes 1 and 4. These same loci also contribute to the development of glomerulonephritis, autoantibody production, and the ability to produce antibody in response to an exogenous agent (immune-response locus). There are other loci where the genetic predisposition has been known to occur and the underlying genes are known. This includes the immunoglobulin locus on chromosome 12 of mouse, which contributes to the immune response. Also, the H2 (MHC) locus on chromosome 17 contributes to development of glomerulonephritis and autoantibody production.

Other genes influence autoimmunity in *lpr/lpr* mice because back-crossing of *lpr/lpr* genes onto different strains of mice results in the development of different types of lymphoproliferative autoimmune disease. Genetic differences between the different strains of *lpr/lpr* mice play a role in determining the levels of autoantibody production, the type and severity of autoimmune disease, and the extent of lymphoproliferation. For example, genes determining the severity of renal disease in mice expressing the *lpr/lpr* gene have been mapped to chromosomes 7 and 12 *(122,123)*, whereas genes associated with the development of arthritis mapped to chromosome 11 are proposed to be inducible nitric oxide synthase (NOS) *(124)*. Heterozygous expression of the *lpr* gene also leads to a less severe form of lymphoproliferative autoimmune disease.

(NZB × NZW) F1 mice exhibit an autoimmune diathesis similar to lupus and have been reported to exhibit a defect in TNF/TNF-R-mediated signaling *(125–127)*. Loci on chromosome 1, also known as *Sle*1, can be demonstrated to cause a lost of tolerance to chromatin autoantigens when expressed on a B-6 background in an interval-specific congenetic strain, B6.NZMc1. The locus on chromosome 4, also known as *Sle*2 is characterized by an intrinsic B-cell hyperresponsiveness to lipopolysaccharide (LPS) and conventional antigens, and heightened, spontaneous B-cell proliferation and IgM secretion in vitro. These results indicate that *Sle*2 contains a gene that leads to spontaneous B-cell hyperactivity in elevated production of B-1-cells. The locus susceptibility on chromosome 7, known as *Sle*3, is associated with amplification of helper-T-cells for humoral autoimmunity. An interval-specific congenetic mouse containing *Sle*3 on chromosome 7 (B6.NZMc7) exhibits a spontaneous expansion of CD4+ T-cells and increased response to T-dependent antigens. These results indicate that *Sle*3 potentates a T-cell responsiveness in general and can predispose to development of spontaneous autoimmunity to a broad spectrum of neutral antigens. It has been proposed that *Sle*3 plays an important role in potentiating the antigen-dependent expansion of helper-T-cells that can drive B-cells to make auto antibodies.

5. Regulation of Apoptosis in Rheumatoid Arthritis

5.1. Apoptosis Defects in Synovial Cells of Patients with Rheumatoid Arthritis

Initial investigations of apoptosis in rheumatoid synovium indicated that apoptotic cells were confined to the synovial lining layer and that infiltrating T-cells express high levels of BcL-2 and were resistant to Fas apoptosis *(130–132)*. Other studies reported decreased expression of Bcl-2 in synovial fluid T-cells and there was no significant difference in Bcl-2 expression and synovial tissue T-cells in RA compared to osteoarthritis (OA) and reactive arthritis *(133,134)*. Soluble Fas, capable of binding Fas ligand and inhibiting Fas apoptosis, is found to be increased in the synovial fluid of patients with RA *(135,136)*. Other investigators reported increased expression of the Fas ligand on activated T-cells in RA synovium *(137–141)*, as well as increased expression of Fas and high sensitivity to apoptosis *(142–147)*. Therefore, most studies support the notion that T-cells in the synovium of patients with RA are activated and correspondingly express increased levels of Fas and the Fas ligand and tend to undergo Fas-mediated apoptosis. However, the question remains whether this apoptosis is appropriately high enough to eliminate T-cells that promote inflammatory disease.

The synovial fibroblast that undergoes hyperplasia in patients with rheumatoid arthritis has been reported to have several defects in Fas, the Fas ligand, apoptosis, and expression of other apoptosis molecules such as p53. Apoptotic synovial lining cells are largely type A (macrophage-like) with little apoptosis of type B (fibroblast-like) synovial cells. These synovial fibroblasts have been demonstrated to be sensitive to apoptosis in an HTLV-1 tax transgenic mouse model when high levels of anti-Fas antibody were injected intra-articularly *(148)*. These experiments were carried out using a novel anti-Fas monoclonal antibody (RK-8), which did not cause significant liver toxicity but can crosslink Fas and induce apoptosis in some strains of mice. Also, transfection of the human Fas ligand into RA synovial fibroblasts that have been transplanted into SCID mice can also produce apoptosis *(149,150)*. Similar results were obtained using anti-Fas monoclonal antibody-inducing apoptosis of human RA tissue engrafted into SCID mice *(151)*. TNFα has been shown to inhibit *(152)* or facilitate *(153)* Fas signaling in human RA synovial fibroblasts. Together, these results indicate that Fas apoptosis signaling may be defective in human synovial fibroblasts and that this signaling can be effected by other cytokines such as TNFα and TGFβ that are present in abundance in the joint tissue *(154)*.

A novel pathway of apoptosis resistance for some synovial cells appear to be the expression of mutant p53 *(155)*. It was hypothesized that free-radical production associated with the highly oxidative metabolism present in the inflammatory and invasive areas of synovium may lead to mutations for the p53 tumor-suppressor gene *(156)*. Therefore, p53 is proposed to be a critical regulator of fibroblastlike synovial cell proliferation, apoptosis and invasiveness. Abnormalities of p53 function might contribute to synovial lining expansion and joint destruction in RA.

5.2. Regulation of Apoptosis Pathways Signaling in RA Synovial Cells

The signaling pathway for Fas in synovial fibroblasts has not been extensively studied but several observations indicate that Fas signaling is downregulated. Fas apoptosis

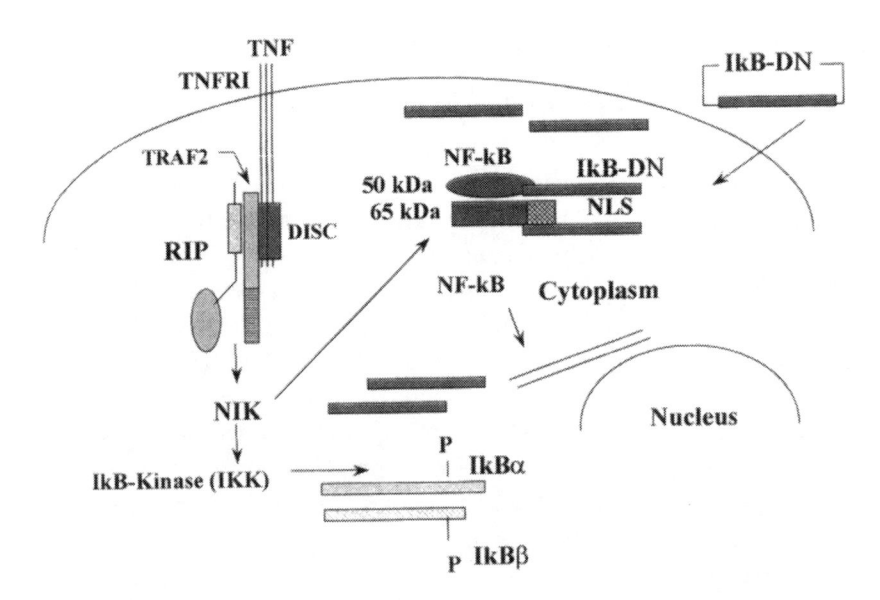

Fig. 8. NF-κB nuclear translocation. Signaling through TNFR1 activates the DISC, and a second pathway leading to activation of NF-κB-inducing kinase (NIK). NIK phosphorylates and activates I-κB kinase, which, in turn, phosphorylates I-κB. This results in dissociation of I-κB-α and -β chains from NF-κB. I-κB-α and -β are degraded in the proteosome and NF-κB is translocated to the nucleus to result in induction of antiapoptosis molecules such as inhibitors of apoptosis (IAPs). Overexpression of an I-κB—dominant negative that lacks the phosphorylation site for I-κB kinase leads to irreversible binding of I-κB to NF-κB and prevents nuclear translocation of NF-κB. This leads to apoptosis of rheumatoid arthritis synovial fibroblasts (RASF) in response to TNFα treatment.

has been shown by one investigator to involve the JUN kinase and the AP1 pathway *(157)*, as well as ceramide signaling *(158)*. Other investigators have found defects of the MAP kinase/kinase to be defective in RA synovial fibroblasts *(159)*. Other pathways of pro- and anti-apoptosis in RA synovial fibroblasts include TNF receptor signaling. TNF receptor signaling can activate a potent anti-inflammatory pathway via NF-κB nuclear translocation *(160,161)*. Analysis of synovium of rats in the Streptococcal cell wall (SCW model) indicated that a mutant form of IκB that prevents nuclear translocation of NF-κB results in enhanced apoptosis of synovium of rats in this model. Other investigators have shown, using an Ad-IκB-dominant negative mutant in human RA synovial cell lines, that blocking of NF-κB nuclear translocation combine with addition of TNFα leads to unopposed activity of the pro-apoptotic pathway and high apoptosis of human RA synovial cells (Fig. 8). Further understanding of the regulation of Fas and TNF-receptor apoptosis pathways in RA synovial fibroblasts should lead to insights to mechanisms to induce apoptosis of these cells and inhibit the synovial hyperplasia characteristic of RA.

5.3. Regulation of Apoptosis as Current Therapy for RA

Most current therapies used for rheumatoid arthritis have been shown to induce apoptosis *(162)*. Chloroquine inhibits growth of human umbilical vein endothelial cells (HUVECS) by induction of apoptosis. This is associated with upregulation of Bcl-X without any change in Bcl-2 *(163)*. The folate antagonist methotrexate (MTX) is used extensively to treat rheumatoid arthritis as well as other chronic inflammatory diseases. MTX exerts an antiproliferative property by inhibition by dihydrofolate reductase and other folate-dependent enzymes. Methotrexate efficiently induced apoptosis of T-cells in a concentration of 0.1–10 µmol. This apoptosis did not depend on Fas or the Fas ligand but required a cell cycle entry. In vitro activation of PBLs from arthritis patients after MTX injection resulted in increased propensity toward apoptosis *(164)*. Phototherapy, useful in the treatment of rheumatic disease, can operate by direct induction of the Fas and Fas ligand system *(165)* and also by Fas-independent apoptosis *(166)*. Soluble TNF-receptor type 2 (Enbrel, Immunex, Seattle, WA) and soluble TNF-receptor type 1 can inhibit later stages of inflammatory disease *(167,168)*. In contrast, we and others have previously shown that TNFα can inhibit development of autoimmune disease and that TNFR1 knockout mice crossed with *lpr/lpr* mice develop an accelerated autoimmune disease *(169,170)*. These different results of TNF are the result of the dual signaling pathway of the TNF receptor. One pathway involves a pro-apoptotic mechanism and acts through TRADD and then FADD and caspase 8, as shown above for Fas. However, this pathway appears to be blocked in RA synovial cells. The second pathway, a pro-inflammatory pathway, is mediated primarily by a nuclear translocation of NF-κB, which induces transcription of pro-inflammatory cytokines as well as transcription of antiapoptosis molecules such as IAP. Sulfasalazine, which is widely used for rheumatoid arthritis as well as inflammatory bowel disease, can induce apoptosis of neutrophils in vitro *(171)*. Neutrophil apoptosis can be blocked by specific inhibitors including a tyrosine kinase inhibitor, protein kinase A inhibitors, and antioxidants. These results indicate that phosphorylation of tyrosine kinase and protein kinase A as well as generations of reactive oxygen species are involved in sulfasalazine-mediated neutrophil apoptosis. Together, these results indicate that a better understanding of apoptosis pathways and better mechanisms to trigger these apoptosis pathways will be beneficial in the treatment of rheumatic diseases.

Acknowledgments

This work was supported in part by the Veterans Administration Merit Review Award, and grants RO1 AG 11653, RO1 AI 42900, and (NO-1 AR-62224) from the National Institutes of Health. The production of transgenic mice at UAB was supported by National Cancer Institute grant CA13148 to the University of Alabama at Birmingham Comprehensive Cancer Center. Hui-Chen Hsu is a recipient of a postdoctoral fellowship from the Arthritis Foundation.

References

1. Nagata, S. and Golstein, P. (1995) The Fas death factor. *Science* **267**, 1449–1156.
2. Itoh, N., Yonehara, S., Ishii, A., et al. (1991) The polypeptide encoded by the cDNA for human cell surface antigen Fas can mediate apoptosis. *Cell* **66**, 233–246.
3. Degli-Esposti, M. A., Dougall, W. C., Smolak, P. J., Waugh, J. Y., Smith, C. A., and Goodwin, R. G. (1997) The novel receptor TRAIL-R4 induces NF-kappaB and protects against TRAIL-mediated apoptosis, yet retains an incomplete death domain. *Immunity* **7**, 813–820.
4. Chaudhary, P. M., Eby, M., Jasmin, A., Bookwalter, A., Murray, J., and Hood, L. (1997) Death receptor 5, a new member of the TNFR family, and DR4 induce FADD-dependent apoptosis and activate the NF-kappaB pathway. *Immunity* **7**, 821–830.

5. Schneider, P., Thome, M., Burns, K., Bodmer, J. L., Hofmann, K., Kataoka, T., et al. (1997) TRAIL receptors 1 (DR4) and 2 (DR5) signal FADD-dependent apoptosis and activate NF-kappaB. *Immunity* **7,** 831–836.
6. Marsters, S. A., Sheridan, J. P., Pitti, R. M., Huang, A., Skubatch, M., Baldwin, D., et al. A novel receptor for Apo2L/TRAIL contains a truncated death domain. *Curr. Biol.* **7,** 1003–1006.
7. Golstein, P. (1997) Cell death: TRAIL and its receptors. *Curr. Biol.* **7,** R750–R753.
8. Wyllie, A. H. (1980) Glucocorticoid-induced thymocyte apoptosis is associated with endogenous endonuclease activation. *Nature* **284,** 555–557.
9. Duke, R. C., Chervenak, R., and Cohen, J. J. (1983) Endogenous endonuclease-induced DNA fragmentation: an early event in cell-mediated cytolysis. *Proc. Natl. Acad. Sci. USA* **80,** 6361–6372.
10. Cohen, J. J., Duke, R. C., Fadok, V. A., and Sellins, K. S. (1992) Apoptosis and programmed cell death in immunity. *Annu. Rev. Immunol.* **10,** 267–271.
11. Savill, J. (1995) The innate immune system: recognition of apoptotic cells, in *Apoptosis and Immune Response*. Wiley–Liss, New York, pp. 341–369.
12. Verhoven, B., Krahling, S., Schlegel, R. A., and Williamson, P. (1999) Regulation of phosphatidylserine exposure and phagocytosis of apoptotic T lymphocytes. *Cell Death Differ.* **6,** 262–270.
13. Bratton, D. L., Fadok, V. A., Richter, D. A., Kailey, J. M., Guthrie, L. A., and Henson, P. M. (1997) Appearance of phosphatidylserine on apoptotic cells requires calcium-mediated non-specific flip-flop and is enhanced by loss of the aminophospholipid translocase. *J. Biol. Chem.* **17,** 26,159–26,165.
14. Golstein, P., Ojcius, D. M., and Young, J. D. (1991) Cell death mechanisms and the immune system. *Immunol. Rev.* 121, 29–65.
15. Surh, C. D. and Sprent, J. (1994) T cell apoptosis detected in situ during positive and negative selection in the thymus. *Nature* **372,** 100–103.
16. Green, D. R. and Scott, D.W. (1994) Activation-induced apoptosis in lymphocytes. *Curr. Opin. Immunol.* **6,** 476–487.
17. Alderson, M. R., Tough, T. W., Davis-Smith, T., et al. (1995) Fas ligand mediates activation-induced cell death in human T lymphocytes. *J. Exp. Med.* **181,** 71–77.
18. Dhein, J., Walczak, H., Baumler, C., Debatin, K. M., and Krammer, P. H. (1995) Autocrine T-cell suicide mediated by APO-1/(Fas/CD95). *Nature* **373,** 438–441.
19. Ju, S. T., Panka, D. J., Cui, H., et al. (1995) Fas (CD95)/FasL interactions required for programmed cell death after T-cell activation. *Nature* **373,** 444–448.
20. Brunner, T., Mogil, R. J., LaFace, D., et al. (1995) Cell-autonomous Fas (CD95)/Fas-ligand interaction mediates activation-induced apoptosis in T-cell hybridomas. *Nature* **373,** 441–444.
21. Zhou, T., Edwards, C. K., III, and Mountz, J. D. (1995) Prevention of age related T cell apoptosis defect in CD2-fas transgenic mice. *J. Exp. Med.* **182,** 129–137.
22. Thoman, M. L., Ernst, D. N., Hobbs, M. V., and Weigle, W. O. T cell differentiation and functional maturation in aging mice. *Adv. Exp. Med. Biol.* **330,** 93–106.
23. Trainor, D. J., Wigmore, A., Chryostomou, J. L., Dempsey, R., Seshadri, R., and Morley, A. A. (1984) Mutation frequency in human T-lymphocytes increases with age. *Mech. Ageing Dev.* **27,** 83–86.
24. Itoh, N. and Nagata, S. (1993) A novel protein domain required for Fas/APO1 (CD95) in yeast and causes cell death. *Cell* **81,** 513–523.
25. Tartaglia, L. A., Ayres, T. M., Wong, G. H., and Goeddel, D. V. (1993) A novel domain within the 55 kd TNF receptor signals cell death. *Cell* **74,** 845–853.
26. Kischkel, F. C., Hellbardt, S., Behrmann, I., Germer, M., Pawlita, M., Krammer, P. H., et al. (1995) Cytotoxicity-dependent APO-1 (Fas/CD95)-associated proteins form a death-inducing signaling complex (DISC) with the receptor. *EMBO J.* **14,** 5579–5588.

27. Grimm, S., Stanger, B. Z., and Leder, P. (1996) RIP and FADD: two "death domain"-containing proteins can induce apoptosis by convergent, but dissociable, pathways. *Proc. Natl. Acad. Sci. USA* **93**, 10,923–10,927.
28. Chinnaiyan, A. M., Tepper, C. G., Seldin, M. F., O'Rourke, K., Kischkel, F. C., Hellbardt, S., et al. (1996) FADD/MORT1 is a common mediator of CD95 (Fas/APO-1) and tumor necrosis factor receptor-induced apoptosis. *J. Biol. Chem.* **271**, 4961–4965.
29. Chinnaiyan, A. M., O'Rourke, K., Tewari, M., and Dixit, V. M. (1995) FADD, a novel death domain-containing protein, interacts with the death domain of Fas and initiates apoptosis. *Cell* **81**, 505–512.
30. Varfolomeev, E. E., Boldin, M. P., Goncharov, T. M., and Wallach, D. (1996) A potential mechanism of "cross-talk" between the p55 tumor necrosis factor receptor and Fas/APO1: proteins binding to the death domains of the two receptors also bind to each other. *J. Exp. Med.* **183**, 1271–1275.
31. Kim, P. K., Dutra, A. S., Chandrasekharappa, S. C., and Puck, J. M. (1996) Genomic structure and mapping of human FADD, an intracellular mediator of lymphocyte apoptosis. *J. Immunol.* **157**, 5461–5466.
32. Boldin, M. P., Goncharov, T. M., Goltsev, Y. V., and Wallach, D. (1996) Involvement of MACH, a novel MORT1/FADD-interacting protease, in Fas/APO-1- and TNF receptor-induced cell death. *Cell* **85**, 803–815.
33. Muzio, M., Chinnaiyan, A. M., Kischkel, F. C., O'Rourke, K., Shevchenko, A., Ni, J., et al. (1996) FLICE, a novel FADD-homologous ICE/CED-3-like protease, is recruited to the CD95 (Fas/APO-1) death-inducing signaling complex. *Cell* **85**, 817–827.
34. Thome, M., Schneider, P., Hofmann, K., Fickenscher, H., Meinl, E., Neipel, F., et al. (1997) Viral FLICE-inhibitory proteins (FLIPs) prevent apoptosis induced by death receptors. *Nature* **386**, 517–521.
35. Medema, J. P., Scaffidi, C., Kischkel, F. C., Shevchenko, A., Mann, M., Krammer, P. H., et al. (1997) FLICE is activated by association with the CD95 death-inducing signaling complex (DISC). *EMBO J.* **16**, 2794–2804.
36. Peter, M. E., Kischkel, F. C., Scheuerpflug, C. G., Medema, J. P., Debatin, K. M., and Krammer, P. H. (1997) Resistance of cultured peripheral T cells towards activation-induced cell death involves a lack of recruitment of FLICE (MACH/caspase 8) to the CD95 death-inducing signaling complex. *Eur. J. Immunol.* **27**, 1207–1212.
37. Vincenz, C. and Dixit, V. M. (1997) Fas-associated death domain protein interleukin-1beta-converting enzyme 2 (FLICE2), an ICE/Ced-3 homologue, is proximally involved in CD95- and p55-mediated death signaling. *J. Biol. Chem.* **272**, 6578–6583.
38. Green, D. R. (1998) Apoptotic pathways, the road to ruin. *Cell* **94**, 695–698.
39. Li, H., Zhu, H., Xu, C., and Yuan, J. (1998) Cleavage of BID by caspase 8 mediates the mitochondrial damage in the Fas pathway of apoptosis. *Cell* **94**, 491–501.
40. Luo, X., Budihardjo, I., Zou, H., Slaughter, C., and Wang, X. (1998) Bid, a Bcl2 interacting protein, mediates cytochrome c release from mitochondria in response to activation of cell surface death receptor. *Cell* **94**, 481–490.
41. Zou, H., Li, Y., Liu, X., and Wang, X. (1999) An APAF-1 cytochrome c multimeric complex is a functional apoptosome that activates procaspase-9. *J. Biol. Chem.* **274**, 11,549–11,556.
42. Green, D. R. and Reed, J. C. (1998) Mitochondria and apoptosis. *Science* **281**, 1309–1312.
43. Hu, Y., Benedict, M. A., Wu, D., Inohara, N., and Nunez, G. (1998) Bcl-XL interacts with Apaf-1 and inhibits Apaf-1-dependent caspase-9 activation. *Proc. Natl. Acad. Sci. USA* **95**, 4386–4391.
44. Medema, J. P., Scaffidi, C., Krammer, P. H., and Peter, M. E. (1998) Bcl-xL acts downstream of caspase-8 activation by the CD95 death-inducing signaling complex. *J. Biol. Chem.* **273**, 3388–3393.

45. Juo, P., Kuo, C. J., Yuan, J., and Blenis, J. (1998) Essential requirement for caspase-8/FLICE in the initiation of the Fas-induced apoptotic cascade. *Curr. Biol.* **8,** 1001–1008.
46. Varfolomeev, E. E., Schuchmann, M., Luria, V., Chiannilkulchai, N., Beckmann, J. S., Mett, I. L., et al. (1998) Targeted disruption of the mouse Caspase 8 gene ablates cell death induction by the TNF receptors, Fas/Apo1 and DR3 signaling and is lethal prenatally. *Immunity* **2,** 267–276.
47. Peter, M. E., Kischkel, F. C., Scheuerpflug, C. G., Medema, J. P., Debatin, K. M., and Krammer, P. H. (1997) Resistance of cultured peripheral T cells towards activation-induced cell death involves a lack of recruitment of FLICE (MACH/caspase 8) to the CD95 death-inducing signaling complex. *Eur. J. Immunol.* **27,** 1207–1212.
48. Kennedy, N. J. and Budd, R. C. (1998) Phosphorylation of FADD/MORT1 and Fas by kinases that associate with the membrane-proximal cytoplasmic domain of Fas. *J. Immunol.* **160,** 4881–4888.
49. Scaffidi, C., Fulda, S., Srinivasan, A., Friesen, C., Li, F., Tomaselli, K. J., et al. (1998) Two CD95 (APO-1/Fas) signaling pathways. *EMBO J.* **17,** 1675–1687.
50. Takahashi, R., Deveraux, Q., Tamm, I., Welsh, K., Assa-Munt, N., Salvesen, G. S., et al. (1998) A single BIR domain of XIAP sufficient for inhibiting caspases. *J. Biol. Chem.* **273,** 7787–7790.
51. Deveraux, Q. L., Roy, N., Stennicke, H. R., Van Arsdale, T., Zhou, Q., Srinivasula, S. M., et al. (1998) IAPs block apoptotic events induced by caspase-8 and cytochrome c by direct inhibition of distinct caspases. *EMBO J.* **17,** 2215–2223.
52. Suzuki, A., Tsutomi, Y., Akahane, K., Araki, T., and Miura, M. (1998) Resistance to Fas-mediated apoptosis: activation of caspase 3 is regulated by cell cycle regulator p21WAF1 and IAP gene family ILP. *Oncogene* **17,** 931–939.
53. Duckett, C. S., Li, F., Wang, Y., Tomaselli, K. J., Thompson, C. B., and Armstrong, R. C. (1998) Human IAP-like protein regulates programmed cell death downstream of Bcl-xL and cytochrome c. *Mol. Cell. Biol.* **18,** 608–615.
54. Farahani, R., Fong, W. G., Korneluk, R. G., and MacKenzie, A. E. (1997) Genomic organization and primary characterization of miap-3: the murine homologue of human X-linked IAP. *Genomics* **42,** 514–518.
55. Griffith, T. S. and Lynch, D. H. (1998) TRAIL: a molecule with multiple receptors and control mechanisms. *Curr. Opin. Immunol.* **10,** 559–563.
56. Cohen, P. L. and Eisenberg, R. A. (1991) Lpr and gld: single gene models of systemic autoimmunity and lymphoproliferative disease. *Annu. Rev. Immunol.* **9,** 243–265.
57. Watanabe-Fukunaga, R., Brannan, C. I., Copeland, N. G., Jenkins, N. A., and Nagata, S. (1992) Lymphoproliferation disorder in mice explained by defects in Fas antigen that mediates apoptosis. *Nature* **356,** 314–317.
58. Nagata, S. and Golstein, P. (1995) The Fas death factor. *Science* **267,** 1449–1156.
59. Itoh, N., Yonehara, S., Ishii, A., et al. (1991) The polypeptide encoded by the cDNA for human cell surface antigen Fas can mediate apoptosis. *Cell* **66,** 233–246.
60. Suda, T., Takahashi, T., Golstein, P., and Nagata, S. (1993) Molecular cloning and expression of the Fas ligand, a novel member of the tumor necrosis factor family. *Cell* **75,** 1169–1178.
61. Takahashi, T., Tanaka, M., Brannan, C. I., et al. (1994) Generalized lymphoproliferative disease in mice, caused by a point mutation in the Fas ligand. *Cell* **76,** 969–976.
62. Lynch, D., Watson, M., Alderson, M. R., et al. (1994) The mouse Fas-ligand gene is mutated in gld mice and is part of a TNF family gene cluster. *Immunity* **1,** 131–136.
63. Wu, J., Zhou, T., He, J., and Mountz, J. D. (1993) Autoimmune disease in mice due to integration of an endogenous retrovirus in an apoptosis gene. *J. Exp. Med.* **178,** 461–468.
64. Adachi, M., Watanabe-Fukunaga, R., and Nagata, S. (1993) Aberrant transcription caused by the insertion of an early transposable element in an intron of the Fas antigen gene of lpr mice. *Proc. Natl. Acad. Sci. USA* **90,** 1159–1163.

65. Zhou, Z., Blüthmann, H., Eldridge, J., Berry, K., and Mountz, J. D. (1991) Abnormal thymocyte development and production of autoreactive T cells in TCR transgenic autoimmune mice. *J. Immunol.* **147,** 466–474.
66. Zhou, T., Cheng, J., Yang, P., Wang, Z., Liu, C., Su, X., et al. (1996) Inhibition of Nur77/Nurr1 leads to inefficient clonal deletion of self-reactive T cells. *J. Exp. Med.* 1879–1892.
67. Zhou, T., Mountz, J. D., Edwards, C. K., Berry, K., and Blüthmann, H. (1992) Defective maintenance of T cell tolerance to a superantigen in MRL-*lpr/lpr. J. Exp. Med.* **176,** 1063–1072.
68. Mountz, J. D., Baker, T. J., Borcherding, D. R., Bluethmann, H., Zhou, T., and Edwards, C. K., III. (1995) Increased susceptibility of Fas mutation MRL-lpr/lpr mice to staphylococcal enterotoxin B-induced septic shock. *J. Immunol.* **155,** 4829–4837.
69. Mountz, J. D., Zhou, T., Long, R. E., Bluethmann, H., Ostergard, W. J., and Edwards, C. K., III. (1994) T cell influence on superantigen-induced arthritis in MRL-lpr/lpr mice. *Arthritis Rheum.* **37,** 113–124.
70. Zhou, T., Edwards, C. K., III, Bluethmann, H., and Mountz, J. D. (1996) Greatly accelerated lymphadenopathy and autoimmune disease in lpr mice lacking tumor necrosis factor receptor I. *J. Immunol.* **156,** 2661–2665.
71. Su, X., Cheng, J., Wang, Z., Zhou, T., and Mountz, J. D. (1998) Autocrine and Paracrine apoptosis are mediated by differential regulation of Fas ligand activity in two distinct human T cell populations. *J. Immunol.* **160,** 5288–5293.
72. Rieux-Laucat, F., Le Deist, F., Hivroz, C., et al. (1995) Mutations in Fas associated with human lymphoproliferative syndrome and autoimmunity. *Science* **268,** 1347–1349.
73. Fisher, G. H., Rosenberg, F. J., Straus, S. E., Dale, J. K., Middleton, L. A., Lin, A. Y., et al. (1995) Dominant interfering Fas gene mutations impair apoptosis in a human autoimmune lymphoproliferative syndrome. *Cell* **81,** 935–946.
74. Sneller, M. C., Wang, J., Dale, J. K., Strober, W., Middelton, L. A., Choi, Y., et al. (1997) Clinical, immunologic, and genetic features of an autoimmune lymphoproliferative syndrome associated with abnormal lymphocyte apoptosis. *Blood* **89,** 1341–1348.
75. Drappa, J., Vaishnaw, A. K., Sullivan, K. E., Chu, J. L., Elkon, K. B., Rajagopal, V., et al. (1996) Fas gene mutations in the Canale-Smith syndrome, an inherited lymphoproliferative disorder associated with autoimmunity. *N. Engl. J. Med.* **335,** 1643–1649.
76. Wu, J., Wilson, J., He, J., Xian, L., Schur, P. H., and Mountz, J. D. (1996) Fas ligand mutation in a patient with systemic lupus erythematosus and lymphoproliferative disease. *J. Clin. Invest.* **98,** 1107–1013.
77. Mountz, J. D., Wu, J., Cheng, J., and Zhou, T. (1994) Autoimmune disease. A problem of defective apoptosis. *Arthritis Rheum.* **37,** 1415–1420.
78. Emlen, W., Niebur, J., and Kadera, R. (1994) Accelerated in vitro apoptosis of lymphocytes from patients with systemic lupus erythematosus. *J. Immunol.* **152,** 3685–3692.
79. Elkon, KB. (1994) Apoptosis in SLE—too little or too much? *Clin. Exp. Rheumatol.* **12,** 553–559.
80. Elkon, K. B. (1994) Apoptosis and SLE. *Lupus* **3,** 1,2.
81. Mysler, E., Bini, P., Drappa, J., et al. (1994) The apoptosis-1/Fas protein in human systemic lupus erythematosus. *J. Clin. Invest.* **93,** 1029–1034.
82. Kovacs, B., Vassilopoulos, D., Vogelgesang, S. A., and Tsokos, G. C. (1996) Defective CD3-mediated cell death in activated T cells from patients with systemic lupus erythematosus: role of decreased intracellular TNF-alpha. *Clin. Immunol. Immunopathol.* **81,** 293–302.
83. Kaneko, H., Saito, K., Hashimoto, H., Yagita, H., Okumura, K., and Azuma, M. (1996) Preferential elimination of CD28+ T cells in systemic lupus erythematosus (SLE) and the relation with activation-induced apoptosis. *Clin. Exp. Immunol.* **106,** 218–229.
84. Kovacs, B., Liossis, S. N., Dennis, G. J., and Tsokos, G. C. (1997) Increased expression of functional Fas-ligand in activated T cells from patients with systemic lupus erythematosus. *Autoimmunity* **25,** 213–221.

85. McNally, J., Yoo, D. H., Drappa, J., Chu, J. L., Yagita, H., Friedman, S. M., et al. (1997) Fas ligand expression and function in systemic lupus erythematosis. *J. Immunol.* **159,** 4628–4636.
86. Sakata, K., Sakata, A., Vela-Roch, N., Espinosa, R., Escalante, A., Kong, L., et al. Fas (CD95)-transduced signal preferentially stimulates lupus peripheral T lymphocytes. *Eur. J. Immunol.* **28,** 2648–2660.
87. Tanaka, M., Itai, T., Adachi, M., and Nagata, S. (1998) Downregulation of Fas ligand by shedding. *Nat. Med.* **4,** 31–36.
88. Aringer, M., Wintersberger, W., Steiner, C. W., et al. (1994) High levels of bcl-2 protein in circulating T lymphocytes, but not B lymphocytes, of patients with systemic lupus erythematosis. *Arthritis Rheum.* **37,** 1423–1430.
89. Ohsako, S., Hara, M., Harigai, M., Fukasawa, C., and Kashiwazaki, S. (1994) Expression and function of Fas antigen and bcl-2 in human systemic lupus erythematosis lymphocytes. *Clin. Immunol. Immunopathol.* **73,** 109–114.
90. Komaki, S., Kohno, M., Matsuura, N., Shimadzu, M., Adachi, N., Hoshide, R., et al. (1998) The polymorphic 43Thr bcl-2 protein confers relative resistance to autoimmunity: an analytical evaluation. *Hum. Genet.* **103,** 435–440.
91. Ohsako, S., Hara, M., Harigai, M., Fukasawa, C., and Kashiwazaki, S. (1994) Expression and function of Fas antigen and bcl-2 in human systemic lupus erythematosus lymphocytes. *Clin. Immunol. Immunopathol.* **73,** 109–114.
92. Rose, L. M., Latchman, D. S., and Isenberg, D. A. (1995) Bcl-2 expression is unaltered in unfractionated peripheral blood mononuclear cells in patients with systemic lupus erythematosus. *Br. J. Rheum.* **34,** 316–320.
93. Georgescu, L., Vakkalanka, R. K., Elkon, K. B., and Crow, M. K. (1997) Interleukin-10 promotes activation-induced cell death of SLE lymphocytes mediated by Fas ligand. *J. Clin. Invest.* **100,** 2622–2633.
94. Mehrian, R., Quismorio, F. P., Jr., Strassmann, G., Stimmler, M. M., Horwitz, D. A., Kitridou, R. C., et al. (1998) Synergistic effect between IL-10 and bcl-2 genotypes in determining susceptibility to systemic lupus erythematosus. *Arthritis Rheum.* **41,** 596–602.
95. Singh, R. R., Hahn, B. H., Tsao, B. P., and Ebling, F. M. (1998) Evidence for multiple mechanisms of polyclonal T cell activation in murine lupus. *J. Clin. Invest.* **102,** 1841–1849.
96. Wu, J., Edberg, J. C., Redecha, P. B., Bansal, V., Guyre, P. M., Coleman, K., et al. (1997) A novel polymorphism of FcgammaRIIIa (CD16) alters receptor function and predisposes to autoimmune disease. *J. Clin. Invest.* **100,** 1059–1070.
97. Herrmann, M., Voll, R. E., Zoller, O. M., Hagenhofer, M., Ponner, B. B., and Kalden, J. R. (1998) Impaired phagocytosis of apoptotic cell material by monocyte-derived macrophages from patients with systemic lupus erythematosus. *Arthritis Rheum.* **41,** 1241–1250.
98. Perniok, A., Wedekind, F., Herrmann, M., Specker, C., and Schneider, M. (1998) High levels of circulating early apoptic peripheral blood mononuclear cells in systemic lupus erythematosus. *Lupus* **7,** 113–118.
99. Kalden, J. R. (1997) Defective phagocytosis of apoptotic cells: possible explanation for the induction of autoantibodies in SLE. *Lupus* **6,** 326–327.
100. Cabrespines, A., Laderach, D., Lebosse, C., Bach, J. F., and Koutouzov, S. (1998) Isolation and characterization of apoptotic nucleosomes, free and complexed with lupus autoantibody generated during hybridoma B-cell apoptosis. *J. Autoimmun.* **11,** 19–27.
101. Casciola-Rosen, L., Rosen, A., Petri, M., and Schlissel, M. (1996) Surface blebs on apoptotic cells are sites of enhanced procoagulant activity: implications for coagulation events and antigenic spread in systemic lupus erythematosus. *Proc. Natl. Acad. Sci. USA* **93,** 1624–1629.
102. Manfredi, A. A., Rovere, P., Galati, G., Heltai, S., Bozzolo, E., Soldini, L., et al. (1998) Apoptotic cell clearance in systemic lupus erythematosus. I. Opsonization by antiphospholipid antibodies. *Arthritis Rheum.* **41,** 205–214.

103. Lorenz, H. M., Grunke, M., Hieronymus, T., Herrmann, M., Kuhnel, A., Manger, B., et al. (1997) In vitro apoptosis and expression of apoptosis-related molecules in lymphocytes from patients with systemic lupus erythematosus and other autoimmune diseases. *Arthritis Rheum.* **40**, 306–317.
104. Utz, P. J., Hottelet, M., Schur, P. H., and Anderson, P. (1997) Proteins phosphorylated during stress-induced apoptosis are common targets for autoantibody production in patients with systemic lupus erythematosus. *J. Exp. Med.* **185**, 843–854.
105. Utz, P. J., Hottelet, M., Le, T. M., Kim, S. J., Geiger, M. E., van Venrooij, W. J., et al. (1998) The 72-kDa component of signal recognition particle is cleaved during apoptosis. *J. Biol. Chem.* **273**, 35,362–35,370.
106. Cheng, J., Liu, C., Koopman, W. J., and Mountz, J. D. (1995) Characterization of human Fas gene. Exon/intron organization and promoter region. *J. Immunol.* **154**, 1239–1245.
107. Cheng, J., Zhou, T., Liu, C., et al. (1994) Protection from Fas-mediated apoptosis by a soluble form of the Fas molecule. *Science* **263**, 1759–1762.
108. Liu, C., Cheng, J., and Mountz, J. D. (1995) Differential expression of human Fas mRNA species upon peripheral blood mononuclear cell activation. *Biochem. J.* **310**, 957–963.
109. Knipping, E., Krammer, P. H., Onel, K. B., Lehman, T. J. A., Mysler, E., and Elkon, K. B. (1995) Levels of soluble Fas/APO-1/CD95 in systemic lupus erythematosus and juvenile rheumatoid arthritis. *Arthritis Rheum.* **18**, 1735–1737.
110. Goel, N., Ulrich, D. T., Clair, W., Fleming, J. A., Lynch, D. H., and Seldin, M. F. (1995) Lack of correlation between serum soluble Fas/APO-1 levels and autoimmune diseases. *Arthritis Rheum.* **38**, 1738.
111. Tokano, Y., Miyake, S., Kayakai, N., et al. (1996) Soluble Fas molecule in the serum of patients with systemic lupus erythematosus. *J. Clin. Immunol.* **16**, 261–265.
112. Jodo, S., Kobayashi, S., Kayagaki, N., et al. (1997) Serum levels of soluble Fas/APO-1 (CD95) and its molecular structure in patients with systemic lupus erythematosus (SLE) and other autoimmune diseases. *Clin. Exp. Immunol.* **107**, 89–95.
113. Nozawa, K., Kayag, N., Tokano, Y., Yagita, H., Okumura, K., and Hasimoto, H. (1997) Soluble Fas (APO-1 CD95) and soluble Fas ligand in rheumatic diseases. *Arthritis Rheum.* **40**, 1126–1129.
114. Rose, L. M., Latchman, D. S., and Isenberg, D. A. (1997) Elevated Soluble Fas production in SLE correlates with HLA status not with disease activity. *Lupus* **6**, 717–722.
115. Bijl, M., van Lopik, T., Limburg, P. C., Spronk, P. E., Jaegers, S. M., Aarden, L. A., et al. (1998) Do elevated levels of serum-soluble Fas contribute to the persistence of activated lymphocytes in systemic lupus erythematosus? *J. Autoimmun.* **11**, 457–463.
116. Kovacs, B., Szentendrei, T., Bednarek, J. M., et al. (1997) Persistent expression of a soluble form of Fas/APO1 in continuously activated T cells from a patient with SLE. *Clin. Exp. Rheumatol.* **15**, 19–23.
117. Al Maini, M. H., Al Nohri, H. A., Richens, E. R., Elajeb, E. M., Al Riyami, B. M., Zhou, T., et al. (2000) Soluble Fas levels—a potential marker of organ damage in SLE. *Lupus* (in press).
118. Gaffney, P. M., Ortmann, W. A., Selby, S. A., Shark, K. B., Ockenden, T. C., Rohlf, K. E., et al. (2000) TWGenome screening in human systemic lupus erythematosus: results from a second Minnesota cohort and combined analyses of 187 sib-pair families. *Am. J. Hum. Genet.* **66**, 547–556.
119. Tsao, B. P., Cantor, R. M., Grossman, J. M., Shen, N., Teophilov, N. T., Wallace, D. J., et al. (1999) PARP alleles within the linked chromosomal region are associated with systemic lupus erythematosus. *J. Clin. Invest.* **103**, 1135–1140.
120. Shai, R., Quismorio, F. P., Jr., Li, L., Kwon, O. J., Morrison, J., Wallace, D. J., et al. (1999) Genome-wide screen for systemic lupus erythematosis susceptibility genes in multiplex families. *Hum. Mol. Genet.* **8**, 639–644.

121. Moser, K. L., Gray-McGuire, C., Kelly, J., Asundi, N., Yu, H., Bruner, G. R., Mange, M., Hogue, R., Neas, B. R., Harley, J. B. (1999) Confirmation of genetic linkage between human systemic lupus erythematosus and chromosome 1q41. *Arthritis Rheum.* **42,** 1902–1907.
122. Gilkeson, G. S., Ruiz, P., Pritchard, A. J., and Pisetsky, D. S. (1991) Genetic control of inflammatory arthritis and glomerulonephritis in congenic lpr mice and their F1 hybrids. *J. Autoimmun.* **4,** 595–609.
123. Watson, M. L., Rao, J. K., Gilkeson, G. S., et al. (1992) Genetic analysis of MRL-lpr mice: relationship of the Fas apoptosis gene to disease manifestations and renal disease-modifying loci. *J. Exp. Med.* **176,** 1645–1654.
124. Weinberg, J. B., Granger, D. L., Pisetsky, D. S., Seldin, M. F., Misukonis, M. A., Mason, S. N., et al. The role of nitric oxide in the pathogenesis of spontaneous murine autoimmune disease: increased nitric oxide production and nitric oxide synthase expression in MRL-lpr/lpr mice, and reduction of spontaneous glomerulonephritis and arthritis by orally administered N^G-monomethyl-L-arginine. *J. Exp. Med.* **179,** 651–660.
125. Drake, C. G., Babcock, S. K., Palmer, E., and Kotzin, B. L. (1994) Genetic analysis of the NZB contribution to lupus-like autoimmune disease in (NZB × NZW)F1 mice. *Proc. Natl. Acad. Sci. USA* **91,** 4062–4066.
126. Kono, D. H., Burlingame, R. W., Owens, D. G., et al. (1994) Lupus susceptibility loci in New Zealand mice. *Proc. Natl. Acad. Sci. USA* **91,** 10,168–10,172.
127. Morel, L., Rudofsky, U. H., Longmate, J. A., Schiffenbauer, J., and Wakeland, E. K. (1994) Polygenic control of susceptibility to murine systemic lupus erythematosis. *Immunity* **1,** 219–229.
128. Theofilopoulos, A. N. (1998) Effector and predisposing genes in lupus. *Lupus* **7,** 575–584.
129. Sobel, E. S., Mohan, C., Morel, L., Schiffenbauer, J., and Wakeland, E. K. (1999) Genetic dissection of SLE pathogenesis: adoptive transfer of Sle1 mediates the loss of tolerance by bone marrow-derived B cells. *J. Immunol.* **162,** 2415–2421.
130. Firestein, G. S., Yeo, M., and Zvaifler, N. J. (1995) Apoptosis in rheumatoid arthritis synovium. *J. Clin. Invest.* **96,** 1631–1638.
131. Salmon, M., Scheel-Toellner, D., Huissoon, A. P., Pilling, D., Shamsadeen, N., Hyde, H., et al. Inhibition of T cell apoptosis in the rheumatoid synovium. *J. Clin. Invest.* **99,** 439–446.
132. Schirmer, M., Vallejo, A. N., Weyand, C. M., and Goronzy, J. J. (1998) Resistance to apoptosis and elevated expression of Bcl-2 in clonally expanded CD4+CD28- T cells from rheumatoid arthritis patients. *J. Immunol.* **161,** 1018–1025.
133. Isomaki, P., Soderstrom, K. O., Punnonen, J., Roivainen, A., Luukkainen, R., Merilahti-Palo, R., et al. (1996) Expression of bcl-2 in rheumatoid arthritis. *Br. J. Rheumatol.* **35,** 611–619.
134. Zdichavsky, M., Schorpp, C., Nickels, A., Koch, B., Pfreundschuh, M., and Gause, A. (1996) Analysis of bcl-2+ lymphocyte subpopulations in inflammatory synovial infiltrates by a double-immunostaining technique. *Rheumatol. Int.* **16,** 151–157.
135. Hasunuma, T., Kayagaki, N., Asahara, H., Motokawa, S., Kobata, T., Yagita, H., et al. (1997) Accumulation of soluble Fas in inflamed joints of patients with rheumatoid arthritis. *Arthritis Rheum.* **40,** 80–86.
136. Aarden, S. M., Smeenk, R. J., and Kallenberg, G. G. (1998) Do elevated levels of serum-soluble fas contribute to the persistence of activated lymphocytes in systemic lupus erythematosis? *J. Autoimmun.* **11,** 457–563.
137. Asahara, H., Hasumuna, T., Kobata, T., Yagita, H., Okumura, K., Inoue, H., et al. (1996) Expression of Fas antigen and Fas ligand in the rheumatoid synovial tissue. *Clin. Immunol. Immunopathol.* **81,** 27–34.
138. Hoa, T. T., Hasunuma, T., Aono, H., Masuko, K., Kobata, T., Yamamoto, K., et al. (1996) Novel mechanisms of selective apoptosis in synovial T cells of patients with rheumatoid arthritis. *J. Rheumatol.* **23,** 1332–1337.

139. Cantwell, M. J., Hua, T., Zvaifler, N. J., and Kipps, T. J. (1997) Deficient Fas ligand expression by synovial lymphocytes from patients with rheumatoid arthritis. *Arthritis Rheum.* **40,** 1644–1652.
140. Asahara, H., Hasunuma, T., Kobata, T., Inoue, H., Muller-Ladner, U., Gay, S., et al. (1997) In situ expression of protooncogenes and Fas/Fas ligand in rheumatoid arthritis synovium. *J. Rheumatol.* **24,** 430–435.
141. Hashimoto, H., Tanaka, M., Suda, T., Tomita, T., Hayashida, K., Takeuchi, E., et al. (1998) Soluble Fas ligand in the joints of patients with rheumatoid arthritis and osteoarthritis. *Arthritis Rheum.* **41,** 657–662.
142. Wakisaka, S., Suzuki, N., Takeba, Y., Shimoyama, Y., Nagafuchi, H., Takeno, M., et al. (1998) Modulation by proinflammatory cytokines of Fas/Fas ligand-mediated apoptotic cell death of synovial cells in patients with rheumatoid arthritis (RA). *Clin. Exp. Immunol.* **114,** 119–128.
143. Sumida, T., Hoa, T. T., Asahara, H., Hasunuma, T., and Nishioka, K. (1997) T cell receptor of Fas-sensitive T cells in rheumatoid synovium. *J. Immunol.* **158,** 1965–1970.
144. Tighe, H., Warnatz, K., Brinson, D., Corr, M., Weigle, W. O., Baird, S. M., et al. (1997) Peripheral deletion of rheumatoid factor B cells after abortive activation by IgG. *Proc. Natl. Acad. Sci. USA* **94,** 646–651.
145. Hasunuma, T., Hoa, T. T., Aono, H., Asahara, H., Yonehara, S., Yamamoto, K., et al. (1996) Induction of Fas-dependent apoptosis in synovial infiltrating cells in rheumatoid arthritis. *Int. Immunol.* **8,** 1595–1602.
146. Nakajima, T., Aono, H., Hasunuma, T., et al. (1995) Apoptosis and functional Fas antigen in rheumatoid arthritis synoviocytes. *Arthritis Rheum.* **38,** 485–491.
147. Sugiyama, M., Tsukazaki, T., Yonekura, A., Matsuzaki, S., Yamashita, S., and Iwasaki, K. (1996) Localisation of apoptosis and expression of apoptosis related proteins in the synovium of patients with rheumatoid arthritis. *Ann. Rheum Dis.* **55,** 442–449.
148. Fujisawa, K., Asahara, H., Okamoto, K., Aono, H., Hasunuma, T., Kobata, T., et al. (1996) Therapeutic effect of the anti-Fas antibody on arthritis in HTLV-1 tax transgenic mice. *J. Clin. Invest.* **98,** 271–278.
149. Okamoto, K., Asahara, H., Kobayashi, T., Matsuno, H., Hasunuma, T., Kobata, T., et al. (1998) Induction of apoptosis in the rheumatoid synovium by Fas ligand gene transfer. *Gene Ther.* **5,** 331–338.
150. Zhang, H., Yang, Y., Horton, J. L., Samoilova, E. B., Judge, T. A., Turka, L. A., et al. (1997) Amelioration of collagen-induced arthritis by CD95 (Apo-1/Fas)-ligand gene transfer. *J. Clin. Invest.* **100,** 1951–1957.
151. Sakai, K., Matsuno, H., Morita, I., Nezuka, T., Tsuji, H., Shirai, T., et al. (1998) Potential withdrawal of rheumatoid synovium by the induction of apoptosis using a novel in vivo model of rheumatoid arthritis. *Arthritis Rheum.* **41,** 1251–1257.
152. Wakisaka, S., Suzuki, N., Takeba, Y., Shimoyama, Y., Nagafuchi, H., Takeno, M., et al. (1998) Modulation by proinflammatory cytokines of Fas/Fas ligand-mediated apoptotic cell death of synovial cells in patients with rheumatoid arthritis (RA). *Clin. Exp. Immunol.* **114,** 119–128.
153. Kobayashi, T., Okamoto, K., Kobata, T., Hasunuma, T., Sumida, T., and Nishioka, K. (1999) Tumor necrosis factor alpha regulation of the FAS-mediated apoptosis-signaling pathway in synovial cells. *Arthritis Rheum.* **42,** 519–526.
154. Kawakami, A., Eguchi, K., Matsuoka, N., Tsuboi, M., Kawabe, Y., Aoyagi, T., et al. (1996) Inhibition of Fas antigen-mediated apoptosis of rheumatoid synovial cells in vitro by transforming growth factor beta 1. *Arthritis Rheum.* **39,** 1267–1276.
155. Firestein, G. S., Nguyen, K., Aupperle, K. R., Yeo, M., Boyle, D. L., and Zvaifler, N. J. (1996) Apoptosis in rheumatoid arthritis: p53 overexpression in rheumatoid arthritis synovium. *Am. J. Pathol.* **149,** 2143–2151.

156. Aupperle, K. R., Boyle, D. L., Hendrix, M., Seftor, E. A., Zvaifler, N. J., Barbosa, M., et al. (1998) Regulation of synoviocyte proliferation, apoptosis, and invasion by the p53 tumor suppressor gene. *Am. J. Pathol.* **152,** 1091–1098.
157. Okamoto, K., Fujisawa, K., Hasunuma, T., Kobata, T., Sumida, T., and Nishioka, K. (1997) Selective activation of the JNK/AP-1 pathway in Fas-mediated apoptosis of rheumatoid arthritis synoviocytes. *Arthritis Rheum.* **40,** 919–926.
158. Mizushima, N., Kohsaka, H., and Miyasaka, N. (1998) Ceramide, a mediator of interleukin 1, tumour necrosis factor alpha, as well as Fas receptor signalling, induces apoptosis of rheumatoid arthritis synovial cells. *Ann. Rheum. Dis.* **57,** 495–499.
159. Han, Z., Boyle, D. L., Bennett, B., Aupperle, K. R., Manning, A. M., and Firestine, G. S. (1998) Activation of JUN kinase (JNK) in rheumatoid arthritis (RA) synoviocytes. *Arthritis Rheum.* **41,** 5136.
160. Miagkov, A. V., Kovalenko, D. V., Brown, C. E., Didsbury, J. R., Cogswell, J. P., Stimpson, S. A., et al. (1998) NF-kappaB activation provides the potential link between inflammation and hyperplasia in the arthritic joint. *Proc. Natl. Acad. Sci. USA* **95,** 13,859–13,864.
161. Zhang, H. G., Zhou, T., Curiel, D. T., and Mountz, J. D. (1998) Increased susceptibility of RA synovial cells to TNFα mediated apoptosis after Ikβ dominante negative gene therapy. *Arthritis Rheum.* **41,** 596.
162. Arend, W. P. and Dayer, J. M. (1995) Inhibition of the production and effects of interleukin-1 and tumor necrosis factor in rheumatoid arthritis. *Arthritis Rheum.* **38,** 151–160.
163. Potvin, F., Petitclerc, E., Marceau, F., and Poubelle, P. E. (1997) Mechanisms of action of antimalarials in inflammation: induction of apoptosis in human endothelial cells. *J. Immunol.* **158,** 1872–1879.
164. Genestier, L., Paillot, R., Fournel, S., Ferraro, C., Miossec, P., and Revillard, J. P. (1998) Immunosuppressive properties of methotrexate: apoptosis and clonal deletion of activated peripheral T cells. *J. Clin. Invest.* **102,** 322–328.
165. Morita, A., Werfel, T., Stege, H., Ahrens, C., Karmann, K., Grewe, M., et al. (1997) Evidence that singlet oxygen-induced human T helper cell apoptosis is the basic mechanism of ultraviolet-A radiation phototherapy. *J. Exp. Med.* **186,** 1763–1768.
166. Ratkay, L. G., Chowdhary, R. K., Iamaroon, A., Richter, A. M., Neyndorff, H. C., Keystone, E. C., et al. (1998) Amelioration of antigen-induced arthritis in rabbits by induction of apoptosis of inflammatory cells with local application of transdermal photodynamic therapy. *Arthritis Rheum.* **41,** 525–534.
167. Elliott, M. J., Maini, R. N., Feldmann, M., et al. (1994) Randomised double-blind comparison of chimeric monoclonal antibody to tumour necrosis factor a versus placebo in rheumatoid arthritis. *Lancet* **344,** 1105–1110.
168. Su, X., Zhou, T., Yang, P., Edwards, C. K., III, and Mountz, J. D. (1998) Reduction of arthritis and pneumonitis in motheaten mice by soluble tumor necrosis factor receptor. *Arthritis Rheum.* **41,** 139–149.
169. Jacob, C. O. and McDevitt, H. O. (1988) Tumour necrosis factor-alpha in murine autoimmune "lupus" nephritis. *Nature* **331,** 356–358.
170. Zhou, T., Edwards, C. K., III, Yang, P., Wang, Z., Bluethmann, H., and Mountz, J. D. (1996) Greatly accelerated lymphadenopathy and autoimmune disease in lpr mice lacking tumor necrosis factor receptor I. *J. Immunol.* **156,** 2661–2665.
171. Akahoshi, T., Namai, R., Sekiyama, N., Tanaka, S., Hosaka, S., and Kondo, H. (1997) Rapid induction of neutrophil apoptosis by sulfasalazine: implications of reactive oxygen species in the apoptotic process. *J. Leukocyte Biol.* **62,** 817–826.

4
Humoral Response

Gary S. Gilkeson

1. Introduction

The humoral immune response is part of both the innate and acquired immune systems with the resulting end product being the production of antibodies by B-lymphocytes. As reviewed in other chapters, the innate response is the frontline nonspecific immune response to foreign antigens. The innate response is composed of a variety of acute-phase reactants, including antibodies. The early innate immune response is independent of T-cell help and is primarily composed of IgM antibodies. Antibodies produced in the innate response are usually highly crossreactive with a number of antigens and of low affinity for any given antigen. Their purpose is to nonspecifically bind all foreign antigens so that they can be presented to the immune system, triggering a secondary, more specific acquired immune response if needed *(1–3)*.

The acquired immune response follows the initial innate response and is almost always T-cell dependent requiring the help of T-cells. There are some antigens that are T independent in that the immune response to them does not require the help of T-cells, so-called T-independent antigens. The majority of acquired secondary immune responses are T dependent *(4–12)*. The secondary response or acquired response is normally composed of IgG antibodies, although some IgM antibodies can be part of a secondary response that is T dependent. The secondary T-cell-dependent immune response is normally more specific and of higher affinity than the primary innate response. The affinity of an antibody for an antigen refers to how tightly the antibody binds to the antigen. Higher-affinity binding normally results in more efficient clearance of the foreign organism or antigen. Normally, the acquired secondary response does not evolve directly from the primary response in that B-cells participating in the acquired secondary response are of a totally different lineage from those in the primary response. Antibodies in the secondary response are also normally highly somatically mutated as described below *(11)*.

Thus, the humoral immune response evolves over time from a relatively nonspecific, low-affinity response to a highly specific high-affinity response to the foreign antigen. Understanding how this process occurs requires a working knowledge of the basic structure of immunoglobulins and the processes resulting in the incredible diversity of antibodies in the immune repertoire. This fundamental knowledge is also essen-

From: *Current Molecular Medicine: Principles of Molecular Rheumatology*
Edited by: G. C. Tsokos © Humana Press Inc., Totowa, NJ

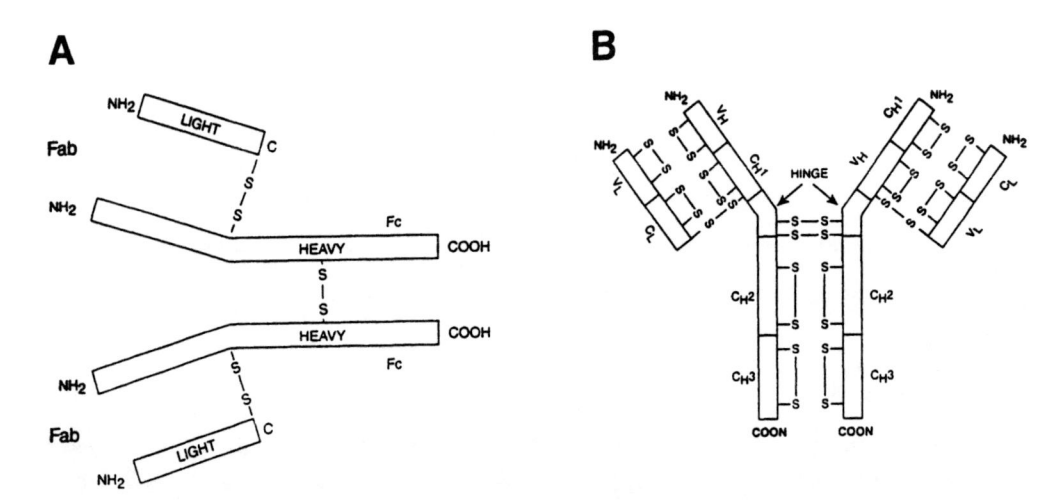

Fig. 1. Immunoglobulin structure. (A) Basic structure with two heavy and two light polypeptide chains linked together by disulfide bonds. The Fab region is involved in antigen binding, whereas the Fc region mediates various effector functions. (B) Increasing detail of IgG molecule showing the domains of both heavy and light chains. The sites of antigen binding involve the amino (NH$_2$)-terminal domains of both the heavy and light chains and are referred to as the variable regions (V$_H$ and V$_L$). The rest of each polypeptide has a relatively constant structure (C$_H$ and C$_L$ domains).

tial for understanding some of the new therapeutic agents that are currently being developed and why some induce an immune response in the patient and others do not. Thus, understanding the differences among a monoclonal antibody, a humanized antibody, and a receptor/Ig conjugate is important if such reagents are to be used appropriately to treat patients.

2. Immunoglobulin Structure

Immunoglobulins or antibodies are the effector arm of B-cell immunity. Immunoglobulins are produced and expressed on the surface of B-cells; poststimulation, some B-cells differentiate into plasma cells and produce immunoglobulin for release into the extracellular space. Immunoglobulins are composed of two sets of paired protein chains: the light chains and the heavy chains (Fig. 1). The light chains and heavy chains are connected through disulfide bonds. A disulfide bond in the hinge region also connects the two heavy chains. Both light and heavy chains contain a variable region and a constant region. The variable regions contain the antigen-binding site and, as suggested by the name, are highly variable from one antibody to another *(1–3)*. Constant regions of the same antibody isotype (*see* Subheading 4.) are similar from antibody to antibody. The constant region of the heavy chain is composed of three to four regions designated CH1–3 or CH4 depending on isotype; IgM and IgD have an additional CH region, CH4. The constant region of the heavy chain defines the isotype of the antibody (i.e., IgG1-4, IgM, IgD, IgA, and IgE) and also determines the effector functions of the antibody. Complement binding, macrophage binding by Fc receptors, bacterial protein binding (i.e., Staphylococcus Protein A) and B-cell superantigen binding all occur in the constant region. Rheumatoid factors bind to the constant region or Fc portion of the

Humoral Response

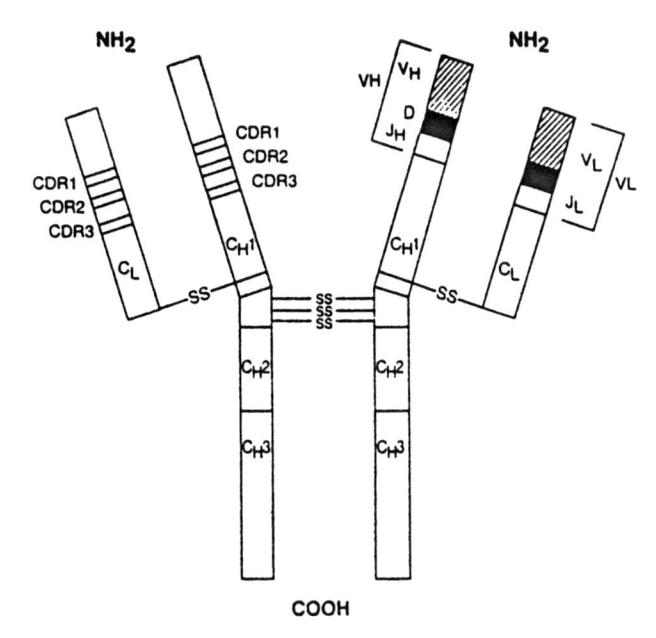

Fig. 2. Structure of the antigen-binding domain. On the left, the hypervariable regions (complementarity-determining regions [CDRs]) of the V_H and V_L domains are shaded. These regions are part of the antigen-binding pocket. The CDRs are separated by intervening segments referred to as framework regions. On the right, the immunoglobulin polypeptide regions are correlated with Ig gene segments (exons), which code for the different domains. Note that the CDR3 region of the variable domains correspond to the V_H–D_H–J_H junctional region of the rearranged heavy-chain gene and the V_L–J_L junctional region of the rearranged light-chain gene.

heavy chain; the self-aggregation of certain cryoglobulins (primarily IgG3) is also dependent on specific sequences within the Fc portion of antibodies (1–3).

Variable regions of the light and heavy chains form the antigen-binding domains known as the Fab. As shown in Fig. 2, the variable regions are composed of segments referred to as framework regions (FR) that separate the complementarity-determining regions (CDRs). Framework regions, as suggested by their name, are relatively constant from antibody to antibody and provide the framework structure for the antigen-binding domain. The complementarity determining regions are highly variable from antibody to antibody and are the primary antigen-binding regions of the antibody. Both the heavy and light chains contain three CDR regions, which are separated by four framework regions. Further details on the molecular characteristics of the CDR regions will be discussed in the next section. Depending on the antigen, binding may occur primarily to the light chain, primarily to the heavy chain, or involve interaction with both the heavy and the light chains (4).

Monoclonal antibodies are derived by fusing a human or mouse B-cell with a myeloma cell, leading to "immortalization" of the B-cell. This B-cell then divides and produces antibody in large quantities that can be harvested for research or therapeutic purposes. Monoclonal antibodies are currently in clinical use as therapeutic agents (i.e., anti-tumor necrosis factor [TNF] antibodies for Crohn's disease). Most of these antibodies are mouse antibodies and they elicit an immune response when injected into humans, as they are foreign proteins. This immune response will neutralize any therapeutic effect of the antibody after the first injection. Strategies to "humanize" these antibodies were developed to prevent the immune response. Partially "humanized" antibodies contain a human constant region with a mouse variable region. Fully "humanized antibodies" are derived by molecular manipulations that replace the human CDRs with the mouse CDRs of the specificity desired. "Humanized" monoclonal antibodies are much less immunogenic than mouse antibodies and can be given repeatedly. An immune response, however, can still develop, even to these hybrid antibodies *(1–4)*.

Antibodies to the variable regions of another antibody are called anti-idiotypes. An antibody idiotype, which is the area of an antibody bound by an anti-idiotype, may consist of a combination of the heavy and light chains or only one chain. The anti-idiotype may or may not block the antigen-binding area of the antibody to which it is directed. Specific idiotypes have been characterized and studied that commonly occur in normal immunity and autoimmunity. Anti-idiotype antibodies are theorized to be part of the control mechanisms of the immune response. Immunization of mice with specific antigens (i.e., arsenic) leads to the production of antibodies bearing a specific idiotype, indicating that most mice respond to immunization with this antigen using antibodies composed of the same immunogloblin heavy- and light-chain variable regions. Similarly, some autoantibody responses (i.e., anti-DNA antibodies) are characterized by the use of specific idiotypes. For example, a number of patients with lupus have anti-DNA antibodies in their serum; some of these antibodies bear a common idiotype, even though the antibodies are derived from the sera of unrelated patients *(13–16)*. These findings suggest that binding to certain antigens requires a specific set of heavy- and light-chain variable regions.

Indeed, one hypothesis for the development of autoimmune disease is a breakdown of the anti-idiotype network *(9)*. According to this hypothesis, everyone makes autoantibodies in response to infections. However, nonautoimmune individuals also make anti-idiotype antibodies that bind and clear the autoantibodies. Autoimmunity develops when the anti-idiotype system breaks down such that autoantibodies are produced without their counteracting anti-idiotypes. One mechanism proposed for the effectiveness of intravenous immunoglobulin (IV Ig) for the treatment of autoimmune disease is that the IV Ig provides the anti-idiotypic antibodies missing in the autoimmune individual. Support for this hypothesis is provided by experiments demonstrating that if serum from normal individuals is treated with high salt, disassociating antibody binding, autoantibodies can then be detected in the normal serum. Anti-idiotype antibodies for known autoantibodies have also been found in IV Ig preparations. Treatment of autoimmune mice with anti-idiotype antibodies for common anti-DNA idiotypes resulted in temporary improvement in renal disease. Other autoantibodies not bearing the idiotype being targeted, however, continued to be produced leading to re-exacerbation of disease. The proposed defect in the anti-idiotypic network may well play a role in autoimmunity, how much of a role is still unknown *(13)*.

3. Molecular Features of Antibodies

Prior to the discovery of the process of genetic recombination, it was believed that each antibody was the product of an individual gene. It became apparent, however, that the human B-cell repertoire contains millions of different antibodies. The genetic material necessary to form these millions of antibodies was calculated to be more than

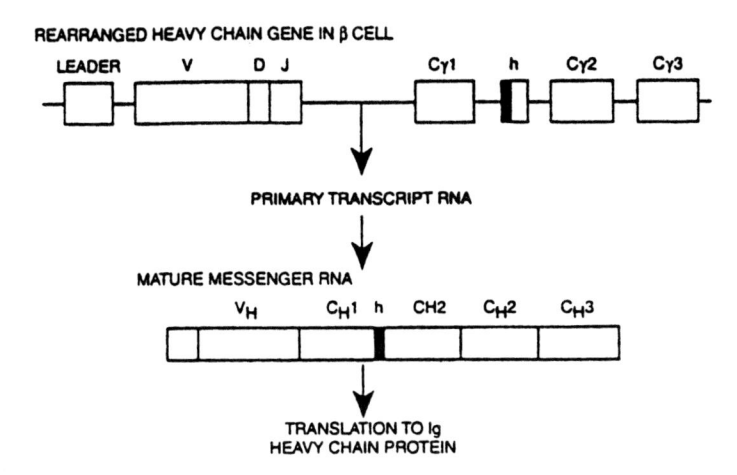

Fig. 3. Immunoglobulin genetic recombination. Corresponding structure of a rearranged IgG heavy-chain gene.

is contained in the total human genome. The concept of genetic recombination was discovered and explained the ability to generate the huge diversity of antibody molecules using limited genetic material *(2)*. As shown in Fig. 3, each antibody is formed by combining several gene segments. This genetic recombination is directed by the gene products of genes called RAG1 and RAG2 (recombinase-activating genes). Without RAG help, neither T-cell receptor or immunoglobulin gene rearrangement occurs. If RAG is deficient, the individual is markedly immune suppressed, as they have neither T-cell or B-cell function *(2–6)*.

The diversity of the antibody repertoire is a combination of genetic recombination, pairing different heavy chains with different light chains, and somatic mutations in the rearranged genes. For light-chain recombination, one of multiple variable region genes (V genes) combines with one of four junctional genes (J genes). This VJ segment, or light-chain variable region, is joined to the constant region gene segment to form the complete light-chain DNA segment. From this DNA segment, a mRNA transcript is made, processed, and then translated into a light-chain protein *(2,5,6)*.

Heavy-chain recombination occurs in a very similar fashion, except that an additional event occurs combining one of many diversity genes (D genes) with a heavy-chain J gene prior to combining with a heavy-chain V gene. The heavy-chain DNA and light-chain DNA are on different chromosomes; thus, the heavy- and light-chain V genes and J genes are different genetic elements. As there are a large number of D genes, the possible combinations of sequences for the heavy chains are increased significantly. The CDR 1,2, and 3 regions of the light chain are all contained within the variable region. In the heavy chain, the CDR1 and 2 are in the variable region sequence; the CDR3 region is formed by combining a D gene and a J gene *(5)*.

Immunoglobulin gene recombination does not occur consistently at the same splice points in the V, D, and J DNA segments. This is best demonstrated in the CDR3 region of the heavy chain. As mentioned previously, the CDR3 region of the heavy chain begins at the junction of the V and D segments. The D gene, however, usually does not splice in directly to the V gene. In a process called N addition, nucleotides (i.e., cytosines, adenosines) are added randomly; any number of nucleotides can be added.

The addition of these N nucleotides is the function of the protein terminal deoxynucleotidyl transferase (TdT) *(5,6)*. Without TdT and N additions, certain V genes favor recombining with specific DJ combinations, thus limiting diversity. The N additions further randomize the combinations of V, D, and J genes by preventing these favored recombinations. D genes are not usually spliced in whole. Thus, anywhere from 1 to 10 D-gene codons can be present in an antibody CDR3. More than one D gene can be present in an antibody CDR3 and, sometimes, the D genes are spliced in backward. N additions add even further diversity in that they may be added as singlets, doublets, or triplets. Because the genetic code is read in threes (i.e., three nucleotides code for one amino acid), if only one or two N additions are made, the reading frame of the nucleotides downstream in the D gene are changed. A similar set of N additions occurs at the DJ junction. Although any number of N additions can be added at either the VD or DJ junctions, the total number added at both ends of the D gene is always divisible by 3, so that the J region is translated in frame. Amino acids critical for antibody structure and function are present in the J segment, necessitating that it be translated in the proper reading frame. Thus, enormous diversity occurs in the CDR3 region of the heavy chain of antibodies, a region that often plays a key role in antibody and autoantibody binding *(5,6)*.

After a functional heavy chain is formed, further recombination of heavy-chain genes does not occur, thus preventing a B-cell from producing more than one heavy chain. This process is called allelic exclusion. If the result of an aberrant recombination event, a nonfunctional heavy chain is formed; the heavy-chain genes on the other parental DNA molecule (termed an allele) become activated, recombine, and form a heavy chain. Prior to the production of light chains in a B-cell, the heavy chains are combined with what are called surrogate light chains; this combination of a heavy chain with a surrogate light chain is expressed on the surface of early B-cells (*see* Chapter 13). There is evidence suggesting there is positive selection of B-cells at the stage of heavy chain/surrogate light-chain expression; the basis of this selection is not known at present.

Except in rare instances, light-chain recombination events occur following the production of a functional heavy chain. Although for the most part, production of one light chain prevents the production of a second light chain; on rare occasions, a B-cell has been shown to be producing two different antibodies composed of the same heavy chain paired with two different light-chains. In both mice and humans, there is substantial room for error in light chain recombination. The kappa gene locus on one allele recombines first; if this recombination is unsuccessful or the light chain is incompatible with the heavy chain (for structural reasons, not all combinations of heavy chains and light chains result in functional antibodies), the second kappa allele recombines. If both kappa rearrangements are unsuccessful, then one of the lambda light-chain alleles recombines, followed by the second if all others fail. Most of the research in this area has been in mice; 95% of mouse immunoglobulin contains kappa light chains. The ratio in humans is kappa predominant but not to the extent that it is in mice *(2,6)*.

Once a functional immunoglobulin is formed, it is expressed on the surface of the B-cell as part of the B-cell receptor complex. The final diversification occurs once the B-cell has left the bone marrow and entered the peripheral circulation. The B-cell, upon encountering antigen, may enter lymph nodes or the spleen and migrate to a germinal center. In the germinal center, with the help of CD4 T-cells, a process called

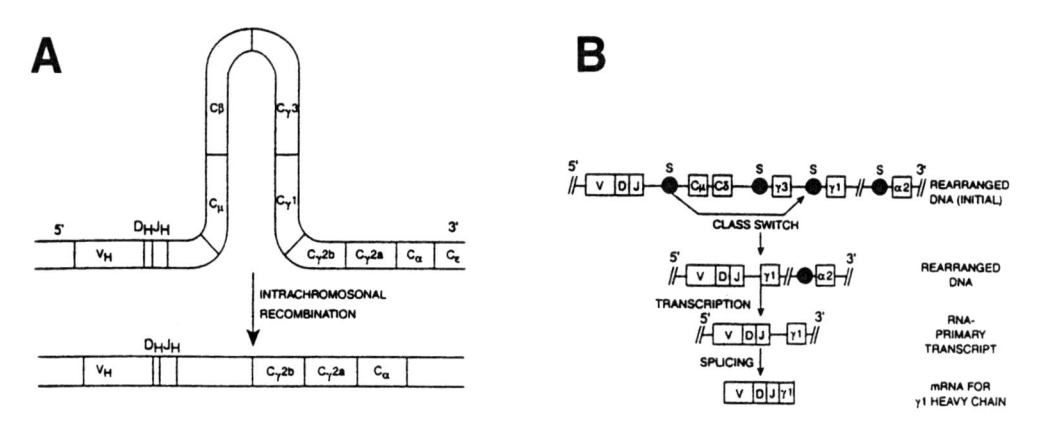

Fig. 4. Isotype switching. Predominant genetic mechanism by which a B-cell switches from production of surface IgM to secrete an IgG, IgA, or IgE molecule. Note that initial rearrangements have taken place to put the V region proximal to the D, J, and Cμ regions. This latter region contains other constant-region gene segments downstream, including Cδ, Cγ3, Cγ1, Cγ2b, Cγ2a, Cα, and Cε. In the process of a VDJ unit rearranging to another C region downstream, the intervening DNA is removed or deleted. (Reprinted with permission from Benjamin, E. and Leskowitz, S. (eds.) (1991) The genetic basis of antibody structure, in *Immunology: A Short Course*, 2nd ed., John S. Wiley & Sons, Inc., New York, p. 92. Copyright 1991 John S. Wiley & Sons, Inc., Reprinted by permission of Wiley-Liss, Inc., a subsidiary of John Wiley & Sons, Inc.)

somatic mutation occurs *(11)*. Somatic mutations result in sequence changes in the DNA coding for the antibody; for example, a cytosine is substituted for an adenosine when the DNA is replicated. Somatic mutations occur more frequently in the CDR regions than the FR regions of antibodies. Some somatic mutations result in a change in the amino acid sequence of the antibody (so-called productive mutations), whereas others do not (silent mutations). Because of changes in the amino acid sequence, somatic mutations may lead to the production of a nonfunctional antibody, may decrease the binding of the antibody to its antigen, or may increase the binding properties (affinity) of the antibody. Through the various recombination events, combining of different heavy chains with different light chains, D gene splicing, N additions, and somatic mutation, a markedly diversified mature B-cell repertoire is formed *(11,12)*.

4. Isotype Switching

Except for rare exceptions noted earlier, a single B-cell makes a single antibody variable region. B-cells can switch the isotype (i.e., switch from IgM to IgG) of the antibody produced or produce antibodies of two different isotypes (IgM and IgD). Although the specificity of the antibody remains the same, the effector function of the antibody is greatly altered. For example, switching to specific IgG isotypes may alter complement fixation or self-agglutination *(10)*.

The process of isotype switching is also a recombinatorial event. As shown in Fig. 4, the VDJ segment of the heavy chain recombines with a constant region further down the DNA strand by looping out the DNA between the desired recombination sites *(2,10)*. The looped-out DNA is then excised and the new VDJ/constant region DNA sequence is transcribed into mRNA, processed, and translated into a functional heavy chain.

Such isotype switching occurs primarily in the periphery following exposure to antigen under the influence of T-cell help. Naive B-cells (B-cells that have not been exposed to their antigen) in the periphery often express both IgM and IgD. This is possible because of alternate splicing of mRNA (i.e., the primary mRNA transcript contains both the IgM and IgD heavy chains). Depending on the splicing of the processed mRNA, the VDJ region will be combined with either an IgM or IgD constant region. Once the B-cell is exposed to antigen and activated, the IgD transcript is no longer expressed on the cell surface and the cell expresses only IgM antibody *(10)*.

In the peripheral immune system (primarily lymph nodes and spleen) isotype switching and somatic mutation occur with appropriate T-cell help. These two processes (isotype switching and somatic mutation), although they occur in the same immunologic compartment and require T-cell help, occur independently, as some isotype-switched immunoglobulins are not somatically mutated, whereas some IgM antibodies are heavily mutated. T-cells direct isotype switching via direct T-cell/B-cell interactions (i.e., CD40/CD40L interaction) and via cytokine secretion. Humans deficient in CD40 are unable to isotype switch to IgG, leading to the "hyper IgM syndrome." These patients are susceptible to a variety of infections. In mice, interferon-γ (IFN-γ) secreted by TH1 T-cells (*see* Chapter 13) induces B-cells to isotype switch to IgG2a and IgG3. Interleukin 13 induces B-cell isotype switching to IgE *(2,10,12)*.

5. Effector Functions

As stated earlier, the effector function of an antibody depends primarily on its isotype. IgM is the first isotype produced and is pentameric (composed of five immunoglobulin molecules). Therefore, IgM is a large molecule that is primarily confined to the intravascular space. It can cross the epithelium and is the most potent isotype for activating complement. It does not cross the placenta nor opsonize (opsonize means enhance the phagocytosis of a cell or bacteria by polymorphonucleocytes or macrophages) bacteria *(1,4)*.

Of the human IgG isotypes, IgG1 and IgG3 fix complement and are therefore able to opsonize bacteria and activate the complement system. They are also powerful sensitizers to induce killing by natural-killer cells. They, as all IgG molecules, actively cross the placenta. IgG2 does not fix complement or activate the complement cascade to any great extent. IgG2 is the primary IgG for binding to T-cell-independent antigens; these include, among other antigens, bacterial polysaccharides. IgG4 is similar in its actions to IgG2, except IgG4 on the cell surface enhances opsonization of that cell *(4)*.

IgA is the primary immunoglobulin in epithelial secretions. IgA is a poor activator of the classic complement cascade but can activate the alternative complement pathway. It is usually secreted as a dimer of immunoglobulin molecules linked by a protein called the secretory piece, which is essential for transepithelial transport. IgE is the primary sensitizer of mast cells with little of no ability to fix complement or opsonize bacteria. It does not cross the placenta but can diffuse into extravascular spaces. IgD has no known effector function at this time *(4)*.

6. Antibody Expression and B-Cell Tolerance

The concept of tolerance is the ability to differentiate between self and non-self. As the recombinatorial events producing antibodies in the bone marrow are random, autoreactive B cells are derived by chance. In the bone marrow, autoreactive B-cells are detected and censored by an incompletely understood mechanism. This censoring occurs by elimination of the B-cell or by rendering the B-cell unresponsive to external stimuli *(8,9)*. This state of unresponsiveness is termed anergy. Whether a B-cell is deleted or anergized depends partially on the affinity of the B-cell receptor for the self-molecule. Thus, if a B-cell has high affinity for a self-protein, it is normally deleted. If the interaction with antigen is less avid, the B-cell is anergized. Most anergized B-cells die soon upon reaching the periphery; on rare occasions, however, they can be reactivated *(8,9)*. In the germinal centers of lymph nodes and the spleen, somatic mutations occur when B-cells are exposed to antigens under T-cell guidance. Some of these somatic mutations can render a previously nonautoreactive cell, autoreactive. These newly derived autoreactive cells are also either anergized and/or deleted. Obviously, the process of tolerance induction is key to maintaining a protective B-cell repertoire without allowing the emergence of autoreactive cells.

Previously, it was felt that all recombinatorial events occurred in the bone marrow or thymus. Recent data suggest, however, that recombinatorial events (i.e., RAG protein expression) also occur in the peripheral immune system. Part of the recombinatorial events occurring peripherally may be the result of "receptor editing." In B-cells, the process of "receptor editing" occurs to allow a B-cell to escape deletion or anergy *(7,9)*. If a particular heavy- and light-chain combination results in autoreactivity of the antibody, the B-cell "receptor edits" to avoid deletion. In this process, the production of the original light chain is turned off and different VJ genes (either V kappa or V lambda) are recombined, leading to the production of a new and different light chain. In many instances, the new heavy/light-chain combination will not be autoreactive, allowing the B-cell to escape censure. A similar process probably occurs in the periphery when a heavy chain or light chain is somatically mutated and acquires autoreactivity. In this instance, receptor editing would occur to offset the acquired autoreactivity. B-cells are also eliminated in the periphery if they do not bind antigen avidly. B-cells condemned for this reason may also receptor edit in an attempt to gain avidity for antigen or acquire a new reactivity. In certain circumstances, it has even been demonstrated that B-cells will switch heavy chains in a final attempt to avoid deletion. This has been primarily demonstrated in the setting of autoimmunity, although B-cells from normal individuals have also been shown to switch heavy chains. The mechanisms, signals, and so forth that activate receptor editing of light or heavy chains are unclear at present *(7,9)*.

7. B-Cell Interactions with Antigen

B-cell interactions with antigen occur through the B-cell receptor (i.e., surface immunoglobulin). An antigen can be of any size or chemical makeup *(3)*. The specific portion of the antigen that an antibody binds is called an epitope. There may be multiple epitopes on one antigen such that antibodies of differing specificity can bind to the same antigen. Immunogens are antigens used for immunization to stimulate an immune response. When a person is immunized with tetanus toxoid, the tetanus toxoid is the immunogen.

Interactions with antigens differ between B-cells and T-cells. Immunoglobulins interact directly with antigens in their native form. As discussed in more detail later,

T-cells interact with antigen only after it has been processed by an antigen-presenting cell (i.e., a macrophage) and then presented to the T-cell on the surface of the macrophage in association with an HLA molecule. Antibody–antigen interactions are similar in many ways to other protein–protein interactions or protein–nucleic acid interactions. Binding can occur on the basis of charge–charge interactions or on the basis of polar interactions. Polar interactions result in hydrogen-bonding between molecules. An example of a charge–charge interaction would be an antibody that contains positively charged amino acids in its CDR regions binding to an antigen composed primarily of negative charges. Constraints on binding are determined by the shape of the binding region because of other amino acids in the framework and CDR regions of the antibodies *(3,4)*. The availability of antigen for binding is also key in antibody–antigen interactions. Thus, a particular epitope may be hidden from the antibody because of its being folded inside the protein. Denaturation and unfolding of the protein would make the epitope available for interaction with the antibody.

A number of antibodies are capable of binding more than one antigen. This multireactivity with more than one antigen is exemplified by anti-DNA antibodies in lupus *(16)*. Many anti-DNA antibodies bind not only DNA but also nucleoproteins such as Sm and histones. Many IgM antibodies are highly polyreactive. These antibodies have antigen-binding sites that are promiscuous and interact with a number of antigens. These IgM polyreactive antibodies are normally of low avidity and are felt to be important in the innate immune response because of their ability to bind a number of antigens.

Antigen–antibody complex formation is influenced by the ratio of antibody to antigen, avidity of antibody–antigen interaction, and antibody isotype. Once the complexes form, they may deposit in tissue, aggregate with other antibody–antigen complexes, bind the complement, or any combination of the three. These various end results of antigen–antibody complexes determine the clinical effect of an antibody–antigen interaction. Thus, the clinical outcome of an antibody–antigen complex that is filtered out of the circulation in the spleen varies markedly from an antibody–antigen complex that binds complement and deposits in the kidney.

8. Maturation of the B-Cell Immune Response

Following initial exposure to an antigen, B-cells specific for that antigen are activated. Under most circumstances, the initial interaction is of low affinity and by itself would not be effective in eliminating an infection. Following this initial activation, some of the naive B-cells transform into plasma cells and secrete immunoglobulin to form the primary immune response. Other B-cells, upon exposure to antigen, become memory B-cells that can be activated upon re-exposure to that antigen.

In the secondary lymphoid organs (spleen and lymph nodes), certain B cells, upon exposure to antigen, proliferate and form germinal centers. In the germinal centers, B-cells are exposed to antigen in the context of T-cell help. With T-cell help, further expansion of the specific reactive B-cell population occurs (a process termed clonal expansion). In conjunction with clonal expansion, the B-cells, with T-cell help through cytokine production, may isotype switch from IgM to IgG, IgA, or IgE. It is during the context of clonal expansion that most somatic mutation occurs *(12)*. As described earlier, somatic mutation results in some B-cell's surface immunoglobulin developing a

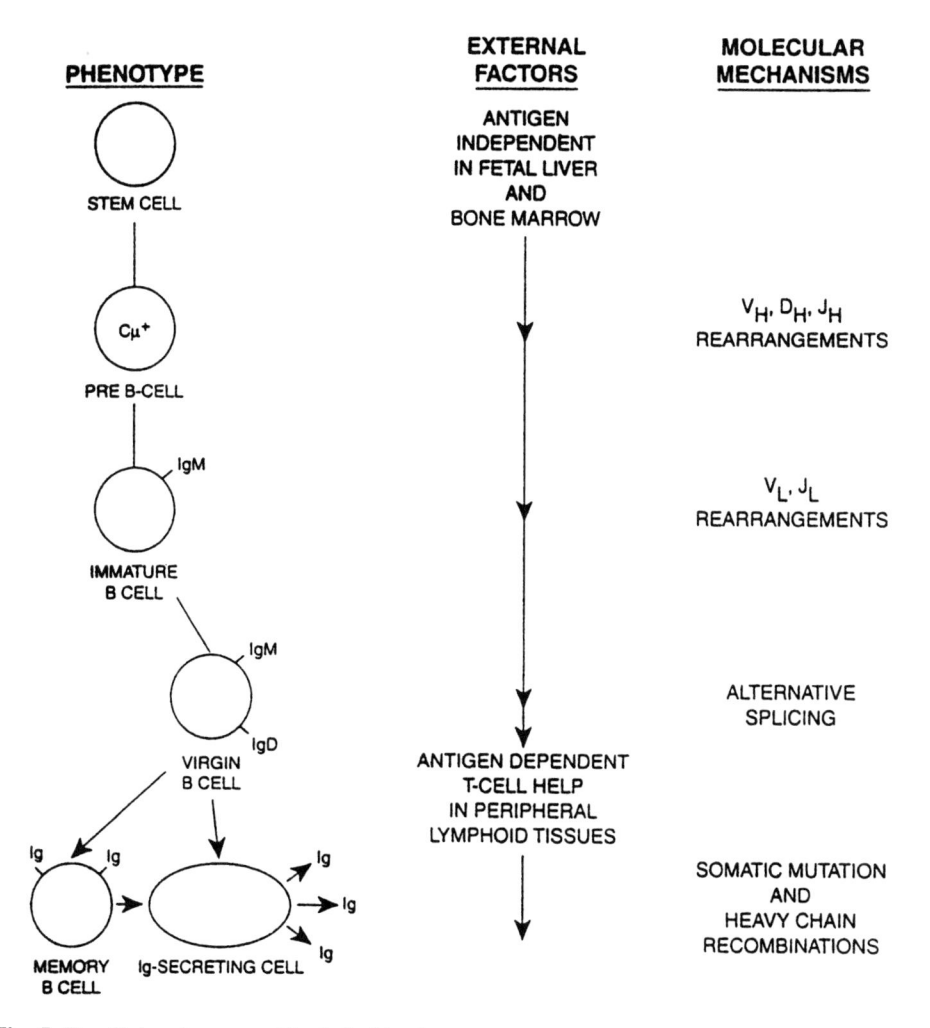

Fig. 5. B-cell development. The left side shows changes in cell-surface Ig expression as B-cells mature and then are stimulated by antigen. Correlation of these developmental events with Ig gene rearrangements is shown on the right side. Note that rearrangements of variable-region gene segments that allow for B-cell development are independent of any antigen interaction and are relatively random.

higher affinity for the antigen than the parent immunoglobulin. The cells with the highest affinity are then selected for further expansion, differentiation into plasma cells, and antibody production. This process is termed B-cell affinity maturation. (*See* Fig. 5.)

9. The B-Cell Receptor

A complex of proteins associates with surface immunoglobulin to form the B-cell receptor (Fig. 6). Two of these proteins are referred to as Igα and Igβ *(3)*. One Igα and one Igβ associate with each heavy chain; thus, the B-cell receptor is composed of one molecule of immunoglobulin and two molecules of Igα and Igβ. Both Igα and Igβ have long tails that extend from the cell surface into the cell cytoplasm. Such intracytoplasmic tails are necessary for signaling inside the cell. A second set of molecules, called the B-cell coreceptor, are present on the cell surface of B-cells and associate

Fig. 6. B-cell receptor. The B-cell receptor is composed of one immunoglobulin molecule and two Iga and two Igb molecules. The Iga and Igb serve to transmit the signal from the surface immunoglobulin intracellularly.

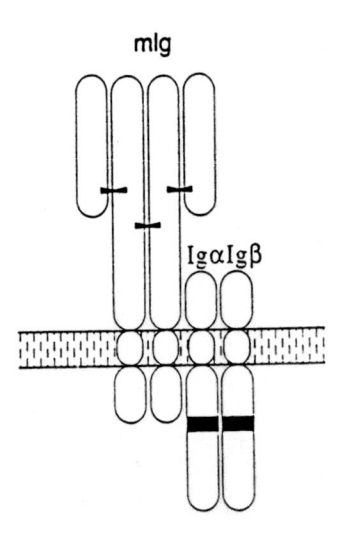

with the surface immunoglobulin. This complex of molecules is composed of proteins CD19, CD2, and TAPA-1 *(3)*. The purpose of this coreceptor appears to be to set the rheostat for B-cell activation. In other words, the coreceptor determines how easy or hard it is for antigen binding to surface immunoglobulin to induce a B-cell response. Antigen binding to surface immunoglobulin thus results in a cascade of intracellular events, modulated by other intracellular signals, leading to B-cell activation and proliferation. Growing evidence suggests that one of the defects in autoimmunity, especially lupus, lies in the altered function of B-cell signaling *(9)*. This concept holds that antigens that signal normal cells to become anergic or to activate the mechanisms for apoptosis are defective in lupus. This defect allows autoantibody-producing B-cells to remain active. The defect is not complete, however, as both B-cell and T-cell censuring functions are, for the most part, intact in lupus. This potential defect in cellular signaling is described in detail in Chapter 20.

10. Autoantibody Production

10.1. Natural Autoantibodies

Defined in the simplest terms, autoantibodies are antibodies that bind self-antigens. It is clear that normal individuals produce autoantibodies and that these self-reactive antibodies play a key role in normal immunity. To understand mechanisms of autoimmunity, the presence of autoantibodies in normals necessitates a scientific differentiation between normal or "natural autoantibodies" and abnormal or "pathogenic" autoantibodies.

Rheumatoid factors (RFs) are prototypic examples of this differentiation. As described earlier, RF are antibodies to the Fc portion of IgG. A significant number of B-cells in normals, when stimulated, produce rheumatoid factors. Indeed, RFs are found in the sera of patients with various inflammatory and infectious diseases; RFs, however, are also thought to be pathogenic in rheumatoid arthritis. Because of their universal presence, RFs almost certainly play a role in normal immunity, perhaps by crosslinking IgG, RF accelerate the early immune response *(14)*.

Features that appear to separate "natural RFs" from "pathogenic RFs" are as follows: (1) isotype—natural RFs are primarily IgM, pathogenic RFs are frequently IgG; (2) affinity—natural RFs are weak binders, pathogenic RF are of high affinity (i.e., bind tightly to IgG); (3) B-cell type—many natural RFs are produced by CD5+ B-cells, pathogenic RFs are produced by CD5– B-cells (*see* Chapter 13 regarding CD5 and B-cells); (4) molecular features—natural RFs are germline encoded (i.e., contain few somatic mutations), whereas pathogenic RFs are highly mutated, suggesting antigen drive (*see* Subheadings 3. and 7.). Similar differentiations are present between "natural" anti-DNA and "pathogenic" anti-DNA. Thus, autoantibodies are not necessarily abnormal. They apparently play a role in normal immunity, likely during the initial phases of an immune response. Binding affinities and specificities allow the differentiation of most natural and pathogenic subsets.

With the advent of techniques for rapid DNA sequencing and techniques that allowed for directed mutation of DNA sequences, molecular features of autoantibodies have been identified. Perhaps the most widely investigated autoantibody response on the molecular level is the anti-DNA response. Studies from a number of laboratories using different murine models of lupus, as well as antibodies derived from humans, have identified a number of molecular characteristics common to most anti-DNA antibodies *(15–17)*.

Although there are frequent exceptions to every rule, VH CDR2, VH CDR3, VL CDR1, and VL CDR3 are the antibody variable regions that interact with DNA. The VH CDR3 region is of particular importance in anti-DNA binding. DNA binding appears to be heavy-chain dominant in that the binding to DNA depends primarily on the heavy chain. The light chain, for most antibodies, affects whether the antibody binds to single-stranded DNA or double-stranded DNA, and the degree of crossreactivity. Most attention in molecular analysis of anti-DNA antibodies has focused on the heavy-chain CDR3 region. Anti-DNA antibodies frequently contain at least one arginine in their VH CDR3 region. As arginines are positively charged, they interact with DNA molecules (DNA is negatively charged) on a charge–charge basis *(16)*. When the arginines are replaced with noncharged amino acids like glycines in an anti-DNA VH CDR3 region, anti-DNA binding is abrogated. Similarly, when arginines are added in the VH CDR3 region of an antibody, anti-DNA binding activity is enhanced. Somatic mutations in anti-DNA antibodies that enhance anti-DNA binding most often occur in the VH CDR2 region and frequently result in the change of a noncharged amino acid to an arginine *(15,17)*. As stated earlier, however, there are frequent exceptions to every rule, including the importance of arginines to DNA binding. Not all anti-DNA antibodies contain arginines in either the VH CDR2 or VH CDR3 and a number of antibodies with arginines in these locations do not bind DNA. "Natural anti-DNA antibodies" do not have a high percentage of arginines in the VH CDR3 region; thus, an increase in VH CDR3 arginines appears to be a feature of only "pathogenic anti-DNA."

Clinically, it has long been recognized that not all anti-DNA antibodies are pathogenic and that not all lupus patients with renal disease have anti-DNA antibodies in their serum. Although there are a number of theories to explain these clinical phenomenon, a number of laboratories have attempted to determine what distinguishes a pathogenic (i.e., glomerular binding) antibody from a nonpathogenic nonglomerular-binding antibody. Unfortunately, there are no universally accepted methods for defining what constitutes a pathogenic antibody. Utilizing a variety of methods to define pathogenicity (primarily binding to glomeruli when injected into normal mice), most of the antibodies characterized to date are highly charged (both negative and positive) in their CDR regions. The need for charged amino acids in binding regions likely reflects the charged nature of glomerular antigens and nucleosomes that deposit in glomeruli. Beyond charge, however, no other defining characteristics have been identified that differentiate pathogenic from nonpathogenic antibodies.

Recently, a number of laboratories have investigated the property of some antibodies to traverse the cell membrane into the cytoplasm and then gain access to the cell nucleus *(15)*. Although this phenomenon was initially described many years ago by Alarcon Sergovia, techniques to study this phenomenon have only recently been developed. Specific sequences were identified that characterize some of these antibodies, including specific nuclear localizing sequences. What role intracellular trafficking has in antibody pathogenicity is still unclear, however, these antibodies will likely be of great use for targeting pharmacologic agents.

There is a less clear understanding of the factors that determine RF activity. Again, however, the VH CDR3 region appears to play a major role in RF activity. TdT-deficient mice, that cannot make N additions, have a decreased ability to produce RFs, implicating sequences in the VH CDR3 in RF activity. When the VH CDR3 region of RF are mutated, RF activity is lost. Finally, long VH CDR3 regions have been implicated in RF activity. In other words, the longer an antibody's VH CDR3 region, the more likely it is to have RF activity. The length of VH CDR3 has also been linked with antibody crossreactivity (i.e., the longer a VH CDR3, the more crossreactive the antibody). Analysis of human RF sequences indicates an additional key role for the Vk CDR3 in RF activity; again, the length of the Vk CDR3 appears important, with longer Vk CDR3 associated with increased RF activity *(14)*.

In summary, there is a significant body of research regarding the characteristics of autoantibodies. Specific characteristics of each autoreactivity have been identified. Perhaps the best summary of these studies, however, is that there is no definitive characteristic that defines every antibody of a given specificity. Insight gained from these studies, however, has led to a number of therapeutic strategies to block autoantibody production and pathogenicity that are now or soon will be in clinical trials.

10.2. B-Cell Repertoire and Autoimmunity

A possible explanation for the production of pathogenic autoantibodies is that the immunoglobulin genes differ between normals and autoimmune individuals. These differences in immunoglobulin genes would result in autoimmune individuals having autoreactive B-cells not present in normal individuals. Animal models provide useful insight into possible differences in B-cell repertoire between normals and autoimmune individuals. Studies of murine models of lupus indicate that there is no difference in immunoglobulin germline gene sequences or expression in autoimmune animals versus normal animals. Additionally, the process of somatic mutation appears to be normally regulated in autoimmunity. Although not complete, similar studies of human immunoglobulin genes and antibody repertoires have found no profound differences in lupus patients versus normals *(16)*.

Current data from transgenic animal studies, however, indicate that autoimmune-prone mice do not properly censure autoreactive B-cells *(18)*. These autoreactive B-cells that are deleted or anergized in normals produce autoantibodies in autoimmune mice; the defect, however, is not global, as lupus mice, for the most part, delete autoreactive B-cells and T-cells normally. Only autoreactive B-cells of certain specificity (i.e., antinucleosomal or anti-DNA) are not properly censured. It is not clear, at present, why the tolerance defect is selective for these antigens. These defects in tolerance induction, however, appear to explain the production of autoantibodies, not differences in immunoglobulin genes between normals and autoimmune individuals *(18,19)*.

10.3. Antigen-Driven Autoantibody Responses

Normal antibody responses follow a pattern of maturation over time and repeated exposures to the inciting antigen. This maturation leads to expansion of B-cells that bind best to the antigen. Somatic mutations within the V regions of the immunoglobulin genes of these B-cells enhance the binding affinity of the antibodies produced *(16,17)*. To determine if autoantibody responses mature in a similar manner to normal antibody responses, a number of cellular and molecular studies were performed. Murine models of lupus were primarily used for these studies, with anti-DNA and RF responses being the most intensively studied.

By sequence analysis, a number of laboratories demonstrated that autoantibodies are the result of clonal expansion of a limited number of B cells whose immunoglobulin genes contain somatic mutations *(16,17)*. Analysis of these immunoglobulin gene somatic mutations suggests that the somatic mutations are not random, but selected for by the stimulating antigen (i.e., DNA). Thus, autoantibody responses are similar to normal antibody responses in their maturation, with preferential expansion of the B-cells expressing the most reactive antibody *(16,17)*. The production of pathogenic autoantibodies appears secondary to a defect in differentiating self from non-self (not a defect in immunoglobulin genes) genetic recombination, or the process of somatic mutation.

11. Summary

The humoral immune response is an integral part of the immune system. It is an incredibly complex system yielding a vast repertoire of antibodies capable of binding and eliminating the millions of foreign challenges presented to it. This huge repertoire and the antigenic challenges presented to it provide a fertile ground for the development of autoreactivity. A number of checks and balances are in effect that prevent clinical autoimmunity in the vast majority of individuals. Autoantibodies are produced and appear to play a key role in normal immunity. It is not definitively clear, but the scientific evidence at present suggests that clinical autoimmunity does not arise from expansion or changes in the "normal autoimmune repertoire". Although we have gained great insight into the makeup and control of the humoral immune response, much remains to be learned, not only about normal immunity but also the defects that allow the humoral immune response to go awry when "pathogenic autoantibodies" are produced.

References

1. Roitt, I. M., Brostoff, J., and Male, D. (eds.), 4th ed (1993) *Immunology.* Mosby, London, Chaps 4 and 6.
2. Blackwell, T. K. and Alt, F. W. (1989) Mechanism and developmental program of immunoglobulin gene rearrangement in mammals. *Annu. Rev. Genet.* **23,** 605–630.
3. Pleiman, C. M., D'Ambrosio, D., and Cambier, J. C. (1994) The B-cell antigen receptor complex: structure and signal transduction. *Immunol. Today* **15,** 393–398.
4. Hahn, G. S. (1982) Antibody structure, function and active sites, in *Physiology of Immunoglobulins: Diagnostic and Clinical Aspects* (Ritzmann, S. E., ed.), Liss, New York.
5. Junkappiller, T. and Hood, L. (1990) Diversity of the immunoglobulin gene superfamily. *Adv. Immunol.* **44,** 1–39.
6. Lewis, S. M. (1994) The mechanism of VDJ joining: lessons from molecular, immunological and comparative analyses. *Adv. Immunol.* **56,** 27–44.
7. Gay, D., Saunders, T., Camper, S., and Weigert, M. (1993) Receptor editing: an approach by autoreactive B cells to escape tolerance. *J. Exp. Med.* **177,** 1165–1173.
8. Hartley, S. B., Cooke, M. P., Fulcher, D. A., Harris, A. W., Cory, S., Basten, A., et al. (1993) Elimination of self-reactive B lymphocytes proceeds in two stages; arrested development and cell death. *Cell* **72,** 325–335.
9. Nemazee, D. (1993) Promotion and prevention of autoimmunity by B lymphocytes. *Curr. Opin. Immunol.* **5,** 866–872.
10. Snapper, C. M. and Mond, J. J. (1993) Towards a comprehensive review of immunoglobulin class switching. *Immunol. Today* **14,** 15–17.
11. Kelsoe, G. (1994) B cell diversification and differentiation in the periphery. *J. Exp. Med.* **180,** 5,6.
12. Berek, C. and Milstein, C. (1988) The dynamic nature of the antibody repertoire. *Immunol. Rev.* **105,** 5–26.
13. Theofilopoulos, A. (1995) The basis of autoimmunity. *Immunol. Today* **16,** 150–159.
14. Cohen, I. R. and Young, D. B. (1991) Autoimmunity, microbial immunity, and the immunological homunculus. *Immunol. Today* **12,** 105–110.
15. Madaio, M. P. and Shlomchik, M. J. (1996) Emerging concepts regarding B cells and autoantibodies in murine lupus nephritis: B cells have multiple roles—all autoantibodies are not equal. *J. Am. Soc. Nephrol.* **7,** 387–396.
16. Radic, M. Z. and Weigert, M. (1994) Genetic and structural evidence for antigen selection of anti-DNA antibodies. *Annu. Rev. Immunol.* **12,** 487–520.
17. Shlomchik, M. J., Mascelli, M. A., Shan, H., Radic, M. Z., Pisetsky, D., Marshak-Rothstein, A., et al. (1990) Anti-DNA antibodies from autoimmune mice arise by clonal expansion and somatic mutation. *J. Exp. Med.* **171,** 265–297.
18. Roark, J. H., Kunts, C. L., Nguyen, K.-A., Caton, A. J., and Erikson, J. (1995) Breakdown of B cell tolerance in a mouse model of systemic lupus erythematosus. *J. Exp. Med.* **181,** 1157–1167.
19. Jacobson, B. A., Panka, D. J., Nguyen, K.-A. T., Erikson, J., Abbas, A. K., and Marshak-Rothstein, A. (1995) Anatomy of autoantibody production; dominant localization of antibody producing cells to T cell zones in Fas-deficient mice. *Immunity* **3,** 509–519.

5
T-Cell Signaling

Gary A. Koretzky and Erik J. Peterson

1. Introduction

In response to an antigenic challenge, peripheral T-lymphocytes are stimulated to produce cytokines, proliferate, and develop effector function. Once the inciting stimulus has been cleared, the vast majority of the antigen-specific responding cells undergo programmed cell death (apoptosis). Failure of T-cell surface receptors to transduce initial activating signals can lead to immunodeficiency, whereas failure of T-cells to undergo apoptosis at the appropriate time may lead to lymphoproliferative disorders. Much insight has been gained in recent years into the molecular mechanisms responsible for both the initial activation response and subsequent cell death. Identification of a number of molecules critical for both responses has led to additional studies in transformed cell lines and experiments utilizing genetically altered mice. Collectively, these approaches have suggested how disruption in signaling pathways in lymphocytes may lead to human disease. In many cases, these suggestions have now been corroborated as mutations in key signaling molecules have been shown to be causal in human immune disorders.

2. Engagement of the T-Cell Antigen Receptor Results in Activation of Protein Tyrosine Kinases

T-Cells sample their environment via a host of cell-surface receptors capable of transducing positive or negative signals. The receptor complex that has received the greatest attention because of its central importance in T-cell activation is the antigen receptor itself (TCR) *(1)*. The TCR is comprised of four heterodimers or homodimers (Fig. 1). Two of these, the α and β chains, arise from rearranging gene segments and provide the antigen recognition function. The other six chains are known collectively as CD3 and are responsible for transducing activation signals. Following antigen binding, the CD3 molecules become phosphorylated on tyrosine residues found within specialized domains known as immunoreceptor tyrosine-based activation motifs (ITAMs) *(2)*. The protein tyrosine kinases (PTK) responsible for ITAM phosphorylation include lck and fyn, two members of the src family. When phosphorylated, these ITAMs become docking sites for other molecules that possess src homology 2 (SH2) domains. One of the key proteins recruited to the CD3 ITAMs is ZAP-70, a PTK belonging to the syk family. When associated with the ITAMs, ZAP-70 becomes accessible for phos-

From: *Current Molecular Medicine: Principles of Molecular Rheumatology*
Edited by: G. C. Tsokos © Humana Press Inc., Totowa, NJ

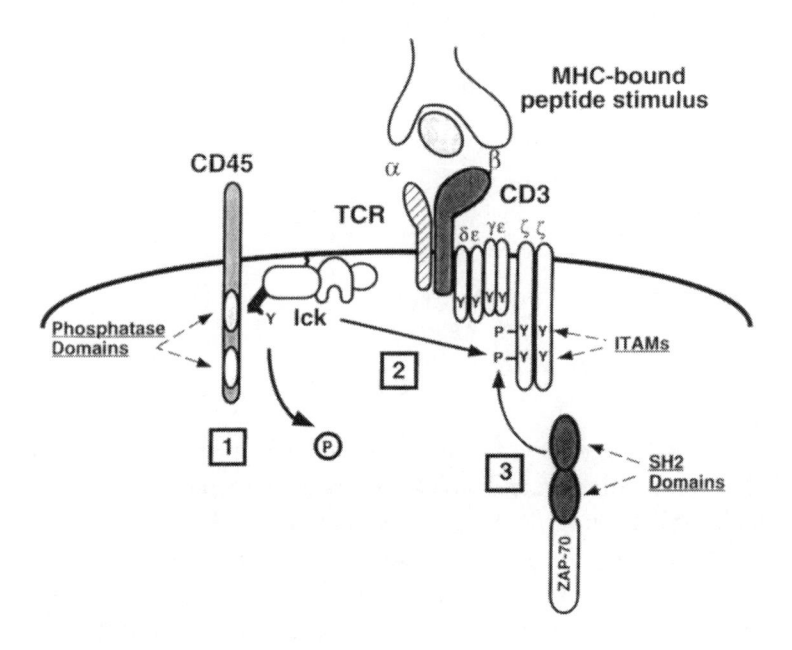

Fig. 1. Membrane-proximal components of TCR signal transduction. The tyrosine phosphatase CD45 dephosphorylates the negative regulatory tyrosine residue on the membrane-associated tyrosine kinase lck, maintaining lck in an open, activatible form *[1]*. Ligation of the TCR brings activated lck into proximity with ITAM-bearing CD3 chains. Lck phosphorylates CD3 complex proteins, including the ζ chain *[2]*. Phosphorylated CD3 chains become sites for recruitment of the cytoplasmic PTK ZAP-70 via tandem SH2 domains *[3]*, allowing activation of ZAP-70.

phorylation by src family PTKs, resulting in an increase in its enzymatic activity. Thus, engagement of the TCR by antigen converts CD3 into an enzymatically active complex capable of further signal propagation.

Evidence for the importance of lck and fyn in the initiation of TCR signaling events has come from studies of cell lines with mutations in these PTKs, as well as mice engineered to be deficient in their expression *(3)*. In experiments utilizing transformed cell lines, it appears that whereas lck expression is an absolute requirement for TCR signaling, fyn plays a less critical role. Experiments using "knockout" mice corroborate this notion. In vivo, both lck and fyn need to be present for optimal TCR function, whereas lck appears to play a more critical role in T-cell ontogeny than does fyn. This is presumably due to the requirement of lck for signal transduction events important for thymocyte maturation. Recently, these findings in mice have been extended to humans in a report demonstrating defective lck protein production in a case of life-threatening immunodeficiency *(4)*.

Much has been learned recently about the regulation of the src family PTKs in T-cells. Early structural work indicated that the enzymatic activity of these proteins is regulated, at least in part, by phosphorylation of a carboxyl-terminal tyrosine *(5)*. When this residue is phosphorylated, an intramolecular interaction occurs, downregulating PTK activity (Fig. 2). Phosphorylation of this tyrosine is regulated dynamically in T-cells by the action of a kinase (CSK) and a phosphatase (CD45), both specific for

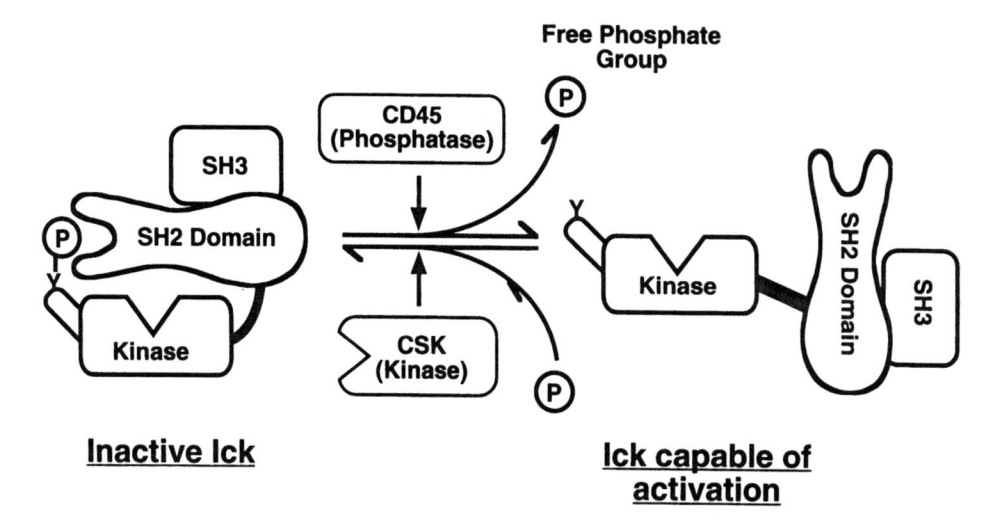

Fig. 2. Tyrosine phosphorylation status determines conformation and activation potential of lck. Three major functional domains of the src-family PTK lck include the kinase, SH2, and SH3 regions. Tyrosine 505, when phosphorylated, forms the basis of an intramolecular association with the lck SH2 domain. The CD45 phosphatase dephosphorylates a regulatory tyrosine residue to maintain lck in an "open" lck conformation and capable of enzymatic activity. CSK counters the CD45 effect through phosphorylation of the same tyrosine and restoration of an inactive, closed conformation.

this residue. Experiments demonstrating the importance of both CSK and CD45 have been performed in mutant cell lines and mice.

Numerous studies demonstrate that all of the biochemical signals known to be important for T-cell activation depend not only on the function of the src family PTKs, but also the recruitment and activation of ZAP-70 (6). Stimulation of the TCR on transformed cell lines lacking ZAP-70 fails to result in signal transduction events. ZAP-70 is known also to play a critical role in signaling events in the thymus during T-cell development. Mice made deficient in ZAP-70 via homologous recombination demonstrate a significant block in thymocyte development. The few ZAP-70-deficient T-cells that transit the thymus and populate peripheral lymphoid organs also show a severe block in activation potential. Most importantly, patients have now been identified who lack functional ZAP-70 protein. These individuals manifest a severe immunodeficiency with loss of the subpopulation of CD8+ peripheral T-cells and a failure of the remaining CD4+ cells to respond to activating stimuli.

3. TCR Signals Downstream of PTK Activation

Following antigenic stimulation and recruitment of ZAP-70 to the CD3 ITAMs, widespread phosphorylation of cellular proteins is observed (7). Insight into the molecular mechanisms important in the regulation of TCR signaling events has come from the identification of many of these TCR-stimulated PTK substrates. One of the first to be characterized was the membrane-associated enzyme phospholipase Cγ1 (PLCγ1) (Fig. 3). When phosphorylated on tyrosine residues, the enzymatic activity of PLCγ1 increases resulting in hydrolysis of membrane-associated phosphatidylinositol

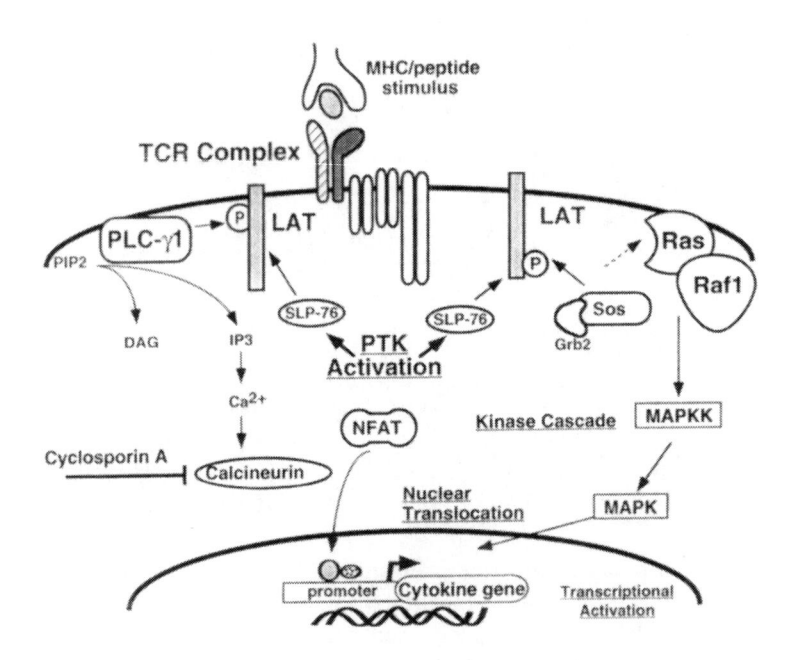

Fig. 3. Signaling pathways activated by TCR engagement. TCR ligation results in activation of PTKs such as ZAP-70 (see Fig. 1). SLP-76 is phosphorylated and associates indirectly with LAT via other adaptor proteins. TCR-inducible phosphorylation of LAT promotes the assembly of other signaling complexes, including recruitment of Grb2/Sos with subsequent Ras activation. Active Ras binds and stimulates the kinase Raf1, which phosphorylates and activates a cascade of serine/threonine kinases, including mitogen-activated protein kinase kinase (MAPKK). Upon phosphorylation and activation, the most membrane-distal component in the cascade, mitogen-activated protein kinase (MAPK), translocates to the nucleus. In a second LAT-related pathway, membrane-bound PLC-γ1, is recruited to LAT and becomes phosphorylated and activated. Hydrolysis of membrane phosphatidyl-inositol bis-phosphate (PIP2) by PLC-γ1 releases diacylglycerol (DAG) and inositol tris-phosphate (IP3). IP3 stimulates an increase in intracellular calcium concentration, which activates the phosphatase calcineurin. Calcineurin dephosphorylates nuclear factor of activated T-cells (NFAT), resulting in NFAT translocation to the nucleus. Transcription factors dependent on MAPK then cooperate with NFAT proteins to upregulate transcription of IL-2 and other activation genes. Cyclosporin A blocks calcineurin function and thus impairs NFAT-dependent transcriptional activation.

4,5 bisphosphate into two intracellular second messengers, diacylglycerol (DAG) and inositol 3,4,5 trisphosphate (IP3) *(8)*. DAG is an activator of members of the protein kinase C (PKC) family of serine/threonine kinases. IP3 interacts with its receptor on endoplasmic reticulum, resulting in the release of calcium into the cytosol. PKC regulates numerous downstream signals important for T-cell activation, including increasing activity of several classes of transcription factors. Similarly, the increase in cytosolic free calcium plays a critical role in signal transduction by increasing the activity of calcineurin, a serine–threonine phosphatase. Calcineurin dephosphorylates nuclear factor of activated T-cells (NFAT), allowing this transcription factor to enter the nucleus, where it upregulates transcription of cytokine and other genes important for T-cell growth and development. The central importance of calcineurin in T-cell activation events is underscored by the fact that this phosphatase is the molecular target for the potent immunosuppressant cyclosporin A. The integration of signals leading to PKC and NFAT is also apparent, as NFAT often acts in concert with PKC-stimulated factors for optimal transcriptional activation.

Stimulation of the TCR also results in activation of the Ras signaling pathway *(9)* (Fig. 3). Ras is a low-mol-wt guanine nucleotide-binding protein that is active when bound to GTP and inactive when bound to GDP. Active Ras stimulates a cascade of protein kinases that, in turn, stimulate the activity of numerous transcription factors. TCR-mediated exchange of GTP for GDP on Ras requires PTK function, although the molecular mechanism coupling PTKs to Ras activation in T-cells remains unclear.

In addition to the phosphatidylinositol and Ras signaling pathways, TCR engagement is known also to activate other second messengers, all of which appear to require prior stimulation of PTKs. In some circumstances, the relevant substrate of the PTKs is not yet known. For other signaling pathways, it is obvious what role the PTKs play because effector molecules critical to initiate those signaling cascades are themselves substrates of the PTKs. One example noted earlier is phosphorylation of PLCγ1. Interestingly, however, even in this circumstance, it appears that phosphorylation of the effector enzyme is not sufficient for optimal activation of the phosphatidylinositol second-messenger pathway, as other PTK substrates seem to play important roles. Therefore, there has been considerable recent interest in identifying novel substrates of the TCR-stimulated PTKs with the hope that these investigations will lead to insight into how the various TCR-stimulated signaling cascades are regulated and integrated.

4. Adapter Proteins Link Signaling Cascades Following TCR Engagement

The first TCR-stimulated PTK substrates identified were components of the TCR complex itself (the ITAMs) or enzymes whose activity is increased upon tyrosine phosphorylation. More recently, it has become appreciated that numerous members of another class of proteins, the adapter molecules, are also substrates of lck, fyn, and ZAP-70. Adapter proteins are molecules with no intrinsic enzymatic activity, but which, through their ability to promote protein–protein interactions, organize complexes of signaling molecules *(10)*. Adapter proteins are characterized by the presence of discrete domains that dictate binding to other proteins. These include src homology 2 (SH2) and phosphotyrosine-binding (PTB) domains capable of interacting with other proteins that are phosphorylated on tyrosine residues; src homology 3 (SH3) domains able to bind other proteins with proline-rich regions; pleckstrin homology domains that encode regions that bind phospholipids; and PDZ domains that bind to regions with defined tryptophan sequences *(10)*.

Efforts to identify substrates of TCR-activated PTKs have led to the identification of several novel members of the adapter family. A number of these proteins have been shown to play essential roles in coupling the TCR with downstream activation. Some adapters act as positive regulators of TCR signaling, whereas others function to interfere with activation events *(11)*. Examples of positive regulators include LAT (linker of activation of T-cells) and SLP-76 (SH2 domain containing leukocyte phosphoprotein of 76 kDa) *(12)*. Both of these adapter proteins are rapidly phosphorylated following TCR engagement and bind to a number of molecules important in signal transduction cascades (Fig. 4).

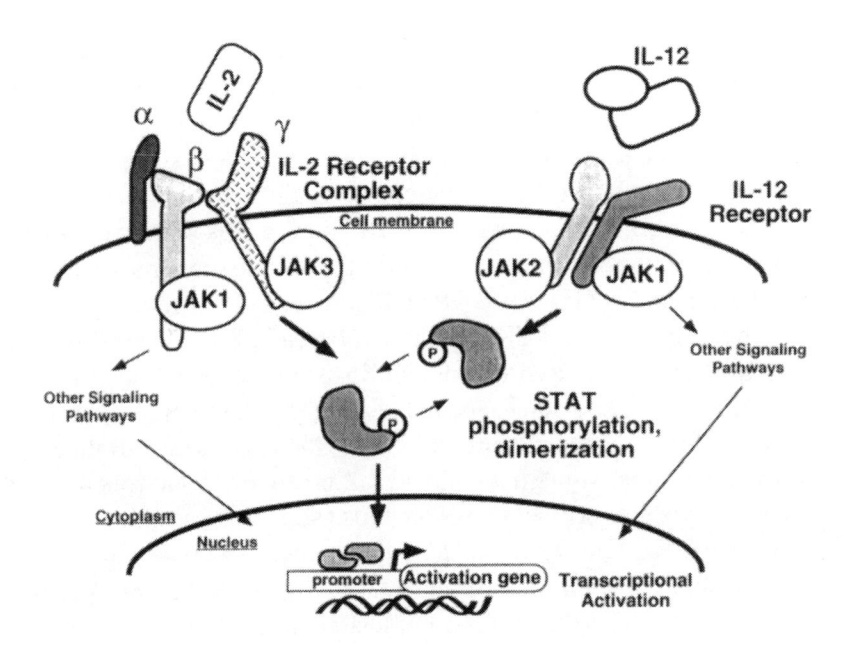

Fig. 4. IL-2 and IL-12 signaling cascades utilize JAKs and STATs. IL-2 binds to activated T-cells through receptor complexes containing combinations of α, β, and γ surface proteins. The β- and γ-chain associated PTKs JAK1 and JAK3 undergo phosphorylation and activation. The JAKs phosphorylate STAT family members, which then dimerize, translocate to the nucleus, and bind response elements in the promoters of target activation genes. IL-12 receptor ligation results in activation of a separate combination of JAK and STAT family members, permitting upregulation of a group of activation genes overlapping with, but distinct from, those genes activated after IL2R ligation.

Several lines of evidence suggest that both LAT and SLP-76 play important roles in T-cell function *(13)*. In one model system, overexpression of mutant variants of LAT result in inhibition of TCR-mediated cellular activation. In other studies, it has been shown that overexpression of wild-type SLP-76 in transformed T-cells augments TCR-stimulated activation of the interleukin 2 (IL-2) gene. In contrast, TCR engagement on a T-cell line lacking expression of SLP-76 fails to induce expression of the IL-2 gene. Furthermore, mice made deficient in SLP-76 expression by gene targeting exhibit a complete block in T-cell maturation, presumably the result of impaired signaling via the pre-TCR on developing thymocytes. The precise mechanism by which SLP-76 or LAT function remains unknown; however, evidence suggests that these proteins bring together effector proteins into larger activation complexes. Although none have yet been identified, it is likely that mutations will be discovered in LAT and/or SLP-76, which are responsible for human immunodeficiency states.

5. Other Signaling Molecules That Interfere with TCR-Mediated Activation Events

In addition to providing insight into the biology of positive regulators of TCR signaling, recent studies have focused on other proteins that function to block downstream events following TCR engagement. Identification of the molecular defects underlying spontaneously occurring animal models of immune dysregulation has provided insight into the complex regulation of lymphocyte activation. "Motheaten" mice are severely immunocompromised animals characterized by uncontrolled growth of macrophagelike cells leading to fatal pneumonitis *(14)*. T-Cell and B-cell growth and function is also abnormal in motheaten animals. The molecular defect underlying the motheaten phenotype is in a cytosolic protein tyrosine phosphatase named SHP-1. SHP-1 plays a critical role in downregulating activation signals in hematopoietic cells by selectively dephosphorylating substrates of the activating PTKs. SHP-1 deficiency allows these substrates to remain phosphorylated on tyrosine residues, thus prolonging the activation signal.

A second example of an inhibitory molecule critical in the regulation of signal transduction pathways is CTLA4, a receptor for ligands expressed on antigen-presenting cells (APCs). In addition to binding CTLA4, these ligands (members of the B7 family of surface receptors) also bind to CD28, an activating coreceptor on T-cells *(15)*. Early in an immune response, T-cells express CD28, but not CTLA4. The presence of B7 family members on the APCs augments their ability to stimulate T-cell effector function through engagement of CD28. Following the initial activation, CTLA4 is induced on the responding T-cells. Because CTLA4 has a higher affinity for the B7 ligands than does CD28, signals are delivered to the T-cell to terminate the response. Although the precise molecular mechanism of CTLA4 action remains unclear, studies in mice made deficient in CTLA4 expression by homologous recombination demonstrate the essential role this negative regulator plays. CTLA4 "knockout" mice demonstrate rampant lymphoproliferation leading to early death because of the failure to downregulate immune responses.

Adaptor molecules may also exert an inhibitory influence upon TCR signaling. For example, cbl is an adapter protein that, like SLP-76 and LAT, is a substrate of TCR-stimulated PTKs. However, unlike SLP-76 and LAT, cbl interferes with TCR-stimulated activation events. Although the precise mechanism of cbl function remains to be elucidated, several lines of evidence suggest that it blocks the ability of the TCR to couple with the Ras signaling cascade *(16)*. Further evidence suggests that cbl plays a physiological role in the development of T-cell anergy (antigen-specific unresponsiveness). Additional evidence for the importance of cbl as a negative regulator comes from studies demonstrating T-cell hyperresponsiveness in mice made deficient in cbl expression through gene targeting.

6. Signaling Through the IL-2 Receptor Leads to Proliferative Responses

The TCR signaling events described in Subheading 5 are important for both the production of IL-2, an essential T-cell growth factor, and for upregulation of the receptor for this important cytokine. Interactions between IL-2 and its receptor then initiate the signals critical for T-cell proliferation. Studies of the IL-2 receptor and the molecules with which it interacts have provided important insights into the signal transduction machinery important for the proliferative phase of lymphocyte activation *(17)*. These molecular studies have been complemented also with experiments in transformed cell lines, genetically manipulated mice, and observations made in human patients with immune dysfunction to provide a more comprehensive understanding of the biology of IL-2 receptor-mediated T-cell growth.

Similar to the TCR, the IL-2 receptor is comprised of a multimeric complex that lacks intrinsic enzymatic function. For IL-2 to bind to T-cells with high affinity, three molecules, receptor α, β, and γ chains, must all be expressed. Interestingly, the γ chain of the IL-2 receptor participates in signal transduction as a component of other cytokine receptors and hence has been designated the "common" γ chain. When IL-2 engages this tripartite receptor, conformational changes occur, allowing the receptor to activate members of another PTK family, the Janus kinases (JAKs) (Fig. 4). JAK activity results in the phosphorylation of a spectrum of substrates including members of the signal transducers and activators of transcription (STAT) family. Phosphorylated STAT molecules dimerize and enter the nucleus, where they participate in transcriptional activation of new genes. Although this pathway describes the most direct connection between IL-2 and the nucleus, IL-2 receptor engagement also stimulates other signaling cascades that modulate the ability of the cell to respond appropriately to its environment.

Mutations in any of the signaling components of the IL-2 receptor pathway lead to dysregulation of T-cell function. This has been studied successfully using cell lines, mutant mice, and cells from patients suffering from severe combined immunodeficiency (SCID). Improved understanding of the signaling pathways initiated by engagement of the IL-2 receptor has enabled precise identification of the molecular defect in many patients with SCID. One immediate benefit of this knowledge is the ability to provide genetic counseling to families with carriers of inherited disorders. Longer-range benefits will involve development of specific therapeutic interventions based on the knowledge of the molecular and biochemical defects causal for these devastating diseases.

In addition to making use of shared receptor elements such as the common γ chain, other members of the cytokine family also make use of similar signal transduction molecules. Thus, as shown in Fig. 4, although interleukin 12 binds to a different cell-surface receptor than does IL-2, it makes use of similar biochemical pathways to initiate cellular activation *(18)*. The precise downstream events elicited by engagement of various activating receptors on the T-cell surface thus requires a complex integration of proximal and distal biochemical signals mediated both by enzymes and a large spectrum of adapter proteins.

7. TCR-Mediated Signaling Also Primes Cells for Apoptosis

Clonal expansion and development of effector function of antigen-specific T-lymphocytes are both required for the appropriate host response to an antigenic challenge. However, once this challenge has been met, the expanded population of activated T-cells must be disposed of to preserve homeostasis of the immune cell compartment and limit potential autoreactivity. Recently, it has become clear that elimination of this expanded population of cells occurs via programmed cell death (apoptosis) and that the death machinery is primed by signals initiated by TCR engagement through a process known as activation-induced cell death (AICD) *(19)*.

Insight into molecular mechanisms of AICD and the contribution of TCR-generated signals has again come from studies of wild-type and mutant cell lines, mutant murine strains, and humans afflicted with immune system disorders. Many studies, described in detail in Chapter 3, have implicated binding of CD95, a member of the tumor necrosis family of receptors, as a required step in AICD. CD95 expression on T-lymphocytes is upregulated following TCR engagement. Interestingly, the protein that activates CD95 (CD95 ligand) is also upregulated following stimulation of the TCR. Recent studies from numerous laboratories indicate that the signal transduction events initiated by TCR ligation, which are critical for upregulation of the CD95 ligand, are very similar to those important for transcriptional activation of cytokine genes, such as IL-2 *(20)*. Thus, it has become clear that when the TCR is bound, the molecules that promote activation and apoptosis are upregulated simultaneously.

Determination of the fate of an individual T-cell depends on the presence or absence of costimulatory signals delivered via receptors such as CD28. These signaling events result in expression of antiapoptotic proteins that function to interdict the default death pathway. Coreceptors such as CD28 are engaged only if the antigenic challenge is presented to the T-cell in the context of an antigen-presenting cell expressing the correct peptide fragment within the major histocompatibility complex groove. Thus, a T-cell whose TCR is triggered inappropriately will be signaled to die, as antiapoptotic signals are not delivered. Additionally, this system ensures that once the inciting antigenic challenge has been met and costimulatory signals are gone, protective proteins will no longer be produced, allowing the default apoptotic pathway to proceed.

Understanding of the role of CD95 and its ligand in directing AICD has been enhanced by the intensive study of two strains of mice with spontaneous mutations in genes in the AICD pathway. These strains, termed *lpr* and *gld*, were long known to exhibit profound disorders in immune cell regulation with severe lymphoproliferation and many features of autoimmunity. Elegant studies suggested that the *gld* mutation is the result of the ligand for the receptor that is abnormal in the *lpr* mouse. Subsequent work demonstrated that the *lpr* mutation resides within the CD95 gene and the *gld* mutation is within the CD95 ligand *(21)*. These studies suggesting a critical role for CD95 and the CD95 ligand as regulators of immune system homeostasis in vivo have been bolstered recently by the identification of mutations responsible for the human autoimmune lymphoproliferative syndrome (ALPS; also known as the Canale–Smith syndrome). This rare disorder is characterized by massive lymphoproliferation and evidence for multiorgan autoimmune phenomena *(22)*. A number of patients who have been studied harbor mutations in one of their two CD95 alleles. Further studies of the protein product of the mutant CD95 gene isolated from many of these individuals indicates that when expressed in a cell-line model, these proteins exert a dominant interfering effect on CD95-mediated apoptosis by inhibiting the ability of CD95 to stimulate signals necessary for apoptosis (Fig. 5). Although these findings suggest that mutations within CD95 play at least one role in the development of the ALPS syndrome, it is also clear that obligate carriers of the mutant CD95 alleles often have no evidence for clinical disease. Thus, a complete understanding of the immune dysfunction associated with the ALPS syndrome will require elucidation of other factors, likely both genetic and environmental, which affect the phenotypic expression of mutant CD95 alleles.

8. Summary

Studies of the biology of signal transduction in the immune system have made us aware of numerous proteins that play critical roles in the regulation of immune cell function. Investigators in many laboratories have applied this knowledge to in vitro molecular studies, experiments using transformed cell lines, and, more recently, to stud-

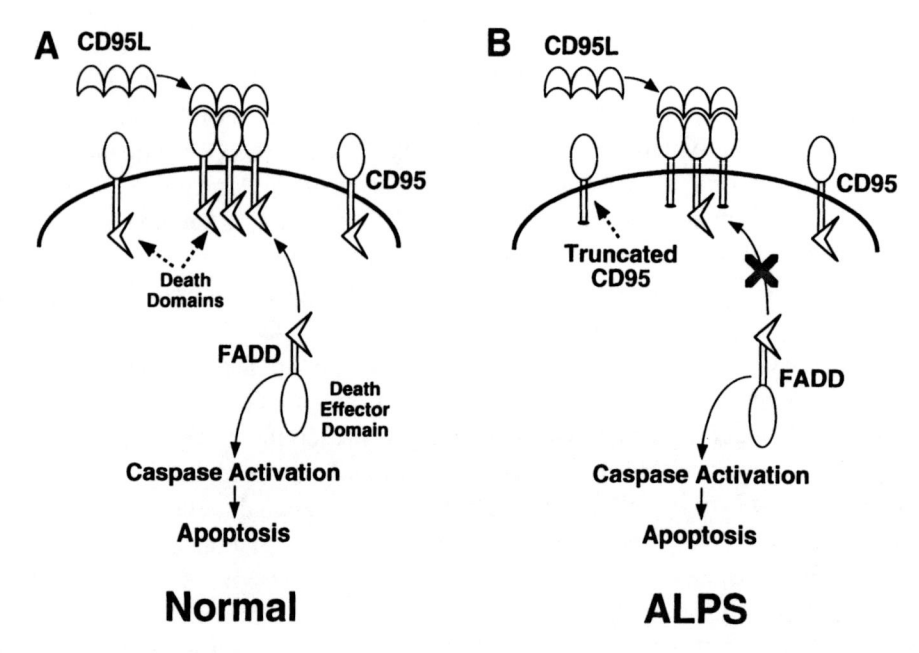

Fig. 5. Autoimmune Lymphoproliferative Syndrome (ALPS) patients exhibit disrupted cysteine protease activation and apoptosis. In the normal T-cell (**A**), trimerized CD95 ligand induces oligomerization of CD95 expressed on the T-cell surface. Cytoplasmic death domains borne by CD95 proteins aggregate and stimulate homotypic association with a death domain within Fas associated Death Domain containing protein (FADD). FADD also contains a death effector domain (DED) which mediates recruitment and activation of members of the caspase family of proteases. Numerous cytoplasmic proteins serve as caspase substrates in a prologue to apoptosis. In ALPS (**B**), mutated CD95 genes encode truncated forms of CD95 lacking the cytoplasmic death domain. The mutant CD95 molecules form CD95L-inducible complexes with wild-type molecules on the T-cell surface and prevent recruitment of FADD to these complexes, thus disrupting downstream apoptotic signaling events.

ies of genetically altered mice to determine the physiological importance of various signaling components in the development, propagation, and termination of immune responses. Importantly, we are now at the point where data derived from studies of molecules, cells, and mice can be applied to human disease, because we are beginning to appreciate the detailed molecular basis of numerous immunologic disorders.

References

1. Weiss, A. and Littman, D. R. (1994) Signal transduction by lymphocyte antigen receptors. *Cell* **76**, 263–274.
2. Flaswinkel, H., Barner, M., and Reth, M. (1995) The tyrosine activation motif as a target of protein tyrosine kinases and SH2 domains. *Semin. Immunol.* **7**, 21–27.
3. Isakov, N., Wange, R. L., and Samelson, L. E. (1994) The role of tyrosine kinases and phosphotyrosine-containing recognition motifs in regulation of the T cell-antigen receptor-mediated signal transduction pathway. *J. Leukoc. Biol.* **55**, 265–271.
4. Goldman, F. D., Ballas, Z. K., Schutte, B. C., Kemp, J., Hollenback, C., Noraz, N., et al. (1998) Defective expression of p56lck in an infant with severe combined immunodeficiency. *J. Clin. Invest.* **102**, 421–429.

5. Thomas, M. L. (1995) Positive and negative regulation of leukocyte activation by protein tyrosine phosphatases. *Semin. Immunol.* **7,** 279–288.
6. van Oers, N. S. and Weiss, A. (1995) The Syk/ZAP-70 protein tyrosine kinase connection to antigen receptor signalling processes. *Semin. Immunol.* **7,** 227–236.
7. Samelson, L. E., Donovan, J. A., Isakov, N., Ota, Y., and Wange, R. L. (1995) Signal transduction mediated by the T-cell antigen receptor. *Ann. NY Acad. Sci.* **766,** 157–172.
8. Berridge, M. J. and Irvine, R. F. (1989) Inositol phosphates and cell signaling. *Nature* **341,** 197.
9. Izquierdo Pastor, M., Reif, K., and Cantrell, D. (1995) The regulation and function of p21ras during T-cell activation and growth. *Immunol. Today* **16,** 159–164.
10. Pawson, T. and Scott, J. D. (1997) Signaling through scaffold, anchoring, and adaptor proteins. *Science* **278,** 2075–2080.
11. Koretzky, G. A. (1997) The role of Grb2-associated proteins in T-cell activation. *Immunol. Today* **18,** 401–406.
12. Peterson, E. J., Clements, J. L., Fang, N., and Koretzky, G. A. (1998) Adaptor proteins in lymphocyte antigen-receptor signaling. *Curr. Opin. Immunol.* **10,** 337–344.
13. Clements, J., Boerth, N., Lee, J. R., and Koretzky, G. A. (1999) Integration of T cell receptor-dependent signaling pathways by adapter proteins. *Ann. Rev. Immunol.* **17,** 89–108.
14. Bignon, J. S. and Siminovitch, K. A. (1994) Identification of PTP1C mutation as the genetic defect in motheaten and viable motheaten mice: a step toward defining the roles of protein tyrosine phosphatases in the regulation of hemopoietic cell differentiation and function. *Clin. Immunol. Immunopathol.* **73,** 168–179.
15. Noel, P. J., Boise, L. H., and Thompson, C. B. (1996) Regulation of T cell activation by CD28 and CTLA4. *Adv. Exp. Med. Biol.* **406,** 209–217.
16. Thien, C. B. and Langdon, W. Y. (1998) c-Cbl: a regulator of T cell receptor-mediated signalling. *Immunol. Cell. Biol.* **76,** 473–482.
17. Leonard, W. J. (1996) The molecular basis of X-linked severe combined immunodeficiency: defective cytokine receptor signaling. *Annu. Rev. Med.* **47,** 229–239.
18. Gately, M. K., Renzetti, L. M., Magram, J., Stern, A. S., Adorini, L., Gubler, U., et al. (1998) The interleukin-12/interleukin-12-receptor system: role in normal and pathologic immune responses. *Annu. Rev. Immunol.* **16,** 495–521.
19. Abbas, A. K. (1996) Die and let live: eliminating dangerous lymphocytes. *Cell* **84,** 655–657.
20. Musci, M. A., Latinis, K. M., and Koretzky, G. A. (1997) Signaling events in T lymphocytes leading to cellular activation or programmed cell death. *Clin. Immunol. Immunopathol.* **83,** 205–222.
21. Nagata, S. (1997) Apoptosis by death factor. *Cell* **88,** 355–365.
22. Drappa, J., Vaishnaw, A. K., Sullivan, K. E., Chu, J. L., and Elkon, K. B. (1996) Fas gene mutations in the Canale-Smith syndrome, an inherited lymphoproliferative disorder associated with autoimmunity. *N. Engl. J. Med.* **335,** 1643–1649.

6
Adhesion and Costimulatory Molecules

Vassiliki A. Boussiotis, Gordon J. Freeman, and Lee M. Nadler

1. Introduction

For successful immune activation, T-cells require two signals. The first signal confers specificity and is mediated by the T-cell receptor (TCR). The second signal, costimulation, is delivered by accessory cell-surface molecules expressed on antigen-presenting cells (APCs). In the absence of costimulation, T-cells enter a state of unresponsiveness termed anergy in vitro and tolerance in vivo *(1,2)*. Anergy reflects the inability of antigen-specific T-cells stimulated through their antigen receptor to mount a secondary antigen-specific response on rechallenge. Tolerance is the identical response reflected in the inability of the intact host to mount an effective secondary antigen-specific response in vivo. Induction of anergy is a dynamic process during which T-cells remain alive yet unreactive toward antigens. T-cell tolerance is defined as the inability of an organism to distinguish foreign from self and can be the result of either deletion or inactivation of the antigen-specific T-cells. Tolerance in the thymus is largely a result of clonal deletion. However, recent studies have demonstrated that T-cell inactivation or anergy is a major mechanism of subsequent tolerance in the peripheral lymphoid tissue.

In recent years, the molecular basis of T-cell trafficking and activation has been unraveled and the various pathways controlling T-cell activation have been defined. A cascade of signaling events directs and regulates the trafficking, homing, and activation of T-lymphocytes after antigenic stimulation. Adhesion receptors include selectins, integrins, and adhesion molecules of the immunoglobulin gene superfamily. Tissue-specific homing receptors direct the tissue-specific trafficking of T-lymphocytes. Costimulatory molecules deliver accessory signals for complete T-cell activation to occur.

2. APC: T-Cell Interactions

Antigen-specific T-cell activation requires interaction of the T-cell with specialized APC. Depending on the microenvironment in which the immune response is initiated, distinct populations of cells serve as APCs *(3)*. For example, in the peripheral blood, dendritic cells, activated B-cells, and monocytes can present antigen, whereas in skin, keratinocytes and Langherhans cells serve this function. Because the major function of

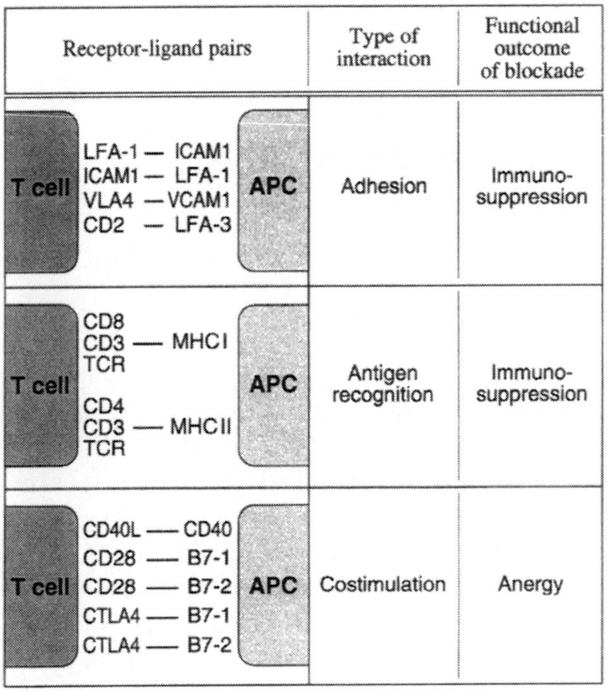

Receptor-ligand pairs	Type of interaction	Functional outcome of blockade
T cell: LFA-1 — ICAM1, ICAM1 — LFA-1, VLA4 — VCAM1, CD2 — LFA-3 — APC	Adhesion	Immuno-suppression
T cell: CD8, CD3 — MHCI, TCR, CD4, CD3 — MHCII, TCR — APC	Antigen recognition	Immuno-suppression
T cell: CD40L — CD40, CD28 — B7-1, CD28 — B7-2, CTLA4 — B7-1, CTLA4 — B7-2 — APC	Costimulation	Anergy

Fig. 1. Receptor ligand pais mediate interactions between activated T cells and APCs. Inhibition of each type of interaction results in an abortive immune response through a different mechanism.

peripheral blood dendritic cells, activated B-cells, and activated macrophages is to process and present antigen, such cells are termed professional APCs (4–6). Other cells (e.g., endothelial cells) can also present antigen under certain conditions (7).

To induce an antigen-specific immune response, T-cells must receive signals delivered by APCs. T-cell–APC interactions can be divided into three stages (Fig. 1) (1) cellular adhesion, (2) TCR recognition of antigen, and (3) costimulation (8–10). Figure 1 summarizes the known cell interaction molecules responsible for progression from one stage to another. In a process termed adhesion, APCs and T cells randomly interact both in circulation and in lymphoid tissues via cell surface ligands and their receptors. These ligands and receptors, referred to as adhesion molecules, may be relatively lineage restricted (e.g., LFA-3 on APC and its receptor CD2 on T-cells) or they may be bidirectional (e.g., ICAM-1 on APC can bind its receptor LFA-1 on T-cells and ICAM-1 on T-cells can bind LFA-1 on APCs). Adhesion appears to be critical for the initiation of T-cell activation because blockade of one or more of the adhesion receptor : ligand pairs completely inhibits a primary immune response. Progression to the next stage, termed antigen recognition, occurs if the APC can process, transport, and present sufficient quantity of the specific peptide antigen in the context of the major histocompatibility complex (MHC). Antigen–MHC will then be recognized by the T-cell via the TCR. Depending on the nature and source of the peptide antigen, endogenous peptides (e.g., derived from intracellular proteins) are generally presented to T-cells coupled to MHC class I (HLA-A, B, or C) cell-surface molecules, whereas exogenous processed peptide antigens (e.g., derived from circulating proteins) are generally presented coupled to MHC class II (HLA-DR, DP, or DQ) cell-surface molecules. Although there is a common TCR/CD3 complex, specific associated recognition structures on T-cells are necessary to interact with the APC class I or class II MHC. Antigens coupled to class I MHC molecules are recognized by TCR/CD3 in the context of an associated CD8 molecule, whereas recognition of antigens coupled to class II requires CD4. This antigen-specific, MHC-restricted interaction initiates a number of complex signaling events. Following ligation of TCR by antigen–MHC, T-cells are competent to respond to a number of potential accessory signals, termed costimulation. Costimulatory molecules provide T-cells with additional signals that reduce the threshold above which the TCR signals can initiate T-cell activation and enhance TCR-induced proliferation. Costimulation by some ligands results in cytokine production that can only be detected at the mRNA level, whereas other costimulatory ligands are capable of inducing significant secretion and accumulation of cytokines.

Each one of these stages of APC–T-cell interactions may be a target of intervention for the modification of the immune response *(11)*. Figure 1 depicts the known interactions between an APC and an antigen specific T-cell and proposes several stages where intervention might result in inhibition of the immune response. It is possible to block either adhesion, TCR signaling, or costimulation. Although each maneuver results in inhibition of T-cell proliferation, the resulting capacity of T-cells to respond to antigen on rechallenge differs significantly. Inhibition of one or more critical adhesion interactions, either by blocking the adhesion ligand or its receptor, completely abrogates the ability of T-cells to receive a signal via their antigen or costimulatory receptor and, therefore, the immune response is totally inhibited. In fact, a blockade of adhesion completely prevents the recognition of antigen. Therefore, these T-cells respond on rechallenge as if they had never before encountered the antigen (i.e., they behave like T cells mounting a primary immune response). Similarly, if adhesion is intact but TCR signaling is prevented, no antigen recognition or proliferation occurs, and rechallenge with antigen after removal of TCR signaling blockade results in a primary type of response. Thus, the functional outcome of blockade of adhesion or TCR recognition is immunosuppression. If these T-cells are withdrawn from such inhibitory conditions, they are again capable of responding to the initial specific antigen. However, if the blockade is at the level of the B7 : CD28 costimulatory pathway, then the outcome is quite different. Under these conditions, T-cells enter a state of long-term antigen-specific unresponsiveness and are incapable of responding on rechallenge with antigen. In summary, a blockade of adhesion or TCR signaling results in immunosuppression, whereas a blockade of costimulation results in anergy.

3. Two-Signal Model for T-Cell Activation

In both murine and human systems, ligation of TCR by antigen induces a number of molecular and biochemical events in the T-cell *(12)*. This TCR-mediated signal, also termed signal 1, is both antigen-specific and MHC restricted, yet fails to induce proliferation and effector function. Therefore, although signaling through the TCR is necessary, it is not sufficient to induce antigen specific T cell activation and cytokine secretion. Most importantly, engagement of TCR by antigen alone not only fails to induce an immune response but also results in a state of antigen-specific unresponsiveness termed anergy *(1,2)*. Anergic T cells are incapable of activating transcription of the IL-2 gene and clonally expanding when restimulated by antigen. In the presence of signal 1 mediated by the TCR, costimulation (termed signal 2), which is neither antigen-specific nor MHC restricted, is necessary to induce productive immunity. In contrast to anergy, productive immunity is characterized by secretion of cytokines, clonal expansion, and generation of effector function of T-cells. The critical nature of this second costimulatory signal in the two-signal model was originally proposed by Bretscher and Cohn *(13)*, later extended by Jenkins and Schwartz, and more recently confirmed in multiple in vitro and in vivo experimental models.

Because the efficient activation of naive T-cells requires the amplification of the TCR signal, an important challenge exists in the elucidation of the mechanisms involved in the initiation of the signals leading to sustained T-cell activation. In fact, it is largely unknown whether the amplification of the TCR signal occurs at a membrane-proximal level as the result of the mobilization and engagement of sufficient "signaling receptors" or in contrast if it occurs as a more downstream event resulting from the integration and magnification of distinct signals transduced to the cell nucleus. Recent studies analyzing the three-dimensional organization at the contact interface during antigen-specific T cell–APC interactions shed some light on the molecular nature of these phenomena *(14,15)*. These studies have clearly shown that the activation of T-cells by APCs induces the formation of segregated clusters of receptors and intracellular proteins, such as TCR/CD3 complexes, LFA-1, talin, PKCθ, lck, and fyn. The formation of these supramolecular clusters (SMAC) is a specific and regulated process initiated by the ligation of the TCR specific to the peptide agonist and seems to be dependent on the presence of accessory events because the receptor engagement by itself is not sufficient to form SMAC. Interestingly, the peptide-engaged TCR/CD3 clusters and the LFA-1 clusters were found to the organized into spatially segregated domains *(15)*. In addition, the accumulation of pairs of both peptide-MHC–TCR and accessory molecules at the APC–T cell contact sites can efficiently amplify weak TCR signals. This accumulation is mediated by the movement of cytoskeleton molecules toward the APC–T cell contact interface, which leads to an increased concentration of molecules such as the receptor pair ICAM-1–LFA-1 interactions, suggesting that the amplification of the TCR signals mediated by these accessory molecules may result from the increased density and engagement of receptor/adhesion-costimulatory molecules at the cell–cell interfaces *(14)*.

Over the past 5 yr, a significant number of molecules expressed on APCs have been identified to have a costimulatory function because they can induce T-cells to proliferate in the presence of a submitogenic TCR signal. Such costimulatory pathways have gained importance in the regulation of the immune response. A major pathway involved in the activation of naive T-cells is the ICAM-1 : LFA-1 (CD54 : CD11a-CD18) pathway. There is increasing evidence that in addition to strengthening the TCR–MHC ligation via their adhesive properties, ICAM-1 binding to LFA-1 can costimulate T-cell proliferation *(8,16)*. Moreover, blockade of the ICAM-1 : LFA-1 interplay results in a significant reduction of T-cell proliferation and interleukin-2 (IL-2) production. Inhibition of signaling through the ICAM-1 : LFA-1 ligand–receptor pair can prolong murine allograft survival. Similar to ICAM-1, LFA-3 costimulation can result in a significant proliferative response. However, although both can act as costimulators, neither ICAM-1 nor LFA-3 induce significant accumulation of IL-2 and are not capable of preventing the induction of antigen-specific anergy *(16)*.

Another important player in the activation of naive T-cells is the interaction between CD40 and its ligand CD40L (CD154) *(17)*. CD40L plays a critical role by inducting and/or upregulating the expression of costimulatory molecules on the APC, which can then costimulate T-cells more efficiently. In fact, it has been demonstrated that CD40L binding by CD40 results in the priming and amplification of antigen-specific CD4+ T-cells and in the activation of professional APCs such as dendritic cells, B-cells, and macrophages. CD40L, a member of the tumor necrosis factor (TNF) family is rapidly induced after TCR ligation and consequent activation of the TCR/CD3 complex *(18)*. It has been suggested that the induction of CD40L on T cells is also mediated by the signal delivered to CD28 by B7-2, which is constitutively expressed at low levels by professional APCs. Early studies examining the contribution of TCR signals, adhesion, and costimulation on the expression of CD40L on T cells showed that TCR ligation by antigen alone is sufficient to induce expression of CD40L. It was also shown that inhibition of CD40–CD40L interactions during antigen recognition results in antigen-specific unresponsiveness. Moreover, B-cells from CD40-deficient mice induced tolerance to allogeneic MHC antigens, which was totally prevented in the presence of anti-CD28 mAbs *(19,20)*. These results suggested that CD40–CD40L interactions are critical for the upregulation of B7 molecules on B-cells that subsequently deliver the costimulatory signals necessary for T-cell proliferation and differentiation. These observations led to a model according to which engagement of TCR by antigen induces CD40L expression on the responding T-cells. Subsequently, expression of CD40L results in engagement of CD40 on B-cells, causing upregulation of B7-1 and B7-2, which trigger T-cells via CD28. It has been also suggested that the CD40 pathway can also directly costimulate T-cells. Therefore, the precise role of the CD40–CD40L interaction in the hierarchy of stimuli required for T-cell activation is still unclear.

The LFA-3 : CD2 (CD58 : CD2) pair represented the major adhesion interaction for resting T-cells and it has been suggested that it acts as a costimulator of naive T-cells. However, some controversy on whether it can induce significant T-cell proliferation and IL-2 production still exists *(21)*. Additional molecules reported as capable costimulators of T-cells include the CD70 : CD27 *(22)*, 4-1BBL : 4-1BB(CDw137) *(23)*, and OX40L : OX40 (CD134) *(24)* pairs and the HSA (CD24) *(25)*, SLAM-1 *(26)*, and CD43 *(27)* molecules. It should be emphasized that soluble molecules such as cytokines can also regulate T cell activation and modulate the outcome of the TCR engagement by (1) delivering costimulatory signals and thereby preventing T-cell unresponsiveness (as in the case of IL-2) *(28)*, (2) inhibiting T cell reactivity (as in the case of tumors growth factor-β [TGF-β]) *(29)*, and (3) deviating the T cell response to specific effector profiles (such as the induction of particular cytokine-secretion patterns) *(30)*.

It is noteworthy that the requirements for the activation of primed T-cells are less restrictive than those of naive T-cells. In fact, the memory antigen-specific and effector T-cells do not require the costimulatory signal for further activation by APCs *(31)*. This has important physiologic relevance because it allows the recognition of target cells expressing the correct agonist peptide–MHC complex even if these cells are not capable of providing costimulatory signals and thereby allows the T-cells to accomplish their effector function.

**Table 1
Members of B7 : CD28/CTLA4 Family**

Name	mol wt (kDa)	Ig structure	Chromosomal localization
B7-1 (CD80)	55	Single IgV and IgC2	3q13.3-3q21
B7-2 (CD86)	80	Single IgV and IgC2	3q13.3-3q21
CD28	44	Single IgV (monomeric or homodimeric)	2q33-34;36
CTLA4 (CD152)	44–48	Single IgV (monomeric or homodimeric)	2q33;6
ICOS	55		?

4. The B7-1(CD80)/B7-2(CD86) : CD28/CTLA4(CD152) Pathway

Among the costimulatory ligand : receptor pairs, B7–CD28 interaction is both necessary and sufficient to provide the requisite costimulatory signal to induce T-cells to produce lymphokines and proliferate *(32–34)*. Since the discovery of the B7 mediated costimulatory pathway 7 yr ago, mounting evidence demonstrates the role of signaling through this pathway in determining immune reactivity versus anergy. Multiple in vivo models clearly demonstrate the role of B7 in the generation of autoimmunity *(35–37)*, tumor immunity *(38–42)*, and allograft rejection *(43)*. Moreover, blockade of the B7 : CD28 costimulatory pathway has been shown to inhibit humoral immunity *(44)*, graft rejection *(45)*, graft versus host disease *(46)*, and ameliorate autoimmune disease *(47,48)*. Therefore, manipulations of this pathway provide great potentials for the induction or prevention of immunity in a variety of clinical settings.

To date, two members of the B7 family, B7-1 (CD80) *(49)* and B7-2 (CD86) *(33,34)*, have been cloned and functionally characterized (Table 1). The genes for both B7 family members are located on human chromosome 3q21 and mouse 16B5. B7-1 and B7-2 are type I membrane proteins with an extracellular domain consisting of one Ig-V-like and one Ig-C-like domain, followed by a transmembrane anchor and a short cytoplasmic tail. B7-1 and B7-2 display 27% amino acid identity in their extracellular domain and even less in other regions. The cytoplasmic domains of B7-1 and B7-2 are markedly different, with the cytoplasmic domain of B7-2 being longer and containing potential sites for phosphorylation by protein kinase C and casein kinase II. Mature B7-1 has 254 amino acids, is heavily glycosylated with 8 potential sites of glycosylation, and has a molecular weight of 45–70 kDa. Mature B7-2 has 304 aminoacids, is heavily glycosylated with 8 potential sites of glycosylation, and has a molecular weight of 60–100 kDa.

B7-1 and B7-2 display a restricted pattern of expression on APCs and, depending on the type of APC, can be induced by a variety of stimuli *(16,50)*. B7-2 is constitutively expressed at moderate levels on dendritic cells and peripheral blood monocytes *(34)*. Interestingly, its expression is not constitutive on lung monocytes *(51)*. On dendritic cells, both B7-1 and B7-2 are upregulated by GM-CSF or CD40L/CD40 signaling. On blood monocytes, B7-1 is induced and B7-2 is upregulated by IFN-γ *(16,50)*. Unlike monocytes and dendritic cells, all other APCs require stimulation for the induction of these molecules. Both B7 molecules are induced in B-cells by crosslinking of CD40, surface Ig, or MHC class II, by bacterial DNA or lipopolysacharide, and their expression is augmented by IL-1, IL-4, IL-5, TNF-α, and TNF-β. After B cell activation, B7-2 is more rapidly expressed than B7-1 and all other APCs display the identical sequence. Memory B-cells constitutively express B7-1 and B7-2 and rapidly upregulate them further after activation, thereby permitting memory B-cells to more rapidly activate T-cells. B7-2 but not B7-1 expression is maintained in terminally differentiated B-cells and myeloma cells. B7-1 and B7-2 are induced in T-cells following activation and are upregulated by IL-7. Other cells also can express B7, including IFN-γ-treated fibroblasts (B7-1), vascular endothelial cells (B7-2), IFN-γ-treated astrocytes (B7-2), and gastric epithelial cells. Adjuvants (e.g., Freund's adjuvant, Neisserial porins) strongly induce B7 expression, providing an important mechanism for the stimulation of an immune response. B7-2 is expressed at sites of inflammation, whereas B7-1 expression is found when chronic inflammation progresses to tissue damage. B7 expression is downregulated by IL-10, TGF-β, ultraviolet light, and crosslinking of the low-affinity IgG receptor CD32, by immune complexes. Certain microorganisms, including Leishmania donovani and Mycobacterium tuberculosis, inhibit B7 expression. Interestingly all the factors that downregulate B7 expression are immunosuppressive. Reduction of B7 costimulatory signals may be, at least in part, a mechanism by which these agents mediate their immunosuppressive function.

In spite of their structural differences, both B7-1 and B7-2 are counterreceptors for two molecules, CD28 and CTLA4. CD28 is expressed exclusively on T-lymphocytes and plasma cells. In the thymus, it is universally expressed on all thymocytes that coexpress CD4 and CD8. In the peripheral blood, CD28 is constitutively expressed on 95% of unactivated CD4+ and 50% of unactivated CD8+ human T-cells, and its expression increases following stimulation with either antigen-specific signals mediated via the TCR or by mitogens. In the mouse, CD28 is expressed on virtually all T-cells. CD28 is the low affinity but major costimulatory receptor for B7-1 and B7-2 because anti-CD28 Fab completely blocks B7-family-mediated costimulation.

A second receptor on T-cells for the B7 family members is CTLA4 *(52,53)*, which is expressed on activated but not resting T-lymphocytes and is the high-affinity receptor for both B7-1 and B7-2. CTLA4 is an oddly expressed protein. Despite good levels of mRNA expression in normal activated T cells, little CTLA4 is expressed on the cell surface, but most is retained within the cell *(53–56)*. CD28 and CTLA4 are also members of the immunoglobulin gene superfamily, but unlike B7-1 and B7-2, they have only a single IgV-like domain. The IgV and IgC domains of B7-1 and B7-2 bind to the same CDR3 and CDR1 regions on CD28 and CTLA4, but the amino acids critical for B7-1 or B7-2 binding are different. The CDR3 loop of CD28 and CTLA4 contains the conserved MYPPPY motif (amino acids 99–104), which is the most critical for both B7-1 and B7-2 binding *(57)*. Although there is limited conservation between the cytoplasmic domains of CD28 and CTLA4, the cytoplasmic domain of CTLA4 displays 100% phylogenetic conservation among human, mouse, and chicken, suggesting a conserved signaling function. Moreover, although the conservation between human and mouse B7-1 is 45% and B7-2 is 50%, the B7 : CD28/CTLA4 pathway can function across species (human, mouse, chicken), suggesting that the ligand-binding site is highly conserved.

A third member of the CD28/CTLA4 family has very recently been identified. In contrast to CD28, this molecule is not constitutively expressed on human *(58)* or murine (Freeman et al., unpublished results) T-lymphocytes but is induced only after activation and is therefore called an inducible costimulator (ICOS). ICOS is a type I transmembrane protein that shares 24% identity with CD28 and 39% identity with CTLA4. The cytoplasmic tail of ICOS has a close resemblance with that of CD28 and CTLA4, but the MYPPPY motif required for binding of CD28 and CTLA4 to their counterreceptors B7-1 and B7-2 is not conserved. Therefore, neither B7-1 nor B7-2 are counterreceptors of ICOS, suggesting that additional members of this family of ligand–receptor pairs are to be identified. ICOS enhances T cell proliferative responses to foreign antigen, upregulates adhesion molecules, and induces effective antibody secretion by B cells. Importantly, in contrast to CD28-mediated costimulation, ICOS does not induce IL-2 secretion but, instead, upregulates secretion of IL-4 and IL-10 *(58)*.

5. Signaling Via the B7-1(CD80)/B7-2(CD86) : CD28/CTLA4(CD152) Pathway and Its Functional Outcome on T-Cells

Initiation of T-cell immune response through the TCR complex is mediated by a complex biochemical cascade initiated by phosphorylation of the TCR complex subunits, activation of proximal protein tyrosine kinases fyn, lck, and ZAP-70, activation of PLCγ1, and hydrolysis of inositol diphosphate to generate inositol triphosphate (IP3) and diacylglycerol (DG). IP3 results in increase of intracellular Ca^{2+} levels and activation of the serine–threonine phosphatase calcineurin, which dephosphorylates the phosphorylated cytoplasmic component of nuclear factor of activated T cells (NF-AT), making it capable of migrating to the nucleus where, with the nuclear fraction of NF-AT, binds on DNA and initiates transcription. Diacylglycerol (DG) activates protein kinase C (PKC) and, therefore, TCR stimulation results in a rapid and marked activation of Ras via both PKC-dependent and PKC-independent mechanisms. Activation of Ras correlates with transcription of the IL-2 gene, the most typical characteristic of T-cell activation (Fig. 2).

B7 bound to CD28 or CTLA4 coassociates on the cell surface with MHC–peptide bound to TCR but engages a distinct signaling pathway. Nevertheless, the TCR, CD28, and CTLA4 signals are all delivered in close proximity in the activation cap between T-cells and APCs. Binding of B7 to CD28, in conjunction with a TCR signal, has multiple effects including stimulation of production of multiple cytokines, including IL-1, -2, -3, -4, -5, -6, -8, -10, and -13, TNF-α, TNF-β, GM-CSF, CSF-1, and IFN-γ *(59)*. B7/CD28 signaling upregulates expression of growth factor receptors including the α and β chains of the IL-2R, and the common γ chain of the IL-2, -4, -7, -13, and -15 receptors *(16,50)*. B7/CD28 signaling also upregulates chemokines including MIP-1α, MIP-1β, and RANTES as well as the chemokine receptor CXCR4. In contrast, B7/CD28 signaling downregulates expression of the chemokine receptors CCR1, CCR2α, CCR2β, and CCR5 *(60)*. B7/CD28 interaction stimulates the production of the antiapoptotic proteins bcl-x_L and bcl-2, leading to enhanced T cell survival *(61–63)*. It also upregulates telomerase expression, thereby contributing to the capacity for T-cell clonal expansion. Interestingly, B7/CD28 interaction upregulates the proapoptotic protein bad *(62)* and also CTLA4, which has a negative regulatory role on T cell clonal expansion *(55,56)*. In addition, B7/CD28 interactions stimulate CD40L expression, permitting

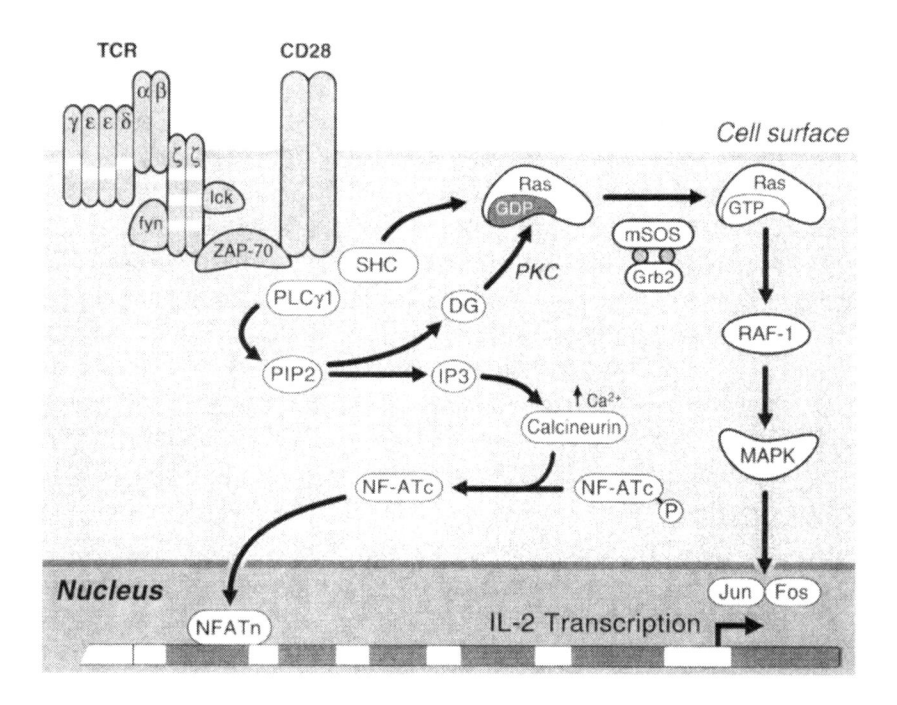

Fig. 2. Successful T cell activation in vitro initiates a cascade of biochemical signaling events that result in transcriptional activation of various genes among which the best studied is the *IL-2* gene.

T-cell help for B-cells. Although some of these proteins can be induced by a strong TCR signal alone, B7/CD28 signaling increases the speed and greatly augments the level of their expression. B7/CD28 interaction lowers the threshold for T-cell activation by approximately two logs of antigen concentration and, therefore, it is most important for the initiation of immune response mediated by low antigen doses or antigens with weak affinity to the TCR.

B7/CD28 interactions are also critical for the differentiation of precursor CD8 T-cells into cytolytic effectors via the induction of cytolytic proteins such as granzyme B *(64)*. Following antigenic stimulation, helper T-cells first upregulate B7 expression on dendritic cells via expression of the CD40L/CD40 pathway. The B7+ dendritic cells then present MHC class I-restricted antigen and B7 to the precursor CTL along with IL-2 produced by helper T-cells, resulting in generation and clonal expansion of antigen-specific CTL. Following the development of cytolytic effectors, B7 expression is not needed on the target cell for CTL killing; however, B7 expression on the target augments cytolysis.

The distinct temporal expression and the induction of B7-1 and B7-2 by different stimulatory signals on APCs suggested that although both bind to CD28, these costimulatory molecules mediate distinct biological functions. Therefore, it was initially hypothesized that B7-2 is critical for the initiation of the immune response, whereas B7-1 is critical for the amplification of the immune response. However, subsequent studies demonstrated more profound differences in the functional outcome of CD28 ligation by B7-1 and B7-2. It was initially shown that treatment with anti-B7-1 or anti-B7-2 mAbs during immunization with proteolipid protein, which induces experimental allergic encephalomyelitis, had a distinct effect on the natural history of the disease, because anti-B7-1 mAb treatment resulted in the generation of effector cells with a Th2 phenotype that prevented the establishment of the disease or abrogated already established disease *(65)*. In contrast, anti-B7-2 mAb treatment resulted in the generation of an effector T-cell population with Th1 phenotype, resulting in increased disease severity. The effect of in vivo treatment with anti-B7-1 or anti-B7-2 mAbs was also examined in the non-obese diabetic NOD murine model *(66)*. That study showed that anti-B7-2 prevented initiation of diabetes, whereas treatment with anti-B7-1 resulted in an increased incidence and accelerated course of the disease. In an in vitro antigen-specific system, it was observed that although both B7-1 and B7-2 equivalently costimulated IL-2 and IFN-γ production, B7-1 was a more efficient GM-CSF costimulator, whereas B7-2 was a more efficient IL-4 and TNF-β costimulator *(67)*. Subsequently, it was shown that B7-1 and B7-2 differentially regulated tumor immunity in various murine models in vivo *(42,68)* and B7-1 but not B7-2 costimulated CD8+ T-cells and generated tumor-specific CTLs in vitro *(69)*. The differential regulation of costimulatory signals on T-cell subpopulations, cytokine secretion, and T-cell subset differentiation by B7-1 and B7-2, when properly utilized, may influence the natural history of autoimmune diseases and the success of tumor antigen vaccination in patients.

CTLA4 has a greater than 100-fold higher avidity for B7 than does CD28 but is expressed only after T-cell activation and at only 2–5% of the level of CD28 cell surface expression *(53)*. Surface CTLA4 is rapidly internalized and most CTLA4 is sequestered inside the cell *(70)*. In contrast to the stimulatory signal delivered by the B7–CD28 interaction, the B7–CTLA4 interaction results in a downregulatory signal *(71,72)*. Crosslinking of CTLA4 results in an active downregulation of TCR and CD28 mediated stimulation, leading to inhibition of IL-2 production and cell-cycle progression and, potentially, to T-cell death *(73–75)*.

Definitive understanding of the role of CTLA4 came from the study of the CTLA4-deficient mouse, which showed massive lymphoproliferation and fatal multiorgan tissue destruction *(76–78)*. Therefore CTLA4-mediated downregulation of autoreactive T-cells appears to be critical for the maintenance of immunologic homeostasis. In these terms, CTLA4 may function in the periphery to downregulate T-cells following antigen exposure and ensure a balanced immune response, or to delete autoreactive T-cells that have not been deleted in the thymus. Either of the potential mechanisms of aberrant T-cell proliferation in the absence of CTLA4 involves B7 : CD28 mediated activation, because it is reversed by CTLA4-Ig. The phenotype of the CTLA4-deficient mouse suggested that triggering CTLA4 could provide a means to regulate activated T-cells mediating autoimmunity and graft rejection.

The differing avidities of B7 for CD28 and CTLA4 and their highly regulated temporal expression has led to a model in which moderate levels of B7 expressed on APCs can engage CD28 on resting T-cells and costimulate T-cell activation. Following activation, the T-cell expresses CTLA4 and CD28, both of which are engaged by B7, but the positive CD28 response dominates. With repeated activation, CD28 expression declines while CTLA4 expression increases. As B7 expression on APCs declines to low levels, all available B7 molecules engage the highly expressed high-affinity receptor CTLA4, leading to downregulation of the T cell response.

CD28 signaling engages multiple intracellular pathways via its short, 41 amino acid long, cytoplasmic tail, containing 4 tyrosines: CD28 crosslinking, by either anti-CD28 mAbs or B7-1, leads to increased phosphorylation of cellular substrates in activated T-cells, including the cytoplasmic domain of CD28. CD28 has been shown to be associated with p72-ITK/EMT kinase, which is rapidly phosphorylated upon CD28 crosslinking. This may lead to the tyrosine phosphorylation of CD28, recruitment of phosphoinositide-3 (PI-3) kinase, and tyrosine phosphorylation of other substrates. However, other studies have shown that CD28 may be primarily phosphorylated by src family kinases, most notably lck, and that ITK binding is a subsequent event dependent on the efficiency of src-mediated phosphorylation of CD28. The same study suggested that PI-3 kinase as well as Grb2/Sos binding to CD28 are also dependent on CD28 phosphorylation by lck. Indeed, several groups have reported that CD28 crosslinking results in a low but consistent lck activation. The significance of lck activation on the CD28-mediated downstream events, more specifically IL-2 gene transcription is still unclear. Stimulation of a lck defective cell line with phorbol ester (PMA) and ionomycin in the presence or absence of CD28 resulted in IL-2 secretion similar to that seen in the wild type, suggesting that lck does not play an obligatory role in CD28 downstream signaling. Moreover, although PI-3 kinase binding on phosphorylated CD28 was initially thought to be of significant importance in CD28 signaling, extensive studies with site-directed mutagenesis have recently shown that PI-3 kinase binding on CD28 is not necessary for CD28-mediated IL-2 secretion. It was recently shown that in the presence of a TCR-mediated signal, CD28 ligation by either B7-1 or B7-2 results in activation of tyrosine phosphorylation of TCR and cytoplasmic proteins and association of TCR with lck and ZAP-70. These biochemical events are critical for the functional outcome of a productive immune response. This observation suggested that although the downstream pathways of TCR and CD28 are distinct, CD28 crosslinking, independent of its downstream events, modifies the initial TCR signal. Therefore, CD28-mediated lck activation may not have a functional role on CD28 downstream signaling, but rather may be important for the initiation of a successful TCR signal.

To date, the molecular and biochemical basis of the differences between B7-1 and B7-2 induced costimulatory signals remains unexplained. B7-1 and B7-2 have the same low affinity for CD28 and high affinity for CTLA4. However, it has been reported that B7-2 binding to CTLA4 displays more rapid dissociation kinetics than B7-1 and that B7-1 and B7-2 utilize different binding determinants of the CTLA4 molecule. More recently it was also shown that the Ig-V domain of B7-2 but not of B7-1 was necessary and sufficient for CTLA4 binding, suggesting that B7-1 and B7-2 may be differentially recognized by their receptors on T-cells. Therefore, a possible explanation for the differences between B7-1 and B7-2 costimulation can be that CD28 engages distinct downstream pathways upon ligation by B7-1 or B7-2, resulting in distinct functional outcomes. Similar observations that differential ligation of the same receptor may lead to activation of distinct pathways and functional outcomes have been reported for the TNF receptor and even for TCR.

Although very intensely studied, the mechanism by which CD28 signaling mediates cytokine gene expression still remains under debate. Most investigators agree that CD28 signaling results in inhibition of the degradation of mRNA of multiple cytokines. It has been shown that CD28 results in increased IL-2 gene transcription and that a CD28-specific NF-κB-like transcription factor (CD28RC) is involved. A more recent analysis demonstrated a role of the CD28 signal transduction pathway in the activation of Jun kinase, which phosphorylates Jun, a component of the AP-1 transcription factor known to bind to several target sequences in the 5' IL-2 gene enhancer. Although MAP kinases ERK1 and ERK2 can be fully activated by TCR stimulation alone, full activation of mitogen activated protein (MAP) kinases that phosphorylate the Jun activation domain JNK1 and JNK2 require both TCR and CD28 signals, suggesting that integration of the signals that lead to optimal T cell activation occurs at the level of JNK activation *(16,50)*.

In contrast to CD28 mediated signaling, much less is known about the signaling pathway mediated via CTLA4. PI-3 kinase binding at the relevant site of CTLA4 cytoplasmic tail has been reported, but the significance of this observation still remains unclear. Importantly, CTLA4 constitutively associates with the protein tyrosine phosphatase syp (and alternative spliced form of SHP-2). Therefore, the downregulatory signal initiated by CTLA4 appears to involve dephosphorylation of substrates and adapter molecules critical for T-cell activation, including TCRζ, SHC, and ZAP-70 *(79)*. However, it is still unclear how binding of the natural ligands B7-1 or B7-2 on CTLA4 activates the CTLA4-associated phosphatase and results in dephosphorylation of the relevant substrates.

6. The Role of CD28 in the Prevention of Anergy and the Initiation of Productive Immune Response

B7-mediated costimulation is sufficient to prevent the induction of anergy in vitro *(80–82)*. In the absence of B7 costimulation, addition of exogenous IL-2 in the presence of a TCR-mediated signal can prevent the induction of the anergic state *(81–83)*. This effect appears to be mediated via the common gamma (γ_c) chain of the IL-2 receptor, because several cytokines that signal via the common γ chain of the IL-2 receptor, including IL-2, IL-4, IL-7, and IL-15, or γ_c crosslinking, can also prevent the induction of T-cell anergy *(28)*.

The role of B7 costimulation in the initiation of a productive immune response was examined by analyzing the proximal biochemical events associated with TCR during the induction of anergy and its prevention by B7-mediated costimulation *(84)*. These studies showed that during the induction of either anergy or productive immunity, protein tyrosine phosphorylation is activated, but distinct patterns are observed. During the induction of anergy, CD3ε is not phosphorylated, whereas TCRζ is only partially phosphorylated and associated with the protein tyrosine kinase fyn but not lck or ZAP-70. In contrast, the induction of productive immunity in the presence of B7-mediated costimulation results in phosphorylation of CD3ε and hyperphosphorylation of TCRζ chains, both of which are associated with lck and ZAP-70. More importantly, during the induction of productive immunity, lck becomes associated not only with TCRζ but also with CD28. Therefore, an intriguing explanation for the requirement of simultaneous ligation of TCR and CD28 to induce biochemical events and functional outcome is that ligation results in coaggregation of these molecules in the T : APC contact patch so that TCR/CD3 and CD28 become components of a supramolecular complex. Under these circumstances, lck becomes activated and associates with both CD28 and TCR, resulting in successful initiation of the TCR-associated downstream signaling events. The previous observation that both antigen and B7 have to be expressed on the same APC to induce an optimal response is consistent with this model *(81,85)*.

7. The Role of CD28 Costimulation in the Maintenance and Downregulation of the Immune Response

Recent reports have also suggested that another role of CD28 costimulation in the functional outcome of the immune response is regulating T-cell survival. In the presence of a TCR signal, CD28 costimulation dramatically upregulates expression of bcl-x_L on T-cells (61). Via heterodimerization with bax, bcl-x_L protects against many forms of cell death, including Fas-mediated apoptosis (86). Both B7-1- and B7-2-mediated costimulation upregulate comparable amounts of bcl-x_L protein that is detectable early after activation. Although CD28 costimulation does not have a significant effect on bcl-2 expression, it results in significant IL-2 accumulation, which can subsequently upregulate bcl-2 expression, providing an additional mechanism for clonal expansion (62,63). Fas and the Fas ligand are rapidly expressed following stimulation on the surface of the T-cells, but no Fas-mediated apoptosis can be induced at less than 48 h of activation. Fas-mediated apoptosis at longer time intervals is temporally associated with downregulation of bcl-x_L protein expression and upregulation of bad. Because the Fas/Fas ligand pathway is the major pathway mediating activation-induced T-cell death in the periphery, CD28 costimulation can maintain adequate numbers of functional T-cells to ensure the successful outcome of a productive immune response. Interestingly, T-cells that are not efficiently stimulated via TCR and CD28 are not capable of undergoing apoptosis via the Fas/Fas ligand pathway (62,87). These observations suggest that in addition to the induction of protective antiapoptotic proteins, the CD28 pathway has an important role in mediating activation-induced cell death by upregulating apoptotic mechanisms.

In addition, successful T-cell activation in the presence of CD28 costimulation results in CTLA4 expression, which, as discussed earlier, activates another potent T-cell downregulatory pathway. It has been previously shown that CD28 pathway induces sphingomyelin hydrolysis (88) and accumulation of ceramide events associated with the initiation of apoptotic cell death mediated by either Fas or TNF-α receptor (89,90). Therefore, CD28-mediated signals could initiate apoptosis, unless the cells are capable of preventing it by other mechanisms, as the upregulation of antiapoptotic proteins. The temporal and tightly controlled expression of these molecules appears to be important for the initiation, maintenance, and dowregulation of a balanced immune response and the control of immunologic homeostasis.

8. Induction of Tolerance In Vivo by Interruption of Costimulation

Several in vivo animal experimental models corroborate the apparent significance of this costimulatory pathway in vivo. The first model demonstrated that the blockade of the B7 : CD28/CTLA4 pathway resulted in long-lasting tolerance to human xenoantigen in mice (45). Human pancreatic islet cells were transplanted under the kidney capsule of artificially induced diabetic mice. Animals were treated with either CTLA4-Ig or control Ig, and the functional outcome was followed by determining blood sugar levels. Infusion of CTLA4-Ig resulted in the normal function of the transplanted human pancreatic islet cells with no histologic evidence of graft rejection. Retransplantation of pancreatic islet cells from the initial donor, not from an unrelated donor, resulted in prolonged graft survival in all animals that had initially been treated with

CTLA4-Ig but not in those treated with control Ig, demonstrating that donor-specific tolerance had developed only in the presence of CTLA4-Ig.

CTLA4-Ig prolonged graft survival in a fully mismatched rat cardiac allograft model *(43)*. In contrast to the pancreatic islet xenograft system, CTLA4-Ig resulted in prolongation of graft survival, but all allografts were finally rejected. The limited effect of CTLA4-Ig in this cardiac allograft experimental model might be the result of the presence of other costimulatory molecules, which might prevent tolerance induction or reverse the already established state of tolerance. Alternatively, failure of tolerance induction might be the result of the lack of antigen recognition because of inadequate antigen-specific stimulation of the host cells, because of the poor APC function of cardiac tissue. To examine this hypothesis, these investigators modified their treatment protocol and administered donor-specific transfusions of peripheral blood mononuclear cells to the host animals prior to the cardiac transplant *(91)*. Subsequently, CTLA4-Ig, infused at the time of transplant not only resulted in prolongation (often indefinite) of cardiac allograft survival but also in suppressed or delayed responses to donor-specific skin grafts, but not to third-party skin transplants. Thus, prior activation of alloantigen-specific T-cells may render them more susceptible to anergization.

Another in vivo murine model investigated the effect of CTLA4-Ig in bone marrow transplant (BMT) between mismatched animals. The BMT of donors and recipients mismatched at both class I and II MHC was undertaken with or without in vivo administration of CTLA4-Ig (46). CTLA4-Ig treatment consistently reduced the incidence of lethal graft versus host disease (GVHD) in recipients although most animals had evidence of subclinical disease. Hematopoietic reconstitution was unaffected in animals under treatment, compared to controls. Later studies from the same group demonstrated that in vivo infusion of recombinant soluble CTLA4-Ig fusion protein in a model of GVHD across major histocompatibility barriers resulted in variable improvement of survival, but not freedom of GVHD, and showed that the in vivo efficacy of CTLA4-Ig was not regulated by T-cell subsets.

A subsequent study further analyzing the role of B7 blockade in GVHD has used a combinatorial approach of blocking the B7/CD28 and the ICAM-1/LFA-1 pathways *(92)*. Because antigen-primed cells might be more susceptible to CD28 : B7 blockade, the study investigated whether CTLA4-Ig alone, anti-LFA1 antibody alone, or the combination of both added to donor–antihost in vitro primed cells could reduce GVHD. To facilitate induction of hyporesponsiveness and to block B7 and ICAM-1 ligands that are upregulated during GVHD, these reagents were also administered to recipients post-BMT. The results demonstrated that CTLA4-Ig plus anti-LFA-1 antibody was highly effective in preventing GVHD-induced lethality. For optimal prevention, both CTLA4-Ig and anti-LFA-1 had to be used in vitro in the context of donor–antihost primed splenocytes and continued in vivo. This in vitro/in vivo combined approach was associated with donor engraftment and recipients were not globally immunosuppressed.

As mentioned earlier, B7 costimulatory molecules can be upregulated upon ligation of the B-cell molecule CD40 with its receptor, CD40L, which is expressed on activated T-cells. However, in addition to being interrelated, the CD28 and CD40 pathways also appear to serve as independent regulators of the T-cell-dependent immune responses *(18)*. This is further supported by the observation that CTLA4-Ig inhibits T-cell responses in CD40L-deficient mice and, conversely, anti-CD40L mAb inhibits T-cell responses and allograft rejection in CD28-deficient mice. Therefore, recent studies have investigated whether simultaneous inhibition of CD40–CD40L and B7–CD28 interactions might be the optimal target for the prevention of graft rejection and GVHD. Simultaneous blockade of CD28 and CD40 pathways resulted in long-term acceptance of skin and cardiac allografts. Blockade of CD28 and CD40 pathways effectively aborted T-cell clonal expansion in vivo, which was not the result of clonal deletion. Instead, these cells were present in vivo, but functionally inactivated. Importantly, consistent with previous in vitro models, the induction of functional inactivation of antigen-specific cells in vivo by blockade of the CD28 and CD40 pathway was inhibited by CsA. Moreover, blockade of the CD28 and CD40 pathways inhibited the development of chronic transplant vasculopathy, which is the main cause of solid-organ transplant failure *(93)*.

Another study examined the effect of inhibition of the CD40/CD40L pathway on the prevention of GVHD *(94)*. Blockade of the CD40/CD40L costimulatory pathway in cultures of CD4+ T-cells from B6 mice used as responders with irradiated T-cell-depleted splenic cells from bm12 mice used as stimulators resulted in host-specific hyporesponsiveness in vitro. Moreover, infusion of the ex vivo tolerized CD4+T-B6 cells in bm12 resulted in 100% survival with a greater than 30-fold reduction in GVHD lethality versus infusion with primed-control B6. More importantly, these ex vivo-tolerized CD4+T-B6 cells, which prevent the induction of GVHD in vivo, have anergy-specific signaling alterations *(95)*.

9. Induction of Antigen-Specific Tolerance Is an Active Signaling Process

Induction of anergy requires protein kinase activation, calcium mobilization, and new protein synthesis, because it is sensitive to cyclosporin A and protein synthesis inhibitors *(1)*. Therefore, induction of anergy is an active biochemical event initiated following TCR ligation by antigen, which however, does not lead to IL-2 secretion. Induction of anergy is associated with lack of activation of lck, ZAP-70, Ras, ERK, JNK, and defective transactivation of the IL-2 enhancer elements AP-1 and NF-AT *(16,96)*. Therefore, the lack of IL-2 transcription in anergy might result from the absence of sufficient positive signals or from the activation of distinct anergizing signals. A novel signaling pathway that results in the active blockade of IL-2 gene transcription in T cell anergy was recently identified (Fig. 3A). Anergic cells have increased phosphorylation of cbl, which coprecipitates with the protein tyrosine kinase fyn, the only proximal protein tyrosine kinase that can be activated in the anergic state. Under these conditions, the adapter protein crkL is associated with phosphorylated cbl and the guanidine nucleotide-releasing factor C3G, which catalyzes GTP exchange on Rap1, a small GTP-binding protein of the Ras superfamily, which is a competitor of Ras *(97)*. Moreover, Rap1-GTP is present in anergic cells. In addition, guanidine nucleotide exchange on Rap1 is mediated by Epac, a novel guanidine nucleotide releasing factor activated by cAMP *(98)*, and cAMP is expressed at high levels in anergic cells *(95)*. The selective efficiency of Rap1 to inhibit IL-2 gene transcription was tested by transfecting recombinant Rap1 cDNA into Jurkat T-cells. Forced expression of even low levels of Rap1-GTP recapitulated the anergic defect, resulting in the blockade of IL-2 transcription. These results show that activated Rap1 functions as a negative regulator of IL-2 gene transcription and may be responsible for the active inhibition of IL-2

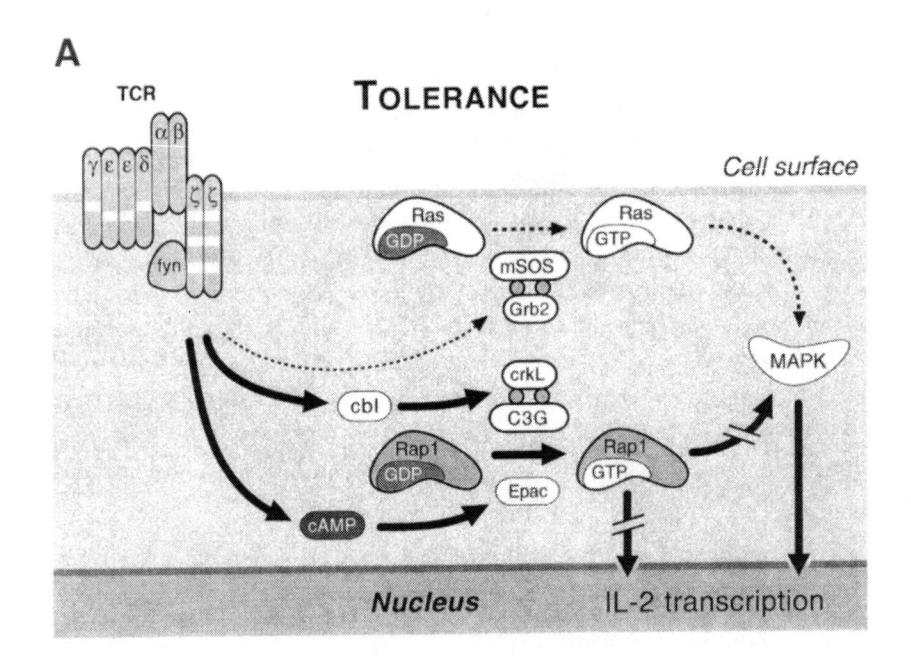

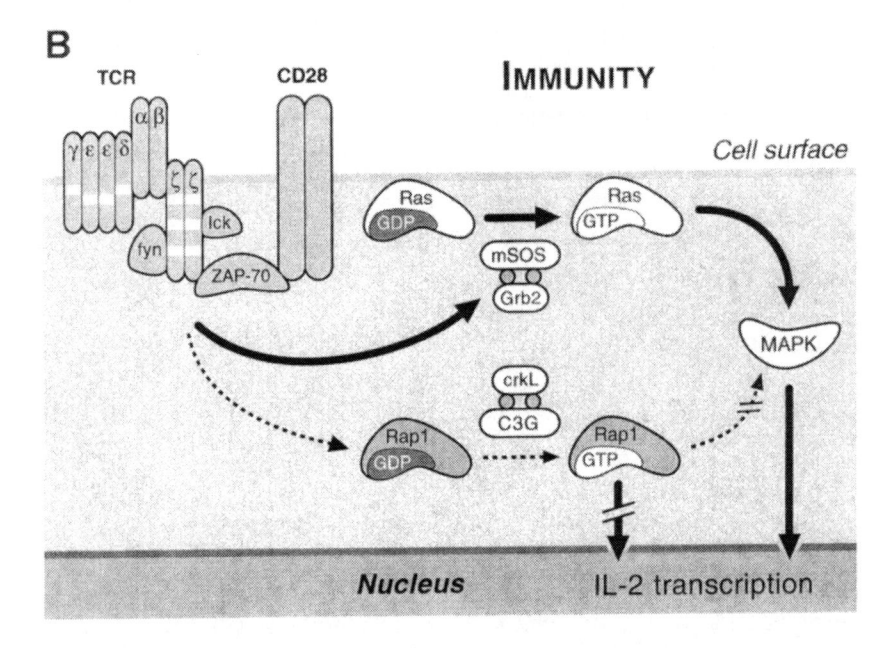

Fig. 3. (A) Numerous in vitro studies have shown that in anergic cells many of the critical signaling events initiated by T cell activation do not occur, whereas other signaling events predominate. Specifically, anergic cells are incapable of activating lck, ZAP-70, phosphorylating the ζ and ε chain of the TCR, activating Ras, JNK and ERK MAP kinases. In contrast, these cells have increased fyn kinase activity, increased concentration of intracellular Ca++, increased phosphorylation of cbl, detectable CrkL-C3G complexes and activation of the GTP binding protein Rap1. (B) Stimulation of T cells via T-cell receptor and costimulatory receptor initiates activation of both Ras and Rap1-GTP binding proteins among which the Ras mediated signaling pathway predominates.

transcription in T-cell anergy. In addition, these results suggest that the key determinant of the functional outcome of TCR-initiated signals that control IL-2 gene transcription is the ratio of Ras-GTP to Rap1-GTP (Fig. 3A,B). Increases of Ras-GTP, which predominates in productive immunity, result in a positive balance and IL-2 transcription (Fig. 3B), whereas predominance of Rap1-GTP, as in the state of anergy, inhibits IL-2 transcription (Fig. 3A). The ability of Rap1 to block T-cell clonal expansion and antagonize TCR-mediated IL-2 transcription suggests that Rap1 may represent a potential target of therapeutic approaches for the modification of T-cell immune responses and the generation of tolerance.

References

1. Schwartz, R. H. (1990) A cell culture model for T lymphocyte clonal anergy. *Science* **248**, 1349–1356.
2. Mueller, D. L., Jenkins, M. K., and Schwartz, R. H. (1989) Clonal expansion versus functional clonal inactivation: a costimulatory signalling pathway determines the outcome of T cell antigen receptor occupancy. *Annu. Rev. Immunol.* **7**, 445–480.
3. Weaver, C. T. and Unanue, E. R. (1990) The costimulatory function of antigen-presenting cells. *Immunol. Today* **11**, 49–55.
4. Steinman, R. M. (1991) The dendritic cell system and its role in immunogenicity. *Annu. Rev. Immunol.* **9**, 271–296.
5. Pierce, S., Morris, J., Grusby, M., Kaumaya, P., Buskirk, A., Srinivasan, M., et al. (1988) Antigen-presenting function of B lymphocytes. *Immunol. Rev.* **106**, 149.
6. Hauser, C. and Katz, S. (1990) Generation and characterization of T helper cells by primary in vitro sensitization using Langerhans cells. *Immunol. Rev.* **117**, 67–84.
7. Shimizu, Y., Newman, W., Tanaka, Y., and Shaw, S. (1992) Lymphocyte interactions with endothelial cells. *Immunol. Today* **13**, 106–112.
8. Springer, T. A. (1990) Adhesion receptors of the immune system. *Nature* **346**, 425–434.
9. Germain, R. N. (1994) MHC-dependent antigen processing and peptide presentation: Providing ligands for T lymphocyte activation. *Cell* **76**, 287–299.
10. Damle, N. K., Klussman, K., Linsley, P. S., and Aruffo, A. (1992) Differential costimulatory effects of adhesion molecules B7, ICAM-1, LFA-3, and VCAM-1 on resting and antigen-primed CD4+ T lymphocytes. *J. Immunol.* **148**, 1985–1992.
11. Guinan, E. C., Gribben, J. G., Boussiotis, V. A., Freeman, G. J., and Nadler, L. M. (1994) Pivotal role of B7:CD28 pathway in transplantation tolerance and tumor immunity. *Blood* **84**, 3261–3282.
12. Weiss, A. and Littman, D. R. (1994) Signal transduction by lymphocyte antigen receptors. *Cell* **76**, 263–274.
13. Bretscher, P. and Cohn, M. (1970) A theory of self–nonself discrimination. *Science* **169**, 1042–1049.
14. Wulfing, C. and Davis, M. M. (1998) A receptor/cytoskeleton movement triggered by costimulation during T cell activation. *Science* **282**, 2266–2269.
15. Monks, C. R., Freiberg, B. A., Kupfer, H., Sciaky, N., and Kupfer, A. (1998) Three dimensional segregation of supramolecular activation clusters in T cells. *Nature* **395**, 82–86.
16. Boussiotis, V. A., Freeman, G. J., Gribben, J. G., and Nadler, L. M. (1996) The role of B7-1/B7-2 : CD28 /CTLA-4 pathways in the prevention of anergy, induction of productive immunity and down-regulation of the immune response. *Immunol. Rev.* **153**, 5–26.
17. Armitage, R. J., Fanslow, W. C., Strockbine, L., Sato, T. A., Clifford, K. N., Macduff, B. M., et al. (1992) Molecular and biological characterization of a murine ligand for CD40. *Nature* **357**, 80–82.

18. Banchereau, J. F., Bazan, F., Blanchard, D., Briere, F., Galizzi, J. P., van Kooten, C., et al. (1994) The CD40 antigen and its ligand. *Annu. Rev. Immunol.* **12,** 881–922.
19. Buhlmann, J. E., Foy, T. M., Arufo, A., Crassi, K. M., Ledbetter, J. A., Green, W. R., et al. (1995) In the absence of CD40 signals B cells are tolerogenic. *Immunity* **2,** 645–653.
20. Hollander, G. A., Castigli, E., Kulbaski, R., Su, M., Burakoff, S. J., Gutierrez-Ramos, J. C., et al. (1996) Induction of alloantigen-specific tolerance by B cells form CD40-deficient mice. *Proc. Natl. Acad. Sci. USA* **93,** 4994–4998.
21. Wingren, A. G., Parra, E., Vaga, M., Kallan, T., Sjogren, H. O., Hedlund, G., et al. (1995) T cell activation pathways: B7, LFA-3, ICAM-1 shape unique T cell profiles. *Crit. Rev. Immunol.* **15,** 235–253.
22. Hintzen, R. Q., Lens, S. M., Lammers, K., Kuiper, H., Beckmann, M. P., and van Lier, R. A. (1995) Engagement of CD27 with its ligand CD70 provides a second signal for T cell activation. *J. Immunol.* **154,** 2612–2623.
23. Vinay, D. S. and Kwon, B. S. (1998) Role of 4-1BB in immune responses. *Semin. Immunol.* **10,** 481–489.
24. Godfrey, W. R., Fagnoni, F., Harara, M. A., Buck, D., and Engelman, E. G. (1994) Identification of human OX-40 ligand, a costimulator of CD4+ T cells with homology to tumor necrosis factor. *J. Exp. Med.* **180,** 757–762.
25. Liu, Y., Jones, B., Aruffo, A., Sullivan, K., Linsley, P., and Janeway, C., Jr. (1992) Heat-stable antigen is a costimulatory molecule for CD4 T cell growth. *J. Exp. Med.* **175,** 437–445.
26. Cocks, B. G., Chang, C.-C. J., Carballido, J. M., Yssel, H., de Vries, J. E., and Aversa, G. (1995) A novel receptor involved in T-cell activation. *Nature* **376,** 260–263.
27. Park, J. K., Rosenstein, Y. J., Remond-O'Donnell, E., Bierer, B. E., Rosen, F. S., and Burakoff, S. J. (1991) Enhancement of T-cell activation by the CD43 molecule whose expression is defective in Wiskott-Aldrich syndrome. *Nature* **350,** 706–709.
28. Boussiotis, V. A., Barber, D. L., Nakarai, T., Freeman, G. J., Gribben, J. G., Bernstein, G. M., et al. (1994) Prevention of T cell anergy by signaling through the γc chain of the IL-2 receptor. *Science* **266,** 1039–1042.
29. Letterio, J. J. and Roberts, A. B. (1998) Regulation of immune responses by TGF-beta. *Annu. Rev. Immunol.* **16,** 137–161.
30. Paul, W. E. and Seder, R. A. (1994) Lymphocyte responses and cytokines. *Cell* **76,** 241–251.
31. Croft, M. (1994) Activation of naive , memory and effector T cells. *Curr. Opin. Immunol.* **6,** 431–437.
32. Linsley, P. S., Brady, W., Grosmaire, L., Aruffo, A., Damle, N. K., and Ledbetter, J. A. (1991) Binding of the B cell activation antigen B7 to CD28 costimulates T cell proliferation and interleukin 2 mRNA accumulation. *J. Exp. Med.* **173,** 721–730.
33. Freeman, G. J., Gribben, J. G., Boussiotis, V. A., Ng, J. W., Restivo, V., Lombard, L., et al. (1993) Cloning of B7-2: a CTLA4 counter-receptor that costimulates human T cell proliferation. *Science* **262,** 909–911.
34. Azuma, M., Ito, D., Yagita, H., Okumura, K., Phillips, J. H., Lanier, L. L., et al. (1993) B70 antigen is a second ligand for CTLA-4 and CD28. *Nature* **366,** 76–79.
35. Guerder, S., Meyerhoff, J., and Flavell, R. (1994) The role of the T cell costimulator B7-1 in autoimmunity and the induction and maintenance of tolerance to peripheral antigen. *Immunity* **1,** 155–166.
36. Harlan, D. M., Hengartner, H., Huang, M. L., Kang, Y. H., Abe, R., Moreadith, R. W., et al. (1994) Transgenic mice expressing both B7 and viral glycoprotein on pancreatic beta cells along with glycoprotein-specific transgenic T cells develop diabetes due to a breakdown of T lymphocyte unresponsiveness. *Proc. Natl. Acad. Sci. USA* **91,** 3137–3141.
37. Verwilghen, J., Lovis, R., De Boer, M., Linsley, P., Haines, G., Koch, A., et al. (1994) Expression of functional B7 and CTLA4 on rheumatoid synovial T cells. *J. Immunol.* **153,** 1378–1385.

38. Chen, L., Ashe, A., Brady, W. A., Hellstrom, I., Hellstrom, K. E., Ledbetter, J. A., et al. (1992) Costimulation of antitumor immunity by the B7 counter receptor for the T lymphocyte molecule CD28 and CTLA-4. *Cell* **71**, 1093–1102.
39. Townsend, S. E. and Allison, J. P. (1993) Tumor rejection after direct costimulation of CD8+ T cells by B7-transfected melanoma cells. *Science* **259**, 368–370.
40. Ramarathian, L., Castle, M., Wu, Y., and Liu, Y. (1994) T cell costimulation by B7/BB1 induces CD8 T cell-dependent tumor rejection: an important role of B7/BB1 in the induction, recruitment and effector function of antitumor T cells. *J. Exp. Med.* **179**, 1205–1214.
41. Matulonis, U., Dosiou, C., Lamont, C., Freeman, G. J., Mauch, P., Nadler, L. M., et al. (1995) Role of B7-1 in mediating an immune response to myeloid leukemia cells. *Blood* **85**, 2507–2515.
42. Matulonis, U., Dosiou, C., Freeman, G. J., Lamont, C., Mauch, P., Nadler, L. M., et al. (1996) B7-1 is superior to B7-2 costimulation in the induction and maintenance of T cell-mediated antileukemia immunity. *J. Immunol.* **156**, 1126–1131.
43. Turka, L. A., Linsley, P. S., Lin, H., Brady, W., Leiden, J. M., Wei, R. Q., et al. (1992) T-cell activation by the CD28 ligand B7 is required for cardiac allograft rejection in vivo. *Proc. Natl. Acad. Sci. USA* **89**, 11,102–11,105.
44. Linsley, P. S., Wallace, P. M., Johnson, J., Gibson, M. G., Greene, J. L., Ledbetter, J. A., et al. (1992) Immunosuppression in vivo by a soluble form of the CTLA-4 T cell activation molecule. *Science* **257**, 792–795.
45. Lenschow, D. J., Zeng, Y., Thistlethwaite, J. R., Montag, A., Brady, W., Gibson, M. G., et al. (1992) Long-term survival of xenogeneic pancreatic islet grafts induced by CTLA4Ig. *Science* **257**, 789–792.
46. Blazar, B. R., Taylor, P. A., Linsley, P. S., and Vallera, P. A. (1994) In vivo blockade of CD28/CTLA4: B7/BB1 interaction with CTLA4-Ig reduces lethal murine graft-versus-host disease across the major histocompatibility complex barrier in mice. *Blood* **83**, 3815–3825.
47. Finck, B., Linsley, P., and Wofsy, D. (1994) Treatment of murine lupus with CTLA4Ig. *Science* **265**, 1225–1227.
48. Milich, D., Linsley, P., Hughes, J., and Jones, J. (1994) Soluble CTLA-4 can suppress autoantibody production and elicit long term responsiveness in a novel transgenic model. *J. Immunol.* **153**, 429–435.
49. Freeman, G. J., Freedman, A. S., Segil, J. M., Lee, G., Whitman, J. F., and Nadler, L. M. (1989) B7, a new member of the Ig superfamily with unique expression on activated and neoplastic B cells. *J. Immunol.* **143**, 2714–2722.
50. Freeman, G. J., Boussiotis, V. A., Gribben, J. G., Sharpe, A. H., and Nadler, L. M. (1998) B7 (CD80 and CD86), in *Encyclopedia of Immunology* (Delves P. J. and Roit I. M., eds.), Academic, London, pp. 304–308.
51. Chelen, C. J., Fang, Y., Freeman, G. J., Secrist, H., Marshall, J. D., Hwang, P. T., et al. (1995) Human alveolar macrophages present antigen ineffectively due to defective expression of B7 costimulatory cell surface molecules. *J. Clin. Invest.* **95**, 1415–1421.
52. Brunet, J. F., Denizot, F., Luciani, M. F., Roux-Dosseto, M., Suzan, M., Mattei, M. G., et al. (1987) A new member of the immunoglobulin superfamily—CTLA-4. *Nature* **328**, 267–270.
53. Linsley, P. S., Brady, W., Urnes, M., Grosmaire, L. S., Damle, N. K., and Ledbetter, J. A. (1991) CTLA-4 is a second receptor for the B cell activation antigen B7. *J. Exp. Med.* **174**, 561–569.
54. Harper, K., Balzano, C., Rouvier, E., Mattei, M. G., Luciani, M. F., and Goldstein, P. (1991) CTLA-4 and CD28 activated lymphocyte molecules are closely related in both mouse and human as to sequence, message expression, gene structure, and chromosomal location. *J. Immunol.* **147**, 1037–1044.

55. Freeman, G. J., Lombard, D. B., Gimmi, C. D., Brod, S. A., Lee, K., Laning, J. C., et al. (1992) CTLA-4 and CD28 mRNAs are coexpressed in most activated T cells after activation: Expression of CTLA-4 and CD28 messenger RNA does not correlate with the pattern of lymphokine production. *J. Immunol.* **149,** 3795–3801.
56. Lindsten, T., Lee, K. P., Harris, E. S., Petryniak, B., Craighead, N., Reynolds, P. J., et al. (1993) Characterization of CTLA4 structure and expression on human T cells. *J. Immunol.* **151,** 3489–3499.
57. June, C. H., Bluestone, J. A., Nadler, L. M., and Thompson, C. B. (1994) The B7 and CD28 receptor families. *Immunol. Today* **15,** 321–331.
58. Hutloff, A., Dittrich, A. M., Beier, K. C., Eljaschewitsch, B., Kraft, R., Anagnostopoulos, I., et al. (1999) ICOS is an inducible T-cell costimulator structurally and functionally related to CD28. *Nature* **397,** 263–266.
59. Thompson, C. B., Lindsten, T., Ledbetter, J. A., Kunkel, S. L., Young, H. A., Emerson, S. G., et al. (1989) CD28 activation pathway regulates the production of multiple T-cell-derived lymphokines/cytokines. *Proc. Natl. Acad. Sci. USA* **86,** 1333–1337.
60. Carroll, R. G., Rilley, J. L., Levine, B. L., Feng, Y., Kaushal, S., Ritchey, D. W., et al. (1997) Differential regulation of HIV-1 fusion cofactor expression by CD28 costimulation of CD4+ T cells. *Science* **276,** 273–276.
61. Boise, L. H., Minn, A. J., Noel, P. J., June, C. H., Accavitti, M. A., Lidsten, T., et al. (1995) CD28 costimulation can promote T cell survival by enhancing the expression of bcl-xL. *Immunity* **3,** 87–98.
62. Boussiotis, V. A., Lee, B. J., Freeman, G. J., Gribben, J. G., and Nadler, L. M. (1997) Induction of T cell clonal anergy results in resistance, whereas CD28 mediated costimulation primes for susceptibility to Fas and Bax mediated programmed cell death. *J. Immunol.* **159,** 3156–3167.
63. Mueller, D. L., Seiffert, S., Fang, W., and Behrens, T. W. (1996) Differential regulation of bcl-2 and bcl-x by CD3, CD28 and IL-2 receptor in cloned CD4+ Helper T cells. *J. Immunol.* **156,** 1764–1771.
64. Guerder, S., Carding, S. R., and Flavell, R. A. (1995) B7 costimulation is necessary for the activation of the lytic function in cytotoxic T lymphocyte precursors. *J. Immunol.* **155,** 5167–5174.
65. Kuchroo, V. K., Das, M. P., Brown, J. A., Ranger, A. M., Zamvil, S. S., Sobel, R. A., et al. (1995) B7-1 and B7-2 costimulatory molecules activate differentially the Th1/Th2 developmental pathways: application to autoimmune disease therapy. *Cell* **80,** 707–718.
66. Lenschow, D. J., Ho, S. C., Sattar, H., Rhee, L., Gray, G., Nabavi, N., et al. (1995) Differential effects of anti-B7-1 and anti-B7-2 monoclonal antibody treatment on the development of diabetes in the nonobese diabetic mouse. *J. Exp. Med.* **181,** 1145–1155.
67. Freeman, G. J., Boussiotis, V. A., Anumanthan, A., Bernstein, G. M., Ke, X.-Y., Rennert, P. D., et al. (1995) B7-1 and B7-2 do not deliver identical costimulatory signals since B7-2 but not B7-1 preferentially costimulates the initial production of IL-4. *Immunity* **2,** 523–532.
68. Gajewski, T. F., Fallarino, F., Uyttenhove, C., and Boon, T. (1996) Tumor rejection requires a CTLA4 ligand provide by the host or expressed on the tumor: superiority of B7-1 over B7-2 for active tumor immunization. *J. Immunol.* **156,** 2909–2917.
69. Gajewski, T. (1996) B7-1 but not B7-2 efficiently costimulates CD8+ T lymphocytes in the p815 tumor system in vitro. *J. Immunol.* **156,** 465–472.
70. Alegre, M. L., Noel, P., Eisfelder, B. J., Chuang, E., Clark, M., Reiner, S. L., et al. (1996) Regulation of surface and intracellular expression of CTLA4 on mouse T cells. *J. Immunol.* **157,** 4762–4770.
71. Walunas, T. L., Lenschow, D. J., Bakker, C. Y., Linsley, P. S., Freeman, G. J., Green, J. M., et al. (1994) CTLA-4 can function as a negative regulator of T cell activation. *Immunity* **1,** 405–413.
72. Krummel, M. and Allison, J. P. (1995) CD28 and CTLA4 have opposing effects on the response of T cells to stimulation. *J. Exp. Med.* **182,** 459–466.

73. Walunas, T. L., Bakker, C. Y., and Bluestone, J. A. (1996) CTLA-4 ligation blocks CD28-dependent T cell activation. *J. Exp. Med.* **183,** 2541–2550.
74. Krummel, M. F. and Allison, J. P. (1996) CTLA-4 engagement inhibits IL-2 accumulation and cell cycle progression upon activation of resting T cells. *J. Exp. Med.* **183,** 2533–2540.
75. Gribben, J. G., Freeman, G. J., Boussiotis, V. A., Rennert, P., Jellis, C. L., Greenfield, E., et al. (1995) CTLA4 mediates antigen-specific apoptosis of human T cells. *Proc. Natl. Acad. Sci. USA* **92,** 811–815.
76. Waterhouse, P., Penninger, J. M., Timms, E., Wakenam, A., Shahinian, A., Lee, K. P., et al. (1995) Lymphoproliferative disorders with early lethality in mice deficient in CTLA-4. *Science* **270,** 985–988.
77. Tivol, E. A., Borriello, F., Schweitzer, N. A., Lynch, W. P., Bluestone, J. A., and Sharpe, A. H. (1995) Loss of CTLA4 leads to massive lymphoproliferation and fatal multiorgan tissue destruction, revealing a critical negative regulatory role of CTLA4. *Immunity* **3,** 541–547.
78. Tivol, E. A., Boyd, S. D., McKeon, S., Borriello, F., Nickerson, P., Strom, T. B., et al. (1997) CTLA4Ig prevents lymphoproliferation and fatal multiorgan tissue destruction in CTLA-4-deficient mice. *J. Immunol.* **158,** 5091–5094.
79. Marenge, L. E., Waterhouse, P., Duncan, G. S., Mittrucker, H. W., Feng, T. S., and Mak, T. W. (1996) Regulation of T cell receptor signaling by tyrosine phosphatase SYP association with CTLA-4. *Science* **272,** 1170–1173.
80. Harding, F. A., McArthur, J. G., Gross, J. A., Raulet, D. H., and Allison, J. P. (1992) CD28-mediated signalling co-stimulates murine T cells and prevents induction of anergy in T-cell clones. *Nature* **356,** 607–609.
81. Boussiotis, V. A., Freeman, G. J., Gray, G., Gribben, J., and Nadler, L. M. (1993) B7 but not ICAM-1 costimulation prevents the induction of human alloantigen specific tolerance. *J. Exp. Med.* **178,** 1753–1763.
82. Tan, P., Anasetti, C., Hansen, J. A., Melrose, J., Brunvard, M., Bradshaw, J., et al. (1993) Induction of alloantigen-specific hyporesponsiveness in human T lymphocytes by blocking interaction of CD28 with its natural ligand B7/BB1. *J. Exp. Med.* **177,** 165–173.
83. Essery, G., Feldmann, M., and Lamp, J. (1988) Interleukin-2 can prevent and reverse antigen-induced unresponsiveness in cloned human T lymphocytes. *Immunology* **64,** 413–417.
84. Boussiotis, V. A., Barber, D. L., Lee, B. J., Freeman, G. J., Gribben, J. G., and Nadler, L. M. (1996) Differential association of protein tyrosine kinases with T cell receptor is linked to the induction of anergy and its prevention by B7 family-mediated costimulation. *J. Exp. Med.* **184,** 365–376.
85. Liu, Y. and Janeway, C., Jr. (1992) Cells that present both specific ligand and costimulatory activity are the most efficient inducers of clonal expansion of normal CD4 T cells. *Proc. Natl. Acad. Sci. USA* **89,** 3845–3849.
86. Boise, L. H., Gonzalez-Garcia, M., Postema, C. E., Ding, L., Lidsten, T., Turka, L. A., et al. (1993) bcl-x, a bcl-2-related gene that functions as a dominant regulator of apoptotic cell death. *Cell* **74,** 597–608.
87. Collette, Y., Benziane, A., Razanajaona, D., and Olive, D. (1998) Distinct regulation of T-cell death by CD28 depending on both its aggregation and T-cell receptor triggering: a role for Fas-FasL. *Blood* **92,** 1350–1363.
88. Chan, G. and Ochi, A. (1995) Sphingomyelin-ceramide turnover in CD28 costimulatory signaling. *Eur. J. Immunol.* **25,** 1999–2004.
89. Dressler, K. A., Mathias, S., and Kolesnick, R. N. (1992) Tumor necrosis factor-α activates the sphingomyelin signal transduction pathway in a cell-free system. *Science* **255,** 1715–1718.
90. Gill, B. M., Nishikata, H., Chan, G., Delovitch, T. L., and Ochi, A. (1994) Fas antigen and sphingomyelin-ceramide turnover-mediated signaling: role in life and death of T lymphocytes. *Immunol. Rev.* **142,** 113–125.

91. Lin, H., Bolling, S. F., Linsley, P., Wei, R. Q., Gordon, D., Thompson, C. A., et al. (1993) Long-term acceptance of major histocompatibility complex mismatched cardiac allografts induced by CTLA4Ig plus donor-specific transfusion. *J. Exp. Med.* **178,** 1801–1806.
92. Blazar, B. R., Korngold, R., and Vallera, D. A. (1997) Recent advanced in graft-versus-host disease prevention. *Immunol. Rev.* **157,** 79–109.
93. Larsen, C. P., Elwood, E. T., Alexander, D. Z., Ritchie, S. C., Hendrix, R., Cho, H. R., et al. (1996) Long-term acceptance of skin and cardiac allografts after blocking CD40 and CD28 pathways. *Nature* **381,** 434–438.
94. Blazar, B., Taylor, P., Noelle, R. J., and Vallera, D. A. (1998) CD4+ T cells tolerized ex-vivo to host alloantigen by anti-CD40 ligand (CD40L : CD154) antibody lose their graft-versus-host lethality capacity but retain normal antigen responses. *J. Clin. Invest.* **102,** 473–482.
95. Boussiotis, V. A., Freeman, G. J., Berezovskaya, A., Grass, I., and Nadler, L. M., unpublished results.
96. Schwartz, R. H. (1997) T cell clonal anergy. *Curr. Opin. Immunol.* **9,** 351–357.
97. Boussiotis, V. A., Freeman, G. J., Berezovskaya, A., Barber, D. L., and Nadler, L. M. (1997) Maintenance of human T cell anergy: blocking of IL-2 gene transcription by activated Rap1. *Science* **278,** 124–128.
98. de Rooij, J., Zwartkruis, F. J. T., Cool, R. H., Nijman, S. M. B., Wittinghofer, A., and Bos, J. L. (1998) Epac is a Rap1 guanidine-nucleotide-exchange factor directly activated by cyclic AMP. *Nature* **396,** 474–477.

7
Transcription Factors

Henry K. Wong

1. Introduction

The plethora of clinical abnormalities seen in rheumatic diseases presents an enormous challenge when one tries to decipher the underlying pathogenetic mechanism of these complex diseases. We know that an imbalance in the immune system is central to the clinical manifestations, as it is the immune products or by-products of cells of the immune system that contribute to the clinical presentation. To gain an understanding in the pathogenesis of rheumatic diseases, an appreciation of the basic mechanism in normal cellular and molecular physiology is essential.

Progress in rheumatic diseases at the molecular level has been advanced so far by identifying potential pathogenic immune cells via molecular markers. This approach has led to improvement in specificity and sensitivity in diagnosis, as certain diseases show repeatable cytokine and autoantibody abnormalities. The complexity of the immune system, where regulation is dependent on concerted interaction from multiple different cell groups whose precise orchestrated effort is required for harmonious normal function, has, nevertheless, challenged research in autoimmune diseases. There are multiple external and internal causes that may impact and lead to an imbalance in the coordination of these players of the immune system. For example, when one cell type loses the music, so to speak, the symphony becomes a cacophony, much like manifestations in the clinical disease.

The dysregulation in different autoimmune diseases has been characterized most extensively at the cellular level. There has been significant progress on the cytokine abnormalities in autoimmune diseases, which affect cells at the level of cell–cell interaction *(1)*. However, a biochemical analysis can be undertaken to focus on the regulatory mechanisms at the intracellular level to understand the basis for the abnormal expression of cytokines and other gene products that are aberrantly expressed in inflammatory disease *(2)*. The study of gene regulation in rheumatic diseases will likely lead to a better understanding of the pathogenesis.

It is becoming evident that numerous cytokines are increased in chronic inflammatory diseases. Some of the lymphokines are expressed systemically in a variety of tissues and some are localized to the tissue with the pathology *(3)*. In rheumatoid arthritis (RA), there is an increase in pro-inflammatory cytokines such as tumor necrosis factor-α (TNF-α), interleukin-1 (IL-1), IL-6, granulocyte macrophage colony stimulating factor (GM-CSF), and IL-8. In addition, inhibitory cytokines IL-12 and IL-10 are also expressed in the synovial spaces, the significance of the imbalance remains an intense area of study. In systemic lupus erythematosus (SLE), there is abnormal lymphokine expression with decreased levels of IL-2 and interferon-γ (IFN-γ), and increased levels of IL-10 and IL-6.

Cytokines play a role in the perpetuation and propagation of chronic inflammation seen in rheumatic diseases. The profile of inflammatory mediators may differ among the different rheumatic diseases, but some common cytokines seem to be the convergent end point of inflammation leading to clinical abnormalities. Inflammation has been characterized by the profound increase in TNF-α and IL-1.

These cytokines are normally regulated by inducible expression in the immune response to infection and tissue injury. When expression is unregulated, disease develops. In chronic inflammation, the level of these cytokines become unbalanced in the location and the type of cells that produce these cytokines. Diseases with aberrant cytokine production include rheumatoid arthritis, inflammatory bowel disease, systemic lupus erythematosus, atopic dermatitis, and scleroderma.

As cytokine expression is under strict regulation to act in specific roles on immediate demand rather than constitutive expression, the level of cytokines is precisely regulated by new mRNA synthesis at the level of transcription. The signal for new synthesis is regulated by molecular switches that bring about the rapid assembly of an active complex at the promoter, the regulatory region of genes. In the nucleus, protein complexes are rapidly assembled at the promoter of cytokine genes that alter the response of the cell and propagate activities that lead to controlled immune responses. As there is aberrant expression of cytokines in autoimmune diseases, the factors that regulate the expression of cytokines may potentially be abnormal by either being decreased, increased, or modified. Understanding the regulation of these transcription factors in rheumatic diseases will shed light on the pathogenesis of these autoimmune diseases.

2. Overview of Transcription

Appropriate regulation of gene expression depends on the precise interpretation of signals encrypted within the nucleotide sequences of the DNA molecule by cellular machinery. Normally, DNA is a double-stranded structure that is highly organized into a compacted state in chromosomes by nuclear histone and nonhistone protein. The DNA is arranged into different levels of chromatin structure that is dependent on nonhistone proteins. To gain access to DNA, the complex levels of organization must be simplified by modification of the histones and their associated proteins. At present, we are only beginning to unravel the regulation of chromatin structure and the relationship to gene expression. An important activity in the regulation of chromatin function is the ability to modify histone proteins by acetylation and deacetylation *(4,5)*.

The process by which mRNA is synthesized from DNA is called transcription. The information in the DNA sequence is deciphered and transcribed onto RNA when the DNA molecule is in the single-stranded form. The DNA strand that has the complementary sequence to the mRNA is the strand that is read by RNA polymerase. Each strand of DNA molecule has a polarity based on the relationship of the linkage of one nucleoside to another through the 3' and 5' carbon molecules of the ribose moiety. One often refers to a position relative to a particular nucleotide that is on the 5' side of the ribose ring as upstream and the 3' side as downstream by convention. In describing genes on DNA, the reference sequence is that of the mRNA.

The control of mRNA synthesis is highly regulated and determined by specific signals in the region of the gene that is 5' to the region that encodes the start of the mRNA (reviewed in refs. 6 and 7). This control region is called the promoter and it is divided into the proximal region and the distal region. The aspect in gene regulation where we have the best understanding is concerning regulatory processes at the sequence level. Dissection at the molecular level has revealed that discrete regions of DNA are separated into segments that have specific functions. The upstream promoter regulatory region is comprised of two regions, the enhancer and the proximal promoter region. This regulatory region resides at the 5' side of the gene and does not encode the protein. The region that is synthesized into RNA is located 3' to the promoter. The RNA produced in the nucleus, nascent heteronuclear RNA, contains both sequences that are necessary for encoding the protein (exons) and also for regions that do not encode protein (introns). To produce the mature mRNA, the nascent RNA undergoes processing by splicing, where the noncoding sequences are cut out to produce the final mRNA.

The regulation of mRNA production can be divided temporally and biochemically into two phases: initiation and elongation. The initiation is the phase that is rate limiting and controls the quantity of mRNA that is produced. Initiation requires the orderly assembly of a large macromolecular complex composed of protein factors that recognize the promoter region followed by the recruitment of the RNA polymerase II enzyme to begin the synthesis of RNA. The first step requires that sequence-specific protein factors bind DNA in the promoter region; these proteins are called transcription factors. Each promoter has recognition sites for different transcription factors and it is the composite of protein factors at the promoter that, in essence, is the language that interprets when the gene is expressed. Each gene, therefore, has a set of sequences that is programmed to be active in certain cells where the transcription factors are present to direct transcription. In regard to the expression of a gene, not all sequences that bind a transcription factor must be occupied and the level of transcription reflects the identity of the sequences and the number of sites occupied in the promoter region.

When the sequence-specific transcription factors assemble appropriately on the DNA, additional second-order general transcription factors are then recruited to form the functional preinitiation complex *(8)*. The formation of this complex depends on protein–protein recognition mediated by the transactivation domain of transcription factors, which is needed to catalyze the association of the general enzymatic transcription machinery, RNA polymerase II complex, to form at the promoter to initiate synthesis of RNA. A diagram of the promoter is illustrated in Fig. 1. Present in most RNA pol II promoters is characteristic nucleotide sequence motif, 5'-TATA-3', located approximately 30 nucleotides upstream (i.e., the 5' side) of the mRNA initiation site. A general transcription factor called the TATA binding factor recognizes this sequence and is essential for proper positioning and initiation. Additional general transcription factors are then assembled in an orderly manner—TFIID, TFIIB, TFIIF, followed by TFIIE and TFIIH (reviewed in ref. 9)—before RNA polymerase II enzyme enters the macromolecular complex to begin RNA synthesis.

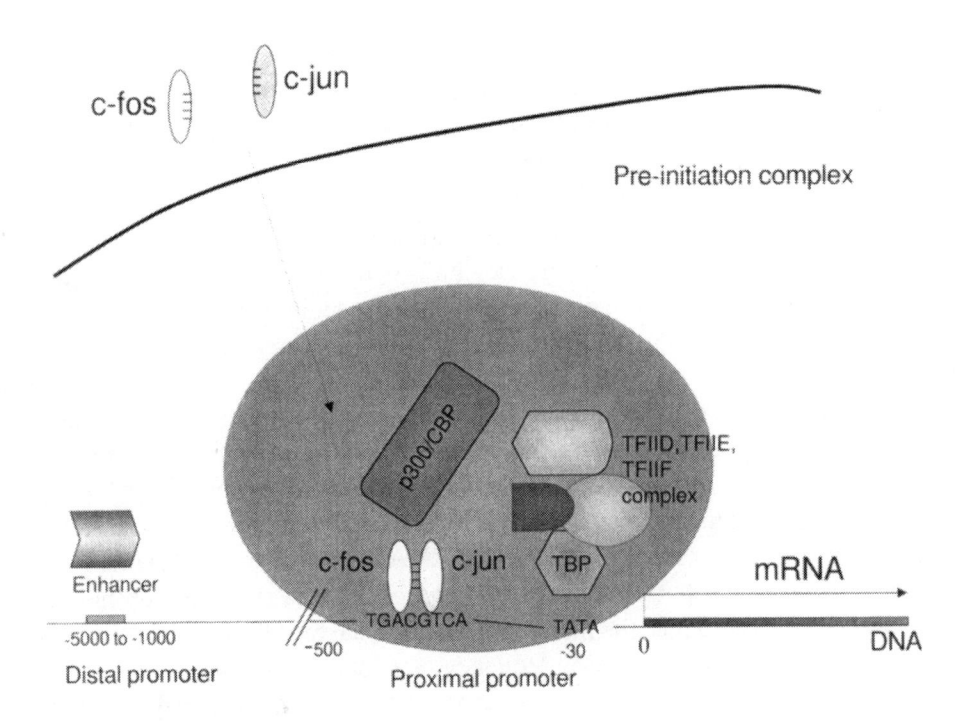

Fig. 1. Diagram of the promoter complex. Typical protein components that assemble at the promoter is shown. The distal promoter contains enhancer sequences, which is recognized by transcription factors that are characterized by their ability to function independent of orientation and position. The proximal promoter contains recognition sequences for transcription factors (e.g., c-fos and c-jun, which makes up AP-1). The orientation and location of these sequences is crucial for the function of AP-1 in the proximal promoter. These factors once situated on DNA then recruit subsequent general transcription proteins to the promoter. The gray circle represents RNA pol II and interacts with the general transcription factors TFIID, TFIIF, and others.

From molecular studies based on genetic engineering to create artificial reporter genes that contain promoters that have been systematically mutated, specific sequences in the promoter that are required for gene expression have been defined. Through the use of transfection studies, a method to introduce the reporter gene DNA into cells, it was determined that only promoters with the proper arrangement of sequences were functional in a particular cell type or in response to a particular stimulus. This suggested that specific proteins recognized the specific sequences in DNA. Having identified specific DNA sequences that are involved in the regulation of gene expression, a search was then undertaken to isolate proteins that recognized and bound to these sequences to gain an understanding of how gene expression is regulated. Biochemical affinity approaches were utilized to purify such DNA-binding proteins to study their role in transcription. When the regulation of these DNA-binding proteins was analyzed, it was found that the function of these proteins was controlled at the level of transcription and posttranslation through modification. Some of these transcription factors are expressed constitutively and some are expressed in an inducible manner. In general, these transcription factors provide a means for the transduction of extracellular signals to the nucleus that initiate a new program of gene products to permanently alter cell phenotype. From studies of the promoters of different genes, specific expres-

Table 1
Common Nucleotide Sequence Motifs in Transcription Regulation

TRE	5'-TGACGTCA-3'	AP-1
CAAT	5'-GGNCAATCT-3'	Oct-1
κB	5'-GGGACTTTCC-3'	NF-κB
CRE	5'-TGACTCA-3'	CREB
ARE	5'-AGGAAAATTTGTTTCA-3'	NF-AT
CCAAT	5'-CCAATT-3'	NF-IL6,C/EBP
GRE	5'-GGTACAnnnTGTTCT-3'	Glucocorticoid receptor
Sp-1	5'-GGGCGGNN-3'	Sp-1 factor

sion of genes have been determined to be regulated through the upstream sequences of the promoters, with the TATA region providing general function for alignment of the RNA polymerase.

The upstream promoter region contains nucleotide sequences that are necessary for specific control of gene expression. The number and the types of sequences present in the promoter are numerous and serves as a code that must be deciphered by the presence of a specific set of transcription factors required for regulating initiation of gene expression. In each promoter, two types of sequences can be identified. There are those that can be found in genes of different tissues. These may serve a general function for basal expression or may serve to coordinate responses in different tissues in response to a common signal. On the other hand, in certain tissues, a recurrent active sequence motif can be identified that are restricted to that tissue type; these are called enhancers because these sequences are responsible for tissue-specific gene expression. (Table 1). The proper combination of transcription factors at the promoter is essential for full-level expression of the gene. In the immune system, there are sequence-specific transcription factors that function in inducible expression of genes, such as cytokine and other genes involved in an inflammatory response. Thus, one view of the promoter is the presence of modular sequences that, in combination, provides the specificity for tissue-specific and temporal regulation. The unique arrangement of protein factors that assemble at the promoter direct the level of gene expression.

Transcription factors are DNA-binding proteins that serve as the interface between the RNA polymerase enzyme and the DNA sequence. When the amino acid sequence of these factors are compared, these factors show distinct structural features that identify them as DNA-binding proteins. From amino acid sequence analysis of many transcription factors, recurring motifs in amino acid sequence hint at an important structural feature. The modular structure of transcription factors suggests that each domain has an unique function. There are protein domains for DNA binding, transactivation, ligand binding, as in the steroid family of hormone receptors; the protein interaction domain such as the leucine zipper and other domains are summarized in Table 2. When these different domains are combined, the functional transcription factor is formed.

3. Transcription Factors Affecting the Immune System and Inflammation: NF-κB, AP-1, NF-AT, STAT, nur77

To determine which factors may be involved in inflammatory diseases, one can examine the transcription factors that regulate products of inflammation and determine

**Table 2
Structural Motifs in Transcription Factor**

Rel proteins: NF-κB, NF-AT
Helix–loop–helix proteins: Myc, MyoD
Leucine zipper proteins: Creb, ATF, Fos, Jun
Homeodomain proteins: Oct-1, Oct-2, Pax family, Hox family
Zinc-finger proteins: Nur77, Egr 1, Krox, GATA family, steroid hormone receptor superfamily
Helix–turn–helix proteins: c-Myb, Ets

whether these are abnormal in inflammatory diseases. These transcription factors binding sites are prominent in the promoters of gene products of inflammation such as cytokines, cell-surface molecules. These are the first genes that are turned on in response to extracellular stimuli to increase the state of the cell to an activated state. Therefore, the activity of these protein factors need to be tightly regulated and any loss of control would lead to abnormal behavior that could change the balance of the immune system. Transcription factors that act rapidly to initiate changes in the pattern of gene expression to respond to foreign agents have common properties. There are several families that have been identified whose regulation is complex and intricate. The members of these families share many features, from structural similarities and, not least of all, their ability to recognize a particular nucleotide sequence. The families to be discussed are the nuclear factor κB (NF-κB), AP-1, STAT, nuclear factor of activated T-cells (NFAT), and Nur77. These are usually present in the preformed state and does not require new protein synthesis to become active, except for AP-1 and Nur77.

In a normal immune response to pathogens, the function of these transcription factors are essential in initiating changes that allow cells to respond appropriately. If the regulation of these transcription factors were to become abnormal, major effects on the immune homeostasis will become evident. Whether the abnormality of transcription factors is primary or secondary, the identification of this abnormality may be the initial step in defining the underlying pathogenic mechanism for the protean manifestation of immune dysfunction in autoimmune diseases.

These transcription factors will be discussed separately, as distinct mechanism are involved in the regulation of each of the respective transcription factor. The role of these factors in inflammation has been well studied and their relation to rheumatic disease remain a nascent area of analysis; nevertheless, from careful analysis of these regulatory factors, insight into the pathogenesis of inflammatory autoimmune diseases will become more apparent.

3.1. Nuclear Factor κB

Nuclear factor κB (NF-κB) was first identified 10 yr ago by Sen and Baltimore in a search for DNA-binding proteins that recognize the kappa enhancer, composed of the core decanucleotide sequence 5'-GGGACTTTCC-3', in the immunoglobulin light-chain promoter *(10,11)*. The original proteins have since been purified from B-cells, sequenced, and found to be expressed in almost all cells. In addition, it is now known that a family of proteins, with each member encoded from a distinct gene, comprise the κB binding activity. Five genetically unique NF-κB genes have been identified and

Table 3
Genes-Regulated by NF-κB

Secreted proteins	
TNF-α	M-CSF
IL-1β	IL-8
IL-2	MIP-1-α
IL-3	MCP-1
IL-6	Gro-α,β,γ
IL-12	Exotoxin
GM-CSF	RANTES
G-CSF	
Inflammatory enzymes	
Inducible NOS	12-lipoxygenase
Phospholipase A2	5-lipoxygenase
Inducible cyclooxygenase 2	
Adhesion molecules	
ICAM-1	E-selectin
V-CAM-1	
Surface receptors	
IL-2 receptor α	CD48
CD11b	Platelet-activating factor
T-cell receptor β chain	
Protooncogenes	
c-myc	ras
p53	

these share similarities by amino acid sequence in a 300 amino acid region termed the rel homology domain. The rel domain was initially identified in drosophila proteins rel and dorsal (12). The κB proteins act as a rapid nuclear genetic signal transducer. The mechanism and activity is so fundamental and ancient that a homologous rel function has been present in living organisms for millions of years, as similar proteins have been identified in fruit flies (dorsal and rel), which binds DNA. In mammals, the NF-κB-related molecules comprise a class of transcription factors involved in ubiquitous regulation of gene expression in the immune system. NF-κB signaling is now known to participate in the initiation of new genetic programs in response to a myriad of extracellular stimuli.

Nuclear factor κB is required for the regulation of numerous genes in the immune and inflammatory responses, intracellular oxidative responses, and other stresses (13). A list of induced genes is presented in Table 3. The NF-κB binding activity is complex and is composed of multiple subunits that combine as homodimers or heterodimers to form the intact NF-κB activity. Two subunits are necessary to form the active DNA-binding complex. The different heterodimer combinations permit control of NF-κB activity by binding sequences with different specificity. These heterodimers can interact with other proteins that form distinct DNA-binding complexes at the promoter. The rel domain contains amino acid sequences that provide the DNA-binding function and the interface for dimerization. Another function, such as the activation of transcription,

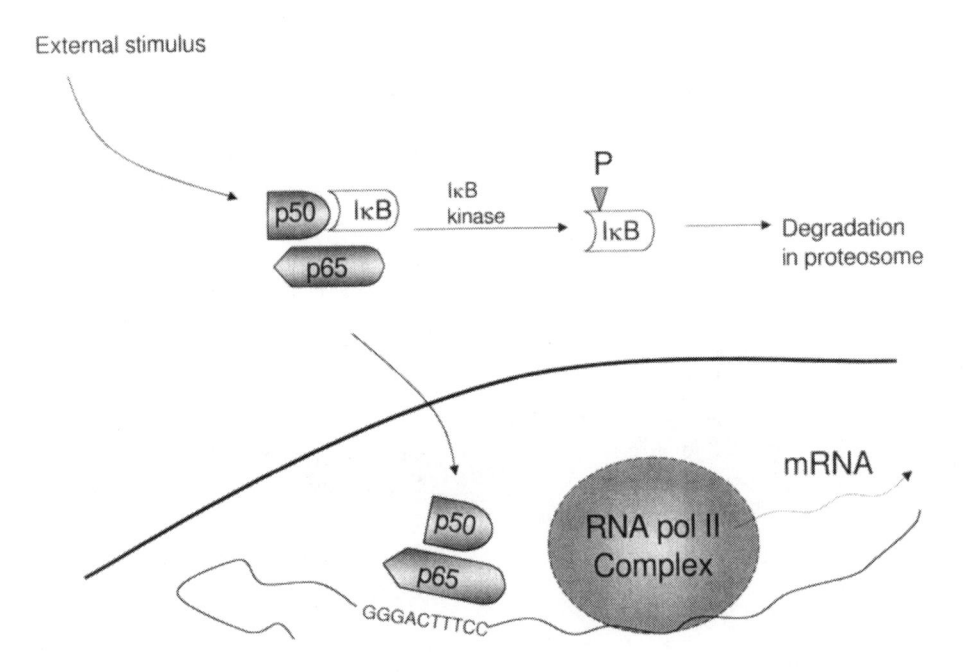

Fig. 2. Model for NF-κB activation. Extracellular signaling induces the activation of a cascade of kinases that then activate IκB kinase which phosphorylates IκB/NF-κB complex located in the cytoplasm. Phosphorylated IκB dissociates from NF-κB, gets ubiquinated, and enters proteosome complexes, where it is degraded. The NF-κB complex then translocates into the nucleus and activate gene expression.

is mapped on a different region of the NF-κB protein, which is present in c-Rel, RelA, and RelB. The smaller NF-κB members, p50 and p52, do not have a protein domain that has transactivation properties. The lack of a positively acting domain in p50 and p52 suggests that these can function in a negative manner when they form homodimers and bind DNA to repress gene expression. Indeed this has been observed in anergic T-cells. When p50 and p52 form heterodimers with other NF-κB family members such as RelA, cRel and RelB, these complexes can activate gene expression.

An important mechanism by which the function of the NF-κB family of proteins is regulated is through subcellular location, by the interaction with inhibitors that prevent nuclear translocation (Fig. 2). There is a family of protein inhibitors, IκB, that acts by directly binding to NF-κB complexes (reviewed in ref. *11*). IκB molecules act by masking the nuclear localization domain of NF-κB complexes. Blocking the recognition of this domain by inhibitor proteins retains the multisubunit NF-κB complex in the cytoplasm. The IκB family consist of numerous members, two members are derived from processing of the NF-κB proteins, p100 and p105, which have a C-terminus region with ankyrin repeats that can sequester NF-κB like the IκB. The other members are the IκB-α, IκB-β, Bcl-3, IκB-γ, and IκB-δ. In total, there are currently 10 members characterized to date.

In response to signals from the cell surface that activate NF-κB, intracellular signaling molecules lead to activation of protein kinase pathways that activate IκB kinase that phosphorylate IκB at serine residues, which leads to further modification of IκB by attachment of marker peptide, ubiquitin, that targets the IκB complex to degradation in proteasomes with the release of NF-κB and the exposure of the nuclear localization domain. The different IκB members are regulated by different IκB kinases and respond to different inducers, thus providing multiple levels of control. Furthermore, the rate of degradation of the IκB members differ and the rate at which these proteins are resynthesize after induction of NF-κB differ. These IκB regulatory differences allows added control in determining which genes are activated. IκB is essential in proper embryonic development and in gene knockout studies, homologous loss of IκB-α leads to death shortly after birth and severe cutaneous inflammation, similar to the histology seen in psoriasis *(14)*.

Processes regulated by NF-κB include apoptosis, increase in cytokine production, and response to external stresses such as ultraviolet (UV) light and oxidative stress. NF-κB is involved in the early response of numerous essential cytokines such as IL-2. Cell-surface markers, such as adhesion molecules ICAM-1, ELAM, and VCAM that play a role in inflammation by recruiting neutrophils, eosinophils, and T-cells to the site of inflammation, are increased by activation of NF-κB. NF-κB does not act alone and this transcription factor interacts with additional rapidly induced and constitutively expressed transcription factor at the promoter to increase expression of target genes.

3.2. Nuclear Factor of Activated T-Cell Family

The proteins of this family of transcription factor initiate response to surface receptors, such as the antigen receptors of T- and B-cells, the Fcε receptor of mast cells and basophils, and receptors on macrophages and natural killer (NK) cells. These receptors activate pathways that increase the intracellular calcium concentrations, which activate the calcium/calmodulin-dependent phosphatase calcineurin that directly activates NFAT by dephosphorylation to induce nuclear translocation and DNA binding (reviewed in ref. *15*) (*see also* Fig. 3). Calcineurin is the target of the immunosuppressant FK506 and cyclosporin. NFAT activity consists of a preformed cytoplasmic component and an induced newly formed component. The induced component is AP-1. The NFAT target DNA sequence contains a κB-like half-site adjacent to an AP-1 site, 5'-(T/A)GGAAAAnnTGAGTCA-3'. There are four members of the NFAT family, which are made from differentially spliced mRNAs. Therefore, each gene can encode for multiple different protein isoforms. These NFAT proteins have amino acid sequences that are similar and likely form a common structural domain, which is required for interacting with calcineurin. This group of proteins share the *Rel* homology domain that exist in the NF-κB proteins. Unlike NF-κB however, NFAT can bind DNA as monomers, whereas NF-κB must bind DNA as dimers. Although Rel domain mediates protein–protein interaction among the NF-κB family members, the NFAT family cannot interact with the NF-κB family as heterodimers. NFAT proteins interact with the bZIP transcription factor AP-1. The affinity of NFAT to DNA can be increased 20-fold by the presence of AP-1 in a cooperative manner. In certain promoters, both NFAT and NF-κB can recognize the same sequence, such as the P sequence of the IL-4 promoter. Unlike the NF-κB proteins, which are expressed almost ubiquitously in different tissues, NFAT expression is more limited and is found most often in cells of the immune system.

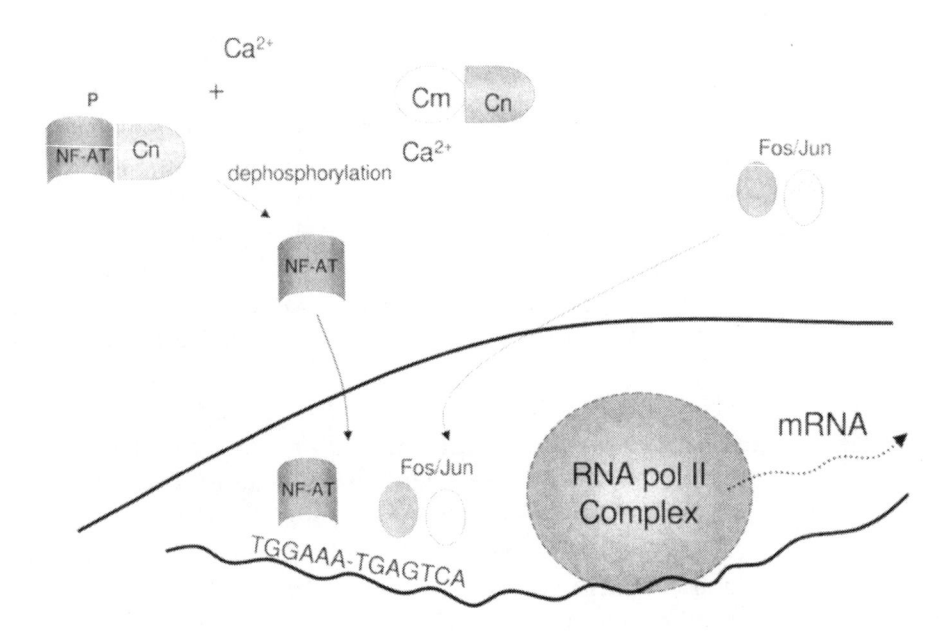

Fig. 3. Model for NF-AT activation. Extracellular signaling leads to increased intracellular Ca^{2+}. Ca^{2+} binds calmodulin (Cm) and leads to the activation of calcineurin (Cn), a phosphatase that dephosphorylate NF-AT. The dephosphorylated NF-AT then translocates into the nucleus and cooperate with AP-1 to activate gene expression.

In the unstimulated state, the NFATp protein is located in the cytoplasm. Upon an appropriate signal with calcium mobilization, the protein is activated by dephosphorylation by the calmodulin-dependent phosphatase whereby NFATp is translocated to the nucleus. In the nucleus, the NFATp interacts with the NFATc to bind DNA and activate gene expression.

NFAT is best defined as T-cell activated factor and is essential in the production of IL-2 in lymphocytes in vitro. In vivo, numerous other transcription factors are essential in IL-2 production, including NF-κB and AP-1. NFAT1 targeted knockout are normal except for mild splenomegaly. These mice are immunocompetent and show no impairment in IL-2, IL-4, TNF-α, or IFN-γ synthesis. When analyzed more specifically with respect to specific responses, these mice have defective immune response with increased Th2 cytokines, IL4, increased eosinophilia, and development of allergic diseases *(16)*.

3.3. AP-1 Family

AP-1 was one of the earliest transcription factor activities studied, being identified as a transcription factor required for activity of the SV40 virus enhancer. The protein components that make up this activity comes from two families, c-fos and c-jun, that are produced from unique genes *(17)*. The c-fos family is composed of c-fos, fosB, fra1 and fra 2. The c-jun family is composed of c-jun, junB, and junD. These two protein families interact by association through a specific alpha helical domain termed the leucine zipper and form dimeric complexes that bind DNA. Fos members can associate only with jun members in a heterodimer complex, whereas jun members can interact with itself to form homodimers, interact with fos to form heterodimers, or interact with another leucine zipper class of transcription factor such as ATF to form heterodimers. The classical AP-1 activity is composed of fos–jun heterodimers. Heterodimers of c-jun with another leucine zipper protein called activating transcription factor (ATF) have a different DNA binding specificity. The AP-1 consensus recognition sequence, 5'-TGACTCA-3', is found in numerous cellular genes that are ubiquitously expressed and precisely regulated. The AP-1 sequence motif is present in the regulatory elements of many genes of the immune system that are induced, one example is IL-2. The AP-1 binding activity is induced rapidly in response to extracellular stimuli mediated by receptors of cytokines, adhesion molecules, and other forms of cellular stresses.

There are distinguishing protein domains from the c-fos and c-jun families defining the bZIP class of transcription factors. This group is identified by two domains. One domain is the basic region, characterized by the presence of amino acids such as arginine and lysine, positively charged in solution. The basic region is required for interaction with DNA and has an overall negative charge. The leucine zipper region mediates protein–protein interaction through hydrophobic domains for dimerization; it is a helical coil that has repeats of leucine residues spaced every seven amino acids apart such that the leucine residues interdigitate to form a stable structure. Proteins with compatible leucine zippers can for homodimers or heterodimers, such as that seen for the c-fos and c-jun families, as described previously.

The regulation of AP-1 occurs at two major levels, the transcriptional level and the posttranslational level. Upon appropriate stimulus, there is rapid transcriptional induction of the c-*jun* and c-*fos* genes to produce high levels of these proteins. Once the proteins are produced, there is modification of these proteins by protein kinases such that the fos–jun complex can activate gene expression in the nucleus. The modification is dependent on the MAP kinase signaling cascade, which is activated by extracellular signals. There are three signaling MAP kinase pathways, extracellular signaling-regulated kinase (ERK), Jun N-terminal kinase (JNK), and the p38 kinases, and these affect the transcriptional regulation of the c-fos and c-jun protein. The JNK pathway phosphorylate c-jun to fully activate c-jun to stimulate gene expression. Finally, the particular combination of fos–jun dimeric complexes contributes to the complexity of fos–jun regulation of gene expression.

AP-1 plays a role in gene expression in many different cells of the immune system in initiating response to stimuli. AP-1 function plays a role in differentiation of CD4 T-helper-cells. Different members of the fos/jun family are present in Th1 or Th2 cells and regulate the expression of genes of these two cell types. Th1 cells express less AP-1 activity, and the proteins that comprise this activity is predominantly c-fos and c-jun. In contrast, Th2 cells express high levels of jun B, c-fos, and c-jun. As different immune diseases or different immune response favor proliferation of one subset of T-helper-cells (for example, lupus is thought to be a Th2 disease with a specific profile of cytokines that shows increased IL-4 and IL-10) the level and composition of AP-1 factors will be different. Measuring the profiles of transcription factor will thus provide a way to predict the response cytokine profile of the cells and may provide a better indicator of disease activity.

AP-1 activity also plays a role in the immunologic property of anergy. Anergy describes a state of T-cells characterized by hyporesponsiveness to antigen. These T-cells do not produce IL-2 nor proliferate in response to antigen. AP-1-specific transcription activation of the IL-2 promoter has been shown to be defective in clonal anergy *(18)*.

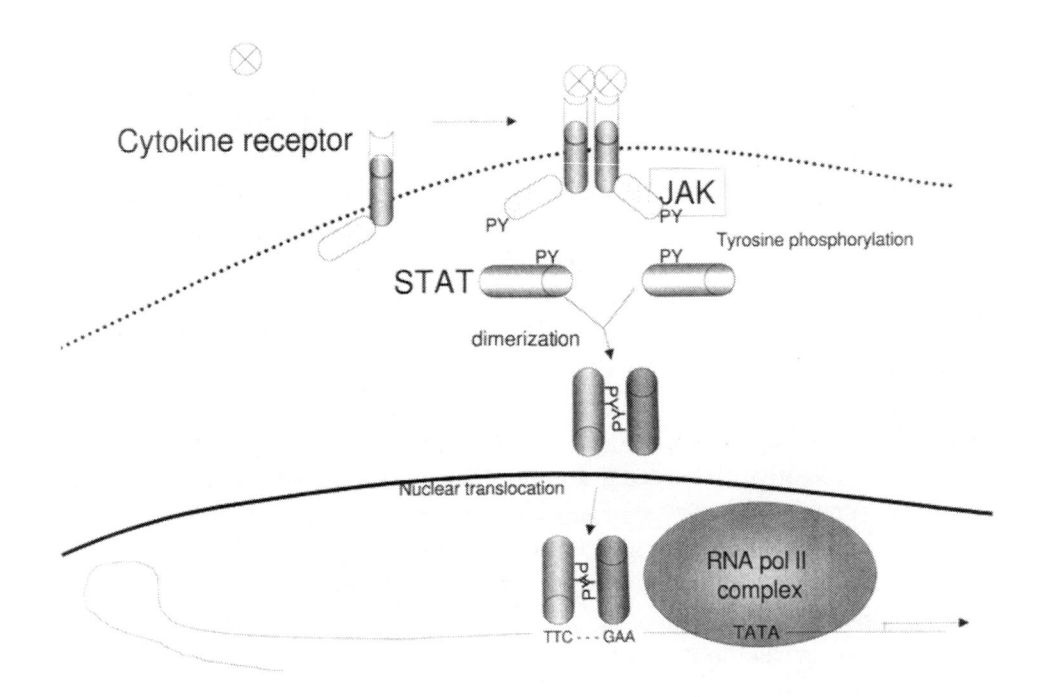

Fig. 4. Model for STAT activation. Signaling pathway for cytokines that interact with Jak kinases are shown. Activation requires dimerization of surface receptor and the juxtaposition of Jak kinases. There is reciprocal phosphorylation of the receptors, followed by tyrosine phosphorylation of STAT (shown as PY). STAT dimerization and nuclear translocation then proceeds rapidly and STAT proteins then bind to target promoters.

3.4. STAT Signaling Transcription Factors

The STAT proteins are composed of a family of immediate acting transcription factors that can act to transduce receptor-initiated signals from the plasma membrane directly to the nucleus (reviewed in refs. *19* and *20*) (*see also* Fig. 4). This process is rapid and STAT proteins can be detected in the nucleus within minutes after activation of a specific cytokine. STAT proteins must therefore exist in a preformed state and no new protein synthesis is required for their activation. Indeed, STATs are appropriately named and is an acronym derived from the initials of Signal Transducer and Activator of Transcription. There are currently seven mammalian proteins, Stat1, Stat2, Stat3, Stat4, Stat5a, Stat5b, and Stat6, and several other insect-related proteins in the STAT family. At the cell membrane, STAT proteins interact with distinct members of the Janus family or Tyk family of tyrosine kinases. Jak kinases, of which there are four members, and Tyk kinases, of which there are two members, interact with the cytoplasmic region of different receptors for cytokines. Upon binding of the cytokine ligand to the respective receptor, the receptor dimerizes and brings the Jak kinase or Tyk kinase together, depending on which receptor system, and leads to their reciprocal phosphorylation of the kinases on tyrosine residues. The phosphotyrosine residue on the kinases provide recognition docking sites for STAT proteins. Upon binding the kinases, the STAT proteins then become the next targets of tyrosine phosphorylation by the Jak or Tyk kinase in the SH2 region. Tyrosine phosphorylated STAT proteins then dissociate from the cell-surface kinases and form dimers with other phosphorylated STAT proteins which becomes activated by cytoplasmic MAP serine kinases at serine residues. The serine phosphorylated activated complex translocates into the nucleus to the promoter of the target genes. The specificity in the STAT arises through the surface receptor kinases with which these proteins interact. Also, STAT proteins can form specific combinations that target the complex to a particular promoter.

STAT proteins have distinct conserved regions that dictate how these proteins interact and function. There is a region required for dimerization of the STAT proteins located at the N-terminus. There is a DNA-binding domain in the middle and an SH2 domain that mediated interaction with phosphotyrosine on kinases and for homodimerization or heterodimerization of tyrosine phosphorylated STAT proteins. Also, there is a region that contains a signal for nuclear localization, which, at present, has not been defined precisely. The transcription activating region is located at the C-terminus and contains a serine residue that must be phosphorylated before the factor is transcriptionally active. The phosphorylation site is likely the recognition target of MAP kinases.

STAT proteins bind to promoters of the genes for IFN, IL-2, IL-4, MHC class II, CD23, and IL-2Rα. The role of STAT proteins in immune function becomes clear in genetic knockout, where a particular Stat expression is lacking. In mice lacking Stat4 and Stat6, T-cells demonstrate an impaired response to IL-12 while showing an enhanced predisposition of T-cells to differentiate into a type 2 phenotype. Stat3 is required for embryonic development. In addition to interacting with cytokine receptor to regulate the immune response, Stat5 can mediate direct signaling by the antigen receptor in T-cells. The TCR ζ chain and Lck tyrosine kinase can appropriately phosphorylate Stat 5 to stimulate genes necessary for proliferation.

3.5. Nur77

Nur77 is a transcription factor with a zinc-finger domain that is induced as an early response gene product after stimulation of the T-cell receptor. It is also known as NGFI-B because it has been identified as a rapidly induced gene in response to nerve growth factor (NGF). This protein is part of the steroid hormone nuclear receptor superfamily, which, structurally, has domains similar to that found in glucocorticoids and retinoid hormone families (21). Nur77 belongs to the orphan receptor subfamily because, unlike steroid or retinoid receptors, the ligand for the orphan receptors has not yet been identified. In general, these nuclear receptors function as dimeric complexes and can form homodimers or heterodimers and recognize specific DNA sequences. There are three structural regions in these receptor proteins, the transcriptional activation region, the DNA-binding region that is composed of zinc-finger motif, and the hormone-binding domain. Nur77 is expressed in the brain and in cells of the immune system. In T-cells, Nur77 has been identified to be important in the upregulation of the *Fas*L gene and is essential in apoptosis. Expression of mutated gene that can inhibit the normal function of Nur77 can prevent the initiation of TCR-induced apoptosis. This protein has been shown to play a role in thymic selection.

4. Transcription Factors Aberrations in Autoimmune Diseases

The role of transcription factors in the pathogenesis of autoimmune diseases remains unclear. Transcription factors may participate in disease potentially as a primary cause or a secondary cause of autoimmune disease. It is clear that these factors play critical roles in the amplification of the inflammatory response through production of cytokines and it is conceivable that a defect in the regulation of essential transcription factor can lead to autoimmune rheumatic diseases. At present, there are no specific transcription factors associated with a primary clinical manifestation. Experimental evidence from genetic knockout studies of transcription factor in mice suggest that abnormalities in transcription factor function can lead to autoimmune disease. In gene knockout experiments of the transcription factor NF-κB, lymphoproliferation has been seen. In mice with Nur77 deficiency, extensive B-cell autoimmunity is observed. Nur77 is required for apoptosis *(22)* and mutations of the Nur77 gene may lead to lymphoproliferation and a defect in the deletion of autoreactive T-cell clones. In contrast, mice that have fos or jun deficiency, for example, do not show significant defects in development or in the immune system.

There are transcription factors that have been identified as nuclear autoantigens and the presence of antibodies against some of them have been associated with clinical manifestations, but the significance of these association to the etiology in rheumatic diseases is unclear. The transcription factor Sp1 has been identified as an autoantigen associated with a malar rash and Raynaud's phenomenon, but not associated with any specific disease *(23)*. Nur77 has been found to be increased in nephritus *(24)* induced by antiglomerular basement membrane antibody. The general transcription factor TFIIB has also been identified as an autoantigen. Another example of a transcription factor that has been described as an autoantigen is NOR90 *(25)*, a transcription factor that regulates ribosomal RNA synthesis and is more abundantly expressed in mitotic cells. NOR90 antibodies have been identified in sera from patients with Sjögren's disease and rheumatoid arthritis. The factors of RNA polymerase II are not prominent nuclear autoantigens. The low frequency of transcription factors as nuclear autoantigen may be the result of the low level of expression of regulatory transcription factors compared to other more abundantly expressed nuclear autoantigens, such as histones, and other structural components that are prominent nuclear autoantigens.

The abnormal expression of transcription factors in autoimmune disease may provide insights into the role of transcription factor in the disease process. In rheumatoid arthritis, there is an increase in the activity of early-response transcription factors in the synovium. AP-1 activity consisting of the c-fos and c-jun proteins is increased in the synovial cells from affected joints of rheumatoid patients *(26)*. The inflamed synovium shows increased AP-1 in the nucleus. Decoy oligonucleotides introduced into synovium that effectively sequesters AP-1 from DNA inhibits inflammation in the murine model of arthritis. In normal immune function, AP-1 is required for the activation of IL-2 in T-cells and other immediate early genes. This transcription factor plays an important role in the regulation of metalloprotease, collagenase, and stromelysin, all genes that have particular relevance in RA. The increased AP-1 may reflect immune activation status or abnormalities in the regulation of this transcription factor.

There are abnormalities in other signaling transcription factors in autoimmune diseases. The activity of STAT proteins has been found to respond to Th2-type cytokines in synovial monocytes, favoring IL-4 and IL-10 *(27)*. The transcription factor that regulates heat shock 70 gene expression is increased in RA synoviocytes *(28)*. The antigen associated with polymyositis/scleroderma can interact with the helix–loop–helix transcription factor E47 and increase the expression of E47 dependent promoter activity *(29)*.

Additional transcription factors, such as Oct-1, has been described to be abnormally increased in peripheral T-cells in Sjögren's syndrome *(30)*. Oct-1 can also be elevated in RA *(31)* in the synovial tissue that is inflamed. NF-κB activity has been found to be increased in synovial cell clones *(32,33)*. In analysis of transcription factor function in lymphocytes from lupus patients, there is decreased expression of NF-κB activity that is consistent with the reported decrease in IL-2 level. Specifically, the p65 RelA subunit is decreased in the majority of lupus T-lymphocytes *(34)*. The significance of these findings is unclear, but the abnormality in transcription factor expression and activity may be important in the pathogenesis of these diseases.

5. Treatment and Transcription

Transcription factors play a vital function in the initiation and the propagation of inflammatory responses. These factors are activated normally during stimulation of the immune response, but they can also be stimulated during autoimmune inflammatory diseases. The transcription factors discussed in this chapter act at crucial steps in the regulation of inflammatory responses and preventing their function in gene expression can impact on the continuation and amplification of inflammation. The most convincing argument for the role of transcription factor in autoimmune rheumatic diseases is the effectiveness of drugs that target these factors. Many potent anti-inflammatory drugs target NF-κB. Aspirin, *N*-acetyl cysteine, and vitamin E inhibit NF-κB activity in vitro. Tepoxalin, a COX inhibitor, blocks NF-κB activity and inhibits transcription of cell-adhesion molecules CD62E, CD11b/CD18, and CD106. Because of the importance of NF-κB, an alternative experimental approach to block expression of NF-κB protein using antisense oligonucleotides for NF-κB genes has shown effectiveness in inhibiting NF-κB activation as a novel approach to control inflammation. The mechanisms by which these anti-inflammatory drugs act are at the level of DNA binding, the level of IκB activation, and the ubiquination and degradation of IκB. The role of steroids will be discussed further in Chapter 28, but, in brief, steroid hormone receptors can antagonize the activity of AP-1 and NF-κB.

NF-κB can be targeted by nonsteroidal anti-inflammatory drugs. In addition to inhibiting the synthesis of cyclooxygenase by-products that have pro-inflammatory effects, salicylates have been demonstrated to block the activation of NF-κB through inhibiting the phosphorylation of IκB to prevent IκB degradation. Other drugs, including pentoxyfyline, salycilates, deferoxamine, curcumin, and sulfasalazine, suppress NF-κB activation by inhibiting the breakdown of IκB through inhibiting the proteasome protein-degradation pathway. The protease inhibitor TPCK prevents IκB-α breakdown and suppresses activation of NF-κB. Over time, other inhibitors of the proteasome pathway may be developed to inhibit modification of IκB, which may have more specific action in the different IκB pathways affected.

Cyclosporin and FK506 control inflammatory diseases by suppressing activation of calcineurin, a calcium-dependent phosphatase involved in the activation of NF-AT. In addition, there is indirect effect on the activation of NF-κB by preventing the nuclear translocation and inhibition of IκB. Gold has been used in the treatment of autoimmune diseases, blistering skin diseases, and RA. This precious metal in salt formulation, aurothiogluconate, has been reported to have inhibitory effects on the DNA binding activity of transcription factors NF-κB and AP-1 *(35)*.

In summary, there has been tremendous advances in understanding the biology of inflammation. Especially fortunate has been the development of molecular biology approaches that permit dissection of nuclear regulatory mechanisms. There is now a convergence in the understanding of nuclear regulation and the mechanisms of potent anti-inflammatory drugs because these drugs target specific pathways that regulate gene expression needed in inflammatory responses. Current studies of regulatory steps in the nucleus in gene expression will lead to the identification of additional compounds that may improve treatment of inflammatory diseases. Developing agents that can target these nuclear signaling pathways will lead to a better treatment of autoimmune diseases.

References

1. Feldmann, M., Brennan, F. M., and Maini, R. (1998) Cytokines in autoimmune disorders. *Int. Rev. Immunol.* **17,** 217–228.
2. Tsokos, G. C. and Liossis, S. N. (1998) Lymphocytes, cytokines, inflammation, and immune trafficking. *Curr. Opin. Rheumatol.* **10,** 417–425.
3. Cutolo, M., Sulli, A., Villaggio, B., Seriolo, B., and Accardo, S. (1998) Relations between steroid hormones and cytokines in rheumatoid arthritis and systemic lupus erythematosus. *Ann. Rheum. Dis.* **57,** 573–577.
4. Wolffe, A. P. and Hayes, J. J. (1999) Chromatin disruption and modification. *Nucleic Acids Res.* **27,** 711–720.
5. Workman, J. L. and Kingston, R. E. (1998) Alteration of nucleosome structure as a mechanism of transcriptional regulation. *Annu. Rev. Biochem.* **67,** 545–579.
6. Hill, C. S. and Treisman, R. (1995) Transcriptional regulation by extracellular signals: mechanisms and specificity. *Cell* **80,** 199–211.
7. Ptashne, M. and Gann, A. (1997) Transcriptional activation by recruitment. *Nature* **386,** 569–577.
8. Tjian, R. (1996) The biochemistry of transcription in eukaryotes: a paradigm for multisubunit regulatory complexes. *Phil. Trans. R. Soc. Lond. B. Biol. Sci.* **351,** 491–499.
9. Buratowski, S. (1997) Multiple TATA-binding factors come back into style. *Cell* **91,** 13–15.
10. Sen, R. and Baltimore, D. (1986) Multiple nuclear factors interact with the immunoglobulin enhancer sequences. *Cell* **46,** 705–716.
11. Baldwin, A. S., Jr. (1996) The NF-kappa B and I kappa B proteins: new discoveries and insights. *Annu. Rev. Immunol.* **14,** 649–683.
12. Ghosh, S., May, M. J., and Kopp, E. B. (1998) NF-kappa B and Rel proteins: evolutionarily conserved mediators of immune responses. *Annu. Rev. Immunol.* **16,** 225–260.
13. Barnes, P. J. and Karin, M. (1997) Nuclear factor-kappaB: a pivotal transcription factor in chronic inflammatory diseases. *N. Engl. J. Med.* **336,** 1066–1071.
14. Attar, R. M., Caamano, J., Carrasco, D., Iotsova, V., Ishikawa, H., Ryseck, R. P., et al. (1997) Genetic approaches to study Rel/NF-kappa B/I kappa B function in mice. *Semin. Cancer Biol.* **8,** 93–101.
15. Rao, A., Luo, C., and Hogan, P. G. (1997) Transcription factors of the NFAT family: regulation and function. *Annu. Rev. Immunol.* **15,** 707–747.
16. Viola, J. P., Kiani, A., Bozza, P. T., and Rao, A. (1998) Regulation of allergic inflammation and eosinophil recruitment in mice lacking the transcription factor NFAT1: role of interleukin-4 (IL-4) and IL-5. *Blood* **91,** 2223–2230.
17. Karin, M., Liu, Z., and Zandi, E. (1997) AP-1 function and regulation. *Curr. Opin. Cell Biol.* **9,** 240–246.
18. Kang, S. M., Beverly, B., Tran, A. C., Brorson, K., Schwartz, R. H., and Lenardo, M. J. (1992) Transactivation by AP-1 is a molecular target of T cell clonal anergy. *Science* **257,** 1134–1138.

19. Leonard, W. J. and O'Shea, J. J. (1998) Jaks and STATs: biological implications. *Annu. Rev. Immunol.* **16**, 293–322.
20. Darnell, J. E., Jr. (1997) STATs and gene regulation. *Science* **277**, 1630–1635.
21. Beato, M., Herrlich, P., and Schutz, G. (1995) Steroid hormone receptors: many actors in search of a plot. *Cell* **83**, 851–857.
22. Woronicz, J. D., Calnan, B., Ngo, V., and Winoto, A. (1994) Requirement for the orphan steroid receptor Nur77 in apoptosis of T-cell hybridomas. *Nature* **367**, 277–281.
23. Spain, T. A., Sun, R., Gradzka, M., Lin, S. F., Craft, J., and Miller, G. (1997) The transcriptional activator Sp1, a novel autoantigen. *Arthritis Rheum.* **40**, 1085–1095.
24. Hayashi, K., Ohkura, N., Miki, K., Osada, S., and Tomino, Y. (1996) Early induction of the NGFI-B/Nur77 family genes in nephritis induced by anti-glomerular basement membrane antibody. *Mol. Cell. Endocrinol.* **123**, 205–209.
25. Fujii, T., Mimori, T., and Akizuki, M. (1996) Detection of autoantibodies to nucleolar transcription factor NOR 90/hUBF in sera of patients with rheumatic diseases, by recombinant autoantigen-based assays. *Arthritis Rheum.* **39**, 1313–1318.
26. Asahara, H., Fujisawa, K., Kobata, T., Hasunuma, T., Maeda, T., Asanuma, M., et al. (1997) Direct evidence of high DNA binding activity of transcription factor AP-1 in rheumatoid arthritis synovium. *Arthritis Rheum.* **40**, 912–918.
27. Wang, F., Sengupta, T. K., Zhong, Z., and Ivashkiv, L. B. (1995) Regulation of the balance of cytokine production and the signal transducer and activator of transcription (STAT) transcription factor activity by cytokines and inflammatory synovial fluids. *J. Exp. Med.* **182**, 1825–1831.
28. Schett, G., Redlich, K., Xu, Q., Bizan, P., Groger, M., Tohidast-Akrad, M., et al. (1998) Enhanced expression of heat shock protein 70 (hsp70) and heat shock factor 1 (HSF1) activation in rheumatoid arthritis synovial tissue. Differential regulation of hsp70 expression and hsf1 activation in synovial fibroblasts by proinflammatory cytokines, shear stress, and antiinflammatory drugs. *J. Clin. Invest.* **102**, 302–311.
29. Kho, C. J., Huggins, G. S., Endege, W. O., Patterson, C., Jain, M. K., Lee, M. E., et al. (1997) The polymyositis-scleroderma autoantigen interacts with the helix-loop-helix proteins E12 and E47. *J. Biol. Chem.* **272**, 13,426–13,431.
30. Flescher, E., Vela-Roch, N., Ogawa, N., Nakabayashi, T., Escalante, A., Anaya, J. M., et al. (1996) Abnormality of Oct-1 DNA binding in T cells from Sjogren's syndrome patients. *Eur. J. Immunol.* **26**, 2006–2011.
31. Wakisaka, S., Suzuki, N., Takeno, M., Takeba, Y., Nagafuchi, H., Saito, N., et al. (1998) Involvement of simultaneous multiple transcription factor expression, including cAMP responsive element binding protein and OCT-1, for synovial cell outgrowth in patients with rheumatoid arthritis. *Ann. Rheum. Dis.* **57**, 487–494.
32. Handel, M. L., McMorrow, L. B., and Gravallese, E. M. (1995) Nuclear factor-kappa B in rheumatoid synovium. Localization of p50 and p65. *Arthritis Rheum.* **38**, 1762–1770.
33. Miyazawa, K., Mori, A., Yamamoto, K., and Okudaira, H. (1998) Constitutive transcription of the human interleukin-6 gene by rheumatoid synoviocytes: spontaneous activation of NF-kappaB and CBF1. *Am. J. Pathol.* **152**, 793–803.
34. Wong, H. K., Kammer, G. M., Dennis, G., and Tsokos, G. C. (1999) Abnormal NF-B Activity in T lymphocytes from patients with systemic lupus erythematosus is associated with decreased p65-RelA protein expression. *J. Immunol.* **163**, 1682–1689.
35. Handel, M. L. (1997) Transcription factors AP-1 and NF-kappa B: where steroids meet the gold standard of anti-rheumatic drugs. *Inflamm. Res.* **46**, 282–286.

8
Immune Complexes

Mark H. Wener

1. Introduction

Antigen–antibody complexes mediate the inflammation and tissue dysfunction associated with many autoimmune rheumatic diseases. Immune complexes (ICs) are strongly implicated in various forms of vasculitis, particularly those associated with immune deposits within tissues. Deposition of ICs within tissues are responsible for many of the major manifestations of systemic lupus erythematosus (SLE), including nephritis and vasculitis. Many types of inflammatory arthritis, including rheumatoid arthritis, are thought to be the result, at least in part, of ICs within joints. This chapter will discuss the role of immune complexes in rheumatic diseases. ICs are strongly implicated in the pathogenesis of a number of nonrheumatic diseases, as well, including various forms of glomerulonephritis and possibly some manifestations of malignancy and infectious diseases (1).

1.1. Basic Immunochemistry of Immune Complexes: The Precipitin Curve

The immunochemistry of immune complexes has been investigated over many decades (2). The classic precipitin curve demonstrates the importance of antigen : antibody ratios in determining the lattice formed by immune complexes in a typical antigen–antibody interaction. Adding increasing amounts of antigen to a constant amount of antibody demonstrates a curve with three general regions: the zone of antibody excess (prozone), the zone of equivalence, and the zone of antigen excess (postzone). In some antigen–antibody systems, the prozone shows an extended region without precipitation. Immune complexes formed in the zone of far antigen or antibody excess are soluble. Large-lattice immune complexes containing IgG, formed at antigen : antibody ratios close to the zone of equivalence, have multiple IgG Fc regions available for interaction with C1q complement proteins, and therefore activate complement efficiently.

The immune-complex lattice structure can be altered if there is interaction with complement proteins, because covalently bound complement peptides sterically inhibit immune-complex interaction and extended lattice formation. Once immune precipitates are formed, their size can be reduced, leading to solubilization of preformed immunoprecipitates via activation of the alternative pathway of complement (3). Activation of the classical pathway of complement can inhibit immune complex growth by

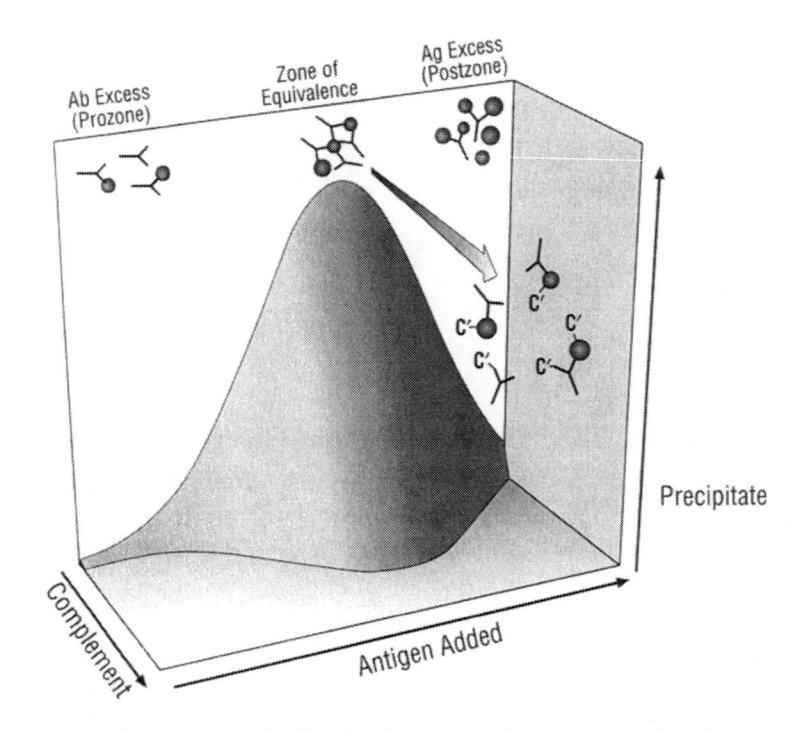

Fig. 1. Modification of precipitin curve or precipitin "surface." In the presence of complement, antigens and antibodies within immune complexes bind complement fragments (**C'**), preventing extension of nascent lattice formation or disrupting lattices, leading to smaller immune complexes. Y = antibody; ● = antigen.

preventing extended lattice formation *(4)*. Thus, in the presence of complement, the precipitin curve can be more properly considered a precipitin "surface," with decreasing precipitate and smaller-lattice immune complexes associated with higher concentrations of complement components (Fig. 1), as well as with antigen or antibody excess. Complement activation thus serves as a negative regulator of immune-complex lattice extension.

1.2. History of Immune Complex Studies

Immune complexes were first implicated in disease by von Pirquet and Schick at the beginning of the twentieth century *(5)*. They hypothesized that serum sickness, characterized by fevers and rashes following repeated doses of horse antitoxin, was caused by the host response to the administered horse serum. Arthus developed the animal model by demonstrating that cutaneous vasculitis and inflammation resulted from immunization of rabbits by injections of horse serum *(6)*. Similarity between the pathological lesions of clinical vasculitis and those of serum sickness was recognized at least as far back as the early 1940s *(7)*. Further development of experimental serum sickness models of glomerulonephritis and vasculitis clarified the potential for circulating immune complexes (antigen–antibody complexes) to cause disease *(8,9)*. Development of immunofluorescence microscopy allowed the demonstration that pathological lesions associated with SLE were characterized by granular deposition of immunoglobulin and complement components, resembling experimental immune-complex disease *(8,10)*. The presence of immune complexes in the circulation of patients with SLE and other rheumatic diseases, as detected by a variety of different techniques, also supported the concept that lupus is an immune-complex disease *(11)*. Other clinical evidence supporting the immune-complex model includes the presence of hypocomplementemia, with activation of the classical pathway of complement in active SLE and resolution of the complement abnormalities during clinical remission. Studies of patients with SLE, rheumatoid arthritis (RA), and mixed cryoglobulinemia from the laboratory of Kunkel provided further clarification of the role of immune complexes in those disorders. Until the discovery of antibodies to neutrophil cytoplasmic antigens and their association with vasculitis, the immune-complex hypothesis was essentially the only mechanism implicated in the pathophysiology of vasculitis. In the early 1980s, evidence could be presented implicating a role for circulating immune complexes in virtually all inflammatory rheumatic diseases *(1)*. Immune complexes are still thought to play a central role in many forms of vasculitis. In recent years, even as the role of genetic factors, cellular mechanisms, infectious etiologies, and cytokines have been the focus of investigation for many rheumatic diseases, the role of circulating immune complexes has remained central to understanding the pathogenesis of some autoimmune rheumatic disorders.

2. Disease Associations
2.1. Immune Complexes and SLE

Active renal SLE is associated with high serum concentrations of antibodies to double-stranded DNA (antidsDNA) and enrichment of anti-DNA within glomerular eluates of patients with SLE, supporting the role of anti-DNA in the pathogenesis of SLE. DNA–anti-DNA immune complexes are thought to be the dominant contributor to immune-complex nephritis in SLE *(10)*. Several investigators have found evidence for circulating DNA–anti-DNA immune complexes and other immune complexes in SLE patients and experimental models (reviewed in ref. *12*).

Antibodies to the collagen-like region of C1q (anti-CLR-C1q) were found to be concentrated within glomerular basement fragments isolated from kidneys of lupus patients *(13)*. Together with data demonstrating a strong association between lupus nephritis and serum levels of anti-CLR-C1q, these data strongly implicate anti-CLR-C1q in the pathogenesis of lupus nephritis. Recent data demonstrates that anti-CLR-C1q tends to be present if there are multiple autoantibodies (including anti-dsDNA, anti-SSA, anti-Sm, and/or others) present and enriched in glomerular basement membrane fragments from kidneys of patients with SLE (Mannik and Wener, unpublished).

Assays for circulating immune complexes have been used to monitor SLE activity. Numerous studies have suggested that immune-complex assays based on C1q and C3 are positive in patients with SLE and can be helpful in assessing disease activity in patients with SLE (reviewed in ref. *12*). Assays for anti-dsDNA and complement components are more widely available than immune-complex assays and are similarly used to monitor disease activity and assist in the diagnosis of SLE; therefore, measurement of immune complexes are not widely used clinically in comparison with those other measurements.

2.2. Immune Complexes and Vasculitis

Using direct immunofluorescence microscopy, immunoglobulins and complement components can frequently be detected in vessels affected by some forms of vasculitis.

In clinical situations, the antibody specificity of the deposited immunoglobulins are rarely determined; therefore, there is rarely direct evidence to conclude the source of the antigens recognized by those antibodies. The pattern of immunoglobulin deposition is most commonly used to infer the mechanism for antibody deposition. Immunoglobulins deposited in a smooth, linear, ribbonlike pattern are presumptively directed against high-density continuous epitopes that are constitutive in the tissues (e.g., glomerular basement membranes in patients with Goodpasture's syndrome), whereas immunoglobulins with a discontinuous, discrete, granular pattern are presumed to be caused by immune complexes.

Immune deposits in tissues are commonly seen in small-vessel vasculitis caused by identified antigens. The most common forms of anaphylactoid purpura (i.e., those vasculitides caused by reactions to drugs such as penicillin) typically will be associated with detectable immune deposits. Similarly, in forms of small-vessel vasculitis associated with chronic infections (e.g., mixed cryoglobulinemia syndrome associated with chronic hepatitis C virus infection), immune deposits are routinely visible in biopsied tissues. Given that the antigens responsible are known to be circulating in blood in fairly high concentrations, the detection of immunoglobulins and complement components in tissues, and the supportive experimental studies demonstrating the responsible antigens in vasculitic lesions, the immune-complex mechanism is strongly supported for these forms of vasculitis. Furthermore, circulating antigen–antibody complexes can be found in plasma in some of these disorders, including the mixed cryoglobulinemia syndrome. This form of vasculitis is clearly immune-complex mediated.

Polyarteritis nodosa (PAN) is associated with hepatitis B virus (HBV) infection in significant numbers of cases, although that association is likely to be less important in the future as immunization prevents spread of HBV infection. The hepatitis B surface antigen together with immunoglobulins and complement components have been described in the vessel wall of tissues involved with vasculitis *(14)*, as well as vessels in some uninvolved tissues. Serum of some patients with PAN have also been found to have positive assays for circulating immune complexes, and the magnitude of elevation has been felt to correlate with disease activity in some cases *(15)*.

Immune-complex deposition probably has a minimal pathogenic role in other forms of PAN, in other vasculitides with primarily medium-sized- and large-vessel involvement, and in Wegener's granulomatosis *(16)*. A minority of these patients have immunoglobulins and complement deposition in tissues by immunofluorescence microscopy. In addition, small-vessel vasculitis cases that are not associated with immune deposits ("paucimmune") are frequently associated with serum antibodies to neutrophil cytoplasmic antigens (ANCA). It has been suggested that ANCA positivity, as found in such diseases as Wegener's granulomatosis, Churg–Strauss syndrome, microscopic polyangiitis, and some cases of PAN, provides an alternative to the immune-complex mechanism of disease *(17)*, despite involvement of small vessels in both immune-complex-mediated vasculitis and ANCA-associated vasculitis. These arguments suggest that small-vessel vasculitis can be associated with either immune complexes or ANCA. Immune complexes have no clear role in larger-vessel vasculitis, such as giant-cell arteritis.

2.3. Immune Complexes and Rheumatoid Arthritis

Rheumatoid factors (RFs) (i.e., antibodies directed against the Fc portion of IgG) can react with IgG and lead to the formation of immune complexes both in vitro and in vivo. High local concentrations of RFs produced within synovium promote immune-complex formation at that site. Activation of complement as well as activation of inflammatory cells via complement and Fc receptors could result. IgG RFs seen in patients with RA and related disorders have the unusual capacity to form aggregates via Fc–F(ab) interactions in the absence of other antigens *(18)*.

IgG, possibly in the form of immune complexes, has been found within articular cartilage of patients with RA, as well as osteoarthritis. Furthermore, immunoglobulins within cartilage are covalently bound to proteoglycans within the cartilage *(19,20)*. These observations support the potential for immune complexes to be present and promoting chronic inflammation within the joint.

In the early 1980s, there was enthusiasm for the measurement of circulating immune complexes as a potential measure of activity in patients with rheumatoid arthritis. Circulating immune complexes were implicated in the polyarthritis associated with infections, such as hepatitis B infection *(21)*. Positive assays for immune complexes were demonstrated in many patients with RA. Enthusiasm was tempered when the many assays correlated only poorly with each other, raising questions about what was being measured and how the results should be interpreted. A systematic study sponsored by the U.S. Centers for Disease Control and the Arthritis Foundation analyzed sera from patients with RA using several different IC assays and compared findings with other clinical laboratory data such as the erythrocyte sedimentation rate and rheumatoid factor measurement *(22)*. The authors found that no single assay was effective at monitoring disease activity and establishing prognosis, although two assays (the fluid-phase C1q assay and the staphylococcal binding assay) were as good as the best of the other laboratory tests (erythrocyte sedimentation rate [ESR], IgG RF) in monitoring disease activity. They concluded that the circulating immune complex measurement had little value in monitoring individual patients with RA.

3. Pathophysiologic Mechanisms
3.1. Immune-Complex Clearance

The mononuclear phagocyte system plays the central role in removing immune complexes from the circulation, with clearance mediated by families of Fc and complement receptors on mononuclear phagocytes, neutrophils, and other cells *(23)*. The presence of C3 receptors on primate erythrocytes but not erythrocytes from other species suggested a trafficking mechanism applicable to humans but not to nonprimate experimental animals *(24,25)*. Immune complexes that had activated complement and bound C3 in the circulation could bind to the complement receptor CR1 on the erythrocyte, and be transported to the liver and spleen while bound to the red cell, and those immune complexes would be phagocytized by cells of the mononuclear phagocyte system, primarily via Fc receptors. A variety of probes of this system have been employed experimentally in humans, including erythrocytes coated with IgG antibodies, aggregated IgG, preformed immune complexes, and antigens infused into preimmunized subjects. Davies et al. have performed studies using several different soluble immune complexes as probes, including tetanus/antitetanus, hepatitis B surface antigen/antibodies, and murine IgG/human anti-mouse IgG *(26)*. The former two types of immune complexes were formed in vitro and then injected into subjects; ongoing studies using the hepatitis IC models indicate that large immune complexes infused into subjects with a normal complement system appear to be carried by erythrocytes to the liver and spleen, whereas complexes that are inefficiently opsonized by complement either because of their small size or because of complement deficiencies are primarily cleared in the liver *(27)*. In other studies, complement depletion led to accelerated clearance of immune complexes by the liver and spleen and might have been associated with increased tissue deposition of immune complexes *(28)*, suggesting that red cell binding of immune complexes could have role in "buffering" excessive loads of immune complexes until they are removed by mononuclear phagocytes. Erythrocyte binding of immune complexes could have a role in immune-complex processing or degradation while on the erythrocyte *(29)*.

Davies et al. *(30)* administered murine IgG and human anti-mouse IgG to study immune complexes formed in vivo, an experiment that might be considered most representative of natural physiology. Patients with ovarian carcinoma were given ^{131}I-murine monoclonal antitumor antibodies and subsequently ^{125}I-human anti-mouse IgG. Immune complexes were large but of a size possibly to be encountered physiologically. Soluble immune complexes formed within 5 min, activated complement, and were cleared with a half-life of 11 min in the liver and without a detectable increase in radioactivity over the spleen. Between 8% and 11% of the total available immune complexes bound to the erythrocyte, and at the time of peak red cell binding, erythrocyte-bound immune complexes constituted approx 20% of total circulating complexes. The majority of soluble immune complexes were cleared by mechanisms that were largely independent of red cells, and the site of clearance of these soluble complexes in the liver differed substantially from the splenic clearance of sensitized erythrocytes that had been previously reported *(31)*.

In SLE patients, several studies have shown that the clearance of antibody-sensitized erythrocytes is slower than the clearance in normal controls and slower in patients with than without active renal disease *(32,33)*. Investigators at Leiden have administered radioiodinated aggregated human IgG (^{123}I-AHG) to SLE patients to explore the fate of circulating soluble immune complexes in patients with SLE. The investigators described an initial rapid clearance and later slower clearance of immune complexes from the circulation (both reported in terms of the time to removal of 50% of the maximum material, $T_{1/2}$). In their first study, the authors reported that the initial-phase $T_{1/2}$ was not significantly different between SLE patients and controls, whereas the second-phase $T_{1/2}$ was prolonged in the patient group *(34)*. In the second study, SLE patients erythrocytes were observed to have a decreased number of CR1, which was associated with less binding of AHG to red blood cells and with a faster initial rate of clearance of AHG (mean half-time to removal was 5.2 ± 0.2 min in patients versus 6.6 ± 0.2 min in controls; $p = 0.01$). The later phase of AHG clearance was similar in patients and controls ($T_{1/2} = 148 \pm 18$ versus 154 ± 20 min). Both the maximum liver uptake and time required to reach the maximum liver uptake were similar in SLE patients and controls. Of interest, the feature most predictive of the rate of AHG clearance in SLE patients was the serum IgG concentration, which was inversely correlated ($r = -0.66$) with the rate of clearance. The authors speculated that the concentration of serum IgG in SLE patients was a primary determinant of the proportion of Fc receptors that were occupied and thereby governed the rate of clearance of AHG *(35)*.

The importance of the rapid, very early removal of immune complexes from the circulation was shown by Schifferli et al. *(36)*, who examined the clearance of immune complexes composed of tetanus toxoid and antitetanus in 4 patients with SLE, as well as 11 other patients and 9 normal subjects. The authors reported that the removal of these large (45 Svedberg units) complexes from the circulation occurred in two phases: a very rapid "trapping" phase which occurred within the first minute, and a monoexponential later phase. In 1 of 9 normal individuals and 11 of 15 patients, over 8% of the injected immune complexes were removed from the circulation ("trapped") within the first minute after administration, a time point and amount removed that could not be attributed to clearance by the liver and spleen, and therefore trapping presumably resulted in deposition of immune complexes in peripheral tissues. This initial trapping was seen in patients with serum complement deficiencies and was associated with lower levels of CR1 on erythrocytes. The later phase of immune complex clearance was monoexponential over the 60 min of measurement, with between 9.9% and 18.7% removed per minute in normals and between 8.6% and 32.2% per minute removed in patients. When opsonized immune complexes that were bound in vitro to erythrocytes via CR1 were injected into patients, there was release of 10–81% of the immune complexes from the erythrocytes within 1 min of injection. The extent of this release was inversely correlated with CR1 number per cell.

Together, these studies of the clearance of soluble immune complexes in SLE patients argue that the hepatic clearance of immune complexes, which governs the late-phase removal of soluble immune complexes, is probably normal in SLE patients. Low CR1 numbers on erythrocytes or profound hypocomplementemia can permit deposition of immune complexes within tissues during the early phase of immune-complex clearance. Reduction in CR1 numbers is an acquired abnormality associated with active SLE *(37)*. It is unclear whether the abnormalities in immune-complex-clearance mechanisms observed in these experiments contribute to immune complex deposition at sites of tissue injury.

More recently, investigations have explored the implications of polymorphisms in various Fcγ receptors with regard to their potential role in clearing immune complexes from the circulation and causing a predisposition to SLE. Lack of the H131 allele of the FcγRIIA, which is responsible for efficient clearance of IgG$_2$-containing immune complexes, has been associated with lupus nephritis in American blacks *(38)*. A report has implicated a functionally important genetic polymorphism of FcγRIIIA as a risk factor for SLE in a genetically diverse group of patients *(39)*.

3.2. Factors Governing Immune Complex Localization: Physicochemical Composition and Site of Formation

Exploration of nonprimate animal models of serum sickness demonstrated that a critical characteristic of circulating immune complexes that governed their clearance and deposition in tissues was their size or the extent of lattice formation. The lattice of an immune complex, defined as the number of antigen and antibody molecules in a given immune complex, governs the number and density of Fc regions in an immune complex and, thereby, its ability to interact with Fc receptors and/or activate Fc-dependent functions. Large-lattice soluble immune complexes (>Ag$_2$Ab$_2$) tended to be cleared rapidly by the mononuclear phagocyte system, primarily by Fc receptors on the Kuppfer cells in the liver. If the mononuclear phagocyte system was saturated or blocked, then these immune complexes would deposit in tissues (e.g., in the mesangial and subendothelial regions of the glomerular basement membrane). In comparison, small-lattice complexes (Ag$_2$Ab$_2$ or smaller) tended to have more prolonged time in the circulation; however, they had a lower tendency to deposit in tissues. Activation of complement proteins was also known to be size dependent, with complement activation occurring much more efficiently with larger-lattice immune complexes. In these rodent experimental systems, complement receptors play a role in removing immune complexes only if the immune complexes are very large (reviewed in ref. *40*).

In experimental models, administration of preformed immune complexes results in mesangial and subendothelial localization of immune complexes within renal glomeruli. Studies in the 1980s using the Heymann model of nephritis, and studies on isolated perfused kidneys emphasized that antibodies and antigens could deposit sequentially in the kidney, with the result that the immune complexes form *in situ* and tend to localize in the subepithelial region of glomeruli, rather than being deposited from circulation *(41)*. Formation of complexes *in situ* can occur because of direct binding of antigens or antibodies, initially because of interaction between the circulating molecule and structures within the kidney. This initial interaction can be relatively weak and/or nonspecific (e.g., because of charge–charge interactions).

Electrical charge on either the antigen or the antibody within the immune complex governs interaction with fixed negative charges on proteoglycans in the basement membrane or in other structures and influences both the deposition and persistence of antigens, antibodies, and immune complexes in tissues. In experimental systems, even a small proportion of positively charged (cationic) antibodies enhance binding and persistence of immune complexes in renal glomeruli *(42)*.

Deposition of antigens or antibodies could be augmented or facilitated also by antigen-specific receptors within the tissues. Particularly relevant for the study of SLE, Emlen demonstrated that immune complexes containing DNA may be removed in part by DNA receptors *(43)*. Several years ago, it was demonstrated in experimental animals that the clearance of immune complexes containing glycosylated antigens was governed in part by specific carbohydrate receptors on hepatocytes *(44)*. A serum carbohydrate binding protein, mannose-binding protein (MBP), may have an important role in clearing immune complexes containing antigens with selected carbohydrate residues. A member of the collagen motif-containing collectin family of proteins, MBP binds terminal mannose, fucose, glucose, fucose, or *N*-acetylglucosamine residues, can activate the classical or alternative pathways of complement *(45)*, activate macrophages via the C1q receptor *(46)*, and serve as an opsonin *(47)*. Recently, it has been shown that genetic polymorphisms responsible for depressed function and serum levels of MBP are associated with SLE in African-Americans *(48)* and other groups *(49,50)*. Furthermore, certain ribonucleoprotein autoantigens, including the U1-specific 68kD and A proteins and the U2-specific B" protein, are glycoproteins, with mannose, glucose, and *N*-acetylglucosamine detected on the 68kD protein *(51)*. Thus, it is conceivable that the clearance of glycoprotein antigens or immune complexes containing such antigens, including the U1-RNP particle, could be influenced by MBP polymorphisms. These considerations suggest that MBP polymorphisms could participate in the pathogenesis of SLE by influencing immune-complex clearance, analogous to the role of polymorphisms in complement components and FcR.

Features on the antibodies within the immune complex can influence the physiology of immune complexes. The isotype of antibodies influences immune-complex handling, because the ability to activate complement influences both the ability to bind to complement receptors as well as to activate inflammatory cascades. AntidsDNA in SLE patients tend to be of subclasses IgG1, IgG2, and IgG3 and tend to be efficient in activation of complement *(52)*. Experimental studies with murine monoclonal IgG3 immunoglobulins have demonstrated that deposition of cryoprecipitating or other self-associating immunoglobulin aggregates, a feature of certain immunoglobulin molecules, may cause glomerulonephritis *(53)*. IgA-containing immune complexes may be cleared by distinct IgA receptors *(54)*.

4. Immune-Complex Rearrangement and Persistence

Circulating immune complexes probably are forming frequently in normal individuals, depending on diet and absorption of antigens from the gut. Only a minority of immune complexes escape uptake by the mononuclear phagocyte system and deposit in tissues, and only a minority of those immune complexes in tissues cause identifiable disease. Many immune complexes that deposit in target organs, such as the kidney, are present only for a few hours and are then cleared. Regions of antigens or antibodies with a strong positive charge can cause a greater persistence of immune complexes in tissues *(42)*. In order to develop immune deposits that are more persistent and visible as typical subendothelial or subepithelial electron-dense deposits within the kidney, immune deposits of small or intermediate size that might deposit from the circulation into tissues must coalesce or rearrange to form larger immune deposits *(55)*. This rearrangement may not occur between immune complexes composed of different antigens or antibodies that do not crossreact, as they would not form a large-lattice immune deposit. Rearrangement of immune complexes may also be associated with movement of deposits within the kidney. In an experimental rat immune-complex model using immune deposits that could be localized by electron microscopy, it could be shown that immune deposits initially were formed and coalesced in subendothelial locations, and then moved to subepithelial locations where they again underwent rearrangement *(56)*. The solubilization of these complexes was associated with binding of C3, and the authors suggested that C3 solubilization of precipitates within the basement membranes facilitated the immune-complex rearrangement.

A hallmark of SLE is the wide variety of antigen–antibody systems within a single individual. Although ample evidence indicates that DNA–anti-DNA comprise the major antigen–antibody system in SLE, other antibodies may also be present and enriched within the glomeruli. For example, glomerular enrichment of antibodies to the SSA/Ro antigen has been described *(57)* and other antibodies are also present (Mannik and Wener, unpublished). What are some of the mechanisms leading to persistence of immune complexes within tissues?

Covalent crosslinking of antigens and antibodies to each other or to tissue antigens in kidneys and articular cartilage has recently been described *(19,58)*. Such covalent bonds on immune complexes within tissues could promote the persistence of immune deposits, leading to chronicity of inflammatory mechanisms at those sites. A mechanism has recently been proposed to explain immune-complex covalent crosslinking *(19)*. Activation of neutrophils leads to formation of reactive oxygen species by neutrophils, and activation of chondrocytes leads to the formation of highly reactive nitric oxide by chondrocytes. These highly reactive molecules were shown to cause covalent crosslinking of antigen–antibody complexes on plastic surfaces. Similar mechanisms could be present in tissues.

4.1. Autoantibodies to the Collagen-like Region of C1q

Antibodies to C1q could also augment aggregation of immune complexes in tissues. Anti-C1q antibodies are found in association with lupus nephritis and are less commonly demonstrable in serum of patients with nonrenal lupus. Rising concentrations of IgG anti-C1q are associated with flares of lupus nephritis, and high levels of anti-C1q are associated with proliferative forms of lupus glomerulonephritis. Antibodies to the collagenlike region of C1q are present and enriched in the glomeruli of many patients with lupus whose kidneys were examined at autopsy, and were associated with proliferative lupus nephritis *(59)*. The fact that these antibodies were released under acid conditions suggests that they were present in the form of immune complexes. Release by DNAse suggests that the immune deposits also contained immune complexes composed of DNA and anti-DNA, which then bound C1q and, in turn, anti-C1q. Together, the clinical associations of anti-C1q with active lupus nephritis and the newer data demonstrating that anti-C1q is present and enriched in glomeruli strongly argue that antibodies to C1q play a pathogenic role in the proliferative forms of lupus nephritis.

By binding to different molecules of C1q that have bound to immune complexes composed of different antigen–antibody systems, antibodies to C1q could promote aggregation of those different types of immune complexes, leading to larger, more persistent, and more pathogenic immune deposits. Preliminary reports indicate that anti-C1q in kidneys from lupus patients tend to be found in patients with multiple autoantibodies identified in the kidney, supporting the idea that anti-C1q could be promoting the aggregation of different antigen–antibody systems (Mannik and Wener, unpublished).

4.2. Tissue Effects of Immune Complexes

Once deposited in tissues, immune complexes cause inflammation. Complement-mediated injury has been considered to be the dominant mechanism responsible. Clinically and experimentally, activation of complement can be demonstrated in serum, at tissue sites, and in urine. The well-known pro-inflammatory chemotactic role of complement fragments is believed to lead to recruitment of inflammatory cells into the lesion. Larger-lattice immune complexes, with a higher density of Fc regions, activate complement more efficiently. Release of pro-inflammatory cytokines from inflammatory cells is also greater for large-lattice immune complexes in synovial fluids than for smaller complexes *(60)*. Nephrotoxic serum nephritis, a form of experimental nephritis probably caused by immune complexes that form *in situ*, could be improved substantially by administration of soluble complement receptor-1-related gene/protein y (Crry), a potent complement inhibitor *(61)*. Overexpression of the Crry protein in a transgenic mouse model also reduced this form of nephritis *(62)*. Depletion of C5a function by antibody *(63)* or through knockout of the C5a receptor gene *(64)* demonstrated dependence of pulmonary immune complex disease on C5a.

Recent information indicates that IgG Fc receptors (FcγR) may have a more important role in mediating immune-complex disease than had been appreciated previously, and complement may mediate less of the inflammation. These data have been reported in a series of papers, largely using mice generated by Ravetch, that lack the transmembrane, signal transducing γ chain that is found on IgG FcRI and FcRIII. In cutaneous Arthus reaction models in those mice, as well as experiments with autoimmune mice crossbred with the Fc receptor knockout mice, neutrophil infiltration and organ dysfunction required intact Fc receptors despite the presence of immune complexes in tissues *(65)*. Furthermore, inflammation was not altered by complement deficiency. The susceptibility to murine lupus nephritis *(66)* and to collagen-induced arthritis was also found to be altered in FcR –/– mice *(67)*, indicating that similar mechanisms were important in these diseases. In a murine model of immune-complex peritonitis, neutrophil migration was attenuated after complement depletion, but totally abolished in mice lacking the FcR γ chain. Additional data suggested that engagement of FcRIII did not lead to neutrophil recruitment, but engagement of FcRI was most important in causing inflammatory exudates *(68)*. It has been proposed that local microenvironments within different tissues could influence expression of FcR on macrophages at different sites, thus modulating the local inflammation and other tissue effects of circulating or deposited immune complexes *(69)*. If FcR activation is more important than complement activation in mediating immune-complex disease, then many additional questions can be raised. For example, could there be steric hindrance by complement fragments in the interaction between immune-complex Fc regions and FcR, thus demonstrating another anti-inflammatory of complement? Does the observed enhanced production of C3 by human mesangial cells *(70)* have pro-inflammatory or anti-inflammatory effects?

Immune complexes themselves have a variety of other immunomodulatory effects. For example, binding of immune complexes to Fc receptors leads to aggregation of those receptors, triggering intracellular signaling pathways *(71)*. Immune complexes have been reported to augment the responsiveness of both B-cells and T-cells to antigen stimulation *(72)*.

4.3. Development of Therapies Based on the Immune-Complex Model

The immune-complex model for the cause of tissue damage in SLE has been the dominant paradigm for several decades, and it remains so. Therapeutic approaches based on this paradigm, however, have been relatively disappointing. For example, whereas plasmapheresis for the treatment of SLE originally met with great enthusiasm, a controlled clinical trial of plasmapheresis in patients with lupus nephritis was unsuccessful *(73)*.

Recently, affinity columns containing silica-bound staphylococcal protein A (SPA) have been approved for use in patients with severe refractory rheumatoid arthritis *(74)*. The rationale for use of SPA immunoabsorbants arises from the observation that IgG within immune complexes binds preferentially to SPA, compared with monomeric noncomplexed IgG. It has been suggested that other mechanisms in addition to immune-complex removal may play a role in the improvement observed (Sasso, personal communication); nevertheless, this successful therapy was developed because of the immune-complex-disease model.

4.4. Importance of Antigen Within Circulating Immune Complexes?

Whereas in the classic serum-sickness immune-complex model, the antigen in the immune complex (often heterologous serum albumin in experimental systems) bears little relevance to the resultant pathology, in SLE and other human immune-complex diseases, the antigen constituents within the immune complex could influence the pattern of clinical sequelae and the risk for cardiovascular disease. For example, recently, antiphospholipid antibodies were found to be enriched in circulating immune complexes in patients with the antiphospholipid syndrome, with or without coexistent SLE *(75)*. In these studies, aliquots of sera that were unfractionated or were fractionated by gel filtration or sucrose density gradients were analyzed for the presence of anti-phospholipid antibodies. The relative concentration of anticardiolipin antibodies was up to 125 times higher in high-molecular-weight fractions, compared with the antibody activity in unfractionated serum. Furthermore, in some sera, minimal levels of anti-phospholipid antibodies were detectable in the unfractionated serum, whereas high levels of antibodies to negatively charged phospholipids were found in the high-molecular-weight fractions. The binding avidity of antiphospholipid antibodies was substantially higher in the immune-complex fractions compared with the unfractionated sera, as assessed by binding curves and elution studies. Different types of immune complexes differ in their ability to bind to and activate platelets *(76)*. Thus, anti-phospholipid-containing immune complexes could augment the tendency of antiphospholipid antibodies to cause thrombosis and enhance vascular disease.

Because antiphospholipid antibodies bind to other families of lipids, including oxidized low-density lipoproteins (LDL) *(77)*, it is possible that the high-molecular-weight antiphospholipid antibodies were part of immune complexes comprised of lipoproteins. Immune complexes containing antibodies to lipoproteins known to be associated with atherogenesis could play a role in development of coronary artery disease. Hasunama et al. found that the anti-cardiolipin cofactor β2-glycoprotein I (β2-GPI) bound preferentially to oxidized plasma lipoproteins, i.e. oxidized [ox]VLDL (very low-density lipoproteins), oxLDL, and oxHDL (high-density lipoproteins), in comparison with the native forms of the lipoproteins *(78)*. Antibodies to β2-GPI bound to the β2-GPI–oxLDL complex. Whereas binding of β2-GPI to oxLDL inhibited the uptake of oxLDL by macrophages, the uptake was enhanced in the presence of immune complexes containing antiβ2-GPI and β2-GPI–oxLDL complexes. Uptake of oxLDL by macrophages predisposes to the formation of foam cells leading to intimal disease and atherosclerosis; thus, the enhanced uptake caused by lipoprotein-containing immune complexes could contribute to accelerated atherosclerosis *(79)* as well as immune-complex disease. Given the growing importance of coronary disease and of the antiphospholipid syndrome in SLE, the role of immune complexes in those manifestations bears further investigation.

5. Clinical Assays for Circulating Immune Complexes

A variety of different assays for circulating immune complexes have been developed, with relatively few used clinically in more than a few laboratories (reviewed in ref. *80*). The most commonly used assays include those based purely on the physical chemistry of immune complexes (e.g., tests depending on polyethylene glycol-induced precipitation or tests for cryoglobulins, i.e., cold-precipitating immunoglobulins), those dependent on binding to C1q, and those detecting the presence of IgG–C3 complexes either by employing cellular C3 receptors (Raji cell assay) or antigenic recognition. A problem with interpretation of results of immune-complex assays is that they can give positive results when antibodies directed against the recognition moieties bind to those moieties as specific antibodies, rather than in antigen-nonspecific immune-complex interactions. For example, with the Raji cell assay, antilymphocyte antibodies from some patients with systemic lupus erythematosus could give a positive result, recognizing antigens on the Raji cell as targets. Use of the C1q solid-phase assay allows autoantibodies directed against C1q to bind and give positive results, even in the absence of immune complexes. Similarly, autoantibodies to C3 components are frequently present in the sera of patients with SLE and related disorders and could lead to positive results in immune-complex assays based on recognition of C3. In the antiC3 assay, serum antibodies directed against the F(ab')2 fragments of antiC3 used to detect the C3-bearing immune complexes have been reported to cause positive assay results. In these examples, the positive results are "false-positive" in that the results are not caused by immune complexes, yet clinically useful results may be obtained (*see* Subheading 2.). However, because the assays may become positive because of the presence of pathologic substances in addition to immune complexes, investigators employing these assays and using them to make conclusions about circulating immune complexes should confirm that immune complexes are responsible for the positive results observed.

One of the challenges of using the clinical assays for circulating immune complexes is that the lack of concordance between the methods has made interpretation of results difficult (*11*). Because of differences in the immunochemical properties of immune complexes and differences in principles of detection with the different methods, these differences may not be unexpected. Furthermore, pathogenically important immune complexes may not be present in the serum specimens usually analyzed, but they may be deposited in peripheral tissues, carried on erythrocytes via their CR1 during their transit through the circulation, or lost during specimen handling. Taylor et al. have provided evidence that the immune complexes bound to circulating erythrocytes may be released into plasma during incubation, whereas they remain on the erythrocytes if serum is the specimen to be analyzed. Furthermore, even attempts to directly quantify erythrocyte-bound IgG, an approach that has the potential to measure immune complexes bound to cells, may be problematic because of the fact that CR1-bound IgG is relatively inaccessible to a variety of probes. Immune complexes contained within cryoglobulins are well recognized as potentially being diminished if the specimen is allowed to cool. Preanalytical factors (i.e., handling of clinical specimens prior to actual assay) and choices of specimen (serum, plasma, or erythrocyte) may substantially influence the results reported from any given patient, and these factors are often not carefully addressed.

5.1. Detection of Immune Complexes: Technical Issues for the Clinician

Analyzing tissue biopsies using direct immunofluorescence microscopy, immunoglobulins and complement components are routinely identified within vessels affected by some forms of vasculitis. The detection of these immune deposits depends in part on technical issues. Biopsy material ideally should be obtained from new "fresh" lesions because immune deposits are transient and may be undetectable in older lesions. A portion of tissue biopsies should be snap-frozen to prevent degradation of immune deposits. For some biopsies, such as small punch biopsies of skin, one specimen may be obtained for routine histology, and a second obtained for freezing and immunofluorescence studies. Specimens should be sent to an experienced laboratory, as background staining, specificity of antibodies, and other factors can influence interpretation of results.

Circulating immune complexes have been measured by a multitude of techniques, few of which are available to most clinicians *(11)*. For the clinician, probably the most important immune-complex assay is the assay for cryoglobulins. The test for cryoglobulins is frequently inaccurate because of problems with specimen handling; for this test, blood should be allowed to remain at 37°C while it clots and should be kept warm while the clot is centrifuged. Phlebotomists and laboratory personnel should be alerted to the possible presence of a cryoglobulin and should be reminded of the special handling requirements.

6. Summary

Inflammation caused by immune complexes in tissues remains the single most important mechanism for clinical manifestations of SLE. Although substantial progress is being made investigating genetic contributions to clearance mechanisms of immune complexes, questions remain about the site and mechanism of immune-complex formation and about factors that influence localization and pathogenicity at different sites. Mechanisms responsible for rearrangement and condensation, the process by which transient, probably nonpathogenic immune complexes become sustained and pathogenic in SLE, also remain largely unexplored. Although the role of anti-DNA as a contributor to lupus immune-complex disease has been studied, the role of other antibodies (such as those directed to nucleoprotein complexes, C1q, and phospholipids) as constituents of immune complexes remains another relatively unexplored area of investigation. The relative role of complement and Fc receptor activation in the pathogenesis of immune-complex disease is controversial. Although immune complexes are one of the fundamental causes of inflammation in autoimmune rheumatic diseases, many mysteries remain concerning their pathophysiology.

Acknowledgments

This work was sponsored partially by NIH grant RO1 AR11476. The author gratefully acknowledges informative and helpful discussions with Mart Mannik and numerous other colleagues concerning this topic. Portions of this manuscript were previously published *(12)* and are used with permission.

References

1. Espinoza, L. R. and Osterland, C. K. (eds.) (1983) *Circulating Immune Complexes. Their Clinical Significance*, Futura Publishing, Mount Kisco, NY.
2. Day, E. (1990) Immune complexes, in *Advanced Immunochemistry*, 2nd ed., Wiley–Liss, New York, pp. 397–467.
3. Czop, J. and Nussenzweig, V. (1976) Studies on the mechanism of solubilization of immune precipitates by serum. *J. Exp. Med.* **143**, 615–630.
4. Johnson, A., Harkins, S., Steward, M. W., and Whaley, K. (1987) The effects of immunoglobulin isotype and antibody affinity on complement-mediated inhibition of immune precipitation and solubilization. *Mol. Immunol.* **24**, 1211–1217.
5. von Pirquet, C. F. and Schick, B. (1905) *Die Serum Krankeit (Serum Sickness)*, F. Deuticke, Leipzig.

6. Arthus, M. and Breton, M. (1903) Lesions cutanees produites par les injections de serum de cheval chez le lapin anaphylactise par et pour ce serum. *Compt Rend. Soc. Biol.* **55**, 817–820.
7. Rich, A. R. (1942) The role of hypersensitivity in periarteritis nodosa. *Bull. Johns Hopkins Hosp.* **71**, 123–140.
8. Dixon, F. J. (1963) The role of antigen–antibody complexes in disease. *Harvey. Lect.* **58**, 21.
9. Germuth, F. G. and Rodriguez, E. (1973) *Immune Complex Glomerulonephritis*, Little, Brown, Boston.
10. Koffler, D., Agnello, V., Thoburn, R., and Kunkel, H. G. (1971) Systemic lupus erythematosus: prototype of immune complex nephritis in man. *J. Exp. Med.* **134**, 169S–179S.
11. Lambert, P. H., Dixon, F. J., Zubler, R. H., Agnello, V., Cambiaso, C., Casali, P., et al. (1978) A WHO collaborative study for the evaluation of eighteen methods for detecting immune complexes in serum. *J. Clin. Lab. Immunol.* **1(1)**, 1–15.
12. Wener, M. H. (1999) Immune complexes and autoantibodies to C1q, in *Lupus Molecular and Cellular Pathogenesis* (Kammer, G. and Tsokos, G., eds.), Humana, Totowa, NJ, 1999. pp. 574–598.
13. Mannik, M. and Wener, M. H. (1997) Deposition of antibodies to the collagen-like region of C1q in renal glomeruli of patients with proliferative lupus glomerulonephritis. *Arthritis Rheum.* **40**, 1504–1511.
14. Gocke, D., Morgan, C., Bombardieri, S., Lockshin, M., and Christian, C. L. (1970) Association between polyarteritis and Australian antigen. *Lancet* **2**, 1149–1153.
15. Leib, E. S., Hibrawi, H., Chia, D., Blaker, R. G., and Barnett, E. V. (1981) Correlations of disease activity in systemic necrotizing vasculitis with immune complexes. *J. Rheumatol.* **8**, 258–265.
16. McCluskey, R. and Fienberg, R. (1983) Vasculitis in primary vasculitides, granulomatoses, and connective tissue diseases. *Hum. Pathol.* **14**, 305–315.
17. Jennette, J. C., Ewert, B. H., and Falk, R. J. (1993) Do antineutrophil cytoplasmic autoantibodies cause Wegener's granulomatosis and other forms of necrotizing vasculitis? *Rheum. Dis. Clin. North Am.* **19**, 1–14.
18. Mannik, M. (1992) Rheumatoid factors in the pathogenesis of rheumatoid arthritis. *J. Rheumatol.* **32(Suppl.)**, 46–49.
19. Uesugi, M., Hayashi, T., and Jasin, H. E. (1998) Covalent cross-linking of immune complexes by oxygen radicals and nitrite. *J. Immunol.* **161**, 1422–1427.
20. Mannik, M. and Person, R. E. (1993) Immunoglobulin G and serum albumin isolated from the articular cartilage of patients with rheumatoid arthritis or osteoarthritis contain covalent heteropolymers with proteoglycans. *Rheumatol. Int.* **13**, 121–129; erratum: *Rheumatol. Int.* (1994), **13**, 214.
21. Onion, D. K., Crumpacker, C. S., and Gilliland, G. C. (1971) Arthritis of hepatitis associated with Australian antigen. *Ann. Int. Med.* **75**, 29–33.
22. McDougal, J. S., Hubbard, M., McDuffie, F. C., Strobel, P. L., Smith, S. J., Bass, N., et al. (1982) Comparison of five assays for immune complexes in the rheumatic diseases. An assessment of their validity for rheumatoid arthritis. *Arthritis Rheum.* **25**, 1156–1166.
23. Frank, M. M., Lawley, T. J., Hamburger, M. I., et al. (1983) Immunoglobulin G Fc receptor-mediated clearance in autoimmune diseases. *Ann. Intern. Med.* **98**, 206.
24. Cornacoff, J. B., Hebert, L. A., and Smead, W. L. (1983) Primate erythrocyte immune complex clearing mechanism. *J. Clin. Invest.* **71**, 236–247.
25. Kimberly, R. P., Salmon, J. E., Edberg, J. C., and Gibofsky, A. (1989) The role of Fc gamma receptors in mononuclear phagocyte system function. *Clin. Exp. Rheumatol.* **7**, S103–S108.
26. Davies, K. A. (1996) Michael Mason Prize Essay 1995. Complement, immune complexes and systemic lupus erythematosus. *Br. J. Rheumatol.* **35**, 5–23.
27. Davies, K., Nash, J., Norsworthy, P., Dell'Agnola, C., Peters, A., and Walport, M. (1997) Model immune complexes which fix complement poorly are cleared primarily in the liver in man. *Arthritis Rheum.* **40**, S163 (abstract).

28. Waxman, F. J., Hebert, L. A., Cornacoff, J. G., et al. (1984) Complement depletion accelerates the clearance of immune complexes from the circulation of primates. *J. Clin. Invest.* **67,** 1329–1340.
29. Medof, M. E. and Prince, G. M. (1983) Immune complex alterations occur in the human red blood cell membrane. *Immunology* **50,** 11–18.
30. Davies, K. A., Hird, V., Stewart, S., Sivolapenko, G. B., Jose, P., Epenetos, A. A., et al. (1990) A study of in vivo immune complex formation and clearance in man. *J. Immunol.* **144(12),** 4613–4620.
31. Frank, M. M., Lawley, T. J., Hamburger, M. I., and Brown, E. (1983) Immunoglobulin G Fc receptor-mediated clearance in autoimmune disease. *Ann. Intern. Med.* **98,** 206–218.
32. Kimberly, R. P., Parris, T. M., Inman, R. D., and McDougal, J. S. (1983) Dynamics of mononuclear phagocytes system Fc receptor function in systemic lupus erythematosus. Relation to disease activity and circulating immune complexes. *Clin. Exp. Immunol.* **51,** 261–268.
33. Van der Woude, F., Van der Giessen, M., Kallenberg, G., Ouwehand, W., Beekhuis, H., Beelan, J., et al. (1984) Reticuloendothelial Fc receptor function in SLE patients. I. Primary HLA linked defect or acquired dysfunction secondary to disease activity. *Clin. Exp. Immunol.* **55,** 473–480.
34. Lobatto, S., Daha, M., Breedveld, F., Pauwels, E., Evers-Schouten, J., Voetman, A., et al. (1988) Abnormal clearance of soluble aggregates of human immunoglobulin G in patients with systemic lupus erythematosus. *Clin. Exp. Immunol.* **72,** 55–59.
35. Halma, C., Breedveld, F., Daha, M., Blok, D., Evers-Schouten, J., Hermans, J., et al. (1991) Elimination of soluble ^{123}I-labeled aggregates of IgG in patients with systemic lupus erythematosus. Effect of serum IgG and number of erythrocyte complement receptor type I. *Arthritis Rheum.* **34,** 442–452.
36. Schifferli, J. A., Ng, Y. C., Paccaud, J.-P., and Walport, M. J. (1989) The role of hypocomplementemia and low erythrocyte complement receptor type 1 numbers in determining abnormal immune complex clearance in humans. *Clin. Exp. Immunol.* **75,** 329–335.
37. Walport, M., Ross, G., Mackworth-Young, C., Watson, J., Hogg, N., and Lachmann, P. (1985) Family studies of erythrocyte complement receptor type 1 levels: reduced levels in patients with SLE are acquired, not inherited. *Clin. Exp. Immunol.* **307,** 981–986.
38. Salmon, J. E., Millard, S., Schachter, L. A., Arnett, F. C., Ginzler, E. M., Gourley, M. F., et al. (1996) Fc gamma RIIA alleles are heritable risk factors for lupus nephritis in African Americans. *J. Clin. Invest.* **97(5),** 1348–1354.
39. Wu, J., Edberg, J. C., Redecha, P. B., Bansal, V., Guyre, P. M., Coleman, K., Salmon, J. E., and Kimberly, R. P. (1997) A novel polymorphism of FcgammaRIIIa (CD16) alters receptor function and predisposes to autoimmune disease. *J. Clin. Invest.* **100,** 1059–1070.
40. Wener, M. and Mannik, M. (1986) Mechanisms of immune deposit formation in renal glomeruli. *Semin. Immunopathol.* **9,** 219–235.
41. Couser, W. G. (1993) Pathogenesis of glomerulonephritis. *Kidney Int.* **42(Suppl.),** s19–s26.
42. Gauthier, V. J. and Mannik, M. (1990) A small proportion of cationic antibodies in immune complexes is sufficient to mediate their deposition in glomeruli. *J. Immunol.* **145,** 3348–3352.
43. Emlen, W. and Burdick, G. (1988) Clearance and organ localization of small DNA anti-DNA immune complexes in mice. *J. Immunol.* **140,** 1816–1822.
44. Finbloom, D., Magilavy, D., Hartford, J., et al. (1981) The influence of antigen on immune complex behavior in mice. *J. Clin. Invest.* **68,** 214.
45. Matsushita, M. and Fujita, T. (1992) Activation of the classical complement pathway by mannose-binding protein in association with a novel C1s-like serine protease. *J. Exp. Med.* **176,** 1497–1502.
46. Tenner, A., Robinson, S., and Ezekowitz, R. (1995) Mannose binding protein enhances mononuclear phagocytic function via a receptor that contains the 126,000 Mr component of the C1q receptor. *Immunity* **3,** 485–493.

47. Kawasaki, M., Kawasaki, T., and Yamashura, I. (1983) Isolation and characterization of a mannose-binding protein from human serum. *J. Biochem.* **94,** 937–942.
48. Sullivan, K. E., Wooten, C., Goldman, D., and Petri, M. (1996) Mannose-binding protein genetic polymorphisms in black patients with systemic lupus erythematosus. *Arthritis Rheum.* **39,** 2046–2051.
49. Davies, E. J., Snowden, N., Hillarby, M. C., Carthy, D., Grennan, D. M., Thomson, W., et al. (1995) Mannose-binding protein gene polymorphism in systemic lupus erythematosus. *Arthritis Rheum.* **38,** 110–114.
50. Davies, E. J., Teh, L. S., Ordi, R. J., Snowden, N., Hillarby, M. C., Hajeer, A., et al. (1997) A dysfunctional allele of the mannose binding protein gene associates with systemic lupus erythematosus in a Spanish population. *J. Rheumatol.* **24,** 485–488.
51. Chen, J. and Agris, P. F. (1992) Small nuclear ribonucleoprotein particles contain glycoproteins recognized by rheumatic disease-associated autoantibodies. *Lupus* **1,** 119–124.
52. Rubin, R., Tank, F., Chan, E., Pollard, K., Tsay, G., and Tan, E. (1986) IgG subclasses of autoantibodies in systemic lupus erythematosus, Sjogren's syndrome and drug-induced autoimmunity. *J. Immunol.* **137,** 2528–2534.
53. Izui, S., Berney, T., Shibata, T., and Fulpius, T. (1993) IgG3 cryoglobulins in autoimmune MRL-lpr/lpr mice: immunopathogenesis, therapeutic approaches and relevance to similar human diseases. *Ann. Rheum. Dis.* **52,** S48–S54.
54. Rifai, A. and Mannik, M. (1984) Clearance of circulating IgA immune complexes is mediated by a specific receptor on Kupffer cells in mice. *J. Exp. Med.* **160,** 125.
55. Mannik, M., Agodoa, L., and David, K. (1983) Rearrangement of immune complexes in glomeruli leads to persistence and development of electron dense deposits. *J. Exp. Med.* **157,** 1516–1528.
56. Fujigaki, Y., Nagase, M., Kojima, K., Yamamoto, T., and Hishida, A. (1997) Glomerular handling of immune complex in the acute phase of active in situ immune complex glomerulonephritis employing cationized ferritin in rats. Ultrastructural localization of immune complex, complements and inflammatory cells. *Virchows Arch.* **431,** 53–61.
57. Maddison, P. J. and Reichlin, M. (1979) Deposition of antibodies to a soluble cytoplasmic antigen in the kidneys of patients with systemic lupus erythematosus. *Arthritis Rheum.* **22,** 858.
58. Mannik, M. (1996) Presence of covalent bonds between immune deposits and other macromolecules in murine renal glomeruli. *Clin. Exp. Immunol.* **103,** 285–288.
59. Mannik, M. and Wener, M. (1997) Deposition of antibodies to the collagen-like region of C1q in renal glomeruli of patients with proliferative lupus glomerulonephritis. *Arthritis Rheum.* **8,** 1504–1511.
60. Jarvis, J. N., Wang, W., Moore, H. T., Zhao, L., and Xu, C. (1997) In vitro induction of proinflammatory cytokine secretion by juvenile rheumatoid arthritis synovial fluid immune complexes. *Arthritis Rheum.* **40,** 2039–2046; erratum: *Arthritis Rheum.* (1998) **41,** 377.
61. Quigg, R., Kozono, Y., Berthiaume, D., Lim, A., Salant, D., Weinfeld, A., et al. (1998) Blockade of antibody-induced glomerulonephritis with Crry-Ig, a soluble murine complement inhibitor. *J. Immunol.* **160,** 4553–4560.
62. He, C., Lim, A., Berthiaume, D., Alexander, J., Kraus, D., and Holers, V. (1998) Transgenic mice overexpressing the complement inhibitor crry as a soluble protein are protected from antibody-induced glomerular injury. *J. Exp. Med.* **188,** 1321–1331.
63. Milligan, M., Schmid, E., Beck-Schimmer, B., Till, G., Friedl, H., Brauer, R., et al. (1996) Requirement and role of C5a in acute lung inflammatory injury in rats. *J. Clin. Invest.* **98,** 503–512.
64. Bozic, C., Lu, B., Hopken, U., Gerard, C., and Gerard, N. (1996) Neurogenic amplification of immune complex inflammation. *Science* **273,** 1722–1725.
65. Sylvestre, D.L. and Ravetch, J. V. (1996) A dominant role for mast cell Fc receptors in the Arthus reaction. *Immunity* **5,** 387–390.

66. Clynes, R., Dumitru, C., and Ravetch, J. (1998) Uncoupling of immune complex formation and kidney damage in autoimmune glomerulonephritis. *Science* **279,** 1052–1054.
67. Yuasa, T., Kubo, S., Yoshino, T., Ujike, A., Matsumura, K., Ono, M., et al. (1999) Deletion of Fcgamma receptor IIB renders H-2(b) mice susceptible to collagen-induced arthritis. *J. Exp. Med.* **189,** 187–194.
68. Heller, T., Gessner, J., Schmidt, R., Klos, A., Gautsch, W., and Kohl, J. (1999) Cutting edge: Fc receptor type I for IgG on macrophages and complement mediate the inflammatory response in immune complex peritonitis. *J. Immunol.* **162,** 5657–5661.
69. Bhatia, A., Blades, S., Cambridge, G., and Edwards, J. C. (1998) Differential distribution of Fc gamma RIIIa in normal human tissues and co-localization with DAF and fibrillin-1: implications for immunological microenvironments. *Immunology* **94,** 56–63.
70. Timmerman, J., Van Gijlswijk-Janssen, D., Van Der Kooij, S., Van Es, L., and Daha, M. (1997) Antigen-antibody complexes enhance the production of complement component C3 by human mesangial cells. *J. Am. Soc. Nephrol.* **8,** 1257–1265.
71. Daëron, M. (1997) Fc receptor biology. *Annu. Rev. Immunol.* **15,** 203–234.
72. Marusic-Galesic, S., Pavelic, K., and Pokric, B. (1991) Cellular immune response to antigen administered as an immune complex. *Immunology* **72,** 526.
73. Lewis, E. J., Hunsicker, L. G., Lan, S. P., Rohde, R. D., and Lachin, J. M. (1992) A controlled trial of plasmapheresis therapy in severe lupus nephritis. The Lupus Nephritis Collaborative Study Group. *N. Engl. J. Med.* **326,** 1373–1379.
74. Wiesenhutter, C., Irish, B., and Bertram, J. (1994) Treatment of patients with refractory rheumatoid arthritis with extracorporeal protein A immunoadsorption columns: a pilot trial. *J. Rheumatol.* **21,** 804–812.
75. Arfors, L. and Lefvert, A. K. (1997) Enrichment of antibodies against phospholipids in circulating immune complexes (CIC) in the anti-phospholipid syndrome (APLS). *Clin. Exp. Immunol.* **108,** 47–51.
76. Pfueller, S. L. and Luscher, E. F. (1972) Review: The effects of immune complexes on blood platelets and their relationship to complement activation. *Immunochemistry* **9,** 1151–1165.
77. Vaarala, O., Alfthan, G., Jauhiainen, M., Leirisalo-Repo, M., Aho, K., and Palosuo, T. (1993) Crossreaction between antibodies to oxidized low-density lipoprotein and to cardiolipin in systemic lupus erythematosus. *Lancet* **341,** 923–925.
78. Hasunuma, Y., Matsuura, E., Makita, Z., Katahira, T., Nishi, S., and Koike, T. (1997) Involvement of β2-glycoprotein I and anticardiolipin antibodies in oxidatively modified low-density lipoprotein uptake by macrophages. *Clin. Exp. Immunol.* **107,** 569–573.
79. Puurunen, M., Manttari, M., Manninen, V., et al. (1994) Antibodies against oxidized low density lipoprotein predicting myocardial infarction. *Arch. Intern. Med.* **154,** 2605–2609.
80. Wener, M. (1997) Tests for Circulating Immune Complexes and Autoantibodies to C1q, in *Manual of Clinical Laboratory Immunology*, 5th ed. (Rose, N. R., de Macario, E. C., Folds, J. D., Lane H. C., and Nakamura, R. M., eds.), American Society of Microbiology, Washington, DC, pp. 208–216.

9
Complement

V. Michael Holers

1. Overview of the Complement System

Complement is a phylogenetically ancient system whose primary roles are to help initiate the immune response to and participate in the clearance of foreign organisms and antigens as well as ischemic and necrotic tissue (reviewed in ref. *1*). However, in humoral autoimmune states, these potent complement effector functions are inappropriately redirected at self tissues. Because of this and the desire to develop complement inhibitors that could be used as therapeutics in these disease states, understanding the specific functions of complement components is necessary.

The complement system consists of >20 proteins that are functionally divided into several categories. The first category consists of activation pathway proteins (*see* Fig. 1 and Table 1) that, together, generate the effector functions of complement described in the chapter (reviewed in ref. *2*). The second category is regulatory proteins (*see* Table 2), which are necessary to control complement activation in the fluid phases as well as on cell membranes (reviewed in refs. *3–5*). The third category is receptors (*see* Table 2) (reviewed in refs. *1* and *6–8*). Complement receptors either help to clear complement-bound targets, transmit signals upon binding of the complement coated targets to cell membranes, or are activated by low-molecular-weight anaphylatoxins C3a and C5a released during complement activation.

2. Mechanisms of Complement Activation

2.1. Classical Pathway

The complement pathway can be initiated by one of three mechanisms. The first is the classical pathway, which is initiated when complement-fixing immunoglobulin (Ig) isotypes recognize their antigens (Ags). In humans, classical pathway complement-fixing isotypes are IgM>IgG3>IgG1>IgG2>>>IgG4. The classical pathway is initiated when the hexameric heads of C1q are bound by complement-fixing isotypes in such a way that the associated C1r and C1s proteases are activated and C4 and C2 are sequentially cleaved and activated. This occurs when either two subunits of the pentameric or hexameric IgM molecules interact with the target Ag, thus generating a site for the globular heads of C1q to interact, or when two individual IgG molecules bind their epitopes in close enough proximity to form a stable C1q interaction site.

The classical pathway can also be activated in the complete absence of any antibody (Ab) directly through the actions of C-reactive protein (CRP) and serum amyloid P

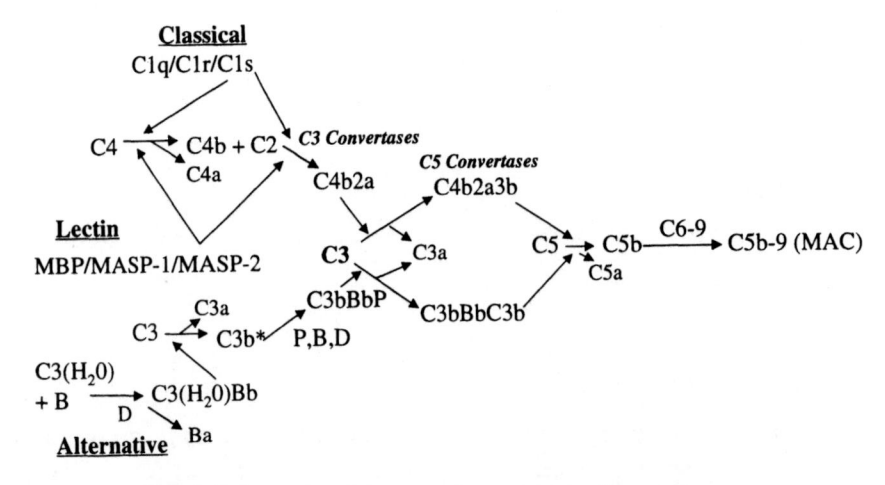

Fig. 1. Schematic of the complement activation pathways.

Table 1
Complement Activation Proteins

Component	Approximate serum conc. (µg/mL)	M_r
Classical pathway		
C1q	70	410,000
C1r	34	170,000
C1s	31	85,000
C4	600	206,000
C2	25	117,000
Alternative pathway		
D	1	24,000
C3	1,300	195,000
B	200	95,000
Lectin pathway		
MBP	150 (very wide range)	600,000
MASP-1	6	83,000
MASP-2	?	52,000
Membrane attack complex (MAC)		
C5	80	180,000
C6	60	128,000
C7	55	120,000
C8	65	150,000
C9	60	79,000

(SAP), two members of the pentraxin family (reviewed in ref. 9). Classical pathway activation occurs when either of these proteins bind nuclear constituents, such as chromatin released from necrotic or dying cells, which then allows C1 to be directly bound and the pathway activated. The classical pathway may also be activated when apoptotic bodies derived from cells directly bind C1q *(10)*.

Table 2
Complement Receptors and Regulatory Proteins

Component	Approximate serum conc. (µg/mL)	M_r
Receptors		
Complement receptor 1 (CR1, CD35)		190,000–250,000
Complement receptor 2 (CR2, CD21)		145,000
Complement receptor 3 (CD11b/CD18)		170,000 (α chain)[a]
Complement receptor 4 (CD11c/CD18)		150,000 (α chain)[a]
C1q receptor C1qR$_P$		126,000
C5a receptor (CD88)		50,000
C3a receptor		60,000
Membrane regulatory proteins		
Decay-accelerating factor (CD55)		70,000
Membrane cofactor protein (CD46)		45,000–70,000
CD59		20,000
Soluble regulatory proteins		
Positive regulation		
Properdin	25	220,000
Negative regulation		
C1-INH	200	105,000
C4BP	250	550,000
Factor H	500	150,000
Factor I	34	90,000
Anaphylatoxin inactivator (carboxypeptidase H)	35	280,000
S protein (vitronectin)	500	80,000
SP-40,40 (clusterin)	60	80,000

[a]Common 95,000 β chain.

2.2. Lectin Pathway

The lectin pathway is a recently described pathway that is initiated by the binding of mannose-binding lectin (MBL) to repeating carbohydrate moieties found primarily on the surface of pathogens (reviewed in ref. *11*). MBL is structurally similar to C1q and is physically associated with proteases called mannose-binding lectin-associated serum protease (MASP)-1 and MASP-2, which are of the same structural family and act like C1r and C1s of the classical pathway *(12,13)*. Similar to C1q, once MBL is bound to its target, MASP-1 and MASP-2 are activated. This results in the cleavage of C4 and C2 and the subsequent activation of C3, which is then followed by the assembly of the remainder of the complement pathway.

2.3. Alternative Pathway

The alternative pathway can be spontaneously activated on surfaces of pathogens that have the proper charge characteristics and do not contain complement inhibitors.

This is due to a process termed "tickover" of C3 that occurs spontaneously and results in the fixation of active C3b on pathogens or other surfaces even in the absence of antibody (reviewed in ref. 2). The alternative pathway can, however, also be initiated by IgA isotype Ab-containing immune complexes, which are found in several human diseases. In addition, activation of the alternative pathway is strongly promoted by substances such as repeating polysaccharides, endotoxin, virally infected cells, yeast cell-wall extracts (zymosan), and cobra venom factor that either present a surface free of regulators or actively exclude serum-regulatory proteins. The alternative pathway is also engaged in a mechanism termed the "amplification loop" (*see* Fig. 1 showing C3b) when C3b is deposited via the classical pathway. Certain autoantibodies, termed C3 nephritic factors (C3Nef), occasionally found in patients also greatly enhance activation of the alternative pathway because they function to stabilize the C3 convertase C3bBbP and do not allow it to spontaneously decay at a normal rate.

2.4. Additional Activation Mechanisms

Other less well-characterized mechanisms underlie activation of complement by biopolymers such as those used in cardiopulmonary bypass and hemodialysis. In addition, several bypass pathways have been described that allow low-level activation of downstream components in the setting of complete C2, C3, or C4 deficiencies.

2.5. Subsequent Activation Steps

The major focus of complement activation is on the C3 protein, as this is the first point at which all three pathways converge. During this process, C4b and C3b become covalently attached to the target or, in the case of C3b, to C4b itself. This "irreversible" marking is possible because these two proteins contain a thioester bond. Lysis of this bond during complement activation allows each of the proteins to form physiologically irreversible ester or amide linkages with target molecules. Subsequent to this step, C5 convertases are formed and C5 is cleaved to C5b and C5a. The membrane attack complex (MAC) is then assembled as C6, C7, C8, and C9 are sequentially added. During this process, the MAC generates hydrophobic patches and can progressively insert itself into an available target membrane or, alternately, is inactivated and becomes a soluble protein complex.

3. Immunobiology of Complement Receptors

3.1. C1q Receptors

C1q that is free of C1r and C1s can interact with a multitude of cell types and has been reported to enhance phagocytosis by polymorphonuclear cell (PMN) and macrophages, increase oxygen radical generation by PMN through a CD18-dependent mechanism, activate platelets, promote Ig production by Staph aureus cowan (SAC)-activated B-cells, and facilitate PMN–endothelial cell binding by increasing E-selectin, ICAM-1 and VCAM-1 expression (reviewed in ref. *11*).

Four receptors for C1q have been described that interact with this protein and other members of the collectin family of which C1q is a member (reviewed in ref. *11*). However, currently only two of the four are believed to actually function as transmembrane receptors. These are C1q receptor-related protein C1qR$_P$ (Table 2) *(14)* and complement receptor type 1 (*see* Subheading 3.2.) *(15)*. Two other "C1q receptors" have been found to be encoded by proteins that are primarily intracellular and, therefore, their contribution to the phenotypic effects described earlier is unclear. Although not yet proven, it is widely thought that other C1q receptors exist and that only some of the members of this family are currently known.

The 126 kD C1qR$_P$ receptor, designated by C1qR$_P$ to reflect its phagocytosis enhancement function, is expressed on myeloid cells (neutrophils and monocytes/macrophages), endothelial cells and platelets. The receptor interacts with C1q collagenlike tails and is physically associated with the more widely distributed molecule CD43, although the functional relevance of this association is not yet known. C1qR$_P$ also binds other collectin family members MBL and SPA. This C1q receptor plays an important functional role by enhancing Fc receptor and complement receptor type 1 (CR1)-mediated phagocytosis. In addition, on endothelial cells, it is apparently involved in the upregulation of adhesion molecules on these cells after interaction with C1q-containing immune complexes.

3.2. Complement Receptor Type 1

Once C3b is bound to a target, it is sequentially cleaved by factor I to the forms iC3b and C3d,g. Like C3b, these forms remain attached to the target through the ester or amide linkage derived from the thiolester bond. CR1 is a relatively widely distributed and clinically important complement receptor (reviewed in ref. 6). CR1 efficiently binds the C3b form in addition to the C4b form of C4, and it has a lower affinity for the iC3b form of C3. As described, CR1 has also been reported to serve as a C1q receptor. In addition to its direct ligand binding, CR1 also exhibits two complement regulatory enzymatic activities. These activities are cofactor activity for factor I-dependent cleavage of C3b and C4b and decay acceleration of the classical and alternative complement pathways.

The structure of CR1 consists of a linear series of structurally related modules designated short consensus repeats (SCR) followed by a transmembrane and short intracytoplasmic domain. SCR-containing proteins such as CR1 are part of a gene family designated the regulators of complement activation (RCA) found on human chromosome 1q3.2 (reviewed in ref. 16). CR1 has four polymorphic structural variants that are believed to vary in size by the inclusion or exclusion of seven-SCR-containing elements called long homologous repeats (LHR). C4b interacts with the most amino-terminal LHR in SCRs 1–4, and C3b interacts with comparable sites in the second and third LHR. This presumably allows the same CR1 molecule to interact with either two to three ligands on the same immune complex or with two individual complexes, thus facilitating the overall interaction of these complexes with cells.

Complement receptor type 1 is expressed on erythrocytes, B-cells, a subset of peripheral T-cells (approx 15%), thymocytes (approx 25%), monocytes, macrophages, neutrophils, follicular dendritic cells (FDCs), eosinophils, glomerular podocytes, and liver Kuppfer cells. Two soluble forms of the molecule have been described. One is in the serum and is believed to be released by proteolytic processing of membrane-bound CR1 from leukocytes; the other soluble form is found in urine and is believed to be released from glomerular podocytes.

Complement receptor type 1 has a number of biologic roles. Erythrocyte CR1 binds large circulating immune complexes that have fixed complement and transports them to the liver and spleen for further processing. CR1 on monocytes, macrophages, and neutrophils promotes the phagocytosis of C3-bound targets. CR1 on FDCs is believed to play a role in the trapping of immune complexes within germinal centers in lymphoid organs, and CR1 on B-cells promotes B-cell activation in addition to facilitating antigen binding and presentation to T-cells. CR1 molecules on erythrocytes are primarily found in clusters, a situation that likely facilitates its role in clearing C3b-bound immune complexes.

Erythrocyte CR1 has also been found to be the polymorphic variant defined by the Knops/McCoy/Swain–Langley/York blood group antigens. In addition, a 6.9-kb *Hin*dIII RFLP has been described that correlates with the levels of expression of erythrocyte CR1 and is believed to mark a genetic element that controls receptor levels on this cell type.

3.3. Complement Receptor Type 2

Complement receptor type 2 (CR2) binds C3d and iC3b forms of C3 and interacts less well with the C3b form (reviewed in refs. *6* and *17*). CR2 is also the Epstein–Barr virus (EBV) receptor and mediates EBV infection and immortalization of B-cells through its interactions with the EBV surface protein gp350/220. Recent studies have also shown that CR2 is a receptor for the important immunomodulatory protein CD23.

Like CR1, CR2 is a member of the RCA family, and its structure consists of a linear series of 15–16 SCRs followed by transmembrane and short intracytoplasmic domains. CR2 mRNA encodes two protein forms that vary by the inclusion or exclusion of a single SCR that is the result of alternative splicing in the CR2 gene; however, this form has an identical affinity for C3d,g and its biologic significance is unknown.

Complement receptor type 2 is expressed on mature B lymphocytes, FDC, a small subset of peripheral T cells, early thymocytes, basophils, keratinocytes, and many types of epithelial cells (nasopharyngeal, oropharyngeal, cervical, lacrimal, and ocular surface). Marginal-zone B-cells express higher levels of CR2, whereas T-cells express approximately one-tenth of normal B-cell levels. A soluble form of CR2 has been detected in serum that is likely shed from the cell surface.

Complement receptor type 2 has a number of biologic roles. On B-cells, CR2 interaction with C3d or mAb mimics promotes B-cell activation by increasing proliferation, Ca_i^{2+}, and c-*fos* mRNA. CR2 associates on B cell membranes with CD19, TAPA-1 (CD81), and Leu-13. It is believed that the association with CD19, itself a potent activating molecule closely linked to B cell membrane IgM Ag receptors, mediates the major effects of CR2 ligation. CR2 also independently associates on the membrane with CR1. CD23 interacts with CR2 to increase production of IgE, rescue germinal center B-cells from apoptosis, and promote T : B-cell adhesion in addition to T-cell activation by B-cell antigen presenting cells. FDC CR2 helps to trap antigen-bearing immune complexes in germinal centers.

3.4. Complement Receptor type 3 and type 4

Complement receptor type 3 (CR3) is a receptor with a rank-order ligand binding of iC3b > C3b > C3d, whereas complement receptor type 4 (CR4) is a receptor with an order of iC3b > C3b (Table 2) (reviewed in ref. *7*). CR3 has many additional ligands, including ICAM-1, factor X, and fibrinogen, among others. CR3 also mediates adherence to plastic and many types of clinically used biomaterials. CR3 and CR4 are members of the integrin family and share common β chains of the β2 form. CR3 and CR4 are expressed on neutrophils, monocytes, macrophages, FDC, a subset of lymphocytes, and eosinophils.

Complement receptor type 3 mediates phagocytosis of C3-bound particles by neutrophils and macrophages, co-associates with Fc receptors on neutrophils, stimulates the respiratory burst and platelet-activating factor (PAF) release in eosinophils, and is physically linked to the cytoskeleton. Of interest, the adhesive characteristics of CR3 are modulated by the interaction of other surface receptors such as ELAM-1 with their ligands, a process known as molecular crosstalk.

3.5. C5a and C3a Receptors

C5a is a potent 74 amino acid fragment of C5 that is released upon activation by the C5 convertases (Fig. 1) (reviewed in ref. 8). C5a, along with the other two anaphylatoxins C3a and C4a, exerts many biologic effects. The C5a receptor is an approx 50 kD transmembrane-spanning protein of the rhodopsin gene family. The C5a receptor is expressed on a variety of cell types, including neutrophils, monocytes, macrophages, eosinophils, subsets of mast cells, hepatocytes, lung vascular smooth-muscle cells, bronchial and alveolar epithelial cells, vascular endothelium, and astrocytes.

The C3a receptor is structurally related to the C5a receptor and is expressed on neutrophils, monocytes, and basophils, in addition to other less well-characterized populations (18). Like the C5a receptor, the C3a receptor is physically associated in the membrane with GTP-binding proteins and exerts its cell-activating effects through pathways involving tyrosine phosphorylation and MAP kinases.

The biologic effects of C4a are less pronounced than C5a or C3a, and the C4a receptor is even less well characterized in humans. Recent studies have suggested that it is expressed on monocytes and causes the release of a protein that inhibits chemotaxis.

3.6. Other Complement Receptors

Reports of receptors for Ba, Bb, factor H, and several other fragments of complement have been published. However, the molecular nature of the receptors is not yet known.

4. Pro-inflammatory and Immunoregulatory Activities of Complement

4.1. Effects of the MAC on Cells

The MAC has two major functions; the first is to lyse or inactivate pathogens that have cell membranes into which the MAC inserts, or to lyse nonnucleated cells such as erythrocytes. The second major function is to act as a signal transducing complex that results in cell activation (reviewed in ref. 5). One outcome of MAC insertion is the initiation of a repair process that attempts to remove the complexes by vesiculation and endocytosis. MAC binding also activates several signal transduction pathways, resulting in increases of arachidonic acid mobilization, generation of diacyl glyceride and ceramide, and activation of protein kinase C, MAP kinases, and Ras. Pro-inflammatory and tissue-damaging phenotypic outcomes following these signaling events include cell proliferation as well as the release of reactive oxygen intermediates, leukotrienes, thromboxane, basic fibroblast growth factor (bFGF), platelet-derived growth factor (PDGF), von Willbrand factor, and GMP-140.

Support for the concept that the MAC plays a major role in human diseases has come from the finding of the MAC (measured by the identification of a neoepitope present only on the intact C5b-9 complex) in relevant tissue sites of neuromuscular diseases such as multiple sclerosis, rheumatoid arthritis, and many forms of glomerulonephritis, including lupus nephritis (reviewed in ref. *4*). Soluble MAC (sC5b-9) has also been identified in many fluids, including urine, in association with complement activation and active inflammation within the tissue of origin.

4.2. Chemotaxis and Inflammatory Cell Activation

The biologic effects of C5a and other anaphylatoxins (in a general order of potency C5a > C3a > C4a) include leukocyte chemotaxis, aggregation of neutrophils and platelets, smooth-muscle contraction, increases in capillary permeability, release of cytokines (such as IL-6, IL-8, and IL-1), generation of leukotrienes and reactive oxygen intermediates, and increased neutrophil–endothelial cell adhesion. The C5aR has been shown to be expressed on hepatic parenchymal cells and mediate changes in acute-phase protein production.

4.3. Phagocytosis

The receptors CR1, CR3, and CR4 play central roles in the clearance of targets by phagocytosis in neutrophils and macrophages (reviewed in ref. *7*). CR3, in particular, is also centrally important as an adhesion receptor whose expression is required for many other phagocytic cell functions.

4.4. Regulation of Humoral Immunity

Recent studies using mice in which the C3 and C4 genes have been inactivated using the "knockout" technique have reinforced the concept that a normal complement pathway is absolutely required for the generation of a normal humoral immune response to T-dependent antigens *(19)*. C3 and C4 act in this fashion in mice via CR2 and CR1 found on B-cells and FDCs, and recent studies have shown that CR2 and CR1 expression is also required in vivo for generation of a normal immune response to T-dependent antigens as well as a robust germinal center phenotype *(20,21)*.

4.5. Other Roles of Complement

As discussed later, complete deficiencies of complement components C1, C4, or C2 strongly promote the development of systemic lupus erythematosus (SLE). Although the basis for this is unclear, recent studies have suggested that CR2 and the C4 component may also play a role in maintaining tolerance to self antigens. The mechanisms proposed are either related to antigen capture in the bone marrow or to enhancing signaling of self-reactive B-cells that normally results in deletion *(22)*. Thus, these results strongly suggest that the early components of the classical complement pathway also play a protective role against the development of autoreactivity.

5. Natural Inhibitors of Complement Activation

Because of the nature of the activation mechanisms, especially the alternative pathway, which allow for a rapid enzymatic amplification of complement, the pathway is tightly controlled by a series of regulatory proteins (Table 2). These proteins are found in the circulation, on cell membranes, and in the interstitial spaces (reviewed in ref. *3*).

Their importance is highlighted by several human diseases caused by genetic deficiencies of inhibitory proteins.

5.1. Membrane Inhibitors

There are two primary classes of intrinsic membrane inhibitors. One is demonstrated by CD59, a glycolipid-anchored protein that acts to block both the initial insertion of C9 into the MAC as well as the subsequent polymerization of C9 (reviewed in ref. *23*). CD59 is a widely distributed protein that is found on the vast majority of cells.

A second class of intrinsic inhibitors is directed at the centrally important step of C3 activation. These proteins include decay-accelerating factor (DAF, CD55) and membrane cofactor protein (MCP, CD46). These proteins act to either dissociate the alternative and classical pathway C3 and C5 convertases (DAF) or to act as a cofactor for serum factor I-mediated cleavage and inactivation of C3b and C4b (MCP). DAF is also glycolipid anchored, whereas MCP is a type I transmembrane protein with alternatively spliced intracytoplasmic sequences. Both proteins have membrane proximal regions with heavy O-glycosylation that contribute to their function. Both are also widely distributed and expressed on almost all cells, with the notable exception that MCP is absent from erythrocytes.

Both DAF and MCP are part of a large family of receptor and regulatory proteins designated the Regulators of Complement Activation (RCA) (Figure 2). This family also includes CR1, CR2, factor H, and the C4-binding protein (C4-bp). These proteins all interact with C3 and/or C4 and are built of a repeating structural motif called a short consensus repeat (SCR). In this regard, CR1 can also serve as an intrinsic regulator and block complement activation using both decay-accelerating and cofactor functions.

The relative importance of these membrane inhibitors is demonstrated by the illness paroxysmal nocturnal hemoglobinuria (PNH). PNH is caused by an acquired somatic cell defect in the biosynthesis of the glycolipid anchor. Patients develop clones of hematopoietically derived cells that lack both CD59 and DAF and present with waves of recurrent hemolysis. Some patients also develop myeloproliferative disorders, but the mechanism is unknown.

5.2. Serum Inhibitors

A centrally important serum complement inhibitor is C1-INH, which is a suicide inactivator of C1r and C1s (reviewed in ref. *24*). Once these proteases are generated, C1-INH binds, inactivates, and restricts their range of activity to the local environment. The importance of C1-INH and its maintenance at a critical level is shown by the phenotype of patients with hereditary angioedema (HAE). These patients have only a heterozygous deficiency, usually with one nonfunctional allele, but exhibit life-threatening angioedema because of the relatively unchecked low-level activation of the classical pathway. This demonstrates the very tight control under which the classical pathway must exist to function normally. Some patients demonstrate an interesting phenomenon of trans-suppression as C1-INH levels are below even that predicted by the heterozygous state. As no individuals who are completely deficient have been described, it is likely that this particular situation is lethal *in utero*.

Factor H and C4-bp are two members of the RCA family that are inhibitors of C3 and C4 activation, respectively. Each is a large protein that has multiple binding sites

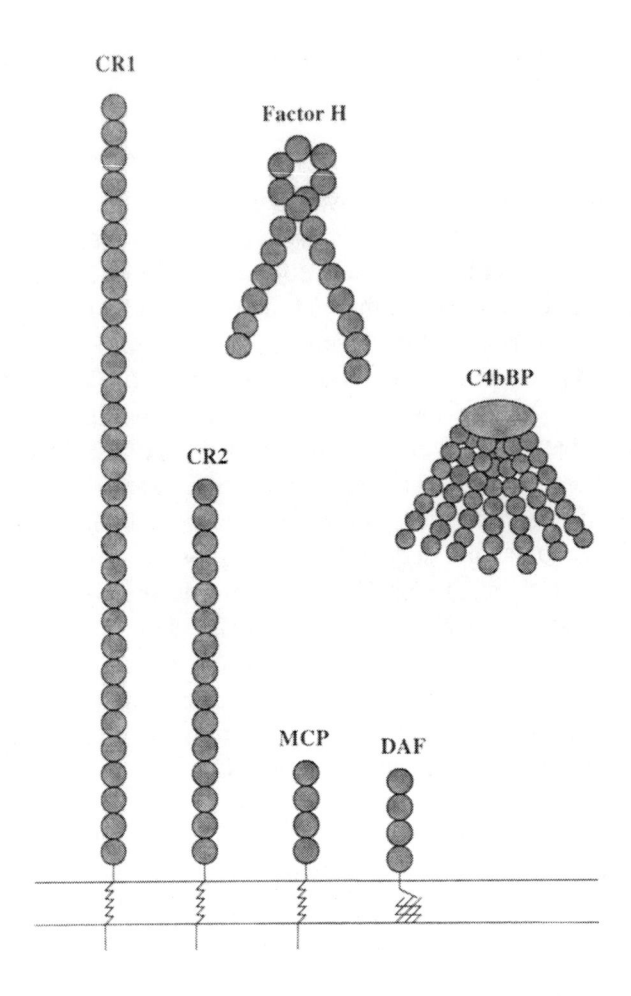

Fig. 2. Schematic diagram of the RCA family members.

and serves as both a decay accelerator and a factor I cofactor for their respective target proteins. These functions allow them, like DAF and MCP, to blocks subsequent activation of the complement pathway.

Factor I is a serum protease with high specificity for C3b and C4b when in the presence of cofactors described above. Factor I can act on C3 and C5 convertases present either in the fluid phase or on cell membranes. Carboxypeptidase H is a serum protein that acts to cleave the carboxy-terminal arginine from C3a and C5a, which inactivates these proteins. S protein and clusterin interact with the MAC and block membrane insertion, thus inactivating this complex.

6. Complement and Human Disease

6.1. Complement and Protection from Infection

A major role of complement is in the protection from infection by pathogens, especially bacteria. This role is especially evident when one examines patients with complement deficiencies (reviewed in ref. 25). Deficiencies of mannose-binding lectin are associated with recurrent childhood infections. Deficiencies of early classical pathway components C1-C4, in addition to predisposing to a SLE-like illness, result in increased susceptibility to many bacterial pathogens, including staphylococcal and streptococcal infections. Also prominent are recurrent Neisserial infections, predominantly in individuals with deficiencies of MAC components but also in patients lacking C2, factor D, or properdin. Further evidence in support of a role for complement has been shown in mouse models where activation of complement by natural Ab has been shown to play a critical role in the protective response to both endotoxin and bacterial pathogens (reviewed in ref. 26).

The necessary role of complement in protecting from infection is also supported by the analysis of individuals with CR3 and CR4 deficiency as part of the disease leukocyte adhesion deficiency (LAD). The deficiency is caused by a number of different mutations within the common β chain and commonly presents with recurrent bacterial infections because of diminished neutrophil activity.

6.2. Complement and Innate Immunity

Complement is now viewed as a major link between the innate immune system, which is an evolutionarily ancient system, to acquired immunity that is provided by T- and B-lymphocytes (27). Acquired immunity is found in vertebrates, whereas complement components and other "pattern recognition" systems of innate immunity are found much earlier in evolution. Complement can be activated in the absence of acquired immunity by mechanisms such as MBL, which itself is a member of an evolutionarily ancient lectin system, as well as the alternative pathway and pentraxins. Some authors include natural IgM Ab as a component of innate immunity, and it is clear from many studies that complement activation is required for the activities of natural Ab. Strong evidence in support of a major role for complement in initiating and propagating the acquired humoral immune system is shown by studies in which mice lacking C4 or C3 demonstrate marked deficiencies in humoral immunity because of a lack of ligation of CR1 and CR2 on lymphocytes (26).

6.3. Complement in Inflammatory and Autoimmune Diseases

Protection from pathogens is a protective and appropriate role for such a potent pathway as complement. However, the complement pathway is often co-opted when humoral, and likely cellular, autoimmunity develops. In this situation, complement-fixing Ig isotypes are directed to self Ags, or immune complexes deposit in sites such as the glomerulus. When these Ig molecules interact with their Ags, C1q is "normally" activated, and the same mechanisms used to attack and inactive pathogens are instead directed at self tissues.

There is strong evidence for a pathogenic role of complement in glomerulopathies, including lupus nephritis, in inflammatory arthritis such as rheumatoid arthritis (RA) and in many other diseases characterized by tissue-specific autoantibodies. With regard to lupus nephritis, the finding of C3 and the C5b-9 MAC in association with glomerular immune deposits and the observations that nephritogenic Abs typically are complement-fixing IgG isotypes support the concept that complement contributes to glomerulonephritis. Patients with active lupus nephritis demonstrate alterations of the complement system typical of chronic activation in vivo (reviewed in ref. 28). Total C3 and C4 serum levels are typically decreased below the normal level, and mean levels of other components such as C1q and C2 are diminished. Serum levels of specific activation fragments are also increased. This includes C4d, C3d and C3c (the fragment of iC3b released when C3d is proteolytically generated), the anaphylatoxins C3a and C5a, Ba and Bb, and the soluble form of the C5b-9 MAC (sC5b-9). Urinary levels of activation fragments such as C3d and sC5b-9 are also increased, likely reflecting local inflammatory disease.

Given this pattern, it is likely that the complement system is activated *in situ* in the glomerulus by immune complexes. Both the classical and alternative pathways contribute to the activation of the MAC in the glomerulus, the classical pathway through immune complexes containing IgM and IgG isotypes, and the alternative pathway through IgA-containing immune complexes and the amplification pathway.

In addition to these changes of complement fragments reflecting activation, changes in complement receptors are also common. CR1 levels on the erythrocytes of patients with SLE have been shown to be substantially decreased. This decrease is believed to lead to abnormal in vivo immune-complex processing in these patients and increased deposition of circulating complexes in the kidney and lung. The decrease in CR1 is believed to be primarily acquired and the result of elevated levels of circulating complexes promoting receptor loss in the reticuloendothelial system, although this point is still controversial. Rare patients with SLE have autoantibodies that interfere with CR1 functions. In patients with SLE, B-cell and neutrophil CR1 levels are also decreased, as are B-cell CR2 levels.

In patients with RA, synovial fluid levels of complement activation fragments such as C5a are also markedly increased. Synovial fluid neutrophils also demonstrate increased CR1 levels consistent with their activated state. Support for a critical role of complement in tissue injury is provided by animal models of RA in which inhibition of complement at the C3 or C5 activation steps blocks the development of inflammatory arthritis.

Substantial experimental and clinical data also support a role for complement in the pathogenesis of other tissue- or organ-specific diseases such as hemolytic anemia, immune thrombocytopenia, and blistering diseases such as pemphigus. In addition, although diseases such as multiple sclerosis and type I diabetes are traditionally viewed as cellular immune diseases, some experiments in murine models suggest that complement may plan an important effector role in tissue damage.

6.4. Complement and Self Tolerance

Although much evidence supports a role for complement in tissue injury in patients with SLE, other observations regarding this disease illustrate that the situation is more complex and that complement activation cannot be considered as simply and only leading to tissue injury. For instance, an SLE-like syndrome, with loss of tolerance manifested by high levels of autoantibodies, is found in patients with relatively rare inherited complete deficiencies of early classical pathway components such as C1 (C1q or C1r/C1s), C4 or C2 *(29)*, as well as in mice with C1q deficiency *(30)*. The incidence of SLE-like disease is higher in C1 deficiency than C4 or C2 deficiency. Although the reasons for these associations are not fully understood and the renal disease in these patients and mice is less severe, these observations have cast some doubt on the importance of classical complement activation as only important in promoting tissue injury in SLE. However, even in these settings, there is abundant alternative pathway complement pathway activation resulting in C5a generation and deposition of C5b-9. Therefore, these latter components still have the capacity to contribute to tissue injury. Support for this is demonstrated by results in mouse models of SLE where treatment with an inhibitory anti-C5 mAb ameliorates disease. Thus, it is possible that inhibition of later MAC function would be protective while earlier components also have a role in maintaining self tolerance that should not be blocked as part of a therapeutic strategy.

6.5. Complement in Ischemia-Reperfusion Injury

Many studies have demonstrated that ischemia-reperfusion injury is at least in part complement mediated *(26)*. This injury occurs when vessels are occluded by injury or thrombosis, or in the setting of cardiopulmonary bypass where the myocardium is ischemic and complement is activated by both endothelium and biopolymers in the oxygenator membrane. Complement is activated by vessel walls because natural IgM Abs react with neoepitopes that are revealed on ischemic endothelium. One source of natural Ab is the $CD5^+$ B-cell subset, but the molecular nature of the neoepitopes is unknown.

6.6. Transplantation and Complement

Complement is a major effector mechanism that limits the success of transplantation. The best evidence of this is found in the hyperacute rejection that follows discordant xenotransplantion with vascularized porcine organs into primates. This rejection occurs in minutes and is accompanied by rapid complement activation, thrombosis, and ischemic death of the organ. In an attempt to remedy this situation, transgenic pigs expressing membrane forms of human DAF, MCP, and CD59 in the transplanted organ have been created. Proof of the role of complement is shown by findings that organs transplanted from these pigs no longer undergo hyperacute rejection.

Whether complement plays a role in failure of allograft transplantation, nonvascularized tissue transplants or in accelerated atherosclerosis that is often found in long-term allografts is unknown, but ongoing studies in murine models should provide important insights into these questions.

6.7. Other Diseases with Possible Complement Roles

In clinically important diseases such as atherosclerosis, complement activation fragments are typically found. Atherosclerotic lesions are characterized by macrophage infiltration, and whether complement activation promotes this in an injurious manner is currently not known.

An additional important illness with a strong potential complement link is Alzheimer's disease *(31)*. In this situation, plaques contain classical and alternative pathway components as well as the MAC. β-amyloid protein can activate in vitro both the classical and alternative pathways in an Ab-independent manner. Again, though, whether this is injurious or an appropriate response to tissue injury is unclear.

6.8. Reproduction

Because the developing fetus is semiallogeneic, a humoral immune response is commonly detected. Membrane complement regulatory proteins are highly expressed at the maternal–fetal interface (reviewed in ref. *32*). Because of this, it is likely that these proteins provide a protective barrier against maternal allo-antibodies directed against the fetus. Whether these regulatory proteins also provide protection against other Ab mediated fetal loss syndromes is currently unknown but is under investigation.

6.9. HIV Infection and Complement

The receptor CR1 on T-cells and thymocytes can interact with complement-opsonized HIV, resulting in CD4-independent infection of these cells (reviewed in ref. *33*). As complement has been shown to be essential for HIV binding to FDC in germinal centers, CR1 may also play an essential role in the retention of HIV in lymph nodes. Other studies have shown that CR2 can mediate complement C3-coated HIV infection of B cells in a CD4-independent manner and, like CR1, may be involved in the complement-dependent binding of HIV to FDC in germinal centers. In addition, CR2 levels are also depressed when cells are infected in vitro with HIV, and patients with HIV demonstrate decreased B cell CR2 levels. Finally, gp120 has been shown to be a complement activator, and HIV-1 itself takes up membrane complement regulatory proteins when it buds from cells. Thus, this virus has many interactions with the complement system.

6.10. Complement Components Acting as Pathogen Receptors

Finally, the complement system is notable because several clinically important pathogens utilize complement proteins as receptors. This includes the Epstein–Barr virus, which utilizes CR2 to infect cells, and the measles virus, which utilizes MCP. DAF is a receptor for several echo viruses, and CR1 is used as a portal of entry by several C3b-coated pathogens.

7. Summary

As discussed in Chapter 30, complement inhibitors are currently under development. As outlined herein in this chapter, the range of potential therapeutic targets is broad, including SLE, RA, ischemia–reperfusion injury, and, most, if not all, autoantibody-mediated diseases. It is very likely that the first complement inhibitors will soon enter the therapeutic arena. These are exciting possibilities, but hopes are tempered by the known role of complement in protection from infection and the potential to alter self tolerance mechanisms when early classical pathway components are blocked.

References

1. Holers, V. M. (1995) Complement, in Principles and *Practices of Clinical Immunology* (Rich, R., ed.), Mosby, St. Louis, MO, pp. 363–391.
2. Muller-Eberhard, H. J. (1988) Molecular organization and function of the complement system. *Annu. Rev. Biochem.* **57,** 321–347.
3. Liszewski, M. K., Farries, T. C., Lublin, D. M., Rooney, I. A., and Atkinson, J. P. (1996) Control of the complement system. *Adv. Immunol.* **61,** 201–283.
4. Morgan, B. P. (1992) Effects of the membrane attack complex of complement on nucleated cells. *Curr. Topics Microbiol. Immunol.* **178,** 115–140.
5. Shin, M. L., Rus, H. G., and Nicolescu, F. I. (1996) Membrane attack by complement: assembly and biology of terminal complement complexes. *Biomembranes* **4,** 123–149.
6. Ahearn, J. M. and Fearon, D. T. (1989) Structure and function of the complement receptors, CR1 (CD35) and CR2 (CD21). *Adv. Immunol.* **46,** 183–219.

7. Brown, E. J. (1991) Complement receptors and phagocytosis. *Curr. Opin. Immunol.* **3,** 76–82.
8. Wetsel, R. A. (1995) Structure, function and cellular expression of complement anaphylatoxin receptors. *Curr. Opin. Immunol.* **7,** 48–53.
9. Gewurz, H., Zhang, X.-H., and Lint, T. F. (1996) Structure and function of the pentraxins. *Curr. Opin. Immunol.* **7,** 54–64.
10. Korb, L. C. and Ahearn, J. M. (1997) C1q binds directly and specifically to surface blebs of apoptotic human keratinocytes. *J. Immunol.* **158,** 4525–4528.
11. Reid, K. B. M. and Turner, M. W. (1994) Mammalian lectins in activation and clearance mechanisms involving the complement system. *Springer Semin. Immunopathol.* **15,** 307–325.
12. Matsushita, M. and Fujita, T. (1992) Activation of the classical complement pathway by mannose-binding protein in association with a novel C1s-like serine protease. *J. Exp. Med.* **176,** 1497–1502.
13. Thiel, S., Vorup-Jensen, T., Stover, C. M., Schwaeble, W., Laursen, S. B., Poulsen, K., et al. (1997) A second serine protease associated with mannan-binding lectin that activates complement. *Nature* **386,** 506–510.
14. Nepomuceno, R. R., Henschen-Edman, A. H., Burgess, W. H., and Tenner, A. J. (1997) cDNA cloning and primary structure analysis of C1qR(P), the human C1q/MBL/SPA receptor that mediates enhanced phagocytosis in vitro. *Immunity* **6,** 119–129.
15. Klickstein, L. B., Barbashov, S. F., Nicholson-Weller, A., Liu, T., and Jack, R. M. (1997) Complement receptor type 1 (CR1, CD35) is a receptor for C1q. *Immunity* **7,** 345–355.
16. Hourcade, D., Holers, V. M., and Atkinson, J. P. (1989) The regulators of complement activation (RCA) gene cluster. *Adv. Immunol.* **45,** 381–416.
17. Cooper, N. R., Moore, M. D., and Nemerow, G. R. (1988) Immunobiology of CR2, the B lymphocyte receptor for Epstein-Barr virus and the C3d complement fragment. *Annu. Rev. Immunol.* **6,** 85–113.
18. Martin, U., Bock, D., Arseniev, L., Tornetta, M. A., Ames, R. S., Bautsch, W., et al. (1997) The human C3a receptor is expressed on neutrophils and monocytes, but not on B or T lymphocytes. *J. Exp. Med.* **186,** 199–207.
19. Fischer, M. B., Ma, M., Goerg, S., Zhou, X., Xia, J., Finco, O., et al. (1996) Regulation of the B cell response to T-dependent antigens by classical pathway of complement. *J. Immunol.* **157,** 549–556.
20. Ahearn, J. M., Fischer, M. B., Croix, D. A., Georg, S., Ma, M., Xia, J., et al. (1996) Disruption of the *Cr2* locus results in a reduction in B-1a cells and in an impaired B cell response to T-dependent antigen. *Immunity* **4,** 251–262.
21. Molina, H., Holers, V. M., Li, B., Fang, Y.-F., Mariathasan, S., Goellner, F., et al. (1996) Markedly impaired humoral immune response in mice deficient in complement receptors 1 and 2. *Proc. Natl. Acad. Sci. USA* **93,** 3357–3361.
22. Prodeus, A., Goerg, S., Shen, L.-M., Pozdnyakova, O. O., Chu, L., Alicot, E. M., et al. (1998) A critical role for complement in maintenance of self-tolerance. *Immunity* **9,** 721–731.
23. Morgan, B. P. and Meri, S. (1994) Membrane proteins that protect against complement lysis. *Springer Semin. Immunopathol.* **15,** 369–396.
24. Davis, A.E. (1988) C1 inhibitor and hereditary angioedema. *Annu. Rev. Immunol.* **6,** 595–628.
25. Figueroa, J. E. and Densen, P. (1991) Infectious diseases associated with complement deficiencies. *Clin. Microbiol. Rev.* **4,** 359–395.
26. Carroll, M. C. (1998) The role of complement and complement receptors in the induction and regulation of immunity. *Annu. Rev. Immunol.* **16,** 545–568.
27. Fearon, D. T. and Locksley, R. M. (1996) The instructive role of innate immunity in the acquired immune response. *Science* **272,** 50–54.
28. Dalmasso, A. P. (1986) Complement in the pathophysiology and diagnosis of human diseases. *CRC Crit. Rev. Clin. Lab. Sci.* **24,** 123–183.

29. Arnett, F. C. (1992) Genetic aspects of human lupus. *Clin. Immunol. Immunopathol.* **63,** 4–6.
30. Botto, M., Dell'Agnola, C., Bygrave, A. E., Thompson, E. M., Cook, H. T., Petry, F., et al. (1998) Homozygous C1q deficiency causes glomerulonephritis associated with multiple apoptotic bodies. *Nature Genet.* **19,** 56–59.
31. Bradt, B. M., Kolb, W. P., and Cooper, N. R. (1998) Complement-dependent pro-inflammatory properties of the Alzheimer's Disease beta peptide. *J. Exp. Med.* **188,** 431–438.
32. Rooney, I. A, Oglesby, T. J., and Atkinson, J. P. (1993) Complement in human reproduction: activation and control. *Immunol. Res.* **12,** 276–294.
33. Dierich, M. P., Ebenbichler, C. F., Marschang, P., Fust, G., Thielens, N. M., and Arlaud, G. J. (1993) HIV and human complement: mechanisms of interaction and biological implication. *Immunol. Today* **14,** 435–440.

10
Eicosanoids and Other Bioactive Lipids

Leslie J. Crofford

1. Introduction

The eicosanoids are a group of compounds derived from the 20 carbon-containing polyunsaturated fatty acid, arachidonic acid (AA) (Fig. 1). The most abundant members of this group of compounds are the prostaglandins (PGs) and leukotrienes (LTs). Eicosanoids were first recognized in the 1930s as the substance in semen that caused contraction of smooth muscle, hence the name "prostaglandin." The structures of the compounds were not identified for another 30 yr, and the biosynthetic pathways were described shortly thereafter *(1)*. The critical importance of PG to inflammatory processes became evident in 1971 when Vane and his co-workers discovered that aspirin and other nonsteroidal anti-inflammatory drugs (NSAIDs) worked by inhibiting the production of PG. The mechanism by which this occurs is through inhibition of cyclooxygenase (COX, PGH synthase), the first enzyme in the committed pathway for prostanoid synthesis *(2)*. The understanding that inhibition of PG synthesis was responsible for the anti-inflammatory, antipyretic, and analgesic effects of NSAIDs was accompanied by the recognition that the common side effects of this class of drugs (gastric ulceration, bleeding, and renal dysfunction) were mechanism based; that is, both the therapeutic effects and the side effects of NSAIDs were the result of inhibition of prostanoid biosynthesis. The duality of PGs as mediators of both physiologic and pathologic functions was clarified when two different isoforms of COX, COX-1 and COX-2, were identified using molecular techniques.

The other abundant types of eicosanoids, the LTs, were originally identified as the slow-reacting substances of anaphylaxis (SRS-A) in guinea pig lung. It is now known that the activity known as SRS-A is mediated by the cysteinyl LTs (LTC$_4$, LTD$_4$, and LTE$_4$). The cysLTs have profound effects on airway smooth musculature and vascular permeability. LTB$_4$ was identified by chemotactic activity for neutrophils, but LTB$_4$ exerts effects on other inflammatory cells as well. LTs are synthesized from AA by 5-lipoxygenase (5-LO), an enzyme whose mechanism of action has recently been clarified *(3)*.

With the advent of molecular techniques applied to the study of the eicosanoids, several breakthroughs in understanding have occurred. It has become clear that there are multiple isoforms of the biosynthetic enzymes, such as COX-1 and COX-2, many

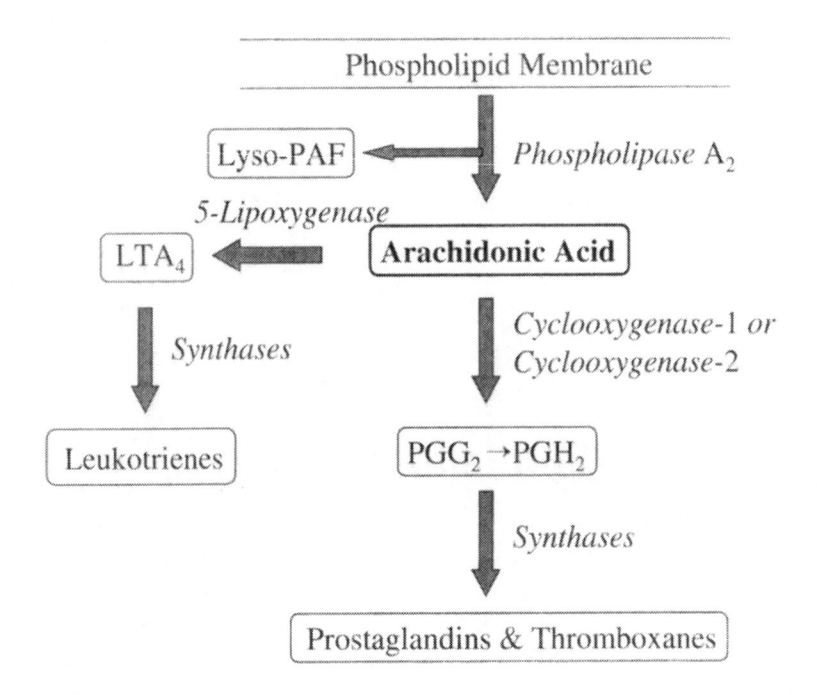

Fig. 1. The arachidonic acid (AA) metabolic cascade. Arachidonic acid is released from phospholipid membranes by phospholipase A$_2$. This also results in formation of lyso-platelet-activating factor (PAF), subsequently leading to synthesis of PAF. Either cyclooxygenase-1 or cyclooxygenase–2 metabolize AA to PGH$_2$, which is then converted to stable prostaglandins or thromboxanes by one of the terminal synthases. Alternatively, AA can enter the lipoxygenase pathway resulting in formation of leukotrienes.

of which are upregulated by cytokines. In addition, receptors have been identified and progress has been made in the understanding of cell-signaling events stimulated by the eicosanoids. Development of pharmacologic compounds that inhibit biosynthesis or action of eicosanoids is based on recent scientific advances and can serve as model for drug development for rheumatic and other types of inflammatory diseases.

2. Phospholipase A$_2$

2.1. Phospholipid Membranes

Eicosanoids are derived from the free fatty acid, arachidonic acid (AA), released primarily from the *sn*-2 position of membrane glycerophospholipids, including phosphatidylinositol (PI), phosphatidlycholine (PC), and phosphatidylethanolamine (PE). Other potential sources of arachidonate include the cholesterol esters or phospholipids of low-density lipoprotein or triglycerides *(4)*. Most AA is likely to derive from the direct action of a group of lipases called phospholipase A$_2$s (PLA$_2$s) *(4)*. However, other phospholipases, including phospholipases C and D, can catalyze AA release by different mechanisms *(4)*.

2.2. Small Secreted Calcium-Dependent PLA$_2$s

There are multiple different forms of PLA$_2$ whose characteristics are detailed in Table 1 *(5,6)*. They were initially characterized as an enzyme activity common to both

Table 1
Characteristics of the Phospholipase A_2 Enzymes

Type	Sources	Location	Size (kDa)	Ca^{2+} Req	S–S Bonds	Molecular characteristics
Venoms		*Small, Secretory, Disulfide Crosslinked*				
I A	Cobras, kraits	Secreted	13–15	mM	7	His–Asp pair active site
II B	Gaboon viper	Secreted	13–15	mM	6	His–Asp pair, carboxyl extension
III	Bees, lizards	Secreted	16–18	mM	5	His–Asp pair
IX	Marine snail	Secreted	14	<mM	6	His–Asp pair
Pancreas						
I B	Pancreas	Secreted	13–15	mM	7	His–Asp pair, elapid loop
Other tissues and cells, venoms						
II A	Rattlesnakes, vipers, human synovial fluid, platelets	Secreted	13–15	mM	7	His–Asp pair, carboxyl extension
II C	Rat/mouse testes	Secreted	15	mM	8	His–Asp pair, carboxyl extension
V	Heart/lung, P388D$_1$ macrophages	Secreted	14	mM	6	His–Asp pair, no elapid loop, no carboxyl extension
X	Lung, spleen, thymus	Secreted	14	mM	8	His–Asp pair, elapid loop, carboxyl extension
		Large, Serine Esterase-type				
IV	Raw 264.7, rat kidney, human U937/platelets	Cytosolic	85	<μM	—	Ser228 in GLSGS consensus sequence, Arg200, Asp549 required; Ser505 phosphorylation site; CaL B domain
VI	P338D$_1$ macrophages, CHO cells	Cytosolic	85	None	—	GxSxG consensus sequence, ankyrin repeats, 340-kDa complex
VII (PAF–Acetylhydrolase)	Human plasma	Secreted	45	None	—	GxSxG consensus sequence, Ser273, Asp296, His351
VIII (PAF–AH isomer IB)	Bovine brain	Cytosolic	29	None	—	Ser47

human pancreatic juice and snake venom that could liberate free fatty acids certain phospholipids from the *sn*-2 position. It has become clear that a large family of enzymes is capable of catalyzing the same reaction. In general, there are two large subgroups within the phospholipase family. The first is a group of small (~14 kDa), extensively disulfide crosslinked, secreted enzymes sharing a high degree of homology. The active site for the small, secreted PLA$_2$s (sPLA$_2$s) is a histidine–aspartate pair of amino acids with a calcium ion in the active site participating in the hydrolysis reaction. Accordingly, these enzymes require high extracellular concentrations of Ca^{2+} for activity. The sPLA$_2$s have no specificity for the presence of AA at the *sn*-2 position. Functionally, this group includes indiscriminate enzymes designed to digest food and kill or injure prey, as well as more selective enzymes that release specific fatty acids during signal transduction and inflammation *(7)*.

The principal small sPLA$_2$ participating in the inflammatory process is type IIA sPLA$_2$, which is widely distributed with variable expression. The enzyme is synthesized as a precursor, then processed in the endoplasmic reticulum. Type IIA sPLA$_2$ expression is induced by pro-inflammatory cytokines, such as interleukin-1 (IL-1) and tumor necrosis factor-α (TNF-α), whereas glucocorticoids inhibit expression *(7)*. The transcriptional regulation of type IIA sPLA$_2$ is similar to that observed for other prostanoid biosynthetic enzymes, including COX-2. In some cell types, a functional linkage between type IIA sPLA$_2$ and COX-2 for catalyzing delayed production of PG after an inflammatory stimulus has been observed *(7)*. Very high concentrations of type IIA sPLA$_2$ are found at inflammatory sites, such a synovial fluid of patients with rheumatoid arthritis. Increased levels of type IIA sPLA$_2$ are also associated with ischemic injury. Lipid peroxidation, caused by ischemia and reperfusion, may increase susceptibility of cellular membranes to PLA$_2$ *(7)*.

2.3. Calcium-Independent PLA$_2$s

The second subgroup of PLA$_2$ enzymes utilize a serine nucleophile contained within an active site characterized by a G-X-S-X-G consensus motif. Enzymatic activity is Ca^{2+} independent. The best characterized is the type IV cytosolic PLA$_2$ (cPLA$_2$) is an 85-kDa enzyme without homology with other PLA$_2$ enzymes *(8)*. cPLA2, in contrast to sPLA$_2$s, has a preference for phospholipids containing arachidonate at the *sn*-2 position. This enzyme is likely to be involved in regulating lipid mediator generation immediately after cell activation *(7)*. Activity of cPLA$_2$ requires translocation and binding to phospholipid membranes *(8)*. Although Ca^{2+} is not required for enzymatic activity, Ca^{2+} is required for translocation and binding to the phospholipid membrane. cPLA$_2$ translocates to membrane vesicles in response to Ca^{2+} in the range found inside cells after mobilization pathways are activated. The nuclear envelope and endoplasmic reticulum (ER) are the primary sites for AA metabolism initiated by cPLA$_2$ in activated cells *(7)*. These are also the primary subcellular locations for the COX enzymes, 5-LO, and some of the terminal synthases. Phosphorylation of cPLA$_2$ is important for maximum in vivo activation *(8)*.

More prolonged increases in cPLA$_2$ levels occur by transcriptional regulation. Although cPLA$_2$ is widely expressed in most tissues at baseline and the promoter has features of a housekeeping gene with no TATA or CAAT elements, expression of cPLA$_2$ can be stimulated by a variety of cytokines and mitogens *(7,8)*. The magnitude of the increase in cPLA$_2$ expression, however, is generally not as large as type IIA sPLA$_2$. There is transcriptional regulation by IL-1 and interferon-γ (IFN-γ), and the presence of two glucocorticoid response elements has led to the suggestion that glucocorticoids may inhibit synthesis. In rheumatoid synoviocytes, cPLA$_2$ is coordinately upregulated with COX-2 in response to IL-1.

Several other Ca^{2+}-independent PLA$_2$s have been identified with diverse functional activities. The best characterized are the platelet-activating factor (PAF)-acetylhydrolases that inactivate PAF and degrade oxidized phospholipids, thereby acting to decrease levels of bioactive and toxic phospholipids *(9)*. In addition, these phospholipases may be important for reincorporation of AA into membrane phospholipids. The PAF-acetylhydrolases will be discussed later.

Arachidonic acid has biologic properties separate from merely providing substrate for eicosanoid biosynthesis. Other roles include regulation of protein kinase C and phospholipase C and modulation of Ca^{2+} flux *(7)*. It is also subject to nonenzymatic oxidation to generate bioactive isoprostanes and isoleukotrienes.

3. Prostaglandin Synthesis and Action
3.1. Cyclooxygenases

The first committed step for prostanoid biosynthesis is the formation of PGH$_2$ by the bifunctional enzyme, PGH synthase, or COX (Fig. 2). COX enzymes are integral membrane proteins that sit within one leaflet of the lipid bilayer of intracellular phospholipid membranes of the nuclear envelope and ER. The cyclooxygenase active site is located in a channel formed in the center of enzyme, allowing the hydrophobic fatty acid substrate access without leaving the membrane. The peroxidation function is located on the outside of the enzyme and appears to be similar in both enzymes *(4)*. Until the mid-1980s, it was thought that the formation of PGs was limited solely by the availability of AA. However, it is now clear that the amount of COX activity is increased substantially in inflamed tissues because of increased expression of the inducible isoform, COX-2 *(10)*.

COX-1 is a continuously transcribed stable message with a promoter region that, similar to cPLA$_2$, lacks a TATA and CAAT elements. There are relatively constant levels of COX-1 in most cell types that provide for homeostatic levels of PG and for acute increases in prostanoid production. COX-2 levels are rapidly upregulated by a variety of stimuli and the mRNA is normally short-lived *(10)*. Pro-inflammatory cytokines, such as IL-1 and TNF-α, are potent inducers of COX-2. Tissue destruction, in part through generation of oxygen radicals by neutrophils, also leads to increased COX-2 expression. Glucocorticoids and those cytokines that restrain inflammation suppress the expression of COX-2.

Animal models of inflammation provide support for the important role of COX-2 in inflammatory processes. Studies indicate that upregulated COX-2 expression is responsible for increased local PG production in animal models of arthritis *(10)*. Similarly, analysis of human synovial tissues in patients with rheumatoid arthritis demonstrates intense COX expression. COX-1 is present predominantly in the synovial lining layer and is not different in osteoarthritis compared with RA. COX-2 is present in immune cells, blood vessel endothelial cells, and sublining synovial fibroblasts. In contrast to COX-1, expression in increased in inflammatory arthritis.

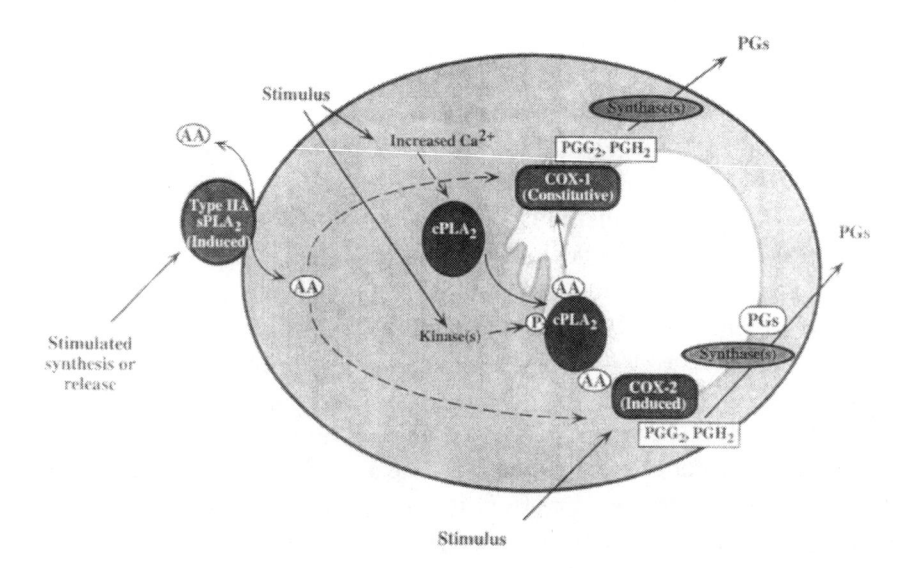

Fig. 2. Pathways for prostaglandin production. sPLA$_2$ is synthesized after stimulation or released from storage granules and secreted. The enzyme associates with cell membranes to release arachidonic acid (AA). cPLA$_2$ is present in the cytoplasm under basal conditions. On stimulation, increased intracellular calcium concentrations promote translocation to the nuclear membrane and activation of kinases leads to phosphorylation of cPLA$_2$, which increases enzyme activity. cPLA$_2$ expression can also be increased after certain stimuli. AA derived from either PLA$_2$ can serve as substrate to COX-1, which is constitutively present in most cells and localized to the endoplasmic reticulum and nuclear membrane. COX-2 expression must be induced, often by pro-inflammatory or mitogenic stimuli. Both COX isoforms catalyze formation of the precursor PG, PGH$_2$. Membrane bound or cytoplasmic synthases convert PGH$_2$ to stable PGs.

COX-2 plays a role in multiple physiologic and pathologic processes other than inflammation (Table 2) *(11)*. COX-2 upregulation is critical for several reproductive processes, including ovulation and implantation. Prostanoids have significant effects on bone remodeling, and it has now been shown that COX-2 is the isoform most responsible for prostanoid production in bone. Although much of the renal PG is derived from COX-1, COX-2 is expressed in several areas of the renal cortex notable the juxtaglomerular apparatus that regulated production of renin *(11)*. Several lines of evidence suggest a role for COX in the pathogenesis of malignancy, particularly colon cancer. Epidemiological studies show a decreased relative risk of colon cancer in individuals taking chronic NSAID therapy. It has now been demonstrated that COX-2 expression is also upregulated in colorectal adenomas and carcinomas in humans *(11)*.

Although regulation of COX-1 and COX-2 expression is quite different, the protein structures and enzymatic functions are remarkably similar. Both enzymes have been crystallized, however, and the few amino acid differences yield structural features sufficient to allow design of pharmaceutical compounds that specifically inhibit COX-2 *(12)*. Early clinical experience with these compounds suggests that the anti-inflammatory, antipyretic, and analgesic effects of nonselective NSAIDs will be preserved, again confirming dependence on the COX-2 isoform. At least some of the COX-1-mediated PG effects, such as normal thrombosis and protection of normal gastric mucosa, are not affected by specific COX-2 inhibitors in early trials *(13)*.

Table 2
Biologic Roles of COX-1 and COX-2

COX-1	COX-2
Homeostatic Functions	Pathologic Functions
Platelet aggregation	Chronic inflammation
Cytoprotection of normal gastric mucosa	Carcinogenesis (colon, ?others)
Renal: blood flow, salt/water	Fever
Vascular homeostasis	Physiologic Functions
Macrophage differentiation	Tissue repair
	Reproduction
	Renal: renin–angiotensin, salt/water
	Bone
	Islet cells
	Vascular homeostasis
	Development
	Kidney
	Brain

3.2. Prostaglandin Synthases

After biosynthesis of PGH_2, this endoperoxide is converted to one of several possible prostanoids by a terminal synthase *(14)*. In general, this process is cell specific with differentiated cells producing only one PG in abundance. Both thromboxane A synthase I and prostacyclin synthase are members of the cytochrome P-450 family *(15)*. Thromboxane (TX) synthase is associated with dense tubular membranes of platelets, the principal source of thromboxane A_2 (TXA_2). PGD_2 and PGE_2 are formed by simple nonoxidative rearrangement *(14)*. It now seems clear that there are different isoforms of these terminal synthases in different cell types. For example, the hematopoietic form of PGD synthase requires glutathione and is homologous to the glutathione S-transferase enzymes *(16)*. The form of PGD synthase found in the brain does not require glutathione and is homologous to the lipocalin superfamily of secretory hydrophobic molecule transporters. There may also be different forms of the PGE synthase. Similar to PGD synthase, both glutathione-dependent and glutathione-independent forms are proposed. The glutathione-dependent enzyme is localized to microsomal membranes and, therefore, topologically associated with COX *(17)*.

3.3. Prostaglandins and Their Receptors

The major PG subclasses are TXA_2, prostacyclin (PGI_2), $PGF_{2\alpha}$, PGD_2, and PGE_2. The prostanoids exert their biological effects by interacting predominantly with cell-surface receptors, although the existence of nuclear receptors for these mediators has been recently demonstrated. The classical prostanoid receptors are cell-surface G-protein-linked receptors. The number of possible G-protein associations that activate a variety of second-messenger systems enhances diversity of PG actions. Study of the biologic effects of ligand–receptor interactions has been hampered by the presence of multiple prostanoid receptors in the same tissues or cells, crossreactivity of different prostanoids with the same receptor, and lack of highly specific antagonists *(15)*.

An exhaustive review of PG actions is beyond the scope of this chapter; however, there are several important points to be made regarding the PGs involved in inflammation. The anti-inflammatory actions of NSAIDs can be mimicked by administration of a monoclonal antibody that neutralizes PGE_2 in an animal model of arthritis, suggesting that PGE_2 has a primary role in the vasodilatation and increased vascular permeability characteristic of the model (18). However, the E-series PGs may also have effects that are predominantly anti-inflammatory; particularly notable are inhibition of several neutrophil functions and monocyte cytokine (19).

At least four different receptors for PGE_2 have been cloned (EP receptors), with the EP3 receptor undergoing alternative splicing at the carboxyl terminus to yield at least three isoforms. The EP receptor subtypes differ in ligand-binding properties, tissue distribution, and potency. The different EP receptors are also coupled to different second-messenger systems. The EP1 receptor is coupled to Ca^{2+} channels and activation results in increased intracellular Ca^{2+} concentration. Both the EP2 and EP4 receptors are coupled to G_s subunits that increase intracellular cAMP, whereas the most abundant EP3 isoform is coupled to a G_i subunit that decrease cAMP concentration (15).

Thromboxane A_2 is produced predominantly in platelets. Interaction with its receptor stimulates platelet aggregation and constriction of smooth muscle. The TXA_2 receptor belongs to the G protein-coupled rhodopsin (G_q)-type receptor that opens Ca^{2+}-activated Cl^- channels on agonist stimulation, suggesting coupling to phosphoinositide metabolism. In platelets, there is increased intracellular Ca^{2+} and activation of phospholipase C after activation of the TXA_2 receptor (15).

Vascular endothelial cells are the major source of PGI_2, however smooth muscle cells also produce this prostaglandin. PGI_2 strongly inhibits platelet aggregation and causes vasodilation. The balance between TXA_2 and PGI_2 play a role in vascular reactivity. The prostacyclin (IP) receptor is rather permissive, binding PGI_2 most avidly, but also binding other prostanoids, most notably PGE_1. Ligand binding stimulates increased intracellular cAMP concentrations suggesting linkage of the receptor to a G_s and stimulation of adenylyl cyclase (15). Other types of IP receptors are suggested by experiments demonstrating a second receptor coupled to phosphoinositide metabolism (15).

Prostaglandin D_2 is formed in a variety of tissues including brain and hematopoietic tissues. Mast cells selectively produce PGD_2 in response to immunological stimuli. PGD_2 produces systemic vasodilation, pulmonary vascular constriction, and bronchoconstriction. Some actions of PGD_2 are mediated through crossreactivity through the TXA_2 and $PGF_{2\alpha}$ receptors. In the central nervous system, PGD_2 is thought to play a role in sleep induction, body temperature, and analgesia (15).

Prostaglandin $F_{2\alpha}$ is formed in multiple tissues and produces bronchoconstriction and constriction of smooth muscle in other tissues. The most prominent action of $PGF_{2\alpha}$ is luteolysis or regression of the corpus luteum. In the corpus luteum, the $PGF_{2\alpha}$ receptor is coupled to phosphoinositide metabolism and activation of protein kinase C (15).

Molecular evolution of prostaglandins and their receptors demonstrates functional clusters. All of the clusters contain PGE receptors, suggesting that the COX pathway may have been initiated as a system composed of PGE and its receptors (20). The earliest divergence is between clusters associated with either an increase or decrease of cAMP, suggested to have arisen as a gene duplication leading to functional divergence. One cluster contains receptors that increase cAMP, including the PGI, PGD, and PGE (subtypes EP2 and EP4) receptors. Another cluster contains the receptor that inhibits adenylyl cyclase and decreases cAMP levels, the EP3 subtype of the PGE receptor. The ancestral EP1 receptor diverged from the EP3 subtype and it functions to increase intracellular Ca^{2+} concentrations rather than altering levels of cAMP. The TXA and PGF receptors appear to have arisen from the EP1 receptor by gene duplication. The ancestral EP3 subtype also acquired, through alternative splicing, functional divergence without duplication. The phylogenetic tree suggests that all the varieties of receptor, and by implication the entire cyclooxygenase pathway, were present before mammalian divergence (20). Lipoxygenase pathway and PAF receptors are not related to the prostaglandin receptors, but to peptide receptors as discussed later (20).

In addition to the classical prostanoid receptors, new evidence is emerging that suggests nuclear receptors for eicosanoids. The candidate receptors identified to date are classified as peroxisome proliferator-activated receptors (PPARs) (21). These nuclear receptors are transcription factors that regulate gene expression of enzymes associated with lipid homeostasis. PPARs complex with the nuclear receptor for 9-*cis*-retinoic acid (RXR) and bind a specific DNA motif termed the PPAR-response element (PPRE). Several eicosanoids, including PGJ_2 and LTB_4, bind to PPARs and affect transcription. PPREs are present in genes involved in the β-oxidation pathway for metabolism of fatty acids. At least one potentially important mechanism underlying PPAR-mediated eicosanoid action is autoregulation of eicosanoid levels through increased synthesis of enzyme-mediating degradation. In addition, PPAR agonists, including PGJ_2, suppress cytokine production.

4. Lipoxygenases, Leukotrienes, and Their Receptors

Lipoxygenases are a family of nonheme iron-containing enzymes that insert molecular oxygen into polyunsaturated fatty acids, including arachidonic acid. The 5-lipoxygenase (5-LO) pathway leads to the formation of leukotrienes (Fig. 3) (21). 5-LO is a bifunctional enzyme. The first product is a fatty acid hydroperoxide (5-HPETE) that is metabolized to LTA_4. Other lipoxygenases (8-LO, 12-LO, and 15-LO) generate HPETEs with molecular oxygen inserted at different sites.

The 5-LO gene lacks typical TATA and CCAAT sequences and has many characteristics of a housekeeping gene. However, certain enhancer elements are present and regulation of 5-LO expression has been described in some cell types. The major mechanism leading to increased production of leukotrienes is mediated by induction of 5-LO activity that occurs through translocation to the nuclear membrane (3). During resting conditions, 5-LO is present in both cytosolic and intranuclear sites. During activation triggered by increased intracellular Ca^{2+} concentrations, 5-LO translocates to the nuclear envelope. An activating protein, termed 5-LO activating protein (FLAP,) is also localized at the nuclear envelope (3). FLAP acts to transfer and present AA to 5-LO, enabling the oxygenation reaction to occur. The gene for FLAP has a TATA box and other regulatory motifs. Regulation of FLAP expression is by different mechanisms than those of 5-LO.

Leukotriene A_4 can be metabolized either by cytosolic metabolism via LTA_4 hydrolase to LTB_4 or conversion by the integral membrane protein LTC_4 synthase to LTC_4. LTB_4 is a potent chemotactic agent for neutrophils. In addition, LTB_4 also enhances neutrophil–endothelial interactions and stimulates neutrophil activation, leading to

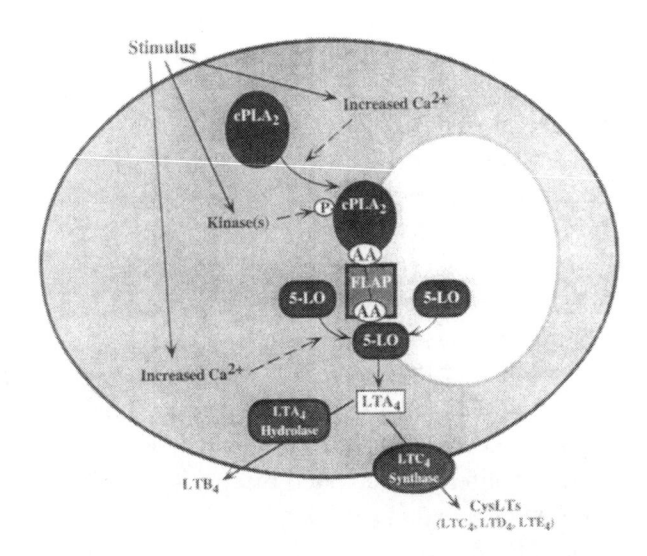

Fig. 3. Synthesis of leukotrienes. Increased intracellular Ca^{2+} causes translocation of $cPLA_2$ to the nuclear membrane and phosphorylation leads to increased enzyme activity. 5-Lipoxygenase (5-LO) also translocates to the nuclear membrane from either the nucleus or cytoplasm. Presentation of AA released from the phospholipid membrane to 5-LO is facilitated by 5-LO-activating protein (FLAP). LTA_4 is the product of 5-LO, which is subsequently metabolized to either LTB_4 or the cysteinyl LTs by their respective synthases.

degranulation and the release of inflammatory mediators. It has also been shown that LTB_4 affects other cells, particularly monocytes and endothelial cells. The range of expression for LTA_4 hydrolase is broader than that of 5-LO. This has led to the suggestion that there may be transcellular metabolism of LTA_4 to LTB_4, particularly in endothelial cells. In fact, LTA_4 hydrolase expression may be regulated by changes in the phosphorylation status of the enzyme in endothelial cells.

The cysteinyl leukotrienes LTC_4, LTD_4, and LTE_4 comprise the slow-reacting substance of anaphylaxis. They are potent bronchoconstrictors, acting on airway smooth muscle. In addition, they are vasodilators, increase vascular permeability, and stimulate mucous secretion in airways.

Both LTB_4 and the cysteinyl LTs act through cell surface receptors. The cysteinyl LTs act through receptors called the cys-LT_1R and cys-LT_2R. LTB_4 acts on a G-protein-coupled receptor (BLTR) originally identified as a chemokine receptor *(22)*. Ligand binding to this receptor mediates increased intracellular Ca^{2+} concentration, accumulation of inositol phosphates, and inhibition of adenylyl cyclase *(22)*. LTB_4 also acts as a ligand for the nuclear receptor, PPARα, as previously noted *(21)*.

5. Other Bioactive Lipids

5.1. Platelet-Activating Factor

Platelet-activating factor (PAF) is generated by an acetyltransferase from lyso-PAF, which is released with arachidonic acid by the action of PLA_2 on membrane phospholipids. PAF is a potent mediator with numerous biological activities related to inflammatory and immune responses. Although originally described as a factor in the blood of animals undergoing anaphylaxis that activated platelets, PAF also activates neutrophils, monocytes, and macrophages. In addition, it causes increased vascular permeability, hypotension, and decreased cardiac output, among other activities *(23)*. There appear to be biologic roles for PAF both in normal physiological events and pathological responses, particularly inflammation and allergy *(23)*.

Platelet-activating factor mediates its biologic activities through interaction with its receptor. As with other bioactive lipids, the PAF receptor belongs to the G-protein-coupled receptor superfamily. The PAF receptor is more closely related to peptide, leukotriene, and lipoxin receptors than to those for prostanoids *(20)*. There appear to be two transcripts for the receptor with identical coding sequences but different promoter regions *(24)*. The PAF receptor may couple to several types of G proteins, possibly G_I and G_q leading to inhibition of adenylyl cyclase and activation of phospholipase C, phospholipase D, mitogen-activated protein (MAP) kinase, and phosphatidylinositol pathways (24).

The enzyme PAF–acetylhydrolase, a member of the PLA_2 superfamily (*see* Table 1) converts the inflammatory mediator back to its biologically inactive form, lyso-PAF. This enzyme is highly specific for phospholipids with short acyl chains at the *sn*-2 position. Presumably, this acts to limit the deleterious effects that may result from excess PAF *(9)*. In fact, recombinant PAF–acetylhydrolase has been shown to decrease vascular leakage and paw edema in animal models of inflammation.

5.2. Lipoxins

Lipoxins are bioactive eicosanoids that modulate immune function. They are generated as a branch of the eicosanoid cascade and appear to function to inhibit many functions of neutrophils in vitro and in vivo *(25)*. Of interest, several novel lipoxins are generated in the presence of aspirin, particularly 15-epi-LXA_4. This species may contribute to the anti-inflammatory actions of aspirin, specifically inhibition of neutrophil migration *(25)*. The actions of lipoxin A_4 (LXA_4) are mediated through a G-protein-linked receptor. The receptor is expressed most abundantly on neutrophils *(25)*. The receptor is more homologous to the chemokine receptors and the LT receptors than to the prostaglandin receptors. In fact, LXA_4 competes for binding with the cysteinyl LTs *(25)*.

5.3. Isoprostanes

Oxygen radicals are implicated in a number of pathophysiological conditions. A central feature of oxidant injury is peroxidation of lipids *(26)*. Isoprostanes are generated in vivo by a nonenzymatic free-radical-induced peroxidation of polyunsaturated fatty acid. In the case of arachidonic acid, four classes of isoprostanes can be produced. Specific structural features distinguishing them from other free-radical-generated products allow for quantitation of oxidant injury during inflammation. Unlike the enzymatic formation of prostaglandins and leukotrienes, which require free arachidonic acid, formation of isoprostanes can occur when the substrate is in the esterified phospholipid form *(26)*. The free isoprostanes are then released by the action of phospholipases *(27)*.

The biologic implications of isoprostane formation are several-fold. Radical oxygenation of the fatty acids located at the *sn*-2 position of phospholipids may create disturbances in cell membrane fluidity and integrity. Isoprostanes themselves exert biological activities. For example, 8-iso-PGF$_{2\alpha}$ is a vasoconstrictor, perhaps acting through the TXA$_2$ receptor *(27)*. 8-Iso-PGF$_{2\alpha}$ is also a potent renal vasoconstrictor *(26)*. Finally, production of isoprostanes may afford a quantitative index of lipid peroxidation as a measure of oxidant stress *(26,27)*.

6. Clinical Implications

Improved understanding of pathways underlying generation and actions of eicosanoids has translated into new therapeutic opportunities. Most relevant to the treatment of inflammatory diseases are the specific inhibitors of COX-2. However, compounds that inhibit the generation and action of leukotrienes have been introduced for the treatment of asthma *(28)*. The specific COX-2 inhibitors are only recently introduced, but several differences from nonspecific inhibitors should be pointed out. First, there is no COX-2 in platelets. The specific COX-2 inhibitors do not alter platelet aggregation and do not inhibit TXA$_2$ release from activated platelets *(13)*. These compounds, therefore, can be used in individuals with other risks for bleeding. They are preferable in situations, such as sports injuries, where pain and inflammation is accompanied by tissue damage. In addition, the risk for gastric bleeding is likely to be augmented by platelet dysfunction when patients are treated with traditional NSAIDs, so the risk of bleeding from gastric sources is likely to be reduced *(12)*. Care should be taken, however, in treating patients at risk for coronary or cerebrovascular thrombosis. The specific COX-2 inhibitors will provide no protection, and low-dose aspirin is advised. The theoretically increased risk for ischemia associated with thromboses because of the imbalance between the vasoconstrictive TXA$_2$, which is COX-1 dependent, and the vasodilatory prostacyclin, which is at least in part COX-2 dependent, has yet to be demonstrated.

Early studies have demonstrated reduced gastric erosions and ulceration as assessed endoscopically *(13)*. These findings are very encouraging that the risk of clinically significant complications of NSAID use, perforation, obstruction, and bleeding, will be reduced with the specific inhibitors of COX-2 *(12)*. Because of the magnitude of chronic NSAID use in the population of patients with arthritis, enormous clinical and economic benefits may accompany reduction of gastrointestinal complications.

References

1. Robinson, D. R. (1997) Eicosanoids and related compounds, in *Arthritis and Allied Conditions*, 13th ed. (Koopman, W. J., ed.), Williams & Wilkins, Philadelphia, pp. 515–528.
2. Vane, J. R. and Botting, R. M. (1996) The history of anti-inflammatory drugs and their mechanism of action, in *New Targets in Inflammation: Inhibitors of COX-2 or Adhesion Molecules* (Bazan, N., Botting, J., and Vane, J., eds.), Kluwar Academic/William Harvey, London, pp. 1–12.
3. Peters-Golden, M. (1998) Cell biology of the 5-lipoxygenase pathway. *Am. J. Respr. Crit. Care Med.* **157,** S227–S232.
4. Smith, W. L. (1992) Prostanoid biosynthesis and mechanisms of action. *Am. J. Physiol.* **263,** F181–F191.
5. Dennis, E. A. (1997) The growing phospholipase A2 superfamily of signal transduction enzymes. *Trends Biochem. Sci.* **22,** 1–2.
6. Dennis, E. A. (1994) Diversity of group types, regulation, and function of phospholipase A2. *J. Biol. Chem.* **272,** 13,057–13,060.
7. Murakami, M., Nakatani, Y., Atsumi, G.-I., Inoue, K., and Kudo, I. (1997) Regulatory functions of phospholipase A2. *Crit. Rev. Immunol.* **17,** 225–283.

8. Leslie, C. C. (1997) Properties and regulation of cytosolic phospholipase A2. *J. Biol. Chem.* **272,** 16,709–16,712.
9. Bazan, N. G. (1995) A signal terminator. *Nature* **374,** 501–502.
10. Crofford, L. J. (1997) COX-1 and COX-2 tissue expression: Implications and predictions. *J. Rheumatol.* **24(Suppl. 49),** 15–19.
11. DuBois, R. N., Abramson, S. B., Crofford, L., Gupta, R. A., Simon, L. S., Van de Putte, L. B. A., et al. (1998) Cyclooxygenase in biology and disease. *FASEB J.* **12,** 1063–1073.
12. Lipsky, P. E., Abramson, S. B., Crofford, L., DuBois, R. N., Simon, L., and van de Putte, L. B. A. (1998) The classification of cyclooxygenase inhibitors (editorial). *J. Rheumatol.* **25,** 2298–2303.
13. Simon, L. S., Lanza, F. L., Lipsky, P. E., Hubbard, R. C., Talwalker, S., Schwartz, B. D., et al. (1998) Preliminary study of the safety and efficacy of SC-58635, a novel cyclooxygenase 2 inhibitor: efficacy and safety in two placebo-controlled trials in osteoarthritis and rheumatoid arthritis, and studies of gastrointestinal and platelet effects. *Arthritis Rheum.* **41,** 1591–1602.
14. Smith, W. L. and DeWitt, D. L. (1995) Biochemistry of prostaglandin endoperoxide H synthase-1 and synthase-2 and their differential susceptibility to nonsteroidal anti-inflammatory drugs. *Semin. Nephrol.* **15,** 179–194.
15. Tanabe, T., Yokoyama, C., Miyata, A., Ihara, H., Kosaka, T., Suzuki, K., et al. (1993) Molecular cloning and expression of human thromboxane synthase. *J Lipid Mediat.* **6,** 139–144.
16. Kanaoka, Y., Ago, H., Inagaki, E., Nanayama, T., Miyano, M., Kikuno, R., et al. (1997) Cloning and crystal structure of hematopoietic prostaglandin D synthase. *Cell* **90,** 1085–1095.
17. Watanabe, K., Kurihara, K., Tokunaga, Y., and Hayaishi, O. (1997) Two types of microsomal prostaglandin E synthase: glutathione-dependent and -independent prostaglandin E synthases. *Biochem. Biophys. Res. Commun.* **235,** 148–152.
18. Portanova, J. P., Zhang, Y., Anderson, G. D., Hauser, S. D., Masferrer, J. L., Seibert, K., et al. (1996) Selective neutralization of prostaglandin E2 blocks inflammation, hyperalgesia, and interleukin 6 production in vivo. *J. Exp. Med.* **184,** 883–891.
19. Weissmann, G. (1993) Prostaglandins as modulators rather than mediators of inflammation. *J. Lipid Mediat.* **6,** 275–286.
20. Toh, H., Ichikawa, A., and Narumiya, S. (1995) Molecular evolution of receptors for eicosanoids. *FEBS Lett.* **361,** 17–21.
21. Serhan, C. N., Haeggstrom, J. A., and Leslie, C. C. (1996) Lipid mediator networks in cell signaling: update and impact of cytokines. *FASEB J.* **10,** 1147–1158.
22. Yokomizo, T., Izumi, T., Chang, K., Takuwa, Y., and Shimizu, T. (1997) A G-protein-coupled receptor for leukotriene B4 that mediates chemotaxis. *Nature* **387,** 620–624.
23. Prescott, S. M., Zimmerman, G. A., and McIntyre, T. M. (1990) Platelet-activating factor. *J. Biol. Chem.* **29,** 17,381–17,384.
24. Shimizu, T. and Mutoh, H. (1997) Structure and regulation of platelet activating factor receptor gene. *Adv. Exp. Med. Biol.* **407,** 197–204.
25. Takano, T., Fiore, S., Maddox, J. F., Brady, H. R., Petasis, N. A., and Serhan, C. N. (1996) Aspirin-triggered 15-epi-lipoxin A4 (LXA4) and LXA4 stable analogues are potent inhibitors of acute inflammation: evidence for anti-inflammatory receptors. *J. Exp. Med.* **185,** 1693–1704.
26. Morrow, J. D. and Roberts, L. J., II (1996) The isoprostanes. *Biochem. Pharmacol.* **51,** 1–9.
27. Rokach, J., Khanapure, S. P., Hwang, S.-W., Adiyaman, M., Lawson, J. A., and FitzGerald, G. A. (1997) The isoprostanes: a perspective. *Prostaglandins* **54,** 823–851.
28. O'Byrne, P. M. (1997) Leukotrienes in the pathogenesis of asthma. *Chest* **111,** 27S–34S.

11

Collagens

Sergio A. Jiménez

1. Introduction

The collagens comprise a family of specialized molecules with common structural features that provide an extracellular framework for all multicellular animals. The collagens are the most abundant body proteins, accounting for more than 20% of total-body mass. At least 20 different collagens (types I to XX) have been identified to date (Table 1) and it is likely that more will be discovered in the future. These different molecules represent homopolymers or heteropolymers of specific polypeptide products of at least 33 different collagen genes.

There is a high degree of specialization in the functions of the various collagens that requires maintenance of a delicate balance in the temporal and spatial expression of each collagen type synthesized in a given connective tissue. In addition, their precise supramolecular organization is essential for the adequate function of the tissues of which they are the principal structural components. The precise regulation of the expression of the genes encoding the various collagens and the numerous posttranslational modifications that occur in the newly synthesized chains (*see* Subheading 5.) allow connective tissue cells in diverse tissues to produce a wide variety of support structures that assemble into specific structures such as ropes (tendons), woven sheets (skin), transparent lenses (the cornea), scaffolds for mineralization (bone), compressible shock absorbers (weight-bearing cartilage), and porous filtering structures (basement membranes).

In addition to structural functions, collagens have been implicated in morphogenesis and in the various complex regulatory processes that occur during growth, development, aging, and tissue repair. Alterations in the structure of collagens resulting from mutations in their corresponding genes or dysregulation of their normal metabolism are involved in the pathogenesis of many disorders, as shown in Table 2.

2. Structural Features *(1–8)*

The definitive structural feature of all collagen molecules is the *triple helix*. This unique protein conformation is the result of the winding of three constituent polypeptide chains of the collagen molecule (known as α chains) around each other. Each chain is coiled into a left-handed helix with about three amino acid residues per turn. The three chains are then twisted around each other into a right-handed super helix to form a rigid structure similar to a thin segment of rope.

From: *Current Molecular Medicine: Principles of Molecular Rheumatology*
Edited by: G. C. Tsokos © Humana Press Inc., Totowa, NJ

Table 1
Collagen Types and Chromosomal Location of the Genes Encoding Their Corresponding α Chains

Protein	Gene	Chromosome
Collagen I	COL1A1	17q21.3-q22
	COL1A2	7q21.3-q22
Collagen II	COL2A1	12q13.11-12
Collagen III	COL3A1	2q24.3-q31
Collagen IV	COL4A1	13q34
	COL4A2	13q34
	COL4A3	2q35-q37
	COL4A4	2q35-q37
	COL4A5	Xq22
	COL4A6	Xq22
Collagen V	COL5A1	9q34.2-q34.3
	COL5A2	2q24.3-q31
Collagen VI	COL6A1	21q22.3
	COL6A2	21q22.3
	COL6A3	2q37
Collagen VII	COL7A1	3p21.3
Collagen VIII	COL8A1	3q12-q13.1
	COL8A2	1p32.3-p34.3
Collagen IX	COL9A1	6q13
	COL9A2	1p32
	COL9A3	20q13.3
Collagen X	COL10A1	6q21-q22.3
Collagen XI	COL11A1	1p22
	COL11A2	6p21.2
	COL2A1	12q13.11-12
Collagen XII	COL12A1	6q12-14
Collagen XIII	COL13A1	10q22
Collagen XIV	COL14A1	?
Collagen XV	COL15A1	9q21-22
Collagen XVI	COL16A1	1p34-35
Collagen XVII	COL17A1	10q24.3
Collagen XVIII	COL18A1	21q22.3
Collagen XIX	COL19A1	6q12-q13
Collagen XX	COL20A1	?

This unique three-dimensional conformation is made possible by a unique amino acid sequence in the polypeptide chains. With the exception of sequences of variable length at the ends of the chains and occasionally interspersed within the triple helix, every third amino acid residue in each collagen chain is glycine. Because the side-chain of this amino acid is a hydrogen atom, glycine is the only residue small enough to occupy the restricted space in which the helical α chains cluster together in the center of the triple helix. Approximately 25% of the residues in the triple helical domains consist of proline and hydroxyproline, amino acids with ring structures that impose

Table 2
Diseases Resulting from Mutations in Collagen Genes or Associated with Alterations in the Synthesis and/or Degradation of Their Corresponding Products

Protein	Disease
Collagen I	Osteogenesis imperfecta, osteoporosis, Ehlers–Danlos syndrome types VIIA, VIIB, rheumatoid arthritis, scleroderma, liver cirrhosis, pulmonary fibrosis, other fibrosing diseases
Collagen II	Several chondrodysplasias, early-onset osteoarthritis, primary generalized osteoarthritis
Collagen III	Ehlers–Danlos syndrome type IV, familial aortic aneurysms, other vascular aneurisms
Collagen IV	Alport syndrome, Alport syndrome with leiomyomatosis
Collagen V	Ehlers–Danlos syndrome types I and III
Collagen VI	Bethlem myopathy
Collagen VII	Epidermolysis bullosa dystrophica
Collagen IX	Multiple epiphyseal dysplasia, early-onset osteoarthritis
Collagen X	Schmid type metaphyseal dysplasia
Collagen XI	Stickler syndrome; Stickler syndrome without ocular lesions
Collagen XVII	Epidermolysis bullosa junctionalis mitis

restrictions on the α-chain conformation and, thereby, strengthen the triple helix and stiffen the collagen molecule. In the most abundant fibril-forming interstitial collagens (types I, II, and III), the triple helical region is approximately 100 nm long and contains about 1000 amino acid residues.

The helical region of the collagen α chain of the fibril-forming collagens can be represented by the molecular formula $(X-Y-Gly)_{333}$, where X and Y are residues other than glycine. In mammalian collagens, about 100 of the X positions are occupied by prolyl residues and about 100 of the Y positions by hydroxyprolyl residues. Hydroxyproline is produced during the collagen biosynthetic process by enzymatic hydroxylation of specific prolyl residues. This complex enzymatic reaction takes place because hydroxyproline cannot be incorporated directly into the nascent collagen polypeptide chain because of the absence of transfer RNA for hydroxyproline. The hydroxylation of peptide-bound prolyl residues involves a specific enzyme, prolyl hydroxylase, which requires O_2, Fe^{2+}, α-ketoglutarate, and ascorbic acid as cofactors. The presence of hydroxyproline residues in the collagen molecule is essential to the maintenance of the collagen conformation, because the hydroxyproline content determines the thermal stability of the collagen triple helix. A decrease in the hydroxyproline content of collagen, as occurs in scurvy, results in unstable molecules that loosen their triple helical conformation at normal body temperatures and, therefore, become susceptible to proteolytic degradation by nonspecific proteases.

The precise sequence of amino acid residues that occupy the remaining X and Y positions differs among the various collagen types. This variability is likely to account for the tissue-specific properties of the collagens of cartilage, skin, basement membranes, and other specialized structures. One characteristic residue that occupies some of these positions is hydroxylysine. Hydroxylysine is also produced by a posttranslational enzymatic hydroxylation of some lysyl residues in the collagen molecules. The responsible enzyme, lysyl hydroxylase, is distinct from prolyl hydroxylase, although it exhibits the same cofactor requirements. Hydroxylysine is involved in many of the subsequent processes of fiber formation and stabilization as a precursor of crosslinking compounds and as a site for attachment of carbohydrate residues. In the latter instance, the hydroxyl group is involved in an *O*-glycoside linkage to a galactose or to glucosyl-galactose.

In the fibril-forming collagens, both ends of the helical region are terminal sequences (telopeptides) that do not have glycine as every third residue and, therefore, lack the triple helical conformation. These regions represent peptide sequences remaining from the proteolytic cleavage of collagen precursors or procollagens after they have been processed by specific procollagen peptidases. These regions have different lengths in the chains of the various collagen types and appear to be important in the formation of supramolecular aggregates as well as in their stabilization. In the non-fibril-forming collagens, one or more non-triple-helical segments, known as NC domains, are intercalated within the triple helix, imparting flexibility to the rigid domain. Variations in the length and location of triple helical regions, known as COL domains, and differences in their primary structure and extent of posttranslational modifications, coupled with variations in the number, location, and length of the NC domains enable the collagens to participate in a vast array of structural complexes.

3. Collagen Polymorphism *(9–22)*

Each collagen type has a unique amino acid sequence and has been firmly identified as a distinct product of one or more collagen genes. The different collagen types can be classified according to their ability to aggregate into highly structured fibrils or to associate with the fibrils of other collagens, to the length of their triple helical domains, and to the presence of intercalated non-triple-helical domains within their triple helical regions (Table 3). The fibril-forming collagens, responsible for the assembly of the extracellular fabric of the major connective tissues, are the most abundant class. A second class comprises the Fibril-Associated Collagens with Interrupted Triple helices (FACIT), and other classes comprise collagens forming specialized structures such as the basement membranes, anchoring fibrils of the dermis, or collagens performing specialized functions such as in the cartilage of the growth plate.

In addition to these molecules that are classified as members of the collagen family, several unrelated proteins contain collagen-like sequences. These sequences presumably enable these molecules to maintain their steric conformation in order to perform their specialized biological functions. For example, the collagenous sequences in the C1q subcomponent of the complement system are thought to provide the molecules with a rigid segment that enables them to self-aggregate, and those in acetylcholinesterase appear to anchor the enzyme to basement membranes. Two protein components of lung surfactant have also been found to contain collagenous sequences that appear to be responsible for the attachment of surface-active phospholipids. Recently, it has been shown that the macrophage-scavenger factor also contains collagenous sequences, although their functional role has not been elucidated.

The structure and supramolecular organization of the various collagens are briefly described in the following subsections and are illustrated in Fig. 1.

Table 3
Genetic Polymorphism of Collagen

Collagen type	Chain composition	Molecular weight (Da)	Tissue distribution
Fibril-forming collagens			
I	α1(I)$_2$, α2(I)	300,000	Skin, bone, tendon, synovium
I trimer[a]	α1(I)$_3$	300,000	Tumors, fetal skin, liver
II	α1(II)$_3$	300,000	Hyaline cartilage, vitreous, nucleus pulposus
III	α1(III)$_3$	300,000	Fetal skin, blood vessels, intestine
V	α1(V)$_2$, α2(V)	300,000	Same as type I collagen
XI	1α, 2α, 3α[b]	450,000	Hyaline cartilage
FACIT collagens			
IX	α1(IX), α2(IX), α3(IX)	500,000	Hyaline cartilage, vitreous, cornea
XII	α1(XII)$_3$	600,000	Same as type I collagen
XIV	α1(XIV)$_3$	Unknown	Skin, tendon
XVI	α1(XVI)$_3$	660,000	Unknown
XIX	Unknown	Unknown	Widespread; restricted to basement membranes
XX	Unknown	Unknown	Widespread; high in cornea
Basement membrane collagens			
IV	Homopolymers or heteropolymers of α1(IV), α$_2$(IV), α$_3$(IV), α$_4$(IV), α$_5$(IV), α$_6$(IV)	450,000	Lamina densa of the basement membrane
VII	α1(VII)$_3$	960,000	Amnion, dermo-epidermal anchoring fibrils
XVII	α1(XVII)$_3$	Unknown	Dermo-epidermal basement membranes
Non-fibril-forming collagens			
VI	α1(VI), α2(VI), α3(V)	570,000	Aortic intima, placenta, skin, kidney, muscle
XIII	Unknown	Unknown	Endothelial cells
Short-chain collagens			
VIII	α1(VIII)$_3$	500,000	Endothelial cells, Descemet's membrane
X	α1(X)$_3$	180,000	Growth plate cartilage
Multiplexins			
XV	α1(XV)$_3$	Unknown	Basement membranes
XVIII	α1(XVIII)$_3$	Unknown	Vasculature

[a]It is not certain whether the α chains forming this collagen are a distinct gene product or are a post-translationally modified form of the α1(I) chain of type I collagen.

[b]The 3 α chains of type XI collagen appear to be a post-translationally modified form of the α1(II) chain of type II collagen.

3.1. Fibril-Forming Collagens

The group of fibril-forming collagens comprises types I, II, III, V, and XI collagens. In electron micrographs, these collagens exhibit a cross-striated pattern with a characteristic 64–67 nm periodicity. The periodicity of the collagen fibril is generated by the

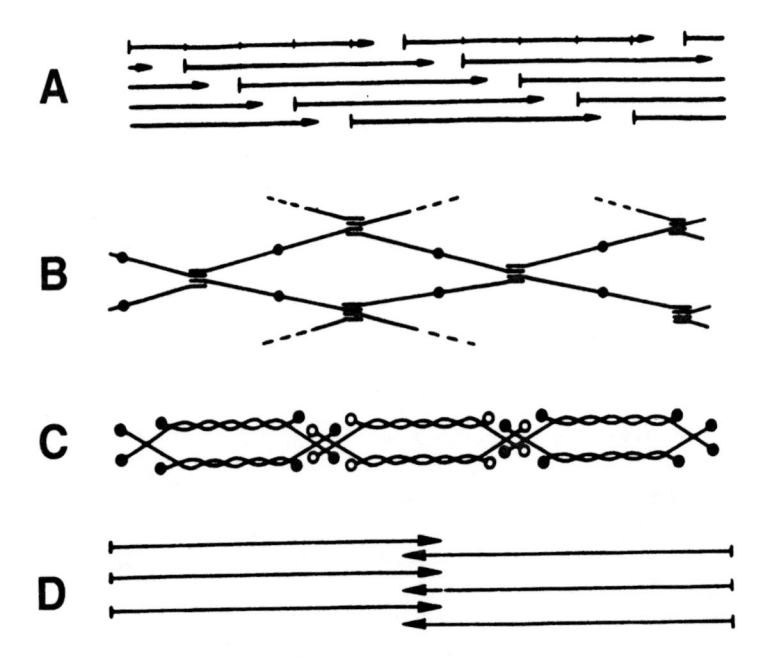

Fig. 1. Diagram showing the macromolecular association of some collagen types. **(A)** Fibrillar collagens I, II, and III. The 300-nm-long rodlike molecules aggregate in a parallel and staggered fashion. These fibrils exhibit in the electronmicroscope a characteristic cross-striation period of 67 nm. Type XI collagen may also form similar fibrillar aggregates. **(B)** Basement membrane type IV collagen. This collagen forms a nonfibrillar network. The molecules aggregate only by their identical ends. Four molecules are held together via the triple helical N-terminus, whereas the C-terminal globular domain connects two molecules with each other. **(C)** Type VI collagen. Dimers are formed by antiparallel and staggered alignment of 105 nm monomers where the 75-nm overlapping helical segments coil around each other. The dimers undergo a symmetrical association into tetramers. Fibrillar structures are formed by end-to-end aggregation. The aggregates are stabilized by disulfide bonds between triple helical segments and globular domains. **(D)** Type VII collagen. The 450-nm-long molecules associate into antiparallel dimeric structures, which show a 60-nm overlap and which subsequently assemble laterally in register. [Adapted from Martin, G. R., Timpl, R., Müller, P. K., and Kühn, K. (1985) The genetically distinct collagens. *Trends Biochem. Sci.* **10,** 285–287.]

packing of the collagen molecules in a precise axial register that is usually described as a near-quarter-stagger with overlap. This axial stagger has been precisely defined at 234 ± 1 residues for type I collagen. At present, the mechanisms responsible for the side-to-side aggregation of collagen molecules, ultimately responsible for the fiber diameter, are not known, although it is likely that the charge profile along the surface of the molecules plays a crucial role. Thus, it is the primary structure of the chains that contains all the information needed to allow the packing of the native molecules into fibers. In addition, some studies have suggested that the ultimate diameter of the collagen fibers may be influenced by the presence of the amino-terminal noncollagenous extensions and by interactions with noncollagenous macromolecules, such as the small proteoglycan decorin. The primary structure also appears to determine the type and number of intermolecular crosslinks that will eventually be formed and the nature of the interaction of the collagen with the other connective tissue components, namely glycoproteins and proteoglycans.

Type I collagen, the most abundant and best characterized mammalian collagen, consists of two identical α1(I) chains and one genetically distinct α2 chain in the molecular form α1(I)$_2$α2(I). This species accounts for about 90% of the collagen in the body and is the major collagenous component of the skin, tendon, bone, synovium, cornea, conjunctiva, and sclera.

A molecule apparently composed of three α1(I) chains has been found in low concentrations in the cornea, skin, embryonic bones and tendons, and rat dentin. This molecular species has also been identified as a product of various cell cultures and tumors. The α chain of this molecular species appears to be identical, by peptide mapping, to the α1(I) chain of type I collagen and gives rise to the nomenclature α1 type I trimer collagen. Although its functional role is not fully understood, this collagen appears in higher concentrations in healing wounds, inflammatory reactions, and embryonic tissues.

Type II collagen is a specific product of chondrocytes and vitreous cells. Its fibers appear much thinner than those of type I collagen in electron micrographs. Type II collagen consists of three identical α chains and is designated α1(II)$_3$. These molecules contain a higher number of hydroxylysine residues and several-fold greater amounts of carbohydrate residues than type I collagen. Several properties of the α1(II) chains of vitreous humor differ from those of the α1(II) chains of cartilage. These differences strongly suggest that type II molecules are not a homogenous population, but they may represent a family of closely related molecules. Furthermore, recent studies of type II collagen transcripts have shown that this collagen exists in at least two distinct molecular species that result from alternative splicing of certain portions of the gene. These isoforms appear to have special functional properties, because they are preferentially expressed in specific tissues at various stages of growth and development.

Type III collagen is frequently coexpressed with type I collagen in the skin, synovium, and vascular wall tissue and is a prominent component of lung interstitium. This collagen contains three identical chains that are readily distinguishable from the previously described fibrillar types and is therefore designated α1(III)$_3$. Unlike the other interstitial collagens, type III collagen molecules contain intrahelical cysteine residues that form interchain disulfide bonds so that the native molecules are disulfide-bonded trimers. The fact that type III collagen forms fibrils of smaller diameter and of different organization than type I collagen suggests that the relative levels of expression of separate collagen genes is an important step in establishing and maintaining the individual characteristics of a particular connective tissue. For example, the relative proportions of type I and type III change drastically in healing skin wounds and in keloid lesions.

Type V collagen is frequently found surrounding fibroblasts, smooth-muscle cells, and other mesenchymal cells. This collagen type contains distinct chains [α1(V), α2(V), and α3(V)], which are minor components found in pepsin digests of the placenta, cornea, skin, and blood vessels and have been identified in surface-associated materials of cells in culture. The type V collagen molecules are comprised of homopolymers or heteropolymers, depending on the tissue of origin. The most common molecular form of type V collagen consists of two α1 chains and one α2 chain. What determines the relative proportion of these chains within the molecule and their exact role in tissue structure or function is not clear.

Type XI collagen is the designation assigned to collagen molecules composed of chains previously known as 1α, 2α, and 3α. Like type II collagen, type XI collagen is a specific constituent of cartilaginous tissues. Type XI collagen molecules are comprised of three chains that retain large globular domains at both ends. There is some controversy regarding the nature of the α3(XI) chain because it is not clear whether it represents a type II collagen chain with extensive posttranslational modifications or a distinct gene product. In most cartilaginous tissues, the proportion of the three chains is equimolar, suggesting that they are arranged in a heterotrimeric structure. It has also been shown that type XI collagen molecules are integral components of the cartilage collagen fibrils and appear to be located in their central axis and it has been suggested that they may play a role in the regulation of the thickness of type II collagen fibrils in cartilage. Despite their prominent presence in cartilaginous tissues, the exact function of type XI collagen molecules has not been determined.

3.2. Fibril-Associated Collagens with Interrupted Triple Helices

These collagens comprise a distinct class of molecules that do not form the characteristic quarter-staggered fibrils of interstitial collagens. This subgroup includes types IX, XII, XIV, XVI, XIX, and XX collagens. Structurally, these collagens contain alternating triple-helical (COL domains) and noncollagenous domains (NC domains) of various lengths and molecular masses and a large amino-terminal NC domain. This structural arrangement provides greater flexibility to these molecules. Topographically, these collagens associate with the fibrils of types I and II collagens and may play important roles in the organization of the matrix in the immediate perifibrillar millieu.

Type IX collagen, the prototype of the FACIT group of collagens is found almost exclusively in cartilaginous tissues. Despite its abundance in cartilage, its function has not been determined. The type IX collagen molecule is composed of three chains, each containing four nonhelical domains alternating with three helical regions. The individual chains are associated by disulfide bonds. The α2 chain of type IX collagen contains a covalently bound glycosaminoglycan and, therefore, can be considered as a proteoglycan core protein. The demonstration of a covalent interaction between a collagen and a glycosaminoglycan molecule in articular cartilage and other hyaline cartilages suggests that type IX collagen may be involved in mediating the interaction of the collagenous matrix with the proteoglycans in these tissues. Rotary shadowing studies have shown that type IX collagen molecules are topographically localized to the surface of cartilage collagen fibrils, surrounding the type II collagen molecules with the COL3 and NC4 domains bent in an angle projecting out of the surface of the fibrils into the surrounding interfibrillar matrix. These studies have led to the suggestion that the NC4 domain of the α1 chain of type IX collagen may be involved in the formation of interfibrillar collagen interactions or in interactions with other components of the articular cartilage matrix. The highly positively charged composition of the NC4 domain may favor the establishment of nonionic interactions with proteoglycans, glycoproteins, or other collagens, thus establishing the interfibrillar "glue" that maintains the structure of articular cartilage matrix. Recent studies have shown that cDNAs corresponding to type IX collagen molecules in the cornea, hypertrophic cartilage of the growth plate, and late developmental stages of the vitreous lack sequences encoding the NC4 domain (short form of type XI collagen). These observations suggest that this NC4 domain may play an important role in determining the structural organization of these tissues, particularly during development.

The search for homologs of type IX collagen in tissues containing type I collagen as their major fibrillar constituent identified molecules with striking similarities to type IX collagen (identically located cysteines and triple helix imperfections). However, further characterization of the intact protein molecule, designated type XII collagen, revealed major differences. *Type XII collagen* is a homotrimer with the molecular structure $\alpha 1(XII)_3$ and contains only two triple helical domains, COL1 and COL2, and three noncollagenous domains. The NH_2-terminal NC3 domain is very large (3×190 kDa). When visualized by rotary shadowing, the type XII collagen molecules have a characteristic morphology with three 60-nm arms projecting from a large central globule and a 70-nm rigid tail. The colocalization of type XII collagen with type I collagen suggests that type XII collagen interacts with fibrils containing type I collagen, although the precise nature of this interaction has not been determined. The homology between the COL1 domains of type IX and type XII collagens suggests that this domain may play a role in this interaction. Recent studies have demonstrated the presence of alternatively spliced transcripts of type XII collagen which appear to be selectively expressed in corneal tissues; however, its function and role in the structure of corneal extracellular matrix remain to be determined.

Another homotrimeric molecule with the characteristic FACIT COL1 domain has been identified in the skin and tendon. Characterization of the molecule at the cDNA and protein levels indicates that it is very similar although clearly distinct from type XII collagen and has been termed *type XIV collagen*. Type XIV collagen has been found mainly in tissues rich in type I collagen, although its presence in type II collagen-containing cartilaginous tissues has also been demonstrated. Type XIV collagen is a disulfide-bonded molecule containing two collagenous domains and three noncollagenous domains. It has also been shown that type XIV collagen may exist in cartilage in a proteoglycan form.

Type XVI collagen was identified in cDNA libraries from human fibroblasts and placenta. Corresponding transcripts have been found in human skin and in cultured lung fibroblasts, keratinocytes, and arterial smooth-muscle cells. The predicted structure for the protein indicates that it contains 10 collagenous domains and 11 relatively short noncollagenous regions. The molecule is very rich in cysteine residues containing 32 residues mainly in the noncollagenous domains. Immunoprecipitation studies have shown that the $\alpha 1(XVI)$ collagen chain is a 220-kDa polypeptide that is secreted as a homotrimer in cultures of dermal fibroblasts and arterial smooth-muscle cells. Its precise function has not been identified, although it has been suggested that it is likely to associate with type I and type III collagen fibrils.

Type XIX collagen was also characterized at the cDNA level. It was first identified in a cDNA library prepared from a human rhabdomyosarcoma. The triple helical region of this collagen appears to contain approximately 1142 amino acids divided into five collagenous domains separated by 22–44 short noncollagenous interruptions. These interruptions are similar in their sequence and location to those found in type XVI collagen. The molecule contains numerous cysteine residues which participate in intrachain disulfide bonds. Although the overall structure and the location of the cysteine residues are similar to those of other FACIT collagens, the genomic structure and the structure of the deduced protein indicate that this collagen represents a novel collagen type. The function of this collagen has not been identified to date. The protein has been found in numerous tissues, but its highest expression appears to be restricted to vascular, neuronal, mesenchymal, and some epithelial basement membranes.

Type XX collagen is a new collagen recently identified while searching the expressed sequence tag (EST) database for molecular species bearing homologies with FACIT collagens. Sequencing of the EST showed that the encoded product was a unique collagen. Type XX collagen contains a domain structure typical of the FACIT collagen subfamily and is very similar to type XIV collagen. Type XX collagen transcripts are widely expressed in connective tissues and have been demonstrated in the tendon, sterna, and calvaria, although their highest expression appears to occur in corneal tissues and in cells derived from corneal epithelium. The function of type XX collagen remains unknown.

3.3. Basement Membrane Collagens

The collagens present in the basement membrane are likely to be responsible for the structural integrity of the membranes and to act as anchors for other extracellular matrix components. At least three collagen types have been identified in the basement membranes. These include types IV, VII, and XVII collagens.

Type IV collagen is the principal component of the basement membrane of renal glomeruli and tubules, and of arterial vessels. Unlike the fibrillar collagens discussed earlier, type IV collagen does not form fibrillar aggregates and appears to be incorporated directly into the basement membrane without prior excision of the pro-peptide extensions.

The structure of this molecular species has been a controversial matter; however, more recent work has identified six distinct α chains that are the products of different genes as the molecular components of type IV collagen. These chains associate to form homotrimers or heterotrimers. Characterization of the structure of type IV collagen has been accomplished by rotary shadowing of intact molecules, demonstrating that these molecules contain several intrahelical noncollagenous domains that probably confer great flexibility to the main body of the molecule. The helical domains of type IV collagen chains display a distinct bend approximately 360 nm from the amino terminal end of the chains. In addition, a large globular domain is present at the carboxy-terminal end of the chains. A large number of cysteine residues are present at both the amino- and carboxy-terminal ends and are involved in intrachain and interchain disulfide bonds.

The molecules of type IV collagen assemble into a very specific supramolecular network formed as a result of the association of similar ends of the molecules. Four molecules are associated through their amino terminal domains distal to the above-described bend, forming a tetrameric pepsin-resistant domain known as the 7S aggregate. The C-terminal globular domains connect two molecules with each other, resulting in a well-organized network arrangement.

Type VII collagen, previously known as "long-chain collagen," is a homotrimeric molecule comprised of chains containing a collagenous helical domain that is at least one and one-half times larger than that of the interstitial collagens (400 nm). The amino terminal ends of each chain fold into separate 36 nm arms and an additional small NC globular domain is present at the carboxy-terminal ends. Type VII collagen molecules form the so-called anchoring fibrils responsible for the attachment of epithelium to stromal tissues, particularly in the epidermal–dermal junction. The type VII collagen molecules interact by antiparallel dimeric arrangement with a 60-nm overlap between the interacting amino-terminal molecular ends. The carboxyl-terminal ends are grouped in a tuft that appears to attach to the basement membrane and to form loops surrounding interstitial collagen fibrils. In the skin, type VII collagen molecules, together with type XVII collagen (*see* the next paragraph) and other molecules, form hemidesmosomes, specialized structures responsible for the attachment of the epidermis to the upper layer of the dermal–epidermal basement membrane.

Type XVII collagen molecules are unique 180-kDa transmembrane molecules involved in the structure of hemidesmosomes. Their unique transmembrane location indicates that they play a crucial role in the attachment of the epidermis to the basement membrane of the skin. The carboxy-terminal end of the molecules is the extracellular domain and is constituted by 13–15 collagenous sequences interrupted by short noncollagenous domains. The amino-terminal ends of the molecule are anchored intracellularly in the cytoplasm of basal keratinocytes.

3.4. Other Non-Fibril-Forming Collagens

Several collagens that do not form the characteristic cross-striated pattern of the fibrillar collagens and that do not appear to have a FACIT molecular structure have been identified. Some of these collagens form highly specialized structures with specific functions, such as the establishment of connections between cell surfaces and the extracellular matrix (type VI collagen).

Type VI collagen consists of chains containing a triple helical collagenous domain flanked by a large globular domain at each end of the chains. The globular domains account for approximately two-thirds of the total chain mass, whereas the collagenous region represents only one-third. Type VI collagen chains have been found distributed in many connective tissues, but are predominantly localized in the skin and may represent the previously described "beaded filaments" found in embryonic tissues as well as in actively involved lesions in scleroderma. The type VI collagen molecules form aggregates comprised of two chains intertwined to form a dimer, and two dimers associated by crisscrossed interactions between their ends to form a tetramer. Tetramers associate by head-to-tail attachment to form long beaded fibrillar structures.

Type XIII collagen is a nonfibrillar collagen of unknown function that has been characterized from analyses of human cDNA and genomic clones. The predicted α1(XIII) collagen polypeptide has been estimated to contain from 526 to 614 amino acids and consists of short N- and C-terminal noncollagenous domains, termed NC1 and NC4, respectively, and three collagenous domains, COL1–3, interrupted by the noncollagenous domains NC2 and NC3. A striking feature of type XIII collagen is that sequences corresponding to nine exons of the human gene undergo complex alternative splicing during the processing of primary transcripts, resulting in remarkable variability in the structures of the COL1, NC2, COL3, and NC4 domains. The functional significance of this complex alternative splicing is not known. *In situ* hybridization experiments with human tissues indicate that type XIII collagen transcripts are found in numerous connective tissues, including the fetal bone, cartilage, intestine, skin, striated muscle, and placenta, although they appear to be expressed in low amounts in virtually all connective tissue-producing cells.

3.5. Short-Chain Collagens

Two distinct collagens characterized by the presence of short triple helical domains have been characterized in vascular tissues and in growth plate cartilage. The two members of this group are type VIII and type X collagens.

Type VIII collagen was originally described as a product of endothelial cells in culture and was termed EC collagen. This collagen is an important component of the corneal endothelium. Type VIII collagen has not been completely characterized, but the molecules appear to be composed of relatively short helical domains, interrupted by protease sensitive, nonhelical domains with large globular domains at each end of the chains. These chains are stabilized by abundant disulfide bonds and the intact molecule appears to have a molecular weight greater than 500 kDa under nonreducing conditions. The type VIII collagen molecules have a dumbbell shape and interact laterally and by their extremities to form regular hexagonal lattices.

Type X collagen is a specific biosynthetic product of growth plate hypertrophic chondrocytes and is almost exclusively found in the regions undergoing endochondral bone formation. The close temporal and topographic relation between initiation of type X collagen synthesis and the onset of tissue calcification suggests that these chains may play a role in the process of endochondral ossification. The type X collagen chains are formed by short (45 kDa), triple helical regions and a 15-kDa globular domain at the amino-terminal end. The triple helical domain appears to be stabilized by disulfide bonds in certain mammalian species such as those present in bovine cartilages. Recent interest has been focused on possible alterations in the metabolism of type X collagen in osteoarthritis since it has been found that in contrast to normal articular cartilage, osteoarthritic cartilage displays the expression of this collagen.

3.6. Multiplexins

A new subgroup of collagenous molecules within the collagen family has been recently established based on their structure. This group comprises collagens *type XV* and *type XVIII*. The genes encoding these two collagens share substantial structural similarities, suggesting that both may be derived from a single ancestral gene. These collagens are localized mainly in the basement membranes and contain a central collagenous domain with multiple interruptions flanked by large amino- and carboxyl-noncollagenous domains. A very high expression of type XVIII collagen has been found in the liver, placenta, kidneys and lungs. Type XVIII collagen is also known as endostatin, a potent inhibitor of *de novo* angiogenesis. Substantial recent interest has been devoted to this molecule as a putative anticancer agent exerting its effects via reduction of the angiogenic process required for tumor growth and metastasis.

4. Collagen Genes (23–34)

The application of recombinant DNA technology has permitted a greater understanding of the initial steps of collagen biosynthesis and has allowed the isolation and characterization of the genes encoding for most of the collagenous molecules described. At least 33 distinct genes encoding for the various collagen chains have been identified and studied to date. These genes are distributed throughout the genome as shown in Table 1. The gene for the pro $\alpha 1$ chain of type I collagen appears to be approximately 18,000 bases long, whereas the gene for the pro $\alpha 2$ chain is much larger, containing approximately 38,000 bases. All collagen genes studied thus far contain coding sequences (exons) interrupted by large, noncoding sequences (introns). The genes encoding most of the collagens, like various other eukaryotic genes, contain numerous regulatory sequences in the 5' region of the gene, including the so-called TATA and CAAT boxes as well as binding sequences for numerous transcription factors, including AP, NF1, CBF, and Sp1. These consensus sequences have been shown to be essential promoter components required for efficient transcription in several other eukaryotic genes. In addition, enhancer sequences, which act as long-range activators of gene transcription, have been identified within the first intron of several collagen genes as well as upstream of the gene.

The genes encoding the chains of the interstitial collagens appear to contain short exons of 54 or 108 bases in length, and it has been suggested that the 54-base exon represents the ancestral collagen gene that has evolved into the present collagen genes by duplication and expansion of the 54-base pair (bp) unit. This appears to be the case for most of the collagens; however, recent characterization of the genes for collagen types VIII, IX, and X demonstrated substantial deviations of this structure, indicating that these genes may represent different families of genes developed by selective pressures exercised during evolution. For example, the gene for the $\alpha 2$ chain of type IX collagen contains the 54-bp coding units only in the central portions of the sequence coding for the triple helix, whereas the genes for types VIII and X collagens contain only four and three exons, respectively, without the 54-bp repeat unit.

5. Collagen Biosynthesis *(35,36)*

The biosynthesis of type I procollagen has been studied in most detail and can be used as an example of a general biosynthetic pathway for all collagens. A general scheme of type I collagen biosynthesis and processing is depicted in Fig. 2. The initial steps of collagen gene expression are extremely complex and involve the initiation of transcription of a particular collagen gene in a collagen-producing cell by mechanisms similar to those of other eukaryotic genes that include a conformational change of condensed chromatin into competent chromatin, the binding of the RNA polymerase transcriptional complex, and the interactions of multiple transcriptional regulatory DNA-binding proteins. The collagen genes are transcribed into a complementary high-molecular messenger RNA (hmRNA). These molecules are then processed to the mature mRNA by a complex series of posttranscriptional modifications, including capping, splicing, methylation, and addition of a polyadenylated tail. Splicing is probably the most important of these reactions because it is responsible for the precise excision of the noncoding, intervening sequences and the exact re-ligation of the remaining sequences that encode the mature protein. Variations in the patterns of splicing (alternative splicing) can result in the production of polypeptide chains with subtle but important structural and functional differences. Thus, alternative splicing appears to provide a versatile mechanism for the generation of a vast molecular diversity of the biosynthesized proteins and may play a crucial role in the temporal and topographic regulation of collagen gene expression. In addition, the genes for certain collagens appear to have more than one transcription initiation site. Selective use of these sites can result in the production of chains with variable lengths and with the inclusion or exclusion of specific molecular domains. The mature mRNA molecules exit the nucleus

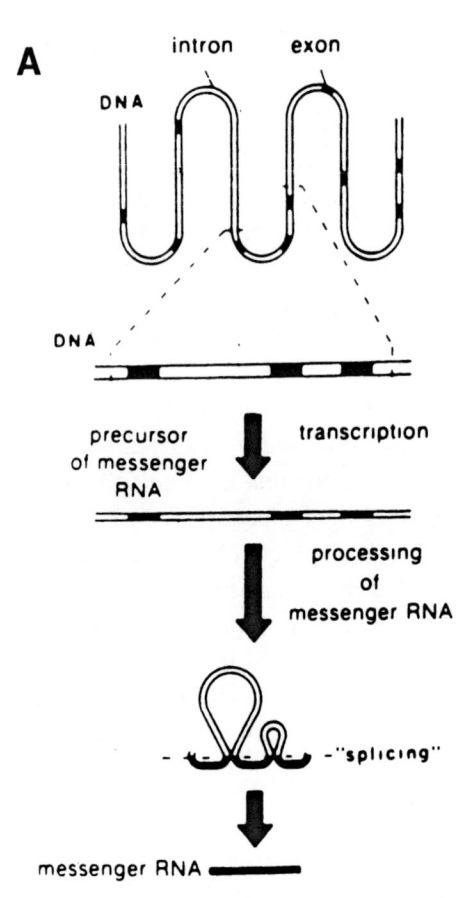

Fig. 2. (A) Intranuclear steps of collagen biosynthesis. The DNA sequences in collagen genes, containing the coding sequences (exons) and the intervening noncoding sequences (introns), are transcribed into a precursor form of the messenger RNA (hmRNA) molecule. The precursor molecule is then processed to functional mRNA by posttranscriptional modifications, including splicing which removes the intervening sequences. (Courtesy of Dr. J. Uitto and colleagues, reproduced with permission of Grune & Stratton.)

and are transported to the rough endoplasmic reticulum where they associate with the polyribosomal apparatus and then undergo translation onto the growing polypeptide chains of the newly synthesized protein.

Studies of the translation of mRNA for type I procollagen in cell-free systems indicate that the molecule is synthesized on the ribosomes as pre-procollagen and each chain contains a short (approximately 20 residue) leader sequence at the extreme amino terminus. This hydrophobic leader sequence is thought to channel the nascent polypeptide through the membrane into the cisternae of the rough endoplasmic reticulum. It is immediately cleaved off by a specific protease to yield procollagen.

Type I procollagen is composed of two pro $\alpha 1$ and one pro $\alpha 2$ chains with estimated molecular weights of about 150 kDa compared with 95 kDa for the corresponding α chains of the fully processed molecule. Each of the pro α chains contains two polypeptide extensions, one at each end of the triple helical region. The amino- and carboxy-terminal extensions are estimated to be 20 kDa and 35 kDa, respectively. The carboxy-terminal ends contain several cysteine residues involved in intrachain and interchain

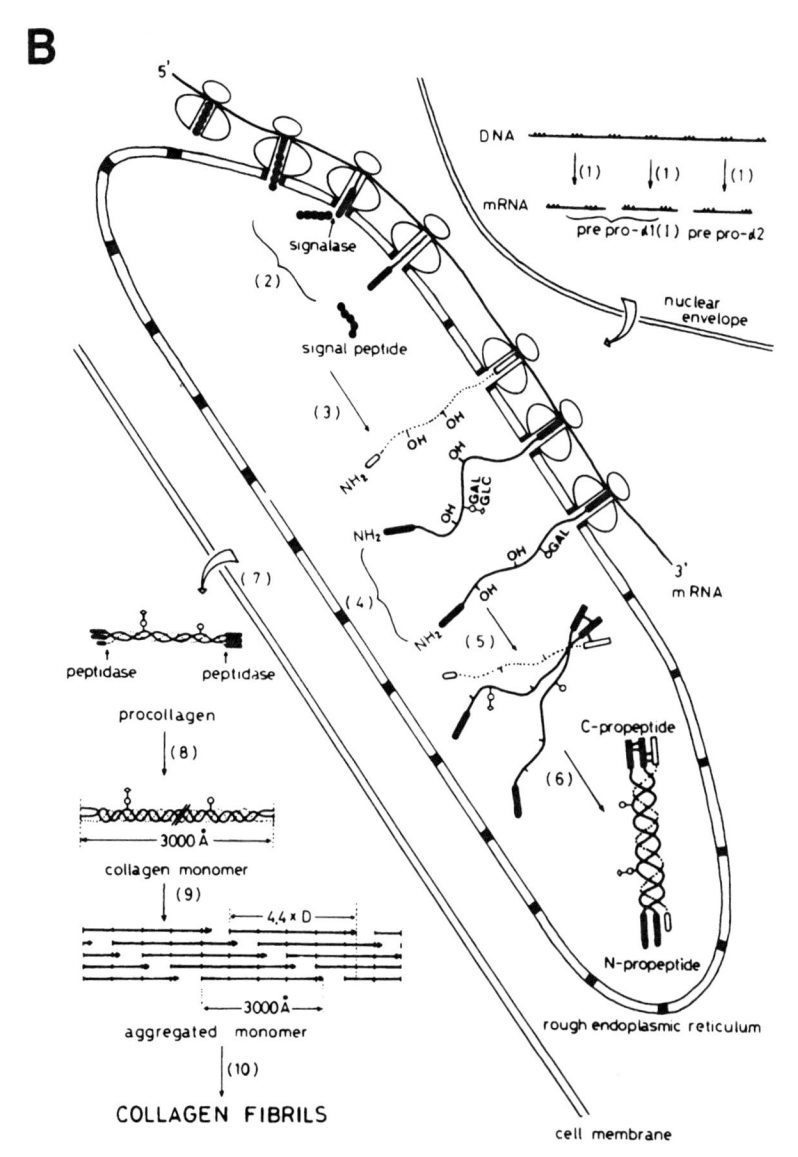

Fig. 2. *(continued)* **(B)** Posttranscriptional steps of collagen biosynthesis. (1) Transcription of collagen genes resulting in synthesis of different mRNAs for each procollagen chain. (2) Translation of the mRNA for each procollagen chain. Procollagen mRNAs are transported from the nucleus to ribosomes lining the rough endoplastic reticulum. The procollagen is depicted as a polypeptide chain having a signal peptide that is cleaved by a signal peptidase. (3) Hydroxylation by peptidyl proline hydroxylase or peptidyl lysine hydroxylase. (4) Glycosylation of hydroxylysyl residues by galactosyltransferase and glucosyltransferase. (5) Formation of the interchain disulfide links in the C-terminal propeptides. (6) Triple helix formation. (7) Secretion. (8) Procollagen-collagen conversion by limited proteolysis (pN-collagen aminopeptidase and pC-collagen carboxypeptidase). (9) Assembly into fibrils by a near-quarter-stagger's shift. (10) Crosslinking of collagen fibrils. (Courtesy of Dr. R. I. Bashey, reproduced with permission.)

disulfide bonds. These extensions, or propeptides, appear to prevent the nonphysiologic formation of collagen fibrils before the molecules reach the extracellular space. They are also involved in directing the proper assembly of the collagen molecules from their constituent chains and in initiation of triple helix formation. Shortly after synthesis of the individual procollagen polypeptide chains, specific association of three chains in a proper ratio (i.e., two pro α1 and one pro α2 chains for type I collagen), formation of disulfide bonds, and triple helix assembly occur. The crucial step of triple helix formation requires an adequate level of proline hydroxylation in order to take place at physiologic temperatures. As mentioned earlier, hydroxyproline-deficient collagen fails to form a stable triple helix at normal body temperatures and undergoes rapid intracellular degradation. Similarly, any excess procollagen chains that are not assembled into a triple helical conformation are degraded intracellularly. The propeptide extensions of newly synthesized procollagen molecules are excised by specific proteases immediately after they are transported into the extracellular millieu. Recent studies have demonstrated that bone morphogenetic protein-1 is the C-proteinase responsible for the processing of the carboxy-terminal extensions of the three major fibrillar procollagen (types I, II, and III) and, thus, it plays a key role in the regulation of deposition of the extracellular matrix in most vertebrate tissues. Some evidence has suggested a role for the cleaved propeptides in feedback inhibition of collagen biosynthesis and in extracellular collagen fibrillogenesis.

During the biosynthetic process, the polypeptide chains of procollagen are subject to at least six different enzyme-mediated modifications prior to secretion. Further posttranslational modifications involving crosslink formation occur extracellularly. These complex enzyme-mediated modifications are not usually found in the biosynthetic pathways of other proteins. Intracellular posttranslational modifications include hydroxylation of proline and lysine, addition of galactose to certain hydroxylysines and of glucose to certain galactose-hydroxylysines, and, finally, extrusion from the cell coupled with proteolytic cleavage of the extension peptides from the amino and carboxy termini of the molecule by specific proteases. The molecule is only secreted after hydroxylation, glycosylation, and triple helix formation are complete. Secretion appears to be a stepwise process, requiring packing into a Golgi vacuole before exocytosis. The posttranslational microheterogeneity resulting from these enzyme-mediated modifications probably represents the fine-tuning that adapts the various collagen molecules for their ultimate biological functions.

Although almost all the procollagens of most tissues are converted to collagen molecules, some unprocessed procollagen molecules may be retained at the cell surface to interact specifically with various structural components of the interfibrillar matrix. Basement membrane procollagens appear to be incorporated into the membrane structure without prior processing.

Processed molecules destined to form extracellular matrix fibrils self-assemble into three-dimensional fibrillar complexes, which are then stabilized by a series of covalent interchain and intrachain crosslinks. Most of these bonds originate from lysine or hydroxylysine and from modified forms of amino acid residues derived by oxidative deamination. Control of the extent of polymerization and of crosslinking is poorly understood, but has multiple and profound effects on the mechanical properties of collagen fibers.

6. Regulation of Collagen Biosynthesis and Gene Expression (37–51)

Under normal conditions, fibroblasts and other connective tissue-producing cells are capable of regulating extracellular matrix production according to the dynamic requirements of processes such as embryogenesis, development, differentiation, and tissue repair.

Remarkable methodologic advances in recent years have resulted in an explosion of knowledge regarding the mechanisms that regulate gene expression in eukaryotic cells. Multiple aspects of the intimate mechanisms responsible for the regulation of expression of the genes encoding for various extracellular matrix proteins have been clarified. These advances will undoubtedly provide light into the mechanisms responsible for the pathologic increase in tissue collagen in fibrotic diseases such as scleroderma or its reduction in diseases such as osteoporosis.

There are three general mechanisms by which the production of collagen can be controlled: (1) modulation of the steady-state level of mRNA; (2) control of mRNA translation; and (3) variation in the fraction of the newly synthesized protein, which is degraded before it is secreted from the cell. In most normal and pathologic conditions, the levels of procollagen or collagen mRNA correlate with the rate of synthesis of the corresponding collagen polypeptides. The steady-state mRNA levels are determined by a delicate balance between the transcription rates of the corresponding genes and the mRNA degradation rates. Transcriptional regulation is, by far, the most important mechanism determining the steady-state collagen mRNA levels; however, under certain conditions, particularly under the influence of growth factors and cytokines, alterations in mRNA stability or in the rates of mRNA degradation may play a substantial role.

Many mechanisms may be responsible for derangement of transcriptional regulation, including mutations in important promoter regulatory regions or in other specialized regulatory elements of the gene. These regulatory elements are also principal targets for the action of promoter-specific transcription factors. The factors may regulate the initiation of transcription of their target genes by possibly controlling the binding of RNA polymerases to pre-existing transcription complexes or by the formation of the transcription complex itself. Alternatively, binding of these transcriptional factors to their cognate DNA sequences or to other transcription factors already bound to DNA may result in bending or looping of the DNA strand, resulting in a modification of the rates of transcription of the corresponding genes. Several transcriptional factors that regulate the levels of expression of various collagen genes have been identified and characterized. They can exert either stimulatory or inhibitory effects on the rates of gene transcription. Some of these trans-acting factors recognize and bind to DNA sequences that are homologous to sequences in other genes, which are targets for transcriptional regulators such as AP1, AP2, NF-1, and the CBF or Sp families of transcription factors. The entire complement of DNA-binding proteins that specifically modulate the transcription of collagen genes has not been determined. The activity of many promoters is also modulated by binding of transcription factors to enhancer elements located either upstream or downstream of the transcription start site. Recent studies of the effects of transcriptional/DNA-binding factors and of their interactions with collagen gene promoter regions or with other regulatory elements indicate that the transcriptional regulation of collagen gene expression is extremely complex and that these interactions will undoubtedly affect the tissue specificity and the levels of collagen production in response to intracellular or extracellular perturbations (Fig. 3).

Posttranslational events may also influence the levels of collagen production. An intriguing control mechanism has been suggested from the observations that the

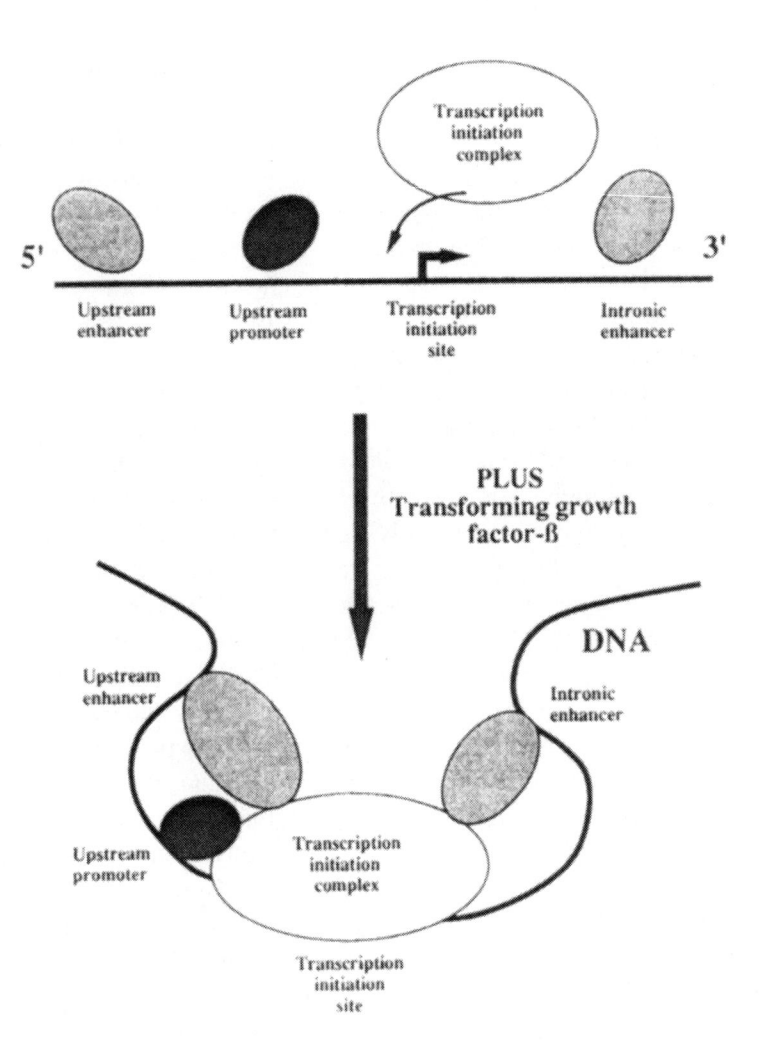

Fig. 3. A simplified view of the regulation of collagen gene transcription. Transcription of the collagen gene is initiated by binding of the transcription initiation complex, which contains RNA polymerase II and various initiation factors, to the DNA *(upper panel)*. This basal level of transcription is markedly stimulated by transforming growth factor-β, which may cause binding of additional transcriptional regulatory factors *(shaded ovals)* to upstream promoter elements and to upstream or intronic enhancer DNA sequences. Binding of the transcriptional factors may result in looping of DNA, allowing distant transcriptional regulatory factors to contact the transcription initiation complex *(lower panel)*. [From Varga, J. and Jimenez, S. A. (1995) Modulation of collagen gene expression: its relation to fibrosis in systemic sclerosis and other disorders. *Ann. Intern. Med.* **122**, 60–62.]

N-propeptides of type I or type III calf collagen can reduce the rate of collagen synthesis when added to cultures of calf dermal fibroblasts and can inhibit the translation of type I procollagen mRNA in a cell-free system. This negative feedback process may be a means whereby the concentration of propeptides in the extracellular matrix can modulate the rate of collagen synthesis at a translation level.

The observation that cultured fibroblasts can degrade a fraction of newly synthesized collagen before it is secreted represents another possible regulatory mechanism.

The fraction of collagen that undergoes such degradation appears to be mediated by lysosomal enzymes and can be increased by a variety of agents that raise the level of intracellular cyclic AMP or cause disruption of triple helix formation. A decrease in the fraction of collagen that is degraded intracellularly could result in a net increase in production of this protein and lead to fibrosis.

In addition to these intrinsic mechanisms of control, it has recently been shown that extrafibroblastic factors may influence the rates of collagen synthesized by these cells. Resident tissue fibroblasts are potential targets for extracellular signaling molecules that can modulate the rates at which collagen genes are expressed. Important physiologic modulators include hormones such as glucocorticoids and various cytokines. Because the development of fibrosis in systemic sclerosis and other fibrosing disorders appears to be preceded by infiltration of affected tissues with mononuclear cells (primarily macrophages and T-lymphocytes), cytokines, and growth factors produced by these cells are candidate-signaling molecules that may account for the upregulation of fibroblast collagen production in these disorders. In other disorders, such as rheumatoid arthritis, cytokines released from inflammatory cells in the synovium may inhibit expression of genes encoding extracellular matrix components and/or stimulate the expression of genes encoding collagenolytic and proteolytic enzymes including various metalloproteinases. Indeed, it has been shown that interferon-γ is one of the most potent inhibitors of collagen production, an effect that appears to occur largely at the transcriptional level, whereas tumor necrosis factors and interleukin-1 are capable of inducing the expression of numerous metalloproteinases.

Of the many cytokines and growth factors that have been shown to stimulate collagen production, transforming growth factor-β has emerged as crucial in tissue repair and fibrosis. This multifunctional cytokine, which has three structurally and functionally similar isoforms, is related to a large superfamily of homologous proteins whose members mediate key events in growth and development. Numerous studies have shed light on the biological activities of transforming growth factor-β involved in connective tissue turnover and the mechanisms of these effects. For example, it has been shown in vitro that transforming growth factor-β stimulates fibroblast production of various collagens. These responses appear to involve the induction or stimulation of gene promoter activity and are associated with increased DNA binding activity by transcriptional factors in the target cells. The identity and function of the collagen promoter–binding proteins activated by transforming growth factor-β are still unknown, although it appears that in the case of the type I collagen genes, their activation may be mediated through the SMAD protein cascade. Because transforming growth factor-β causes both sustained stimulation of collagen production and autoinduction of its own synthesis, a brief exposure of fibroblasts to this growth factor may result in persistent alteration in their biosynthetic phenotype. Exogenous administration of transforming growth factor-β in vivo has been shown to accelerate the healing of incision wounds, and endogenous production of transforming growth factor-β induced by targeted gene transfer has been shown to cause glomerulosclerosis when expressed in the kidney, and medial hyperplasia when expressed in arteries. On the other hand, antagonists of transforming growth factor-β prevent fibrosis. For instance, neutralizing transforming growth factor-β activity with specific antibodies inhibited scar formation in healing dermal wounds and prevented the development of carotid intimal hyperplasia following balloon angioplasty. Another growth factor, which has been recently implicated in the pathogenesis of tissue fibrosis, is connective tissue growth factor. This 38-kDa polypeptide is expressed in tissues undergoing active repair and remodeling and its production is stimulated by transforming growth factor-β. Connective tissue growth factor appears to function as a downstream mediator of transforming growth factor-β effects on connective tissue cells.

Currently, only circumstantial evidence implicates transforming growth factor-β in the formation of tissue fibrosis in systemic sclerosis. Increased expression of transforming growth factor-β has been shown by immunohistochemical methods and by *in situ* hybridization in the skin of patients with early systemic sclerosis but not in that of healthy controls. However, fibroblasts in tissues undergoing inflammation and remodeling are probably sequentially or simultaneously exposed to numerous cytokines and growth factors. These polypeptides may interact with each other and may modulate target cell responsiveness to other cytokines by various mechanisms. It is, therefore, the total cytokine and growth factor context that determines how a given cell responds to a specific signal.

In light of the rapid progress being made in understanding the biology of physiologic and pathologic tissue repair processes, the importance of delineating the molecular mechanisms of fibroblast signaling and regulation of collagen gene expression has become apparent. Numerous processes such as receptor and ligand interactions, intracellular pathways that are activated after signaling, and the mechanisms of induction or activation DNA-binding transcriptional factors by transforming growth factor-β and other cytokines and growth factors still need to be elucidated. The importance of these studies must be emphasized, as each of these steps is a potential target for highly specific therapeutic interventions. Novel antifibrotic strategies evolving from a precise understanding of these processes may provide potent therapies for systemic sclerosis and other diseases that are accompanied by pathologic tissue fibrosis. Alternatively, inhibition of expression of the genes encoding extracellular matrix degradative enzymes or interruption of their cytokine-mediated activation may lead to novel and effective treatments for diseases characterized by excessive extracellular matrix degradation such as rheumatoid arthritis.

References

1. Beck, K. and Brodsky, B. (1998) Supercoiled protein motifs: the collagen triple-helix and the α-helical coiled coil. *J. Struct. Biol.* **122**, 17–19.
2. Brodsky, B. and Ranshaw, J. A. (1997) The collagen triple-helix structure. *Matrix Biol.* **15**, 545–554.
3. Gay, S. and Miller, E. J. (1983) What is collagen, what is not. *Ultrastruct. Pathol.* **4**, 365–377.
4. Gordon, M. K. and Olsen, B. R. (1990) The contribution of collagenous proteins to tissue-specific matrix assemblies. *Curr. Opin. Cell Biol.* **2**, 833–838.
5. Mayne, R. and Burgeson, R. E. (eds.) (1987) *Structure and Function of Collagen Types*. Academic, New York.
6. Miller, E. J. (1985) The structure of fibril-forming collagens. *Ann. NY Acad. Sci.* **460**, 1–13.
7. Prockop, D. J. and Kivirikko, K. I. (1995) Collagens: molecular biology, diseases, and potentials for therapy. *Annu. Rev. Biochem.* **64**, 403–434.
8. Rosenbloom, J., Harsch, M., and Jimenez, S. A. (1973) Hydroxyproline determines the denaturation temperature of chick tendon collagen. *Arch. Biochem. Biophys.* **158**, 478–484.

9. Brown, J. C. and Timpl R. (1995) The collagen superfamily. *Int. Arch. Allergy Immunol.* **107**, 484–490.
10. Bruckner, P. and van der Rest, M. (1994) Structure and function of cartilage collagens. *Microsc. Res. Tech.* **28**, 378–384.
11. Burgeson, R. E. (1993) Type VII collagen, anchoring fibrils, and epidermolysis bullosa. *J. Invest. Dermatol.* **101**, 252–255.
12. Eyre, D. R., Wu, J. J., Woods, P. E., and Weis, M. A. (1991) The cartilage collagens and joint degeneration. *Br. J. Rheumatol.* **30**, 10–15.
13. Fichard, A., Kleman, J. P., and Ruggiero, F. (1995) Another look at collagen V and XI molecules. *Matrix Biol.* **14**, 515–531.
14. Fukai, N., Apte, S. S., and Olsen, B. R. (1994) Nonfibrillar collagens. *Methods Enzymol.* **245**, 3–28.
15. Martin, G. R., Timpl, R., Müller, P. K., and Kühn, K. (1985) The genetically distinct collagens. *Trends Biochem. Sci.* **10**, 285–287.
16. Mayne, R. and Brewton, R. G. (1993) New members of the collagen superfamily. *Curr. Opin. Cell Biol.* **5**, 883–890.
17. Pihlajaniemi, T. and Rehn, M. (1995) Two new collagen subgroups: membrane-associated collagens and types XV and XVII. *Prog. Nucleic Acid Res. Mol. Biol.* **50**, 225–262.
18. Pulkinen, L. and Uitto, J. (1998) Hemidesmosomal variants of epidermolysis bullosa. Mutations in the α6β4 integrin and the 180-kD bullous pemphigoid antigen/type XVII collagen genes. *Exp. Dermatol.* **7**, 46–64.
19. Shaw, L. M. and Olsen, B. R. (1991) FACIT collagens: diverse molecular bridges in extracellular matrices. *Trends Biochem. Sci.* **16**, 191–194.
20. Sutmuller, M., Bruijn, J. A., and deHeer, E. (1997) Collagen types VIII and X, two non-fibrillar, short-chain collagens. Structure homologies, functions and involvement in pathology. *Histol. Histopathol.* **12**, 557–566.
21. Thomas, J. T., Ayad, S., and Grant, M. E. (1994) Cartilage collagens: strategies for the study of their organization and expression in the extracellular matrix. *Ann. Rheum. Dis.* **53**, 488–496.
22. van der Rest, M. and Garrone, R. (1991) Collagen family of proteins. *FASEB J.* **5**, 2814–2823.
23. Dalgleish, R. (1988) Collagen gene structure. *Biochem. Soc. Trans.* **16**, 661–663.
24. Jacenko, O., Olsen, B. R., and LuValle, P. (1991) Organization and regulation of collagen genes. *Crit. Rev. Eukaryote Gene Express.* **1**, 327–353.
25. Krieg, T., Hein, R., Hatamochi, A., and Aumailley, M. (1988) Molecular and clinical aspects of connective tissue. *Eur. J. Clin. Invest.* **18**, 105–123.
26. Kuivaniemi, H., Tromp, G., and Prockop, D. J. (1997) Mutations in fibrillar collagens (types I, II, III and XI), fibril-associated collagen (type IX), and network-forming collagen (type X) cause a spectrum of diseases of bone, cartilage, and blood vessels. *Hum. Mutat.* **9**, 300–315.
27. Lee, B., D'Alessio, M., and Ramirez, F. (1991) Modifications in the organization and expression of collagen genes associated with skeletal disorders. *Crit. Rev. Eukaryote. Gene Express.* **1**, 173–187.
28. Olsen, B. R. (1995) Mutations in collagen genes resulting in metaphyseal and epiphyseal dysplasias. *Bone* **17**, 45S–49S.
29. Olsen, B. R. (1995) New insights into the function of collagens from genetic analysis. *Curr. Opin. Cell Biol.* **7**, 720–727.
30. Rimoin, D. L. (1996) Molecular defects in the chondrodysplasias. *Am. J. Med. Genet.* **63**, 106–110.
31. Sado, Y., Kagawa, M., Naito, I., Ueki, Y., Seki, T., Momota, R., et al. (1998) Organization and expression of basement membrane collagen IV genes and their roles in human disorders. *J. Biochem.* **123**, 767–776.
32. Sandell, L. J. (1996) Genes and gene regulation of extracellular matrix proteins: an introduction. *Connect. Tissue Res.* **35**, 1–6.

33. Sandell, L. J. and Boyd, C. D. (eds.) (1990) *Extracellular Matrix Genes*. Academic Press, New York.
34. Vuorio, E. and deCrombrugge, B. (1990) The family of collagen genes. *Annu. Rev. Biochem.* **59,** 837–872.
35. Peltonen, L., Halila, R., and Ryhanen, L. (1985) Enzymes converting procollagens to collagens. *J. Cell Biochem.* **28,** 15–21.
36. Ramirez, F., Boast, S., D'Alessio, M., Prince, J., Su, M. W., and Vissing, H. (1989) Molecular pathobiology of human collagens. *Connect. Tissue Res.* **21,** 79–88.
37. Adams, S. L. (1989) Collagen gene expression. *Am. J. Respir. Cell Mol. Biol.* **1,** 161–168.
38. Bienkowski, R. S. and Gotkin, M. G. (1995) Control of collagen deposition in mammalian lung. *Proc. Soc. Exp. Biol. Med.* **209,** 118–140.
39. Bornstein, P. (1996) Regulation of expression of the α1(I) collagen gene: a critical appraisal of the role of the first intron. *Matrix Biol.* **15,** 3–10.
40. Bornstein, P. and Sage, H. (1989) Regulation of collagen gene expression. *Prog. Nucleic Acid Res. Mol. Biol.* **37,** 67–106.
41. Bornstein, P., Horlein, D., and McPherson, J. (eds.) (1984) *Regulation of Collagen Synthesis, Myelofibrosis and the Biology of Connective Tissue.* Alan R. Liss, New York.
42. Brenner, D. A., Rippe, R. A., Rhodes, K., Trotter, J. F., and Breindl, M. (1994) Fibrogenesis and type I collagen gene regulation. *J. Lab. Clin. Med.* **124,** 755–760.
43. Freundlich, B., Bomalaski, J. S., Neilson, E., and Jimenez, S. A. (1986) Regulation of fibroblast proliferation and collagen synthesis by cytokines. *Immunol. Today* **7,** 303–307.
44. Jimenez, S. A., Freundlich, B., and Rosenbloom, J. (1984) Selective inhibition of human diploid fibroblast collagen synthesis by interferons. *J. Clin. Invest.* **74,** 1112–1116.
45. Jimenez, S. A., Hitraya, E., and Varga, J. (1996) Pathogenesis of scleroderma. Collagen. *Rheum. Dis. Clin. North Am.* **22,** 647–674.
46. Karsenty, G. and Park, R. W. (1995) Regulation of type I collagen genes expression. *Int. Rev. Immunol.* **12,** 177–185.
47. Raghow, R. and Thompson, J. P. (1989) Molecular mechanisms of collagen gene expression. *Mol. Cell Biochem.* **86,** 5–18.
48. Slack, J. L., Liska, D. J., and Bornstein, P. (1993) Regulation of expression of the type I collagen genes. *Am. J. Med. Genet.* **45,** 140–151.
49. Trojanowska, M., LeRoy, E. C., Eckes, B., and Krieg, T. (1998) Pathogenesis of fibrosis: type I collagen and the skin. *J. Mol. Med.* **76,** 266–274.
50. Varga, J. and Jimenez, S. A. (1995) Modulation of collagen gene expression: its relation to fibrosis in systemic sclerosis and other disorders. *Ann. Intern. Med.* **122,** 60–62.
51. Varga, J., Rosenbloom, J., and Jimenez, S. A. (1987) Transforming growth factor β (TGFβ) causes a persistent increase in steady state amounts of type I and type III collagens and fibronectin mRNAs in normal human dermal fibroblasts. *Biochem. J.* **247,** 597–604.

II
CELLULAR MECHANISMS IN RHEUMATIC DISEASES

12

T-Lymphocytes

Nilamadhab Mishra and Gary M. Kammer

1. Introduction

All hematopoietic cells are derived from pluripotent stem cells, which give rise to the principal lineages of lymphoid and myeloid cells. The common lymphoid progenitor has the capacity to differentiate into either T-lymphocytes or B-lymphocytes, depending on the microenvironment to which it homes. In humans, T-cells develop in the thymus, whereas B-cells evolve in fetal liver and bone marrow. The T-lymphocyte pool is established in the thymus early in life and is maintained throughout life by antigen-driven expansion of naive peripheral T-cells into memory cells that reside primarily in lymphoid organs.

Mature T-cells constitute 70–80% of normal peripheral blood lymphocytes. However, only 2% of total-body lymphocytes circulate in peripheral blood at any time. T-cells comprise 90% of thoracic duct lymphocytes, 30–40% of lymph node cells, and 20–30% of splenic lymphoid cells. In lymph nodes, T-cells occupy deep paracortical regions and surround B-cell germinal centers; in the spleen, T-cells are located in the periarteriolar regions of the white pulp.

T-cells are the primary effectors of cell-mediated immunity. As such, they regulate other T-cells, B-cells, and antigen-presenting cells (APCs) by direct cell-to-cell contact and the production of cytokines.

2. T-Lymphocyte Ontogeny

2.1. T-Lymphocyte Subpopulations

Mature T-cells are identified by the CD3 complex of transmembrane receptors expressed on their cell-surface (Fig. 1). CD is an abbreviation for cluster of differentiation or designation, which is a systematic nomenclature for the identification of cell-surface receptors by monoclonal antibodies. Of these receptors, the CD3 ε chain is most commonly used to identify mature T-cells. T-cells are comprised of two principal subpopulations: (1) a subset bearing the CD4 coreceptor that provides helper function for B-cell maturation and antibody production and (2) a subset bearing the CD8 coreceptor that mediates cytotoxicity against tumor cells and virally infected cells. Both CD4 and CD8 are often referred to as coreceptors because of the functions they subserve in cell–cell contact with APCs, such as macrophages or dendritic cells. CD4

From: *Current Molecular Medicine: Principles of Molecular Rheumatology*
Edited by: G. C. Tsokos © Humana Press Inc., Totowa, NJ

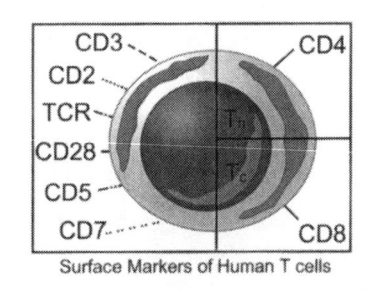

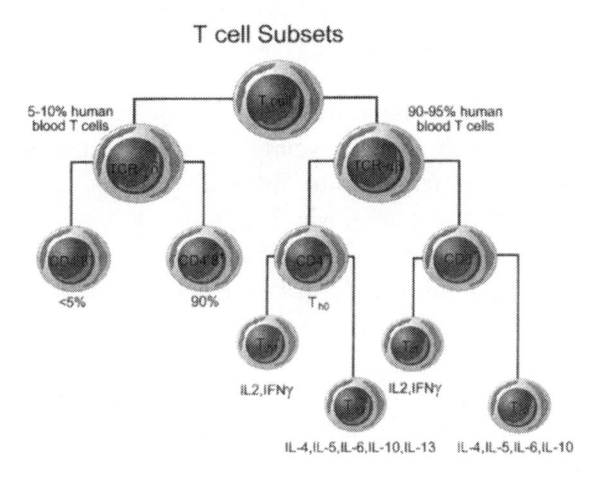

Fig. 1. **(A)** Surface markers of human T-cells. **(B)** T-cell subsets. T-cells can be subdivided into different subsets based on the expression of the T-cell receptor (TCR-αβ or TCR-γδ). TCR αβ cells express either CD4 or CD8. CD4 T-cells can be further subdivided into Th1 and Th2 and CD8 to Tc1 and Tc2 population based on their profiles of cytokine production.

and CD8 are utilized as markers for each subpopulation and are identified by specific monoclonal antibodies. The biological significance of CD4 and CD8 depends on their capacity to bind to nonpolymorphic regions of class II and class I molecules, respectively, on APCs in order to identify self and to initiate signal transduction. Each subset also expresses multiple other cell-surface receptors, which will be described later.

2.2. Thymocyte Development

The thymus develops from the third pharyngeal pouch as an epithelial rudiment of endodermal origin. Migration of stem cells into the thymus is not a random process; instead, it results from chemotactic signals periodically released from the thymic rudiment.

The thymus is organized as lobules. Each thymic lobule has cortical and medullary regions where epithelial cells, macrophages, and bone-marrow-derived interdigitating cells, rich in major histocompatibility complex (MHC) class II receptors, are found. Differentiation of T-cells depends on their direct interactions with these cell types. The thymic subcapsular region is the first to be colonized by stem cells arriving from the bone marrow. These cells gradually develop into large, actively proliferating, self-renewing lymphoblasts that generate the thymocyte population. Phenotypic analysis

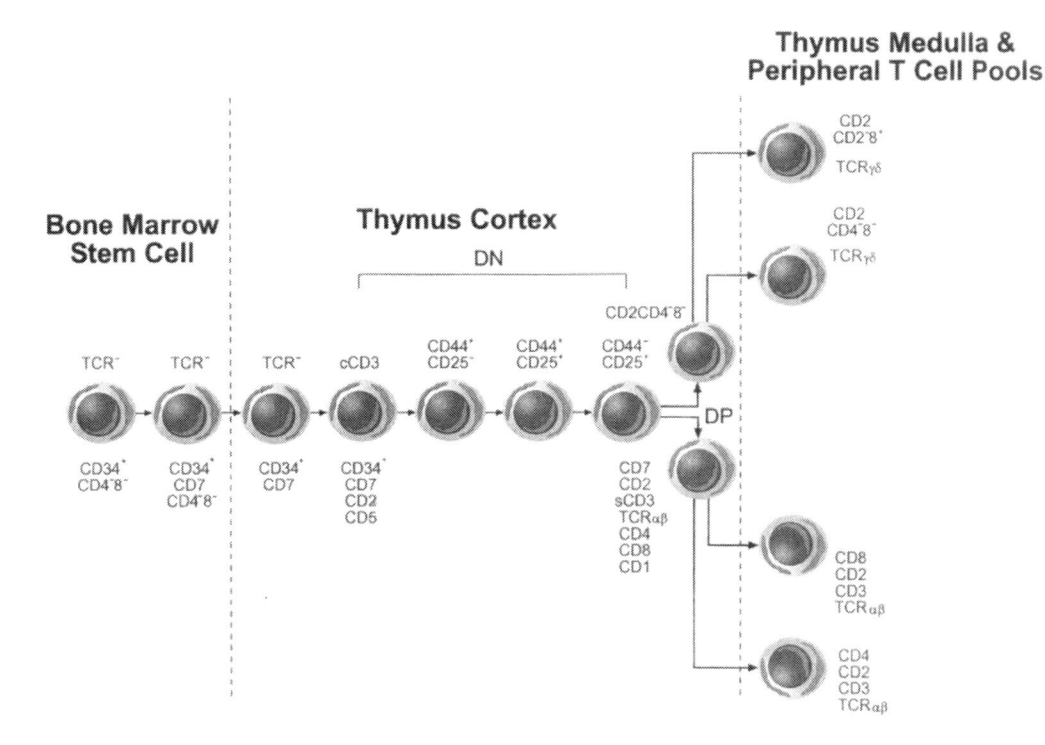

Fig. 2. Stages of thymocyte development. Progenitor cells migrate from the bone marrow to the thymus. sCD3: surface CD3 expression; cCD3: cytoplasmic CD3 expression; DN: double negative; DP: double positive.

has revealed a succession of cell-surface phenotypes during T-cell maturation. This systematic and progressive phenotypic evolution appears to occur in three stages *(1,2)*.

2.2.1. Stage I (Early) Thymocytes

These thymocytes express CD7, CD2, CD5, and CD44 (Fig. 2). In addition, proliferation markers, including CD71 (transferrin receptor) and CD38 (a marker common to all early hematopoietic precursors), are expressed at this stage. However, none of these proliferation markers is T-lineage-specific. In this stage, thymocytes are double-negative (DN) cells that lack expression of both the CD3/TCR complex and the CD4 and CD8 coreceptors. Later, DN cells express Rag1 and 2 genes, rearrange the TCRβ gene, and express CD4 and CD8 coreceptors to become double-positive (DP) cells *(1,3)*.

2.2.2. Stage II (Intermediate or Common) Thymocytes

Stage II thymocytes account for approximately 85% of lymphoid cells in the thymus. These DP cells are characterized by the appearance of additional surface markers, including CD1 (Fig. 2). DP thymocytes make up the bulk of cells in the thymic cortex; these cells have a life-span of 3–4 d, with 25–33% of them being replaced each day. As T-cell development progresses, thymocytes migrate from the cortex to the medulla. Three critical processes occur at this stage: (1) rearrangement of the T-cell receptor-α (TCR-α) gene; (2) positive and negative selection through interaction with MHC molecules on epithelial cells; and (3) evolution of single-positive (SP) CD4 helper (Th) and CD8 cytotoxic (Tc) cells in the thymic medulla (Fig. 2) *(1–3)*.

2.2.3. Stage III (Mature) Thymocytes

Stage III thymocytes undergo major phenotypic changes: (1) loss of CD1; (2) expression of cell-surface CD3 that is associated with the high-density αβ TCR; and (3) completion of switch from DP to SP cells expressing CD4 or CD8. At this stage, the majority of thymocytes lack both CD38 and CD71 and are virtually indistinguishable from mature, circulating T-cells. Moreover, stage III thymocytes express the receptor, CD44, which mediates transvascular migration and homing to peripheral lymphoid tissue. The adhesion molecule, L-selectin, also becomes expressed during this period *(1–4)*.

2.3. Thymocyte Education: Positive Selection

Developing thymocytes that recognize foreign peptides in association with self-MHC molecules are selected to survive; the remainder undergoes apoptosis or programmed cell death. Positive selection ensures that only thymocytes expressing TCRs with moderate affinity for self-MHC are allowed to mature. Thymocytes displaying very high or very low receptor affinities for self-MHC undergo apoptosis, dying in the cortex.

Positive selection appears to be mediated through thymic epithelial cells. As a part of this positive selection process, Tc cells are selected for recognition of class I MHC molecules, whereas Th cells are selected for recognition of class II MHC molecules *(5)*.

If developing thymocytes with receptors that recognize self-peptides associated with self-MHC molecules were to mature in the thymus and migrate to peripheral lymphoid tissues, autoimmunity would develop. This process is prevented by negative selection in the thymus.

2.4. Thymocyte Education: Negative Selection (Central Tolerance)

Negative selection leads to the elimination of developing thymocytes that react strongly with self-peptides bound to self-MHC molecules in the thymus. In other words, only thymocytes that fail to recognize self-antigen can proceed to maturity. Unlike positive selection, which occurs mainly on the surface of thymic epithelial cells, negative selection occurs predominantly on the surface of APCs, including dendritic cells or macrophages that originate in the bone marrow and migrate into the thymus *(5)*.

The mechanisms responsible for thymic education are incompletely understood. In both cases, however, programmed cell death appears to be triggered to eliminate potentially autoreactive T-cells. Several hypotheses have been proposed to account for thymic education. One recent hypothesis, referred to as the *avidity model of thymocyte selection*, proposes that, to a large extent, positive and negative selection represent qualitatively different responses to different intensities of signaling through the TCR *(6)*. Avidity is the product of the affinity of the TCR for a given peptide–MHC complex and the densities of the TCR and the peptide–MHC complex. The overall strength of signaling in a T-cell is proportional to TCR occupancy, which, in turn, reflects both the number of TCRs engaged and their affinity for binding the antigen–MHC complex. Below a certain level of TCR occupancy, an effective signal is not initiated. According to the avidity model, a moderate level of occupancy provides a positive signal that promotes thymocyte growth and maturation, whereas excessive occupancy (above a certain, undefined threshold) causes cell death by apoptosis. Thymocytes whose receptors bind strongly to self-peptide MHC complexes in the medulla would thus be eliminated (i.e., negative selection), whereas those that give weak but perceptible binding to the same complexes in the cortex would be positively selected. We do not yet know, in biochemical terms, exactly what constitutes the critical difference between the survival signal delivered by low-avidity TCR binding and the apoptotic signal triggered by high-avidity interactions. Nevertheless, the avidity model offers a plausible schema by which TCR–MHC interactions could guide both positive and negative thymic selection.

Recently, the vav protein has been associated with defective selection. p95vav is an intracellular rho family GTP/GDP exchange factor that is required for efficient TCR signaling and thymopoiesis in mice. TCR transgenic mice that lack p95vav have a profound defect in positive selection and a less dramatic impairment in negative selection. Interestingly, vav-deficient thymocytes show impaired calcium mobilization in response to TCR stimulation, suggesting a mechanism by which the mutation may affect development *(5)*.

2.5. TCR Diversity Generation in the Thymus

T-cells have to recognize a diverse variety of different antigens. To accomplish this task, T-cells have evolved two combinations of transmembrane receptors, termed α,β and γ,δ, to comprise the TCR and enhance diversity. The genes of αβ and γδ TCRs undergo somatic recombination during thymic development to produce functional genes for the different T-cell receptors. The β and δ chains are encoded by V, D, and J segments. The α and γ chains use only V and J segments. The first TCR genes to rearrange during thymocyte development encode the γ chains; this is followed by rearrangement of the β- and α-chain genes. Through a random assortment of different gene segments, a large number of productive rearrangements can be made. Thymocytes that make nonproductive rearrangements are destroyed. Remarkably, more than 95% of the cells produced die before they are able to mature and migrate to peripheral lymphoid organs. This waste is the result of a stringent selection process that operates during T-cell development to ensure that only cells with potentially useful receptors survive *(1)*.

3. T-Cell Migration from the Thymus

The vast majority of T-cells released by the thymus consist of mature CD3, CD4, and CD3, CD8 cells. These cells are fully functional at the time of exit. Thymic emigrants appear in thoracic duct lymph within a few hours and migrate rapidly to the spleen and lymph nodes. The total number of cells released by the thymus per day is quite low.

The thymus is a conspicuously large organ during young age. Release of T-cells from the thymus is maximal in young age. However, it begins to atrophy at the time of puberty. Thymic atrophy is progressive and reaches its nadir in old age. Outputs of mature T-cells tend to decline with age and concomitant thymic atrophy, reaching very low levels in old age.

4. T-Cell Effector Functions

4.1. Th Functions

The Th cells express the CD4 coreceptor on their cell surface. Unlike Tc cells, these cells do not act directly to kill infected cells or to eliminate microorganisms. Instead, they stimulate macrophages and other phagocytic cells, enhancing their capacity to

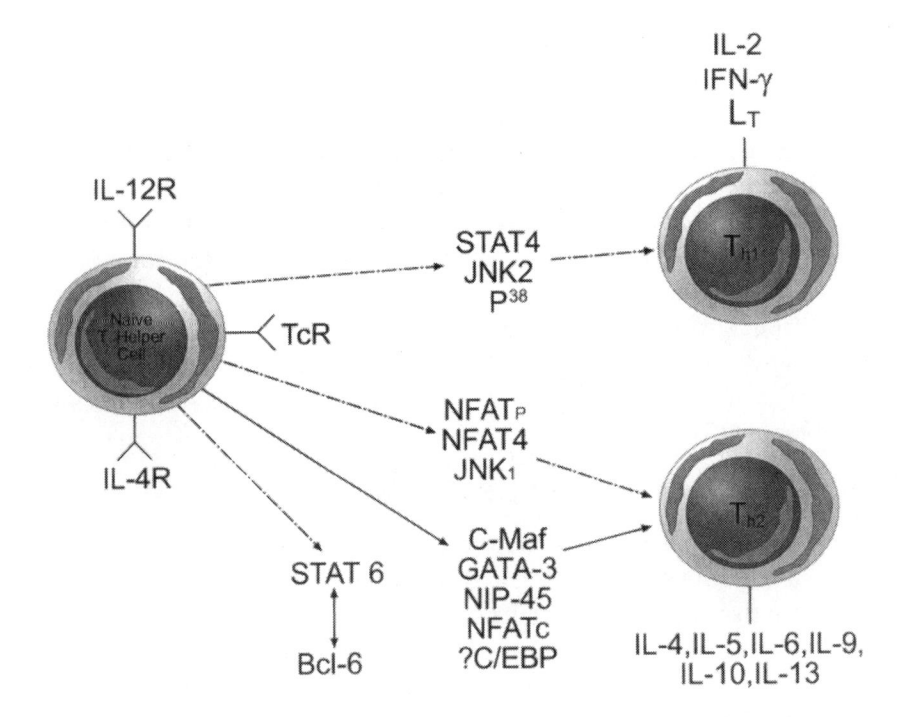

Fig. 3. Transcription factors that control Th lineage commitment. (Modified from ref. 3, with permission.)

phagocytose and destroy pathogens. Th cells are activated by binding antigenic peptides bound to class II MHC on the surface of APCs via TCRα,β. Once activated, CD4 Th1 cells produce cytokines, particularly interleukin-2 (IL-2), that induce entry into the cell cycle and mitogenesis. This enlarges the clone of T-cells responsive to the antigen (ag). IL-2 and other cytokines can also induce maturation and antibody production by B-cells by both membrane-bound and secreted signals. A principal membrane-bound signaling molecule is CD154 (CD40 ligand), which is expressed on the surface of activated, but not resting, Th cells. CD154 is recognized by CD40 on the B-cell surface. The interaction between CD154 and CD40 is required for activated Th cells to stimulate B-cells to proliferate and mature into memory and antibody-secreting cells. Cytokines secreted by Th2 cells, such as IL-4 and IL-6, bind to specific receptors, initiating intracellular signaling events that promote B-cell proliferation and maturation and, in some cases, class switching of antibody (e.g., IgM → IgG) *(7)*.

Naïve CD4 Th precursor cells may secrete IL-2, interferon-γ (IFN-γ), and IL-4. Because such cells secrete cytokines that derive from both Th1 and Th2 cells, they are often referred to as Th0. Th1 cells secrete IL-2, IFN-γ, transforming growth factor-β (TGF-β), and tumor necrosis factor-β (TNF-β), and commonly function to provide help for Tc cells and macrophages. Th2 cells, by contrast, secrete IL-4, IL-5, IL-6, IL-10, and IL-13 and promote help to B-cells and eosinophils (Figs. 1 and 3). This differentiation is highly dependent on the presence of certain cytokines and their downstream signaling transcription factors. As shown in Fig. 3, Th1 and Th2 subsets utilize IL-12/stat4 and IL-4/stat6, respectively, in their development *(2,3,8,9)*.

4.2. Tc Lymphocytes (CTL)

Cytotoxic lymphocytes (CTL) are immunized T-cells whose role in the immune response is to kill allogeneic targets, virus-infected cells, intracellular bacterial pathogens, and tumor cells. CTL activity has been detected in two principal subsets: (1) CD8 T-cells recognizing peptide antigens of 9–10 amino acids in length presented by MHC class I molecules and (2) TCRγδ T-cells exhibiting cytolytic activity against bacteria-pulsed targets. Similar to CD4 T-cells, CD8 T-cells can be divided into two subsets: Tc1 and Tc2, based on cytokine production. Tc1 cells produce IFN-γ and IL-2, whereas Tc2 cells produce IL-4, IL-5, IL-6, and IL-10. These cytotoxic memory cells are stable and retain their cytokine pattern.

Cytotoxic T-cells directly kill infected target cells that display fragments of microbial protein on their surface. Some of the microbial proteins that are synthesized in the cytosol of the target cell are degraded by proteasomes; from there, peptide fragments are pumped by an ABC transporter into the lumen of the endoplasmic reticulum (ER), where they bind to class I MHC molecules. The peptide–MHC complexes are then transported to the target cell surface, where they can be recognized by cytotoxic T-cells *(10)*.

T-cells appear to kill infected target cells by at least three discrete mechanisms: secretion of cytotoxic cytokines (such as TNF-α and IFN-γ) and calcium-dependent and calcium-independent contact-dependent cytotoxicity. The calcium-dependent pathway relies on the secretion of cytotoxic granules onto the surface of the target cell and is, therefore, known as the granule exocytosis pathway. The calcium-independent pathway causes target death via interaction with the Fas ligand (FasL) on the CTL and the Fas receptor (FasR) on the target cell *(11)*.

4.2.1. Killing by Cytotoxic Granules (Early Form of Cytotoxicity)

Cytotoxic lymphocyte granules and their constituent proteins are synthesized 24–48 h after stimulation via the TCR. Perforin is an integral cytotoxic protein that is similar to some of the terminal components of the complement cascade. It can polymerize in the presence of calcium to form channel-like structures comprised of 10- to 20-nm pores in target cell membranes. These perforin pores are not sufficient to kill nucleated target cells, which have the ability to repair membranes and thereby avoid osmotic lysis. The other key granule components are the granzymes, granzyme B and granzyme A, which are neutral serine proteases that pass through the channel formed by perforin to the inside of the cell. After entering to the target cell, granzymes translocate to the cytoplasm of the cell, where they act on specific substrates involved in the ultimate death of the cell and/or they are transported to the nucleus, where they may directly cleave and activate death substrates. As an Aspase, Granzyme B activates most procaspases. It also activates caspases 3, 6, 7, 8, and 9. Whether granzyme B activates the caspase pathway to induce rapid target cell death or whether granzyme A is the critical granzyme that is responsible for this process remains unknown. This perforin/granzyme system is dominant in CD8, but not CD4, CTLs *(10,11)*.

4.2.2. Killing by the FasL–Fas Pathway

Antigen recognition stimulates CTLs to express FasL, a member of the tumor necrosis factor (TNF) family. The interaction of FasL with FasR induces apoptosis in Fas-expressing cells. This is the late form of cytotoxicity in CD8 CTLs and is the second mechanism of cytotoxicity in perforin-deficient CTLs. CD4 CTLs deficient in FasL allow approximately 30% of animals mismatched at MHC class II to survive, suggesting that this pathway is important for CD4 CTL-mediated cytotoxicity. Based on the limited lysis of selected target cells, it is estimated that the perforin mechanism is responsible for approximately two-thirds of killing activity and the Fas system for the remaining one-third *(10–12)*.

4.2.3. Killer Cell Inhibitory Receptor Expression by CTLs

Killer cell inhibitory receptors (KIRs) are a new family of MHC class-I-specific receptors. They were initially discovered on natural-killer (NK) cells. KIRs allow NK cells to identify and lyse cells that do not express sufficient amounts of MHC class I molecules. CD8+ T-cells principally express KIRS; these receptors also appear to inhibit TCR-mediated functions. KIR expression on mature NK cells appears to be constitutive, whereas it can be induced on T-cells. It is not clear whether KIRs, once expressed, remain stable until cell death or whether these receptors are downregulated. KIR expression might play a physiological role in preventing CTLs from crossreacting with self-antigens, and their defective expression could be involved in autoimmune diseases caused by autoreactive CTLs. The other side of the coin is the inability of KIRs expressed on CTLs to control viral infections or tumor growth effectively. Different cytokines regulate KIR expression on T-cells. TGF-β and IL-10 induce KIR expression, whereas IL-4, IL-6, IL-7, IL-12, and IFN-γ do not. The discovery of KIRs on T-cells has uncovered new frontiers in immunology *(11–13)*.

4.3. Memory T-Cells

Immunological memory is possibly the single most universally recognized characteristic of the immune system. Memory cells are lymphocytes derived from a population of naïve, resting cells, selected by antigen from the recirculating pool and stimulated to proliferate to allow rapid response and longer life. There are three important factors of the memory response: accelerated speed, increased size and persistence. T-cell memory can involve both CD4 and CD8 T cells. Memory T-cells differ from virgin T-cells in their surface phenotype. Various cell-adhesion molecules have also been proposed as markers of memory, including leukocyte-function-associated molecule 1 (LFA-1), LFA-3, CD2, intercellular adhesion molecule 1 (ICAM-1), very late antigen 4 (VLA-4), reduced L-selectin expression, and increased CD44 expression (Fig. 4). LFA-1 and CD2 appear to play fundamental roles in facilitating cell–cell interactions (e.g., between T-cells and APCs). LFA-1 binds to ICAM-1, whereas CD2 binds to LFA-3. CD44 and VLA4 bind to components of the extracellular matrix and have been implicated in T-cell homing. Other molecules, such as CD45 and CD28 receptors, modulate signals initiated at the TCR and, therefore, play integral roles in early signaling events in the plasma membrane *(14)*.

At present, the most reliable method of identifying naïve cells from memory cells is by the CD45 isoform expressed on the cell surface (Fig. 4). Resting CD4 T-cells expressing a high-molecular-weight CD45 isoform, $CD45R^{hi}$, are induced by mitogen or Ag to switch to expression of a restricted isoform of low molecular weight, $CD45R^{lo}$. Depending on the specificity of the monoclonal antibodies used, $CD45R^{hi}$ (naïve) T-cells are identified as $CD45RA^+$, and $CD45R^{lo}$ (memory) T-cells are $CD45RA^-$ (CD45R0). There are two distinct, but lineage related, subsets of CD4 memory T-cells. Ag-primed $CD45R^{lo}$ memory T-cells provide the rapid response kinetics and follow

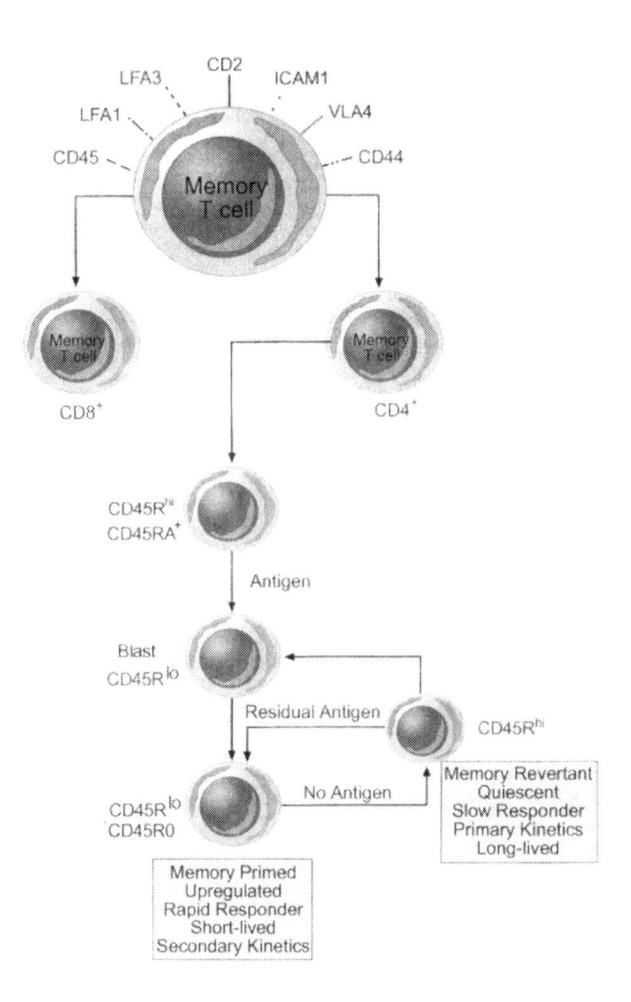

Fig. 4. Memory cells can be subdivided to CD8 memory T-cells and CD4 memory T-cells. There are two distinct subsets of CD4 memory T-cells: CD45R^{lo} and CD45R^{hi}. Naïve CD45R^{hi} CD4 T-cells proliferate in response to Ag, undergo blast transformation, express the CD45R^{lo} phenotype, and become memory primed. This phenotype is unstable and dependent on Ag. In the absence of Ag, memory T-cells revert to expression of the CD45R^{hi} isoform and become quiescent. These revertant memory T-cells resemble naïve T-cells in all respects.

specific migratory routes. In addition, these cells are strictly dependent on Ag and are short-lived. CD45R^{hi} revertant memory T-cells are derived from the CD45R^{lo} subsets, but are quiescent, resemble naïve CD4 T-cells, and show increased Ag-specific precursor frequency and a capacity for longer life. CD45R^{hi} revertants are capable of responding only with primary kinetics, but they ensure that immunological memory endures beyond the life of the antigen.

Naïve and memory T-cells exhibit different properties. Memory T-cells function less effectively than naïve T-cells in responding to alloantigens, but provide strong helper function for B-cell antibody production. In addition, the memory T-cell phenotype tends to resemble Th2 cells because they preferentially release IL-4. Moreover, naïve and memory T-cells migrate by different pathways: memory T-cells by the extravascular route and naïve T-cells by crossing high endothelial venules (HEVs) of lymph nodes. Unlike short-lived virgin T-cells, which exist for a matter of weeks, memory T-cells are long-lived, capable of self-renewal, and persist for years. Memory cell survival appears to depend on the presence of Ag *(14)*.

4.4. γδ T-Cells

About 5% of mature T-cells do not express a TCR α/β dimer. These cells have a second form of TCR, composed of a CD3 complex together with a dimer of polypeptides designated γ and δ. Interestingly, the first T-cells to mature during fetal development are γδ T-cells. Typical γδ cells are CD4$^-$8$^-$, although a small proportion are CD4$^-$8$^+$. These cells are relatively rare in the lymphoid tissue, including the thymus, but are conspicuous in epithelial tissues such as the skin, gut, and genitourinary tract. Unlike αβ T-cells, γδ cells show a curious propensity for reacting to heat-shock proteins *(1,2)*.

Human γδ T-cells bearing the TCR Vγ9Vδ2 isotype are of especial interest because they respond to both naturally occurring and synthetic, nonpeptidic phosphoags that are quite different from lipids, superags, or classical peptides that trigger αβ T-cells. Moreover, Vγ9Vδ2 T-cells react strongly against certain lymphoma cells, suggesting a possible crossreactivity between microbial and tumor-associated Ags. The cell-surface expression of inhibitory MHC class I receptors (INMRs) (predominantly the CD94–NKG2-A complex) on 80% of circulating human γδ T-cells is substantially higher than that on 4% αβ T-cells from the same donors. It is noteworthy that only functionally mature Vγ9Vδ2 T-cells express one or more types of INMRs.

The γδ T-cells may guide the establishment of acquired immunity through cytokine and chemokine secretion. Triggering CD94–NKG2-A interferes with γδ T-cell proliferation to bacterial or viral Ags as well as with the synthesis of cytokines. The cytotoxic activity of γδ T-cells also involves the recognition of HLA class I molecules. INMRs may set a higher TCR activation threshold, which helps regulate their reactivity toward self-Ags.

Control of Vγ9Vδ2 T-cell activation requires coordinated interactions of the stimulatory (CD3–Vγ9Vδ2 TCR) and inhibitory (CD94–NKG2-A) receptors with their ligands. CD94 engagement facilitates the recruitment of SHP-1 phosphatase to the TCR/CD3 complex and affects phosphorylation of Lck and Zap-70 kinases. The cytoplasmic tail of the CD94-associated NKG2-A C-type lectin contains two immunoreceptor tyrosine-based inhibitory motifs (ITIMS). Tyrosine phosphorylation of ITIM(s) by a protein tyrosine kinase(s) (PTK) results in binding of this region to a negative regulatory molecule containing a SH2 domain, such as SHP-1. This interrupts the flow of downstream activation signals. Coaggregation between CD3–Vγ9Vδ2 TCRs and INMRs is required for the inhibition of cell activation, suggesting that INMRs may be phosphorylated by a PTK associated with the CD3–Vγ9Vδ2 TCR complex, although coupling of INMRs to PTKs cannot be excluded.

The γδ T-cells regulate the initiation, progression, and resolution of immune responses triggered by infectious etiologies. In particular, strong γδ T-cell responses have been demonstrated in many viral infections, suggesting that antiviral immunosurveillance may be one of the primary γδ T-cell functions. For example, human γδ T-cells lyse human immunodeficiency virus (HIV)-infected targets and are capable of suppressing viral replication in vitro. In vivo, major changes in γδ T-cell numbers and functions have been repeatedly observed in acquired immune deficiency syndrome patients. In many of them, these changes occur at early stages of HIV infection. Transient increases of γδ cell numbers have also been observed in the peripheral blood of healthy donors exposed to *Mycobacterium tuberculosis* (MTbc)-infected patients, but not in the blood of chronically ill tuberculosis patients, indirectly suggesting a protective role of these cells. γδ T-cell responses are markedly increased in primary MTbc-infected children in comparison with age-matched controls. This increase in γδ T-cell reactivity typically subsides after successful antibiotic therapy, suggesting that persistent exposure to mycobacterial ags is required for the maintenance of γδ T-cell activation in vivo *(13,15)*.

5. Nuclear Events in the T-Cell

The cascade of early biochemical events that follows binding of different extracellular ligands to T-cells ultimately trigger a genetic program for growth and expression of differentiated functions *(16)*. As part of this program, small quiescent T-cells are transformed into lymphoblasts with increases in cellular and nuclear size, a more prominent Golgi apparatus, and a polyribosome-rich cytoplasm. On the molecular level, these morphological and functional changes are accompanied, and apparently caused by, a coordinated sequential activation of previously silent genes. These transcriptional events culminate in the initiation of DNA synthesis approximately 24 h after initial triggering *(4)*.

Among the de novo-induced genes during T-cell activation, some may encode products associated with cell-cycle progression and, thus, may be common to many cell types. Others are unique for T-cells and are associated with specific immunological functions of these cells. More than 70 gene products are regulated during the early and late phases of T-cell activation. Induction of the majority of these genes is resistant to, and in many instances are augmented by, the protein synthesis inhibitor cycloheximide. Regulated genes in T-cells have been divided into immediate (e.g., independent of protein synthesis), early (e.g., protein synthesis dependent, but induced prior to onset of proliferation), and late (e.g., following initiation of cell division). Among the regulated genes studied more extensively during T-cell activation are the cell-cycle-regulated protooncogenes, *c-fos*, *c-myc*, *c-myb* and some of the genes related to the specific functions of T-cells, including IL-2, IL-2Rα, IL-3, -4, -5, -6, NF-IL6, NFAT, and NF-κB *(17)*. c-*fos* is the earliest identified gene induced during T-cell activation during the early stage of transition from the G0–G1 phase of the cell cycle (Fig. 5). Its mRNA can be detected as early as 10–15 min after stimulation, peaks after approximately 30 min, and declines to undetectable levels by 1–2 h. c-fos protein dimerizes with jun family proteins, forming activator protein 1 (AP1) transcription factor; this factor plays a central role in the activation of the IL-2 gene via its binding to the IL-2 promoter. By contrast, transcriptional activation of *c-myc* and *c-myb* are slower than that of *c-fos* (Fig. 5). IL-2 readily induces their mRNAs during the G1–S phase transition *(18)*. Three to five days after stimulation of T-cells with Ag or mitogen, genes encoding RANTES, perforin, granzyme A and B, and 519/granulysin are upregulated. Little is known regarding the mechanisms of these late-expressing genes. Early activated nuclear factors, such as NFAT and NFIL6, are switched by the later activated factors, R(A) FLAT and R(C) FLAT, which regulate the RANTES promoter. The T-cell

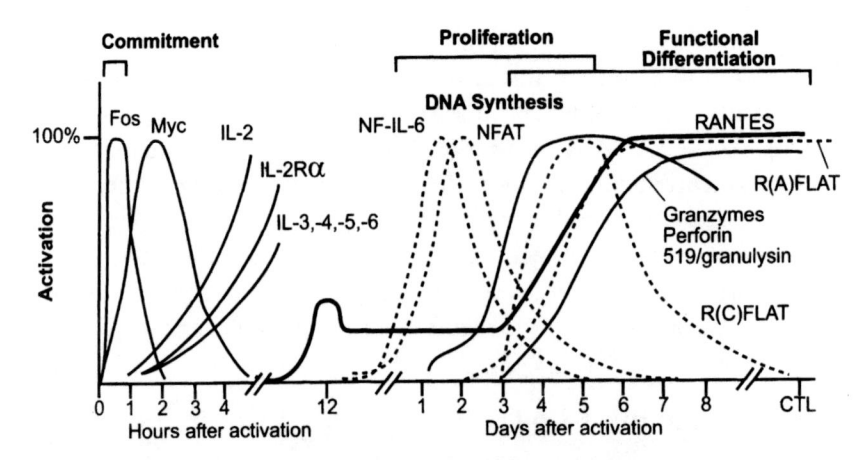

Fig. 5. Nuclear events in T-cell activation. Immediate activators are c-fos, myc, and IL-2. NF1L-6 and NFAT are early activators. RANTES, perforin, granzymes and 519/granulysin are upregulated late after T-cell activation. A switch in transcriptional regulatory factors, R(C) FLAT to R(A)FLAT, accompanies the onset of functional differentiation of T-cells. (Modified from ref. *18*, with permission.)

progresses from the early to late activation process (Fig. 4). What causes this switch to occur? It has been suggested that early transcription factors may be responsible for upregulation of late transcription factors in a cascade of genetically regulatory events. Various cytokines that accumulate during the immune response may upregulate the late factors while actively downregulating early transcription factors. Alternatively, late activated transcription factors may be released from repression via mechanisms that are independent of early transcription factors.

References

1. Lydyard, P. and Grossi, C. (1996) Development of the immune system, in *Immunology*, 4th ed. (Roitt, I., Brostoff, J., and Male, D., eds.), Mosby, Barcelona, pp. 10.2–10.14.
2. Killeen, N., Irving, B. A., Pippig, S., and Zingler, K. (1998) Signaling check points during the development of T lymphocytes. *Curr. Opin. Immunol.* **10**, 360–367.
3. Glimcher, L. H. and Singh, H. (1999) Transcription factors in lymphocyte development—T and B cells get together. *Cell* **96**, 13–23.
4. Alberts, B., Bray, D., Lewis. J., Raff, M., Roberts, K., and Watson, J. D. (1994) The immune system, in *Molecular Biology of the Cell*, 3rd ed. Garland, New York, pp. 1234–1245.
5. Jameson, S. C., Hogquist, K. A., and Bevan, M. J. (1995) Positive selection of thymocytes. *Annu. Rev. Immunol.* **13**, 93–126.
6. Williams, O., Tanaka, Y., Tarazona, R., and Kioussis, D. (1997) The agonist-antagonist balance in positive selection. *Immunol. Today* **18**, 121–126.
7. Weigle, W. O. and Romball, C. G. (1997). CD4+ T cell subsets and cytokines involved in peripheral tolerance. *Immunol. Today* **18**, 533–538.
8. Tsokos, G. C., Kovacs, B., and Liosis, S. N. C. (1997) Lymphocytes, cytokines, inflammation, and immune trafficking. *Curr. Opin. Rheumatol.* **9**, 380–386.
9. Clevers, H. and Ferrier, P. (1998) Transcriptional control during T cell development. *Curr. Opin. Immunol.* **10**, 166–171.
10. Murry, J. S. (1998) How the MHC selects TH1/TH2 immunity. *Immunol. Today* **19**, 157–163.

11. Shresta, S., Pham, C. T. N., Thomas, D. A., Graubert, T. A., and Ley, T. J. (1998) How do cytotoxic lymphocytes kill their targets. *Curr. Opin. Immunol.* **10,** 581–587.
12. Mingare, M. C., Moretta, A., and Moretta, L. (1998) Regulation of KIR expression in human T cells: a safety mechanism that may impair protective T cell response. *Immunol. Today* **19,** 153–157.
13. Stenger, S. and Modlin, R. L. (1998) Cytotoxic T cell responses to intracellular pathogens. *Curr. Opin. Immunol.* **10,** 471–477.
14. Bell, E. B., Sparshott, S. M., and Bunce, C. (1998) CD4+ T-cell memory, CD45R subsets and the persistence of antigen—a unifying concept. *Immunol. Today* **19,** 60–64.
15. Stenger, S. and Modlin R. L. (1998) Cytotoxic T cell responses to intracellular pathogens. *Curr. Opin. Immunol.* **10,** 471–477.
16. Dayal, A. K. and Kammer, G. M. (1996) The T cell enigma in lupus. *Arthritis Rheum.* **39,** 23–33.
17. Altman, A., Coggeshall, K. M., and Mustelin, T. (1990) Molecular events mediating T cell activation. *Adv. Immunol.* **48,** 227–360.
18. Ortiz, B. D., Nelson, P. J., and Krensky, A. M. (1997) Switching gears during T-cell maturation: RANTES and late transcription. *Immunol. Today* **18,** 468–471.

13
B-Lymphocytes

Robert F. Ashman

1. Introduction

B-Lymphocytes ("B-cells") look exactly like T-lymphocytes by common histologic techniques. Yet they are a distinct cell lineage, distinguished from T-cells by (1) their development, (2) their ability to synthesize immunoglobulin (no other cell does this), (3) their display of Ig molecules on their plasma membrane, where they serve as an identifying marker for B-cells as well as the B-cell's receptor for specific antigens, (4) their precise anatomic location within lymphoid tissue, (5) their ability to capture antigens that bind to their surface Ig, and present them to CD4+ T-cells as peptide–class II major histocompatibility (MHC) complexes, thus activating the T-cells, and (6) their ability to evolve into "memory cells" that ensure that a second exposure to antigen will trigger a more effective antibody response than the first exposure ("immunologic memory").

2. Development

The purpose of B-cells is to make antibody, and the purpose of antibody is to recognize foreign antigens and tag them for destruction by phagocytes. The surface Ig of a B-cell reacts with the same foreign epitope as the antibody it will eventually produce, a relationship that explains why the antibody response is specific for the antigen that triggered it. Of course, the unique antigen-binding property of an antibody implies that antibodies differ from each other in the amino acid sequence in their combining sites (Chapter 4), and because gene sequence determines protein sequence, it also implies that mature B-cells must express different Ig genes. How is it possible for an organism to devote to Ig sequences enough DNA to enable it to react to an antigenic universe of over a million epitopes? The answer lies in the ingenious sequence of gene rearrangements that define the stages of B-cell development, as well as generating the diversity of antibodies. B-Cells and T-cells begin to diverge at the lymphoid stem-cell stage in the bone marrow, beginning a sequence of events (Fig. 1) that will produce a population of tens of thousands of B-cell clones, each one expressing Ig molecules that recognize a particular epitope. Driven by interleukin-7 from marrow stomal cells, first the heavy-chain (H) chromosome rearranges, splicing a particular V_H, D_H, and J_H to the $C\mu$ gene segment (details in Chapter 4), and splicing the "membrane terminus" with its transmembrane segment to the C end of the $C\mu$ segment. Transcription then begins, followed by μ-chain translation. These pre-B-cells are recognizable by the presence of

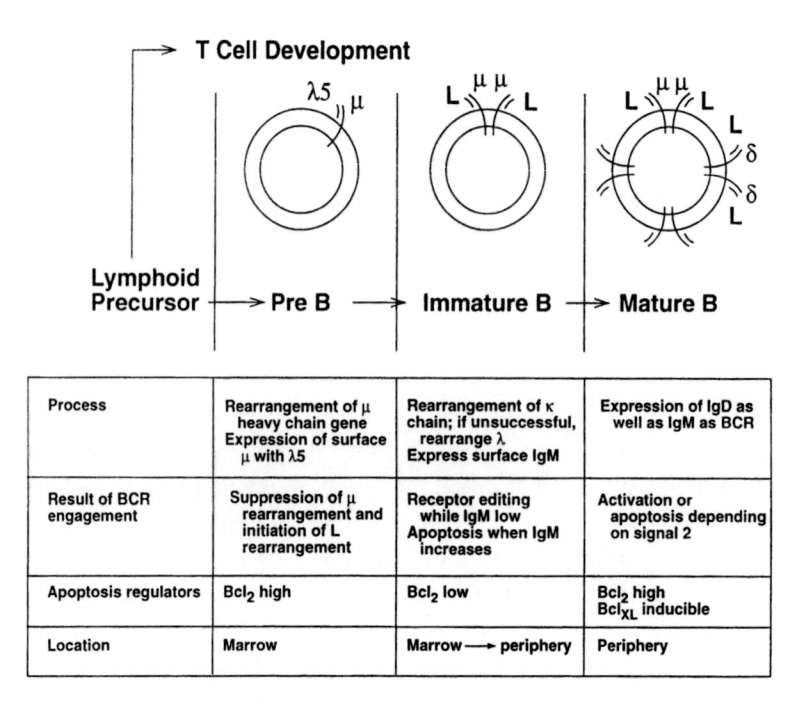

Process	Rearrangement of μ heavy chain gene Expression of surface μ with λ5	Rearrangement of κ chain; if unsuccessful, rearrange λ Express surface IgM	Expression of IgD as well as IgM as BCR
Result of BCR engagement	Suppression of μ rearrangement and initiation of L rearrangement	Receptor editing while IgM low Apoptosis when IgM increases	Activation or apoptosis depending on signal 2
Apoptosis regulators	Bcl_2 high	Bcl_2 low	Bcl_2 high Bcl_{XL} inducible
Location	Marrow	Marrow → periphery	Periphery

Fig. 1. B-Cells develop mainly in the bone marrow from a lymphoid precursor cell in the fetal liver. The stages of development are defined by the rearrangement of the Ig genes, with surface expression of the gene products also assisting in identification. Bcl_2 and Bcl_{XL} are apoptosis-protective molecules. When their expression is low, the B-cell is susceptible to apoptosis induced by a signal through its B-cell receptor (BCR).

the μ chain attached to membranes in the cytoplasm, without the light (L) chain. However, the pre-B-cell expresses a small amount of its μ chain on its surface, bound to an invariant L-chain-like molecule called "surrogate L chain" or λ5. Engagement of this pre-B-cell receptor triggers the rearrangement of the L-chain gene so a whole mature IgM molecule can be expressed on the membrane, and rearrangement of the H-chain gene stops, excluding transcription of the second H-chain chromosome (1). Thereafter, Ig containing the same L and VDJ_H characterizes all the future progeny of that B-cell, from the immature stage on (Fig. 1).

3. B-Cell Activation

Surface Ig is the antigen receptor of the mature B-cell, sometimes abbreviated BCR in parallel to the T-cell receptor, TCR. Mature naive B-cells (i.e., those that have not yet interacted with antigen) express surface IgM and IgD as their BCRs (Fig. 1). Much research has been devoted to discovering functional differences between surface IgM and IgD without clear answers. Either isotype of BCR can transmit a partial activation signal (signal 1) to the B-cell when engaged by antigen or anti-Ig. However, although signal 1 alone from typical protein antigens may be sufficient to activate certain early genes (e.g., c-myc and class II MHC), it only achieves full activation of RNA and DNA synthesis in a small minority of B-cells. Indeed, it is more likely that signal 1 alone will result in apoptosis (programmed cell death, Chapter 3), an effect that may play a role in self-tolerance.

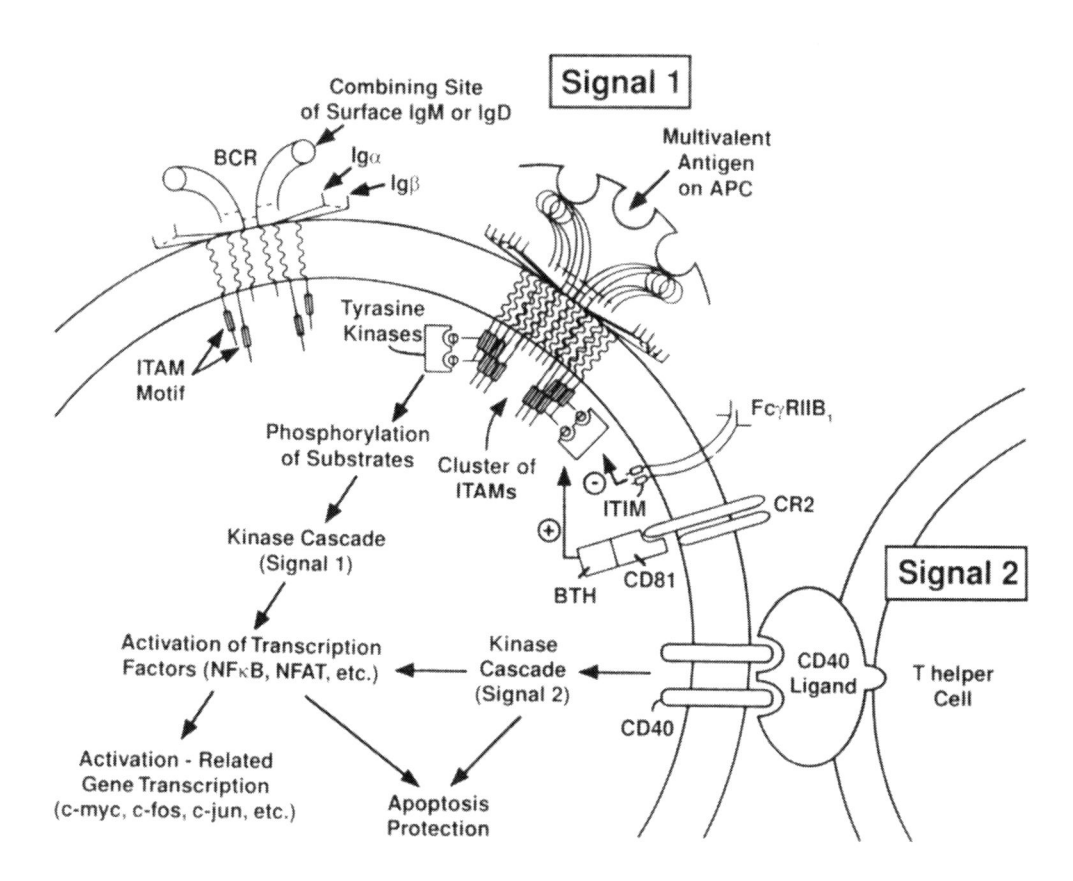

Fig. 2. The mature B-cell expresses on its membrane multiple copies of IgM and IgD molecules, all of which bind the same antigen because they contain the same combining site structure. These Ig molecules are the B-cell receptors for antigen (BCR). When BCR are bound by protein antigen on the surface of an antigen-presenting cell (APC), or by a carbohydrate antigen which is intrinsically multivalent, BCRs are clustered. Thus, the Igα and Igβ signaling molecules bound to the BCRs are also clustered, initiating a signal transduction pathway (signal 1) culminating in the transcription of genes needed for proliferation. Signal 1 can be inhibited by pulling the IgG Fc receptor, FcγRIIB, into the cluster, and enhanced by pulling in the complement (C3) fragment receptor CR2. Because B-cells and T helper cells often encounter their antigen on the same APC, the T-cell can give signal 2 to the B-cell also. A critical component of signal 2 is the CD40 signal, which is sufficient to drive proliferation but also inhibits apoptosis.

4. B-Cell Signal 1 (Fig. 2)

Although it may not be necessary for rheumatologists to know in detail the current status of the rapidly evolving field of signal transduction, certain concepts appear to be firmly established:

1. Signal cascades begin when an external ligand binds the exterior domain of an intrinsic membrane protein (receptor), which creates a high local concentration of a protein region called an activation motif on the cytoplasmic side of the membrane *(2)*.
2. This cluster of motifs bind a cluster of intracellular proenzymes, activating them.
3. Commonly, these proenzymes are kinases that add phosphate groups to specific sites (tyrosines, serines, or threonines) on specific protein substrates. Others are phosphatases

that take off phosphate groups. Often, the degree and location of phosphate groups determines the activity or inactivity of enzymes. Examples of kinases phosphorylating themselves have been shown, introducing an amplification step.

4. Some of the participating molecules are not enzymes, but "adapter proteins" that bind two or more molecules together so that enzyme can find the substrate.
5. Reaction pathways diverge, and converge with pathways initiated by other membrane receptors.
6. Receptors that initiate inhibitory pathways also exist. In B-cells, a prominent example is the B-cell isoform of the IgG–Fc receptor (FcγRIIB). This Fc receptor is included in the BCR cluster whenever the external ligand is an IgG-containing immune complex, because such complexes contain free-antigen epitopes, free-antibody combining sites, and the Fc of IgG. The cytoplasmic tail of FcγRIIB has an Ig transduction inhibition motif (ITIM) that recruits phosphatases that reverse early steps in BCR signal transduction *(3)*.
7. Surface proteins that enhance the BCR signal also exist. One example is the B-cell/dendritic cell complement receptor CR2, which consists of CD19, CD21, and CD81, the protein that links it to the B-cell tyrosine kinase (BTK). CR2 binds the complement fragment iC3b in immune complexes and also is the means by which Epstein–Barr virus selectively infects B-cells. Coengagement of CR2 and BCR allows an equivalent BCR signal with less than one-thousandth as much antigen *(4)*. When BTK is genetically missing, B-cell development stops at the pre-B-cell state [X-linked hypogammaglobulinemia, *(5)*].
8. Prominent among the results of signal cascades are the initiation of transcription of a set of genes whose products usher the cell into a round of proliferation, (examples: c-myc, fos, jun-B) and another set coding for costimulatory molecules such as class II MHC and B7.1/7.2.
9. So how does signal 1 begin in the B-cell *(2)*? Both the IgM and IgD BCRs have transmembrane (TM) segments, but the cytoplasmic tails of both the μ and δ chains are too short to have a signaling function of their own (Fig. 2). However the TM of μ and δ each bind noncovalently to other membrane proteins called Igα and Igβ, which have much larger cytoplasmic tails. Their cytoplasmic tail (CY) contains a sequence motif called ITAM (immunoreceptor tyrosine activation motif) similar to those of CD3ζ in T-cells (Chapter 5), which has affinity for the "SH$_2$ domain" of tyrosine kinases (TK) of the src family such as fyn, blk, and lyn and also syk, the B-cell homolog of zap70 (Chapter 5). When antigen binding to the BCR external domain induces clustering of BCR, these ITAM motifs of Igα and Igβ are also clustered on the underside of the membrane. The more ITAMS are clustered, the more effectively they recruit SH$_2$-bearing TKs to the membrane, and activate them, starting a "signal transduction cascade" of sequential events (Fig. 2).

5. Signal 2

How then does the B-cell acquire the "signal 2" needed for full activation? Very briefly, in a normal T-dependent immune response to a foreign protein antigen administered intramuscularly, the sequence of events is likely to be as follows: (1) Antigen from lymph is trapped by dendritic cells or macrophages (antigen presenting cells) in lymphoid tissues, digested, and presented to CD4+ helper T-cells as peptide–MHC class II complexes. B-Cells themselves can present antigen, but only the antigen their BCR recognizes, whereas macrophages and dendritic cells can present any antigen. Effective presentation also requires B7 (costimulator) expression. (2) The helper T-cell reacts to B7 through its CD28, and to peptide–MHC through its TCR. Having received the two signals it requires for activation, the T-cell then provides the B-cell with its signal 2 in the form of the CD40 ligand (a membrane protein), which interacts with the

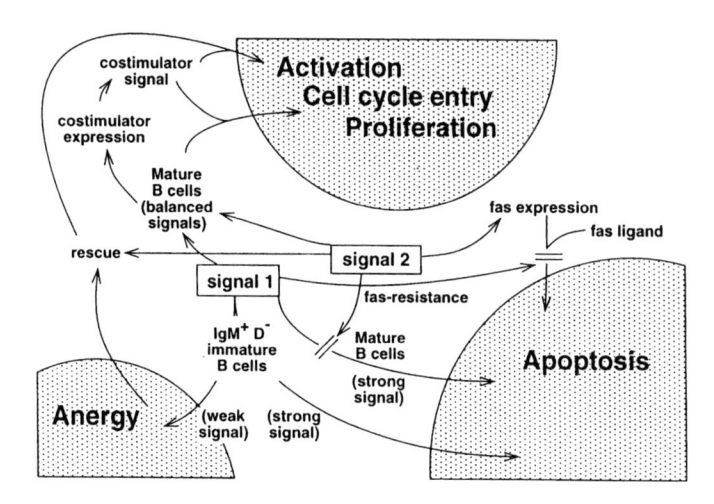

Fig. 3. A mature B-cell receiving both signal 1 and signal 2 in balance goes into the cell cycle, and if these signals continue, rounds of proliferation ensue, especially if the costimulator CR2 can be engaged. Excess of signal 1 over signal 2 results in apoptosis. Immature B-cells are less responsive to signal 2 and also less likely to acquire it, so after an encounter with antigen, they are especially likely to die or to survive with crippled signaling machinery (anergy). In the early stages of such an encounter, signal 2 can rescue anergic cells and block apoptosis. However, signal 2 also induces fas, thus promoting the later elimination of activated B-cells through fas-mediated apoptosis.

B-cell's CD40, and cytokines (especially interleukin-2 [IL-2] in humans and IL-4 in mice). These components of signal 2 also initiate signal transduction cascades through different receptors: CD40 and the IL-2 or IL-4 receptor. There is convergence of the CD40 and BCR pathways on the transduction of some of the same activation-associated genes, but signal 2 pathways also have other effects. For example, they inhibit programmed cell death (apoptosis), ensuring that a higher proportion of B cells survive to enter cycle and proliferate, whereas an isolated signal 1 is more likely to favor apoptosis (Fig. 3). The end result is selective expansion of the B-cell population whose BCR recognizes this particular foreign protein and the production of antibody to that protein. The relationship between the antigen specificity of the BCR and the eventual products of the immune response, antibody and memory B cells, assures the specificity of the response.

A second special result of signal 2, not shared by signal 1, is the induction of expression of fas (CD95), a membrane molecule that serves as an apoptosis trigger on both B- and T-cells (Chapter 3). Activated T-cells also express the ligand for fas. When the fas ligand engages fas, the fas-expressing cell dies by apoptosis. Thus activated T-cells can kill activated B-cells or T-cells. However, signal 1 confers on B-cells a brief period of resistance to fas-mediated apoptosis. These relationships illustrate how a balance between signal 1 and signal 2 favors survival long enough for the immune response to take place, but, afterward, apoptosis, perhaps as a result of the inevitable later signal imbalance, corrects the B-cell population back toward its original size (Fig. 4).

Each step in the activation pathways of signal 1 and signal 2 provides potential targets for therapeutic agents yet to be developed, which will be intended to manipulate the balance among the resting state, proliferation, and apoptosis in B cells responding

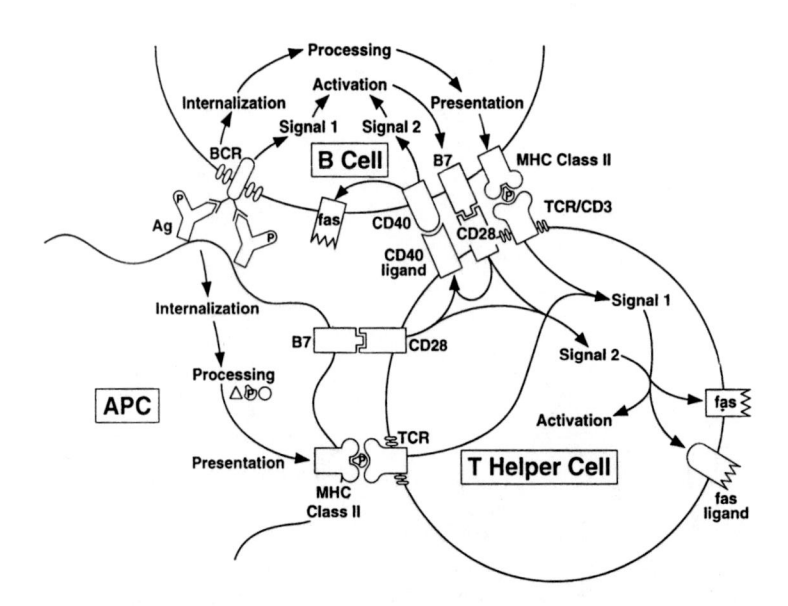

Fig. 4. In a typical T-dependent immune response, protein antigen is captured by antigen-presenting cells (APC). Intact antigen molecules bunched on the APC surface engage the BCR, generating signal 1 in the B cells. At the same time, the APC processes the antigen and mounts its peptides on MHC molecules so as to provide signal 1 to T-cells through their TCR. Although only a tiny fraction of the T- and B-cell population recognize this antigen, their chances of meeting and interacting are greatly increased because they are interacting with the same APC. Thus, the T-cells recognizing peptide "P" can receive a TCR-mediated signal 1 not only from the APC but also from any B-cell whose BCR recognizes an epitope on the antigen. By providing both signal 1 and signal 2 to each other, interacting T- and B-cells enhance each other's activation status. However, fas expression is also enhanced by activation, rendering both cells susceptible to later fas-mediated apoptosis, an event that controls the size of the proliferating clones.

to vaccination or cancer (where we would want more activation) and autoimmunity (where we would want more apoptosis).

The following two sections place this series of B-cell activation events in their anatomic context.

6. The Itinerary of an Activated B-cell

The initial activation of the naive mature B-cell (the interaction of macrophage, T-cell, and B-cell) often takes place in the T-dependent areas of lymph nodes or spleen or in the follicle's marginal zone *(6)* (*see also* Fig. 5, step one). Antigen is accumulated by follicular dendritic cells (FDCs), which possess the costimulatory molecules needed for effective presentation of antigen. The "mutually activating cognate interaction" of T- and B-cells takes place on the surface of the FDC. The B-cell that has been activated by signal 1 + signal 2 then homes into primary follicles and begins to divide. Soon, the follicle assumes the differentiated appearance of a secondary follicle (germinal center) with a light zone and a dark zone in standard Hematoxylin & Eosin-stained sections because of a difference in the density of nuclei (Fig. 5, step 2). In the dark zone the rapidly dividing B-cells temporarily lose their apoptosis protection (bcl$_2$, bcl$_{XL}$, *see* Chapter 3) and become especially vulnerable to apoptosis. They also rapidly mutate

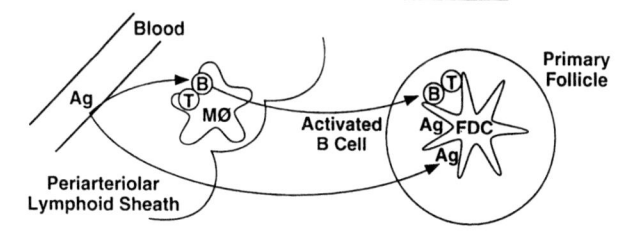

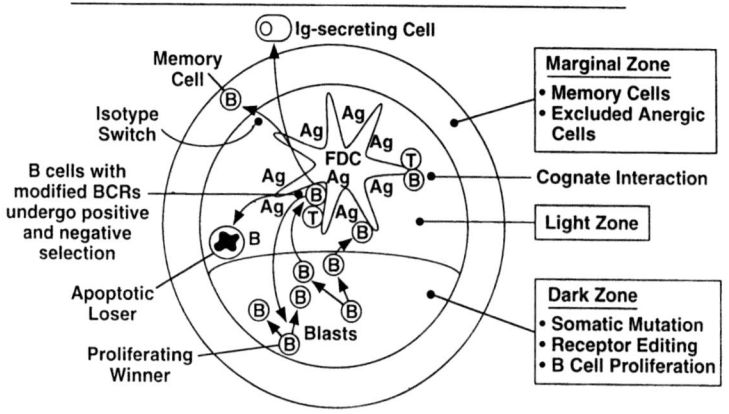

Fig. 5. In Step 1, antigen from the circulation enters the periarteriolar lymphoid sheath of the spleen and is trapped by antigen presenting cells (Mφ = macrophage, FDC = follicular dendritic cell). The primary response takes place as a cognate interaction among T-, B-, and FDC antigen-presenting cells. B-cells stimulated by CD40 ligand are admitted to the primary follicle where they begin to proliferate. As the clones of B-cells reacting to the antigen expand, they compress the cells of the primary follicle into the marginal zone. Soon, a dark zone packed with rapidly proliferating B-cells can be distinguished from a light zone that also contains FDCs and T-cells, and we recognize a germinal center (Step 2). B-cells are restimulated in the light zone, move to the dark zone for a bout of somatic mutation, receptor editing, and proliferation, then move back to the light zone, expressing altered BCRs. If the altered BCR has lost affinity for the antigen, the B-cell dies by "spontaneous" apoptosis, whereas if its new BCR reacts with self Ag, it dies by an excess of signal 1 over signal 2. However, if its new BCR has a higher affinity for Ag, it will be stimulated longer, and its progeny may become the dominant clone (affinity maturation), contributing most of the Ig-secreting cells from that germinal center. Signal 2 also drives the isotype switch, so that memory cells also derive from the dominant clone. Different germinal centers evolve different dominant clones reacting with the same antigen, contributing to the heterogeneity of antibody in the blood.

regions in their Ig genes coding for sequences that determine antigen binding (somatic hypermutation). In the light zone there is a high concentration of specialized highly branched, B7-rich FDCs displaying both whole antigen (for B-cells) and peptide–MHC class II (for T-cells). A small minority of the somatically mutated B-cells that gained higher affinity for the antigen in the dark zone now compete especially successfully for antigen and T-cell help on the light-zone FDC (another round of signal 1 + signal 2), returning to the dark zone to divide ever more vigorously and mutate some more. There is evidence that dark-zone B-cells may also edit their receptors to generate new specificities. With continued stimulation, one or two high-affinity clones begin to dominate in each follicle. However, the majority of B-cells with mutated Ig genes lose binding affinity for the original antigen and these undergo apoptosis as a result of signal deprivation. If they have mutated so as to acquire affinity for a crossreacting self antigen, they undergo apoptosis as a result of signal 1 (self antigen) without signal 2 (insufficient T help). After a few cycles like this, the selected B-cell clones still proliferating in response to T-dependent antigen give rise to two products: (1) differentiated IgM-secreting cells, which in the spleen migrate into the red pulp through the marginal zone, and in lymph nodes station themselves near venules. Ig-secreting cells are end-stage cells which will ultimately lose their sensitivity to apoptosis-protective signals and die. (2) The second is a population of "memory cells" bearing high-affinity BCRs ready to react to the next dose of the same antigen. These stay mostly in the marginal zone of the follicle, and in response to cytokines (IL-4, IL-5, IL-2, IFN-γ, IL-6), they rearrange their Ig-H genes to splice the clone's chosen VDJ to a C gene segment downstream of Cμ and Cδ, perhaps Cγ (for IgG1) or Cα (for IgA). IL-4 is especially necessary for the switch to Cε (for IgE). "Switched" memory B-cells are recognized by their display of these new Ig classes as BCRs. Such cells respond to the next dose of antigen by secreting the same Ig class they are displaying as their BCR, always with the same L chain and the same VDJ_H, thus retaining high affinity for the same antigenic epitope.

What happens to these events if the signal 2 pathway is permanently blocked? Patients with mutant nonfunctional CD40 molecules show (1) low resting and antigen-induced levels of the switched isotypes (IgG, A and E), (2) high levels of IgM, (3) poor memory B-cell function, and (4) poor germinal center formation. This condition is called "humoral immune deficiency with hyper-IgM" *(5)*.

7. B-Cells as Antigen-Presenting Cells

Effective function of antigen-presenting cells is the key to an effective immune response, including the antibody response. "Professional" antigen-presenting cells (mainly macrophages and dendritic cells) have the ability to capture antigen from their environment, internalize it, and digest it in a special endosomal compartment. Those antigen peptides that fit the groove of its class II MHC do so, and migrate to the cell surface to turn on a T helper cell. APC also must display costimulator molecules (B7.1 and B7.2) to function. B-Cells are equipped to do all of this, except that only antigens recognized by its BCR get into the cell (Fig. 4). Thus, the epitopes recognized by the B- and T-cell engaged in cognate interaction are commonly different, but derive from the same antigen molecule. B-Cell epitopes are restricted to the outside of the native antigen molecule, whereas T-cells can recognize peptides from the inside or outside.

Rheumatoid factor (RF) is an antibody to human IgG that is present in high titer in rheumatoid arthritis and certain other chronic inflammatory states (Chapter 21), but can be made by normal individuals. BCRs with RF activity are surprisingly common in the normal B-cell repertoire, for an autoantibody. One attractive explanation is that having anti-Ig B-cells is an advantage because they are much less restricted in their antigen-presenting activity than normal B-cells, being able to trap and present any antigen present in IgG-containing immune complexes. RF-containing complexes also often activate complement well, thus engaging the CR2 costimulator mechanism *(4)*.

8. B-Cell Tolerance

The ability to distinguish self from non-self and avoidance of autoimmune responses are among the most famous properties of the immune system, yet this distinction is far from absolute, despite several semiredundant mechanisms that favor self-tolerance. Indeed, there is an inherent conflict between the advantage of maintaining as diverse a BCR repertoire as possible on the one hand, so as to respond effectively to every pathogen, and the advantage of restricting the BCR repertoire, so as to avoid crossreaction with a substantial universe of self-antigens on the other. The solution to this dilemma is a compromise, in the form of a series of "gates," each of which incompletely screens out B-cells that recognize self:

1. Receptor editing. At the stage immediately after expression of the first small amounts of surface IgM, engagement by (self) antigen triggers the reexpression of L-chain recombination, leading to the expression of new antigen specificities. By losing affinity for self antigen, such clones may then proceed toward maturation (Fig. 1).
2. Negative selection in the bone marrow. The IgM$^+$ IgD$^-$ B-cells, which express an intermediate amount of BCR, then go through a phase when they are not yet fully sensitive to "signal 2" and are vulnerable to apoptosis from a strong signal 1 (Fig. 3). The likelihood of encountering a self antigen rather than a foreign antigen is high at that stage, so the frequency of B-cells specific for self decreases sharply at the transition to mature B-cells.
3. Immature B-cells with intermediate or full amounts of BCR that have received a dose of signal 1 too weak to cause apoptosis may nevertheless have their BCR signaling apparatus partially disabled and become incapable of responding in future to a dose of signal 1 that would normally be effective. We call such B-cells "anergic." They can be rescued from anergy only by extrahigh doses of signal 2 (Fig. 3).
4. B-Cells that have become anergic by encounter with self antigen suffer the further disadvantage that they cannot gain admission to the follicles where rescue signals are available, as long as any fully activated B-cells are competing with them.
5. While B cells are dividing and somatically mutating in the light zone of follicles, as a "side effect" of generating higher-affinity BCRs to improve the quality of the secondary response, new anti-self BCRs may also be generated. However, light-zone B-cells are especially vulnerable to apoptosis from signal 1 without signal 2, which helps to reduce the anti-self B-cell population in the periphery.

The safeguards against autoimmune B-cells thus remain incomplete because of the necessity of maintaining a large enough repertoire to repel pathogens. When the exact epitopes recognized by the B-cells of different individuals are studied in detail, one finds immuno-dominant epitopes to which the majority react, but also a wide variety of reaction patterns to minor epitopes, reflecting the diversity of the inherited class II MHC molecules that present different peptides to T-cells. Several examples teach us that attaching an extra T-cell epitope to a selfantigen so as to engage nontolerant T-helper-cell clones frequently is all that is needed to trigger an autoantibody response. Thus, autoimmune B-cell clones are available, and although their numbers are small, they can be expanded with optimal stimulation. In general, lack of T help provides a more significant barrier to autoimmunity that the lack of autoreactive B-cells. As we age, responding repeatedly to foreign antigens, some of which crossreact with self, the prevalence and amount of autoantibodies (including antinuclear antibody and rheumatoid factor) normally increases.

9. B-Cell Population Dynamics

Even in adult life, the bone marrow normally releases a great excess of immature B cells into the periphery (about 5×10^7 per day), whereas only about 10^6 per day reach maturity (i.e., express a high IgD/M ratio) or find their home in lymphoid organs. There is evidence that mature B-cells out of contact with lymphoid organs or CD40 ligand undergo apoptosis, so homing of the new B-cells to lymphoid organs is literally a race against death. Once comfortably ensconced in a lymphoid organ, mature naive B-cells may live for several months. Experiments in which Ig genes may be acutely disrupted in adult animals indicate that the slow loss of naive B-cells is greatly accelerated if BCR expression is removed, suggesting that a low level of BCR stimulation may contribute to survival *(7)*.

10. T-Independent Versus T-Dependent Antigens

Most protein antigens have only one copy of each epitope per molecule, so that unless they are aggregated, they can only engage one BCR molecule at a time. They activate B-cells largely indirectly through a helper T-cell, so we call them T-dependent antigens. By capturing antigen, internalizing it, and presenting its peptides to a T-cell, the B-cell may earn a dose of signal 2 sufficient for activation, even if signal 1 is minimal. Another class of antigens is T-independent because they have multiple copies of the same epitope on each molecule and can send an extrastrong signal 1 (as illustrated in Fig. 1). Polysaccharides and complex lipids (such as lipid A of endotoxin) are in this class, and they can drive B-cells to produce IgM, with just a little IgG. However, because the class switch, somatic mutation, affinity maturation, and memory cell production are driven mainly by signal 2, T-independent immune responses lack these features. To a T-independent antigen, subsequent responses resemble the primary IgM response. In contrast, second and later responses to the same T-dependent antigen show these features: (1) an earlier response; (2) a lower antigen requirement; (3) progressive dominance of high-affinity clones; (4) switch to IgG, IgA, or IgE antibody, and (5) generation of more memory cells expressing these isotypes, with high-affinity BCRs.

The IgM secreting cells differ from mature B-cells in having prominent endoplasmic reticulum (ER) and Golgi apparatus, as one would expect of any protein-secreting cell. However, IgM-secreting cells rarely are as swollen with ER and ribosomes as cells secreting the "switched isotypes" that predominate in secondary responses (plasma cells). With their excentric nuclei, such cells may be prominent in the red pulp of the spleen or the hilum of lymph nodes where their products have direct access to venous blood. They are also prominent in the inflamed synovium of rheumatoid arthritis. The plasma cell is an "end-stage" cell, meaning that it undergoes apoptosis rather than evolving into another cell type.

11. CpG Oligonucleotides Activate B-Cells

B-Cells contribute to our natural immunity by virtue of their unique proliferative response to bacterial DNA, not shared by other cell types and not elicited by mammalian DNA. Bacterial DNA differs from mammalian DNA especially in the frequency of a motif "not C, unmethylated C, G, not G." Synthetic oligonucleotides containing this motif are among the most powerful B-cell mitogens known *(8)* by virtue of their ability to inhibit apoptosis while they drive B-cells into cycle, apparently activating transcription of many of the same genes that are activated by CD40 ligand and BCR. Because they also stimulate transcription of the IL-12 gene in macrophages, they generate TH1-type response on the T-cell side. Because they enhance the immune response to antigens given simultaneously, they can serve as useful adjuvants in a variety of immunization protocols. Thus, in a bacterial infection, it is thought they may provide an early warning to jump-start the immune system.

12. Cytokine Secretion

Although one normally thinks of T-cells and macrophages as the principal source of cytokines, activated B-cells can contribute, especially with IL-6, representing an autostimulatory loop. IL-6, together with other inflammatory cytokines (TNFα and IL-1), travels hormonelike through the circulation, acting on the brain to induce fever and on the liver to induce the production of acute-phase reactants.

13. Summary

The main function of the B lymphocyte is to make antibody. The main function of antibody in host defense is to usher foreign substances and pathogens toward destruction and elimination from the body. But, antibodies to self antigens characterize several autoimmune rheumatic diseases where they are important to diagnosis, prognosis, and (in some cases) pathogenesis. The sequence of events in B-cell development appears to be arranged so that the specificity of the response is maintained and so that responses to foreign antigens are favored over autoimmunity. Activation of B-cells to antibody secretion is a multistep process. Except in the case of rare T-independent antigens (mainly carbohydrates), B-cell responses involve interaction with T-cells and APCs (principally macrophages and dendritic cells). Although it is convenient to segregate these steps into signal 1 (through the BCR, normally initiated by antigen) and signal 2 (from a T helper cell), each of these signals has many steps that are subject to regulation by costimulatory and inhibitory pathways initiated through other receptors. The complexity of these pathways, together with the fact that survival requires balance between signal 1 and signal 2, provides many potentially testable hypotheses regarding the regulation of autoimmunity, as well as potential targets for new therapeutic strategies in rheumatic disease.

References

1. Ehlich, A., Martin, V., Muller, W., and Rajewsky, K. (1994) Analysis of the B-cell progenitor compartment at the level of signal cells. *Curr. Biol.* **4,** 573–583.
2. Buhl, A. M. and Cambier, J. C. (1997) Co-receptor and accessory regulation of B-cell antigen receptor signal transduction. *Immunol. Rev.* **160,** 127–138.
3. Cambier, J. C. (1997) Positive and negative signal co-operativity in the immune system: the BCR, Fc gamma RIIB, CR2 paradigm. *Biochem. Soc. Trans.* **25,** 441–445.
4. Fearon, D. T. and Carter, R. H. (1995) The CD19/CR2/TAPA-1 complex of B lymphocytes: linking natural to acquired immunity. *Annu. Rev. Immunol.* **13,** 127–149.
5. Conley, M. E. (1994) X-linked immunodeficiencies. *Curr. Opin. Genet. Dev.* **4,** 401–406.
6. Rajewsky, K. (1996) Clonal selection and learning in the antibody system. *Nature* **381,** 751–758.
7. Rajewsky, K. (1993) B-Cell lifespans in the mouse—why to debate what? *Immunol. Today* **14,** 40–43.
8. Krieg, A. M., Yi, A.-K., Matson, S., Waldschmidt, T. J., Bishop, G. A., Teasdale, R., Koretzky, G. A., and Klinman, D. (1995) CpG motifs in bacterial DNA trigger direct B-cell activation. *Nature* **374,** 546–549.

14
Monocytes and Macrophages

James M. K. Chan and Sharon M. Wahl

1. Introduction

Rheumatoid arthritis (RA) is a disease characterized by an inflammatory response within the joint resulting in cartilage and bone destruction. Infiltration of mononuclear cells, including monocytes and macrophages, in synovial tissues is characteristic of RA. The role of macrophages is essential in the development of a normal inflammatory immune response and host defense. In addition to their functions against infectious agents and tumor cells, and as antigen-presenting cells, macrophages secrete and respond to multiple cytokines and other mediators that control key events in the initiation, resolution, and repair processes of inflammation and the immune response (Table 1). Although macrophages are essential for these events in innate and adaptive host defense, persistent activation of this population may have negative consequences.

Macrophages have the ability to initiate and sustain or to suppress an immune response, because of their ability to produce and secrete a wide range of regulatory molecules. This dual functioning of macrophages, namely at an early stage to enhance host defense and at a later stage to dampen the immune response, suggests that any imbalance between these functions could contribute to disease manifestations.

The resolution of acute inflammation is characterized by the clearance of neutrophils and macrophages and the restoration of tissue architecture. However, in a number of disease processes, inflammation does not resolve. Rather, it persists and is often associated with tissue degradation, fibrosis, and, possibly, loss of tissue or organ function, as exemplified by glomerulonephritis, rheumatoid arthritis (RA), and other chronic inflammatory diseases. Although macrophages are able to promote wound healing, continued macrophage accumulation is also a hallmark of chronic and pathologic inflammation. By the release of enzymes, proinflammatory cytokines, presentation of antigens to T-cells, and recruitment of additional inflammatory cell populations, macrophages can influence pathways leading to tissue damage. In this chapter, we will focus on this population of cells and its contribution to inflammation as well as their pivotal role in the pathogenesis of rheumatoid arthritis.

2. Macrophages in Inflammation

Stemming from marrow myeloid precursors, circulating blood monocytes emigrate across the endothelium and are distributed to different tissues where they mature and

From: *Current Molecular Medicine: Principles of Molecular Rheumatology*
Edited by: G. C. Tsokos © Humana Press Inc., Totowa, NJ

**Table 1
Monocyte/Macrophage Functions
in Inflammation, Immune Responses, and Repair**

Chemotaxis
Phagocytosis
Release of reactive oxygen (O_2, H_2O_2) and nitrogen (NO) intermediates
Microbicidal activity
Antitumor activity
Antigen presentation to lymphocytes
Production of cytokines (*TNF-α, *IL-1, *IL-6, *TGF-β, *OSM, *IL-10 and IL-18)
Inflammatory mediators: prostaglandins, MMPs
Angiogenesis
Tissue repair: production of growth factors (FGF, PDGF, VEGF, TGF-β)

Note: Asterisk denotes cytokines discussed in text.

reside as resident tissue macrophages. It has long been recognized that macrophages isolated from different anatomical sites are heterogeneous, in part because they adapt to the local microenvironmental influences by developing attributes that enable them to perform functions relevant to their host tissue (1). Local macrophages are recruited in addition to the recruitment and accumulation of blood monocytes through their response to multiple chemotactic factors that vary with the stimulus. Consequently, within an inflammatory site, various functionally and phenotypically heterogeneous populations of inflammatory mononuclear phagocytes may be found, dependent on the nature of the injury and the time during its evolution.

Knowledge of what controls macrophage activation and function within an inflammatory site is crucial for our understanding and control of inflammatory diseases. Macrophage functions are influenced by numerous factors including T-cell-derived cytokines such as interferon-γ (IFN-γ). Recently, using bone-marrow-derived macrophages, it was determined that these macrophages became programmed by the first cytokine to which they were exposed, and that once initiated, the programming rendered the macrophages hyporesponsive to alternative programming stimuli (2). Surprisingly, these results suggested that, at least in these experimental conditions, macrophage activity was not determined by the sum of the activities of the cytokines to which they were exposed, but rather by the initial cytokine contact.

Although macrophage functions are clearly aberrant in chronic inflammatory lesions, abnormalities in myeloid lineage bone marrow cells from RA patients have also been reported. Among these are the presence of unusual myeloid cell populations, elevated numbers of myeloid precursors cells and very high colony stimulating factor (CSF; see Subheading 11.) activity in bone marrow, particularly adjacent to inflamed joints (3). Whether the presence of these abnormalities is a result of the disease or contributes to the disease in human is currently unknown. However, studies carried out using an autoimmune mouse strain, the MRL/lpr mice, indicate dysfunction among the leukocyte populations. These mice have been widely studied as a model of systemic lupus erythematous (SLE) and are characterized by dysregulated T-cells, B-cells, and macrophages, which disrupt the immune system. Among macrophages, aberrant production or expression of H_2O_2, interleukin-1 (IL-1), class II antigen, tumor necrosis factor-α

(TNF-α), and IL-6, fosters autoimmune-like pathology. Clearly, macrophages represent one of the most influential populations of cells, not only in physiologic inflammation and the immune response, but also, under conditions where the delicate balance between pro-inflammatory and anti-inflammatory signals is toppled, macrophages become key players in orchestrating tissue destruction and/or fibrotic sequelae. As such, these cells also have emerged as targets for anti-inflammatory therapy.

3. Origin of Macrophages in RA

The noninflamed synovial intima is a thin layer of cells (normally one to two cells in depth) that lines the intra-articular space and is composed of the bone-marrow-derived type A macrophage-like cells and the local mesenchymal-type B fibroblast-like cells. In RA, the synovium changes dramatically and is characterized by an increase in lining-layer thickness and significant infiltration of inflammatory cells. The lining layer may undergo marked thickening up to 20–30 cells thick, and within the sublining area, an increase in vascularity and an inflammatory infiltrate including macrophages and T cells becomes evident.

Synovial macrophage-like cells may originate locally, but also have a bone marrow origin during inflammation *(4)*, involving the emigration of monocytes from the circulation. It has been widely accepted that monocyte-derived macrophages have limited proliferative potential and a variable life-span under normal, steady-state conditions. Tissue macrophages are typically replenished by the migration of monocytes from the circulation into tissues and serous cavities, followed by their differentiation and maturation into resident or exudate macrophages. Based on this concept, most macrophages, including resident macrophages in tissues and macrophages recruited to inflammatory sites, are considered to be maintained by the influx of monocytes from circulation.

In addition to the influx of circulating monocytes, local proliferation may also contribute to the rapid expansion of the macrophage population at a site of inflammation. Recent reports suggest that local macrophage proliferation occurs and that recruitment is not a prerequisite for resident macrophages to acquire the characteristics of differentiated inflammatory macrophages. The recruitment of precursor cells, such as colony-forming cells, to an inflamed site could also act as a local source for macrophage expansion *(5)*. In this regard, both GM-CSF and M-CSF (*see* Subheading 11.), growth factors for monocytic cells, have been found in rheumatoid synovial tissues and fluids. The accumulation of macrophages within the synovium likely includes both recruitment and local proliferation.

4. Leukocyte Trafficking

The rapid increase in cell numbers at a site of inflammation involves the migration of blood leukocytes across the endothelium into the tissue. This process involves the interaction of leukocytes with adhesion molecules expressed on endothelium of blood vessels. Inflammatory mediators (*see* Subheadings 7., 8., and 12.) activate the expression of these molecules on endothelium for which leukocytes have complementary inducible receptors. Four superfamilies of adhesion molecules are described according to their structural similarities, these include the integrins, the immunoglobulinlike proteins (intercellular adhesion molecules-1 and –2 [ICAM-1, ICAM-2] and vascular cell adhesion molecule [VCAM], the selectins (L-, P- and E-selectin), and mucin-like selectin ligands (reviewed in refs. 6 and 7). Together with the actions of chemotactic signals generated from a site of inflammation, adhesion enables leukocytes to initially "roll" along endothelial cells at the site of inflammation against the concentration gradient of chemotactic signals (i.e., migrate toward the highest concentration of the stimuli.)

Transient adhesion of circulating leukocytes, particularly neutrophils, is initially mediated by the selectin family of adhesion molecules and their corresponding counter-receptors or ligands. This phenomenon is typically referred to as *rolling* because of the behavior of leukocytes on the surface of the endothelial lining. Expression of P-selectin is rapidly increased on the plasma membrane of endothelium after stimulation by inflammatory mediators such as thrombin, platelet-activating factor, and cytokines *(8)*. P-selectin interacts with P-selectin glycoprotein ligand (PSGL-1), a member of the mucin family that is expressed on neutrophils. P-selectin on endothelium and L-selectin on neutrophils establish contact between neutrophils and the endothelium.

The transmigration of leukocytes from vessel to subvascular tissue proceeds with the activation of additional adhesion molecules, the leukocyte integrins (Fig. 1). Integrins are membrane proteins composed of one of multiple α-subunits and one of several β-subunits. Concurrent with the increased expression of integrins and thus integrin-mediated adhesion, selectin interactions are downregulated. These processes lead to the arrest of leukocyte rolling by close and stable cell–cell adhesion between leukocytes and endothelial cells and, hence, facilitates transmigration of leukocytes through endothelial tight junctions and the subsequent migration into tissue spaces under the control of chemotactic factors *(6,8)*. Binding of lymphocytes and monocytes that express β1 integrins (including very late antigen-4, VLA-4, or α4β1) to the endothelium adhesion molecule VCAM-1 is promoted by the cytokine IL-1, which induces VCAM-1 expression. β1 integrins interact not only with endothelial cell adhesion molecules, but also with extracellular matrix molecules, including fibronectin, facilitating movement of leukocytes from the vasculature into the subvascular space and the site of tissue inflammation. In this regard, interruption of this process with synthetic fibronectin peptides that bind to and block leukocyte β1 receptors inhibits adhesion to endothelial cells and to matrix molecules and inhibits macrophage signal transduction *(9)*. Using a streptococcal-cell-wall (SCW)-induced rodent model of acute and chronic erosive arthritis, the fibronectin peptides, delivered systemically, effectively ameliorated recruitment, inflammation, and tissue destruction *(10)*.

In addition to its role in adhesive events, the integrin αvβ3, is involved in angiogenesis *(11)*. Angiogenesis, the formation of new blood vessels, is one of the earliest histopathologic findings in RA. This process is thought to play a role in maintaining local inflammation by feeding the growing tissue (pannus), and also the supply of immune cells. Furthermore, it is also a source of delivery and transport of pro-inflammatory cytokines and chemokines. Macrophages contribute to this process via the release of angiogenesis-promoting factors such as VEGF, FGF, and PDGF. In theory, blockage of angiogenesis should downregulate or inhibit persistent inflammation. The benefit of agents that suppress neovascularization in arthritis was first demonstrated *(12)* by using the fumagillin derivative AGM-1470 (TNP-470). This compound, which is toxic to proliferating endothelial cells, prevented arthritis and reversed established disease in both adjuvant arthritis and collagen-induced arthritis (CIA) in rats. In addition to

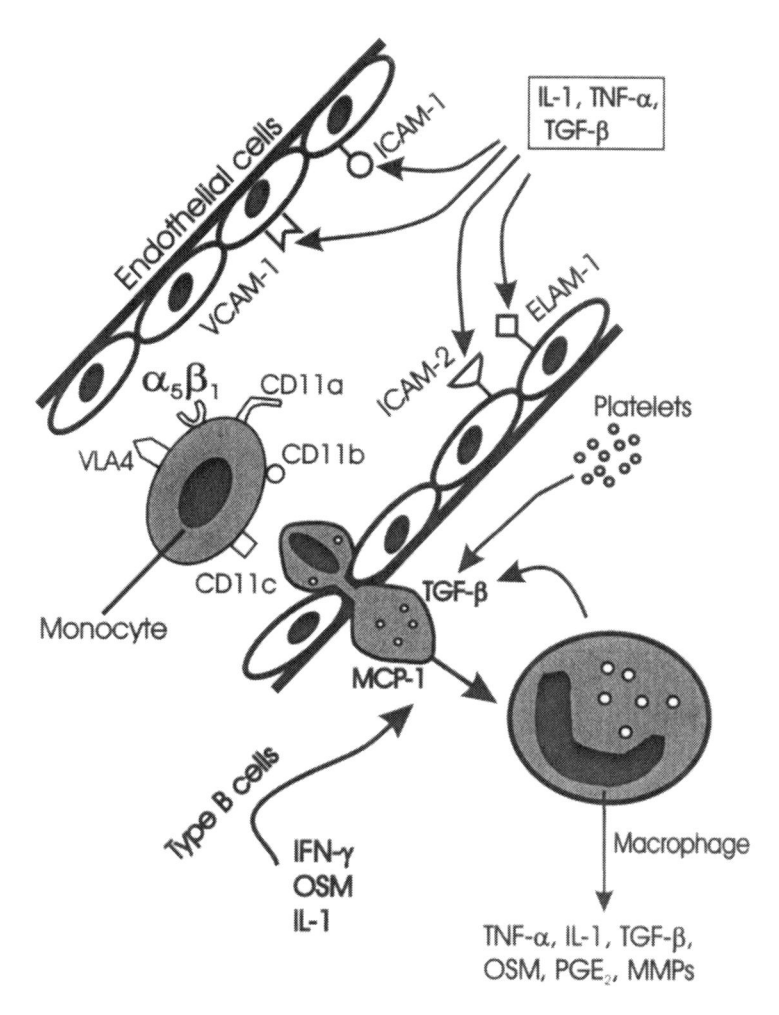

Fig. 1. Monocyte/macrophage trafficking. The interaction of monocyte/macrophages with adhesion molecules (endothelial leukocyte adhesion molecule-1 [ELAM-1], vascular cell adhesion molecule-1 [VCAM-1], intercellular adhesion molecule-1,2 [ICAM-1,2], very late antigen 4 [VLA-4], CD11a,b,c/CD18 (β2 integrins), in response to chemoattractants such as monocyte chemotactic protein 1 (MCP-1) and TGF-β.

reduced inflammation, bone and cartilage damage were also suppressed. A cyclic peptide antagonist of αvβ3 delivered in an antigen-induced arthritis model in rabbits likewise promoted vascular apoptosis, to inhibit synovial angiogenesis and arthritic sequelae *(13)*.

The migration of monocytes (Fig. 1) from the circulation to synovial tissue is also mediated by the interactions between β2 integrins (α-subunit: CD11a, b, or c, β-subunit: CD18) expressed on their surface and their counter-receptors on the endothelial cells (ELAM-1, VCAM-1, ICAM-1, and ICAM-2), under the influence of monocyte chemoattractants. The essentiality of these adhesive interactions is evident in gene-targeted mice lacking specific adhesion molecules or their cognate ligands. Such mice have provided important information concerning the role of these molecules in adhesion, recruitment, and inflammatory processes (reviewed in ref. *14*).

In addition to localization of blood leukocytes through adhesive interactions, directed migration to an inflammatory site is dependent on chemotactic stimuli. A plethora of leukocyte chemoattractants may be released at a site of inflammation including transforming growth factor-β (TGF-β), C5a, bacterial products (FMLP) and chemokines. Chemokines represent a growing superfamily of chemotactic proteins. Based on their protein structures, several groups have been identified, but the CXC (structure with one amino acid between two cysteines) chemokines and the CC (two adjoining cysteines) chemokines are the most studied. CXC chemokines, such as IL-8, are primarily chemotactic for neutrophils and also lymphocytes, whereas CC chemokines, such as monocyte chemotactic peptide-1 (MCP-1), RANTES, and macrophage inflammatory peptides (MIP-1α and MIP-1β) preferentially attract monocytes and lymphocytes. Confirming this specificity, MCP-1- and CCR2 (the MCP-1 receptor)-deficient mice have reduced macrophage recruitment and inflammation in induced peritonitis, delayed-type hypersensitivity reactions, and pulmonary granulomatous response compared with their wild-type/normal controls. In a mouse model of nephrotoxic serum nephritis using MCP-1-deficient mice *(15)*, it was reported that tubular injury in MCP-1-deficient mice was markedly reduced compared to MCP-1-intact mice. Thus, blockage of MCP-1 expression could be considered as a therapeutic strategy for the treatment of chronic inflammatory diseases.

In the SCW-induced arthritis rat model, which includes an acute-phase inflammation where neutrophils are the predominant infiltrating cell type, followed by a chronic phase of mononuclear cell infiltration, it was shown (J. Zagorski, unpublished data) that the kinetic expression of several chemokines correlated with the cell-specific recruitment characteristic of the biphasic inflammation, although redundancies were apparent. These results suggested a direct link between chemokine expression and the evolution of pathology in this model, pointing to therapeutic possibilities with the blockage of chemokine activity. In fact, a study *(16)* using CINC (cytokine-induced neutrophil chemoattractant) receptor antagonist reduced neutrophil influx and reduced inflammation in vivo.

In addition to leukocyte trafficking, some adhesion molecules may also be involved in recognition and signal transduction in leukocytes *(6,9)*. Activated leukocyte cell adhesion molecule (ALCAM or CD166) is a divalent cation-independent ligand for CD6. CD6 is expressed on the majority of T-cells and a subset of B-cells, as an adhesion molecule associated with the immune response. A role for CD6 in the primary immune response has been suggested by studies showing that CD3+ and CD6− peripheral blood cells are less alloreactive than CD6+ peripheral blood T-cells. Furthermore, the prevention of CD6–ALCAM interactions by anti-CD6 mAb inhibits the autoreactive responses of cloned T–cells in autologous mixed lymphocyte reactions *(17)*. ALCAM expression on blood monocytes was inducible in vitro by M-CSF, GM-CSF, and IL-3, and M-CSF neutralizing antibody significantly inhibits this in vitro induction *(18)*. Furthermore, ALCAM is constitutively expressed on CD14+ RA synovial fluid (SF) cells, and anti-M-CSF antibody significantly inhibited culture-induced expression of ALCAM on SF CD14+ cells. From the same study, it was reported that ALCAM was expressed on type A synovial cells from all RA patients compared to lower levels associated with OA. From these observations, it was postulated that ligation of CD6 by monocyte/macrophage ALCAM may foster activation and perpetuation of autoreactive T-cells in RA synovium.

5. Involvement of Monocytes/Macrophages in RA

Currently, the pathogenesis of RA is considered to be initiated by T-cells, but orchestrated by macrophages and fibroblasts. From chronic RA patients, the relatively low levels of T-cell-derived cytokines in serum and synovial fluid, in contrast to those derived from macrophages, the progressive invasion of rheumatoid synovium in the absence of significant number of T-cells *(19)*, and the incomplete responses of T-cell-targeted therapies suggest that these cells may be less important as effectors in RA, but are instrumental in the initiation of the disease. This is supported by the finding of increased numbers of PBMC (peripheral blood mononuclear cells) secreting IL-2 and IFN-γ from patients with early-onset synovitis *(20)*.

As in other inflammatory lesions, there are abundant data to support the involvement of macrophages in RA. One of the key functions of these cells is the removal of foreign substances from synovial fluid. Such foreign substances would first encounter the lining layer and activate this cell population, resulting in the induction of inflammatory mediators, which recruit inflammatory cells during the early phase of arthritis. Infiltrating inflammatory cells and recruited cells in the sublining and lining regions show hyperplasia shortly after arthritis induction and likely represent a source of pro-inflammatory and tissue-damaging mediators such as cytokines and metalloproteinases.

Consistent with this concept, in a murine model of arthritis *(21)*, depletion of synovial lining phagocytic cells before the induction of arthritis resulted in decreased polymorphonuclear neutrophils (PMN) infiltration and reduced cartilage damage. It was suggested that the absence of these lining cells led to less production of chemotactic factors, and thus the subsequent reduced PMN infiltration. Using a similar approach of phagocytic lining cell depletion, the pro-inflammatory cytokine IL-1 was markedly diminished along with reduced cell influx. These studies and others suggest that the synovial phagocytic cells contribute to the onset of synovitis.

A positive correlation between macrophages and articular destruction has also been established, because only synovial macrophage numbers (both lining and sublining macrophages) reportedly correlated with knee pain and radiologic course of articular destruction *(22,23)*. The identification of the macrophage-like type A lining cells, in addition to infiltrating cells and fibroblasts, as a source of matrix metalloproteinases, also suggested their involvement in matrix degradation. In addition to the positive correlation between the number of macrophages and articular destruction, there was also a positive correlation between the expression of IL-6 and TNF-α (both products of macrophages) and scores for knee pain *(23)*.

In an in vitro study *(24)* comparing cartilage degradation between synovial fibroblasts from RA and osteoarthritis (OA) patients, direct fibroblast–macrophage contact was not necessary for cartilage destruction, whereas the fibroblasts had to be in contact with cartilage to mediate degradation. The macrophage cytokines, TNF-α, IL-1β, and IL-6, could effectively activate the synovial fibroblasts to mediate cartilage destruction. In this experimental system, anticytokine antibodies which neutralize TNF-α, IL-1β, or IL-6 were inhibitory, supporting a role for macrophages in controlling cartilage degradation by activation of fibroblasts. Antibodies against T-cell cytokines, IFN-γ, IL-2,

IL-10 and had little or no effect on the degradation process. Because macrophages and their products appear to support the evolution of inflammatory pathology in the synovium, the subsequent section focuses on some of these products and their potential activities in synovitis.

6. Monocyte/Macrophage Products in Arthritic Joints

In a setting like the RA joint, the interactions among different cells and their products (e.g. cytokines, prostaglandins, MMP, and enzymes) are multifactorial and complex. There appears to be a cytokine network operating within inflamed joints, with pro-inflammatory and anti-inflammatory actions operating at the same time. Many of these products are from synovial macrophages and fibroblasts, but also from T- and B-lymphocytes and monocytes. The balance or imbalance between these two arms of action will determine the outcome of an inflammatory reaction. An array of cell products, typically associated with activated macrophages, has been detected in RA joints (*see also* the review in ref. 25). These include tumor necrosis factor-α (TNF-α), interleukin-1 (IL-1), oncostatin M (OSM), granulocyte–macrophage colony-stimulating factor (GM-CSF), macrophage colony-stimulating factor (M-CSF), transforming growth factor-β (TGF-β) and interleukin-10 (IL-10), several of which are being considered as targets for therapy and are highlighted in this review (Fig. 2).

7. Tumor Necrosis Factor-α

Tumor necrosis factor-α is a cytokine which has multiple proinflammatory effects (Table 2) and is mainly a product of macrophages and fibroblasts, in which its mRNA and protein are strongly expressed in inflamed synovial tissue and/or synovial fluid. The fact that it is detected at the cartilage–pannus junction suggests its further involvement in cartilage degradation *(25)*. TNF-α has multiple pro-inflammatory activities as summarized in Table 2 and is an upstream trigger of a cytokine cascade. TNF-α also releases nuclear factor κB (NFκB), a DNA-binding transcription factor, from its cytoplasmic inhibitor enabling it to translocate to the nucleus where it binds to the promoters of many proinflammatory genes including TNF-α and IL-6. TNF-α concentrations are increased in the synovial fluid of patients with active RA, and increased plasma levels are associated with joint pain *(26)*. TNF-α and IL-1 synergistically stimulate fibroblast proliferation and increase secretion of IL-6, GM-CSF, and the matrix metalloproteinase (MMP) collagenase. Naturally occurring antagonists of TNF-α include its soluble receptors, p55 and p75, and it is probable that an imbalance between TNF-α and its soluble receptor (TNFR) contributes to inflammation in RA. In this regard, one report suggested that the serum TNF-α/TNFR ratios in RA patients were not increased proportionally, compared to healthy individuals *(27)*.

Considerable evidence for a role of TNF-α in the pathogenesis of arthritis was initially derived from animal studies that also revealed that inhibiting this cytokine ameliorates certain aspects of the disease process. For example, transgenic mice overexpressing TNF-α spontaneously develop destructive arthritis typified by cartilage destruction, bone erosion, and leukocyte infiltration, which is preventable by the administration of neutralizing anti-TNF-α monoclonal antibodies (mAb) *(28)*. The observation that these mice develop arthritis, but apparently no other symptoms, would suggest that the joint tissue is extremely sensitive to the pro-inflammatory effect of TNF-α. In several

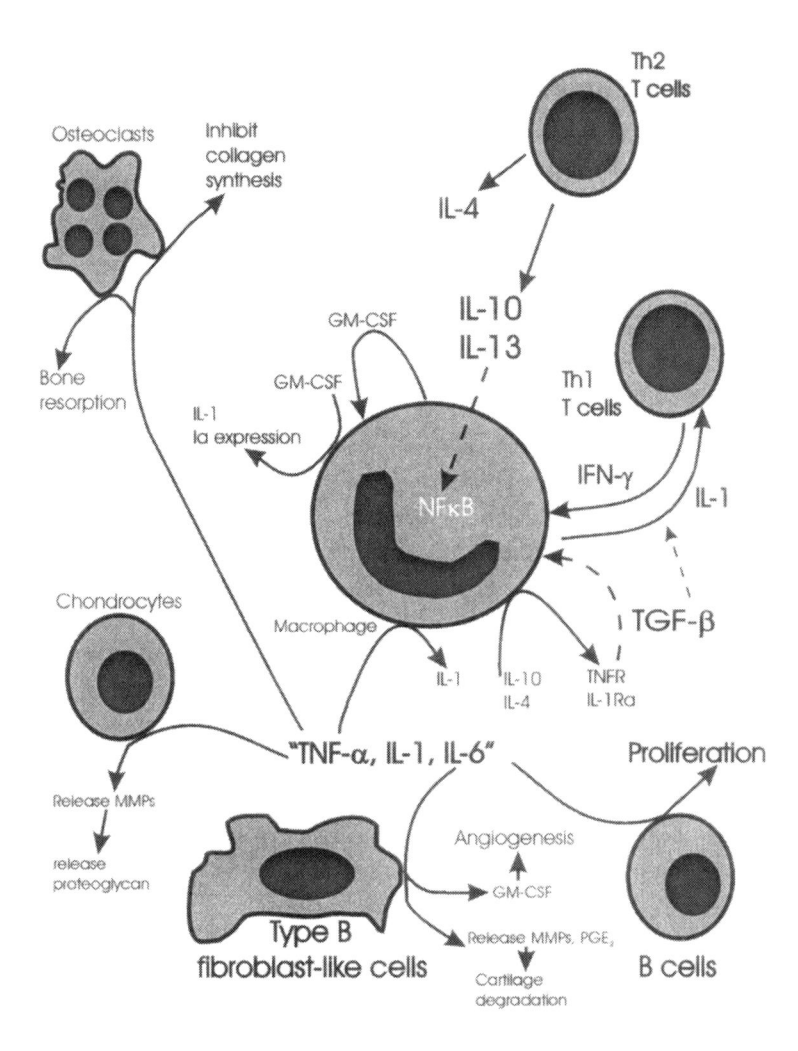

Fig. 2. A summary of cytokine network within rheumatoid synovium. The interaction among different cytokines *(see text)* with an emphasis on the pro-inflammatory roles of TNF-α, IL-1, and IL-6, and the potential anti-inflammatory functions of IL-10, IL-4, and TGF-β. Stimulatory (———) and inhibitory (- - - -) effects of cytokines on different cell types in RA synovium.

Table 2
Biologic Effects of TNF-α in RA

↑ Release of matrix metalloproteinases from neutrophils, fibroblasts, and chondrocytes
↓ Collagen synthesis in osteoblasts
↑ Proteoglycan release
↑ Expression of endothelial adhesion molecules (ICAM-1, ELAM-1/E-selectin and VACM-1)
↑ Pro-inflammatory cytokine release, such as IL-1 and IL-6
↑ Collagenase production
↑ PGE_2 production
↑ Bone resorption, ↓ bone formation
↑ PMN phagocytic activity, degranulation, production of reactive O_2 species

Table 3
Biologic Effects of IL-1 in RA

↑ Expression of endothelial adhesion molecules (ICAM-1, ELAM-1, and VCAM-1)
↑ Release of matrix metalloproteinases
↑ PGE_2 production
↑ GM-CSF and IL-6 production by synovial cells
↓ Collagen type VI mRNA production by fibroblasts
↑ pannus formation, ↑ type B-cells proliferation angiogenesis

experimental arthritis models, the administration of neutralizing anti-TNF-α mAb greatly reduced the severity of the disease. Because there appears to be a hierarchy within the cytokine network with TNF-α in a controlling position, antagonizing TNF-α is considered a promising approach to disease treatment. Recently, clinical trials in humans using an anti-TNF-α mAb, cA2, have provided promising therapeutic results (for a review, *see* ref. 25) with downstream decreases in serum IL-6, C-reactive protein, IL-1β, and soluble CD14 *(29)*. In addition to the changes in the cytokine levels, cA2 treatment also downregulated VCAM-1 and E-selectin expression by endothelial cells; serum levels of E-selectin and ICAM-1, but not VCAM-1, were also reduced by the treatment *(30)*. The major contribution of TNF-α to rheumatoid pathogenesis has recently been upheld by clinical studies in which a recombinant human p75 TNFR : Fc fusion protein improves inflammatory symptoms of RA *(26)*. Moreover, gene transfer of the p75 TNFR : Fc fusion protein is being explored in rodent arthritis models (Chan et al., unpublished data).

8. Interleukin-1

Interleukin-1 is a proinflammatory cytokine that exists in two forms, IL-1α and IL-1β, which bind to the same receptors and share many activities (Table 3). Relatively low doses of IL-1 inhibit chondrocyte proteoglycan synthesis, whereas higher IL-1 levels effect proteoglycan degradation. Furthermore, the ability of IL-1 to induce fever and to promote the production of acute-phase proteins by hepatocytes contributes to the systemic manifestations of RA. Experimentally, both intra-articular injection and systemic administration of IL-1 induce and/or accelerate the development and progression of the disease. Conversely, inhibitors of IL-1 ameliorate both early and late stages of arthritis, compared to anti-TNF-α treatment, which was most effective shortly after disease onset *(31)*. The naturally occurring IL-1 inhibitor, the interleukin-1 receptor antagonist (IL-1ra), is produced in equivalent amounts to IL-1 in normal synovium, whereas in RA, the balance shifts toward IL-1, thus favoring the inflammatory process. IL-1ra binds to IL-1 receptors to compete with IL-1α or IL-1β, but has no agonist activity. The inhibition of IL-1-induced cellular responses in T-cells, fibroblasts, and chondrocytes in vitro requires a 10- to 100-fold excess of IL-1ra, because the target cells are extremely sensitive to IL-1, with only 2–5% of available receptors needing to be occupied for a cellular response. As monocytes mature and become macrophages in vitro, their IL-1 production decreases and their IL-1ra production increases *(32)*. Synovial macrophages of RA or OA subjects appear to be the primary IL-1ra-expressing cells, which suggests that the body attempts to mount its own response against inflammation as a mechanism for the resolution of the disease process; however, in the case of RA, the levels of IL-1ra seem insufficient to resolve the inflammation.

To embellish the inadequate endogenous levels of the IL-1 receptor antagonist, the inhibitor has been administered therapeutically in experimental models and in human trials. IL-1ra administration in arthritic mice resulted in both reduced synovial inflammatory cell infiltration and cartilage damage. In rats, IL-1ra cDNA was transduced into synoviocytes, which were then engrafted in ankle joints of animals with SCW arthritis, resulting in significant suppression in the severity of recurrence of arthritis *(33)*. These studies not only highlight the therapeutic potential of IL-1ra but also point to its predominant preventive role in cartilage-destructive processes. Although animal models predicted its therapeutic efficacy *(31,34)*, only recently have human clinical trials been performed to support its effectiveness *(35)*. Moreover, because inhibition of either IL-1 or TNF-α has beneficial effects, but is not curative, combined inhibition of IL-1 and TNF-α is being considered for more effective resolution of inflammatory pathology.

9. Oncostatin M

Oncostatin (OSM), a cytokine produced by monocytic cells, has only recently been associated with synovial pathogenesis. OSM is produced by activated monocytes and is related to a cytokine family that includes LIF, G-CSF, and IL-6. Quantitatively, there are significantly higher levels of OSM in RA joints than in OA or normal joints *(36)*. The OSM concentration in synovial fluid appeared to correlate significantly with the synovial fluid white cell count *(37)*. Using immunolocalization, tissue macrophages in deeper synovial tissue were identified as a source of OSM in inflamed joints. Synovial macrophages isolated from RA joints have been shown to produce OSM spontaneously *(36)*. OSM promotes further monocyte recruitment by stimulating synovial fibroblasts, together with IL-1α, to secrete the chemokine, MCP-1 *(38)*.

The process of collagen degradation represents the consequence of elevated matrix metalloproteinases (MMPs) derived from macrophages and fibroblasts. The MMPs are a family of enzymes that can degrade all the components of the extracellular matrix, however, their activity depends on the relative balance between MMP levels and their naturally occurring inhibitors, the so-called tissue inhibitors of metalloproteinases (TIMPs). OSM induces similar amounts of MMP-1 (interstitial collagenase) and TIMP-1 from human cartilage in vitro, but in combination with IL-1α, it induces high levels of MMP-1 and inhibits TIMP-1, resulting in collagen release from cartilage. MMP-1 and MMP-13 (collagenase 3) are both upregulated in response to IL-1α and TNF-α.

10. Interleukin-6

Interleukin-6, present at high levels in the synovial fluid from RA patients, is a cytokine produced by monocytes, T-lymphocytes, and synovial fibroblasts, often in response to TNF-α and IL-1 and a link in the cytokine cascade. IL-6 shares some biologic activities to those of TNF-α and IL-1 (Tables 1 and 2), except has not been shown to stimulate prostaglandin E_2 (PGE_2) and collagenase production in chondrocytes and synovial fibroblasts. Another important function of IL-6 is its ability to increase B-lymphocyte proliferation and immunoglobulin production, which may foster elevations in rheumatoid factor. Because IL-6 induces T-cell proliferation and differentiation *(39)*, it likely affects persistence of the autoimmune-based synovial response. By inducing osteoclast differentiation from hematopoietic precursors and stimulating the growth of synovial fibroblasts, IL-6 may represent an important target. As an indicator of disease activity, the synovial fluid IL-6 levels reportedly correlate with the intensity of the lining layer cellularity.

In one recent report, the administration of mAb against the IL-6 receptor (MR16-1) significantly suppressed murine collagen-induced arthritis *(40)*, but the time of administration was crucial. Only the administration on d 0 or d 3 after the initial immunization with bovine type II collagen (CII) resulted in the suppression of arthritis. Inhibition of IL-6 also reduced the production of IgG anti-CII antibody and the responsiveness of splenic lymphocytes to CII. Antibody treatment on d 21 was ineffective, suggesting that, in the later disease phase, IL-6 may be less important. Gold and cyclosporine, both used in the treatment of RA, apparently inhibit IL-6 production. In IL-6-gene-deleted mice, no collagen-induced arthritis could be induced, nor were anti-CII antibodies produced *(41)*.

11. The Colony-Stimulating Factors GM-CSF and M-CSF

Colony-stimulating factors (CSFs), initially characterized and identified by their ability to stimulate in vitro colony formation by hematopoietic progenitor cells, are present in rheumatoid joints *(42,43)*. Produced by multiple cell populations including T-lymphocytes, cultured synovial macrophages, synovial fibroblast-like cells, and chondrocytes, GM-CSF promotes granulocyte and macrophage development from their precursor cells, whereas M-CSF regulates growth, differentiation, and function of mononuclear phagocytes. GM-CSF also enhances differentiated functions of mature effector cells, notably degranulation of neutrophils, cytokine expression, and tumor-cell killing by macrophages. However, the functions of the CSFs are not limited to myeloid cells, because GM-CSF stimulates human endothelial cells to migrate and proliferate and induces differentiation of dendritic cells, critical in antigen presentation. Importantly, GM-CSF also upregulates MHC class II expression by synovial macrophages to enhance antigen presentation *(43)*. Thus, the presence of GM-CSF and M-CSF in the rheumatoid joint may induce differentiation of myeloid cells to increase the number of mature macrophages and to sustain and activate this population in the inflamed synovium. Consistent with this concept, CSFs, in particular GM-CSF, exacerbated the disease process in a CIA model in mice *(44)*, whereas in GM-CSF-deficient mice, no disease developed *(45)*.

12. Transforming-Growth Factor-β

Although platelets represent the most concentrated source of TGF-β (20 mg/kg), activated lymphocytes, macrophages, neutrophils, and synovial fibroblasts also generate TGF-β and respond to TGF-β. With the production of TGF-β by multiple cell types at a site of inflammation, an autocrine and paracrine system likely exists for the continued production of TGF-β. TGF-β plays a role in leukocyte recruitment and activation on one hand, and facilitates healing by promoting fibroblast recruitment and matrix synthesis on the other *(46)*. TGF-β was originally identified as the most potent chemoattractant for monocytes with activity in the femtomolar concentration range and also has chemotactic activity for neutrophils and T-cells. TGF-β also enhances mononuclear phagocyte recruitment by modulation of integrin expression, augmenta-

Table 4
Systemic Versus Local Effects of TGF-β

Systemic	Local
↓ Adhesion	↑ adhesion
Reduce chemotactic gradient	TGF-β chemotactic gradient
Inhibition of recruitment	Leukocyte activation
Inhibition of selectins	Fibroblast accumulation
Inhibit immune-cell proliferation	Stimulate matrix production
	Matrix accumulation
	Inhibition of MMP
	Induces TIMP

tion of monocyte-matrix adhesion, enhancement of matrix-specific collagenase secretion, and chemotaxis *(47)*. TGF-β augments resting monocyte mRNA levels for IL-1, TNF-α, platelet-derived growth factor (PDGF), IL-6, and basic fibroblast growth factor (bFGF), which may, in turn, trigger the production of TGF-β from an array of cell types, in a cyclic feedback loop.

Transforming growth factor-β can be both pro- and anti-inflammatory; it typically stimulates resting cells, but its immunosuppressive qualities are most evident on activated cell populations. TGF-β antagonizes the ability of IL-1 to induce lymphocyte proliferation, reduces IL-1 receptor expression, and induces IL-1ra in macrophages. Taking advantage of its ability to inhibit inflammatory cells once they are activated, TGF-β has been explored as a therapeutic agent in arthritis models. TGF-β1 counteracted IL-1-induced inhibition of articular cartilage proteoglycan synthesis and stimulated restoration of the cartilage matrix by increasing chondrocyte proteoglycan synthesis. This protective role of TGF-β1 was observed in young mice (12 wk old), but not in old mice (18 mo old) *(48)*. TGF-β has different effects on inflammatory responses, depending on its local or systemic administration (Table 4), but when delivered systemically, it interrupts the inflammatory process *(46,47,49)*. In recent reports, systemic delivery of TGF-β protein *(50)* or TGF-β gene-transferameliorated rodent arthritis *(51)*. One target for elevated circulating TGF-β may be endothelial cells, because TGF-β inhibits their E-selectin expression to block adhesion and localization of leukocytes to the site of inflammation. Moreover, leukocytes are normally sensitive to a concentration gradient of chemotactic signals emanating from the site of inflammation, and the presence of elevated TGF-β in the circulation could eliminate such an outward gradient and thus contribute to the reduction in leukocyte infiltration.

Consistent with these observations, induction of oral tolerance to inhibit arthritis is associated with increased levels of TGF-β. Oral administration of cartilage-derived type II collagen ameliorates arthritis in animal models *(52)*, as does oral administration of SCW *(53)*. Oral administration of antigen to develop oral tolerance induces enhanced production and systemic routing of TGF-β to favor its potent immunosuppressive actions. The level of circulating TGF-β induced by oral administration of antigen was shown to be inversely proportional to TNF-α levels and to the articular index of the disease *(53)*. Upregulated IL-10, considered an anti-inflammatory cytokine, also occurred in SCW-tolerized spleen cell cultures and, interestingly, anti-TGF-β neutralizing mAb downregulated SCW-specific IL-10 production. These data suggested that the induction of IL-10 in this animal model may be, in part, regulated by TGF-β.

13. Interleukin-10

Interleukin-10, a potent anti-inflammatory cytokine produced by monocytes/macrophages and human Th2-type T-cells and B-cells induces anergy of human CD4+ T-cells in vitro. It regulates B7 costimulatory molecules, while suppressing IFN-γ production by inhibiting IL-12, to favor Th2 cell differentiation. Because IL-10 is able to downregulate the antigen-presenting function of synovial macrophages, even when they are efficiently activated (54), IL-10 may be instrumental in interrupting chronic activation. Not only does IL-10 downregulate TNF-α and IL-1 production, but it also enhances IL-1ra and soluble TNF receptor release from macrophages, the net effect of which is suppression of inflammatory sequelae. Moreover, because IL-10 inhibits NFκB, multiple downstream events become interrupted. A number of genes involved in inflammation and immune surveillance share a DNA-binding motif for this transcription factor. In unstimulated cells, NFκB is sequestered in the cell cytoplasm via its association with the inhibitory protein IκB (inhibitor of NFκB). During cell activation, such as by TNF or IL-1, IκB is phosphorylated and released, activating NFκB, which is translocated to the cell nucleus. Once in the nucleus, it binds to gene promoters to trigger transcription of adhesion molecules and cytokines. Thus, inhibition of NFκB has become recognized as an anti-inflammatory target (55).

Interleukin-10 and the Th2 cytokine, IL-4, share an ability to reduce expression of multiple cytokines including TNF and IL-1 (Fig. 2) (56–58). IL-4 also promotes monocyte apoptosis favoring resolution of inflammation (59). In the absence of IL-10, the IL-10-deficient mice are not only growth retarded and anemic but develop a chronic inflammatory bowel disease resembling Crohn's disease (60). On the other hand, injection of recombinant IL-10 is anti-inflammatory, protecting mice from lethal endotoxemia. IL-10 also suppresses established CIA (61,62), whereas the neutralizing antibody to IL-10 increases the severity of arthritis (63). Combined treatment with IL-10 and IL-4 in a mouse model of arthritis resulted in a profound amelioration of the disease when compared to IL-10 or IL-4 treatment alone (64). This synergistic effect warrants further exploration.

14. Summary

Cells of the mononuclear phagocytic lineage play a crucial role either in the prevention or in the evolution of synovitis and tissue destruction. Macrophages in inflamed synovium are a source of an array of pro-inflammatory cytokines that function as components of a cytokine network. These cytokines operate within an autocrine and paracrine system in the joint and, in excess, may function as endocrine molecules (e.g., IL-1 induces fever). Macrophage-derived cytokines orchestrate the participation of multiple cell types (fibroblasts, chondrocytes, osteoclasts) and together, these cells are responsible for matrix degradation and tissue destruction. Although anti-inflammatory cytokines (IL-10 and IL-4) and cytokine antagonists (TNFR and IL-1ra) are released into the joint in an attempt by the host to counteract the effects of excess pro-inflammatory cytokines, it is likely that the persistent imbalance of this relationship is responsible for the pathophysiologic events in RA. With the accumulating foundation of knowledge concerning the cytokine network within the inflamed synovium, a number of therapeutic approaches have emerged. In general, these approaches focus on blocking the action of pro-inflammatory cytokines and/or increasing anti-inflammatory cytokine levels. Furthermore, interrupting leukocyte recruitment by targeting chemokines and/or adhesion molecules, as well as angiogenic pathways, offers additional avenues for blocking the pathophysiologic events leading to unrelenting inflammatory destruction.

References

1. Henson, P. M. and Riches, D. W. (1994) Modulation of macrophage maturation by cytokines and lipid mediators: a potential role in resolution of pulmonary inflammation. *Ann. NY Acad. Sci.* **725**, 298.
2. Erwig, L.-P. and Rees, A. J. (1999) Macrophage activation and programming and its role for macrophage function in glomerular inflammation. *Kidney Blood Press. Res.* **22**, 21.
3. Hamilton, J. A. (1993) Rheumatoid arthritis: opposing actions of haemopoietic growth factors and slow-acting anti-rheumatic drugs. *Lancet* **342**, 536.
4. Bresnihan, B. (1992) The synovial lining cells in chronic arthritis. *Br. J. Rheumatol.* **31**, 433.
5. Chan, J., Leenen, P. J. M., Bertoncello, I., Nishikawa, S.-I., and Hamilton, J. A. (1998) Macrophage lineage cells in inflammation; characterization by colony-stimulating factor-1 (CSF-1) receptor (c-Fms), ER-MP58, and ER-MP20 (Ly-6C) expression. *Blood* **92**, 1423.
6. Wahl, S. M., Feldman, G. M., and McCarthy, J. B. (1996) Regulation of leukocyte adhesion and signaling in inflammation and disease. *J. Leukocyte Biol.* **59**, 789.
7. Ali, H., Haribabu, B., Richardson, R. M., and Snyderman, R. (1997) Mechanisms of inflammation and leukocyte activation. *Med. Clin. North Am.* **81**, 1.
8. Springer, T. A. (1994) Traffic signals for lymphocyte recirculation and leukocyte emigration: the multistep paradigm. *Cell* **76**, 301.
9. McCarthy, J. B., Vachhani, B. V., Wahl, S. M., Finbloom, D. S., and Feldman, G. M. (1997) Human monocyte binding to fibronectin enhances IFN-γ-induced early signaling events. *J. Immunol.* **159**, 2424.
10. Wahl, S. M., Allen, J. B., Hines, K. L., Imamichi, T., Wahl, A. M., Furcht, L. T., et al. (1994) Synthetic fibronectin peptides suppress arthritis in rats by interrupting leukocyte adhesion and recruitment. *J. Clin. Invest.* **94**, 655.
11. Brooks, P. C., Clark, R. A., and Cheresh, D. A. (1994) Requirement of vascular integrin alpha v beta 3 for angiogenesis. *Science* **264**, 569.
12. Peacock, D. J., Banquerigo, M. L., and Brahn, E. (1992) Angiogenesis inhibition suppresses collagen arthritis. *J. Exp. Med.* **175**, 1135.
13. Storgard, C. M., Stupack, D. G., Jonczyk, A., Goodman, S. L., Fox, R. I., and Cheresh, D. A. (1999) Decreased angiogenesis and arthritic disease in rabbits treated with an alphavbeta3 antagonist. *J. Clin. Invest.* **103**, 47.
14. Ley, K. (1995) Gene-targeted mice in leukocyte adhesion research. *Microcirculation* **2**, 141.
15. Tesch, G. H., Schwrting, A., Kinoshita, K., Lan, H. Y., Rollins, B. J., and Kelly, V. R. (1999) Monocyte chemoattractant protein-1 promotes macrophage-mediated tubular injury, but not glomerular injury, in nephrotoxic serum nephritis. *J. Clin. Invest.* **103**, 73.
16. Zagorski, J. and Wahl, S. M. (1997) Inhibition of acute peritoneal inflammation in rats by a cytokine-induced neutrophil chemoattractant receptor antagonist. *J. Immunol.* **159**, 1059.
17. Singer, N. G., Richardson, B. C., Powers, D., Hooper, F., Lialios, F., Endres, J., et al. (1996) Role of the CD6 glycoprotein in antigen-specific and autoreactive responses of cloned human T lymphocytes. *Immunology* **88**, 537.
18. Levesque, M. C., Heinly, C. S., Whichard, L. P., and Patel, D. D. (1998) Cytokine-regulated expression of activated leukocyte cell adhesion molecule (CD 166) on monocyte-lineage cells and in rheumatoid arthritis synovium. *Arthritis Rheum.* **41**, 2221.

19. Cunnane, G., Hummel, K. M., Muller-Ladner, U., Gay, R. E., and Gay, S. (1998) Mechanism of joint destruction in rheumatoid arthritis. *Arch. Immunol. Therap. Exp.* **46,** 1.
20. Kanik, K. S., Hagiwara, E., Yarboro, C. H., Schumacher, H. R., Wilder, R. L., and Klinman, D. M. (1998) Distinct patterns of cytokine secretion characterize new onset synovitis versus chronic rheumatoid arthritis. *J. Rheum.* **25,** 16.
21. van Lent, P. L. E. M., Holthuysen, A. E. M., van Rooijen, N., van de Loo, F. A. J., van de Putte, L. B. A., and van den Berg, W. B. (1998) Phagocytic synovial lining cells regulate acute and chronic joint inflammation after antigenic exacerbation of smouldering experimental murine arthritis. *J. Rheumatol.* **25,** 1135.
22. Mulherin, D., Fitzgerald, O., and Bresnihan, B. (1996) Synovial tissue macrophage populations and articular damage in rheumatoid arthritis. *Arthritis Rheum.* **39,** 115.
23. Tak, P. P., Smeets, T. J. M., Daha, M. R., Kluin, P. M., Meijers, K. A. E., Brand, R., et al. (1997) Analysis of the synovial cell infiltrate in early rheumatoid synovial tissue in relation to local disease activity. *Arthritis Rheum.* **40,** 217.
24. Scott, B. B., Weisbrot, L. M., Greenwood, J. D., Bogoch, E. R., Paige, C. J., and Keystone, E. C. (1997) Rheumatoid arthritis synovial fibroblast and U937 macrophage/monocyte cell line interaction in cartilage degradation. *Arthritis Rheum.* **40,** 490.
25. Brennan, F. M., Maini, R. N., and Feldmann, M. (1998) Role of proinflammatory cytokines in rheumatoid arthritis. *Springer Semin. Immunopathol.* **20,** 133.
26. Moreland, L. W., Baumgartner, S. W., Schiff, M. H., Tindall, E. A., Fleischmann, R. M., Weaver, A. L., et al. (1997) Treatment of rheumatoid arthritis with a recombinant human tumor necrosis factor receptor (p75)-Fc fusion protein. *N. Engl. J. Med.* **337,** 141.
27. Robak, T., Gladalska, A., and Stepien, H. (1998) The tumor necrosis factor family of receptors/ligands in the serum of patients with rheumatoid arthritis. *Eur. Cytokine Network* **9,** 145.
28. Keffer, J., Probert, L., Cazlaris, H., Georgopoulos, S., Kaslaris, E., Kioussis, D., et al. (1991) Transgenic mice expressing human tumor necrosis factor: a predictive genetic model of arthritis. *EMBO J.* **10,** 4025.
29. Lorenz, H. M., Antoni, C., Valerius, T., Repp, R., Grunke, M., Schwerdtner, N., et al. (1996) In vivo blockade of TNF-alpha by intravenous infusion of a chimeric monoclonal TNF-alpha antibody in patients with rheumatoid arthritis. Short term cellular and molecular effects. *J. Immunol.* **156,** 1646.
30. Tak, P. P., Taylor, P. C., Breedveld, F. C., Smeets, T. J. M., Daha, M. R., Kluin, P. M., et al. (1996) Decrease in cellular and expression of adhesion molecules by anti-tumor necrosis factor α monoclonal antibody treatment in patients with rheumatoid arthritis. *Arthritis Rheum.* **39,** 1077.
31. Joosten, L. A., Helsen, M. M., van de Loo, F. A., and van den Berg, W. B. (1996) Anticytokine treatment of established type II collagen-induced arthritis in DBA/1 mice. A comparative study using anti-TNF alpha, anti-IL-1 alpha/beta, and IL-1Ra. *Arthritis Rheum.* **39,** 797.
32. Arend, W. P. and Jean-Michel, D. (1990) Cytokines and cytokine inhibitors or antagonists in rheumatoid arthritis. *Arthritis Rheum.* **33,** 305.
33. Makarov, S. S., Olsen, J. C., Johnston, W. N., Anderle, S. K., Brown, R. R., Baldwin, A. S. J., et al. (1996) Suppression of experimental arthritis by gene transfer of interleukin 1 receptor antagonist cDNA. *Proc. Natl. Acad. Sci. USA* **93,** 402.
34. Henderson, B., Thompson, R. C., Hardingham, T., and Lewthwaite, J. (1991) Inhibition of interleukin-1-induced synovitis and articular cartilage proteoglycan loss in the rabbit knee by recombinant human interleukin-1 receptor antagonist. *Cytokine* **3,** 246.
35. Bresnihan, B., Alvaro-Gracia, J. M., Cobby, M., Doherty, M., Domljan, Z., Emery, P., et al. (1998) Treatment of rheumatoid arthritis with recombinant human interleukin-1 receptor antagonist. *Arthritis Rheum.* **41,** 2196.
36. Okamoto, H., Yamamura, M., Morita, Y., Harada, S., Makino, H., and Ota, Z. (1997) The synovial expression and serum levels of interleukin-6, interleukin-11, leukemia inhibitory factor, and oncostatin M in rheumatoid arthritis. *Arthritis Rheum.* **40,** 1096.

37. Hui, W., Bell, M., and Carroll, G. (1997) Detection of oncostatin M in synovial fluid from patients with rheumatoid arthritis. *Ann. Rheum. Dis.* **56,** 184.
38. Langdon, C., Leith, J., Smith, F., and Richards, C. D. (1997) Oncostatin M stimulates monocyte chemoattractant protein-1- and interleukin-1-induced matrix metalloproteinase-1 production by human synovial fibroblasts in vitro. *Arthritis Rheum.* **40,** 2139.
39. Akira, S., Taga, T., and Kishimoto, T. (1993) Interleukin-6 in biology and medicine. *Adv. Immunol.* **54,** 1.
40. Takagi, N., Mihara, M., Moriya, Y., Nishimoto, N., Yoshizaki, K., Kishimoto, T., et al. (1998) Blockage of interleukin-6 receptor ameliorates joint disease in murine collagen-induced arthritis. *Arthritis Rheum.* **41,** 2117.
41. Alonzi, T., Fattori, E., Lazzaro, D., Costa, P., Probert, L., Kollias, G., et al. (1998) Interleukin 6 is required for the development of collagen-induced arthritis. *J. Exp. Med.* **187,** 461.
42. Isomaki, P. and Punnonen, J. (1997) Pro- and anti-inflammatory cytokines in rheumatoid arthritis. *Ann. Med.* **29,** 499.
43. Alvaro-Gracia, J. M., Zvaifler, N. J., and Firestein, G. S. (1989) Cytokines in chronic inflammatory arthritis. IV. Granulocyte/macrophage colony-stimulating factor-mediated induction of class II MHC antigen on human monocytes: a possible role in rheumatoid arthritis. *J. Exp. Med.* **170,** 865.
44. Campbell, I. K., Bendele, A., Smith, D. A., and Hamilton, J. A. (1997) Granulocyte-macrophage colony stimulating factor exacerbates collagen induced arthritis in mice. *Ann. Rheum. Dis.* **56,** 364.
45. Campbell, I. K., Rich, M. J., Bischof, R. J., Dunn, A. R., Grail, D., and Hamilton, J. A. (1998) Protection from collagen-induced arthritis in granulocyte-macrophage colony-stimulating factor-deficient mice. *J. Immunol.* **161,** 3639.
46. Wahl, S. M. (1994) Transforming growth factor β: The good, the bad, and the ugly. *J. Exp. Med.* **180,** 1587.
47. Wahl, S. M. (1992) Transforming growth factor beta (TGF-β) in inflammation: a cause or a cure. *J. Clin. Immunol.* **12,** 61.
48. van Beuningen, H. M., van der Kraan, P. M., Arntz, O. J., and van den Berg, W. B. (1994) In vivo protection against interleukin-1-induced articular cartilage damage by transforming growth factor-β1: age-related differences. *Ann. Rheum. Dis.* **53,** 593.
49. McCartney-Francis, N. L. and Wahl, S. M. (1994) Transforming growth factor β: a matter of life and death. *J. Leukocyte Biol.* **55,** 401.
50. Brandes, M. E., Allen, J. B., Ogawa, Y., and Wahl, S. M. (1991) Transforming growth factor β1 suppresses acute and chronic arthritis in experimental animals. *J. Clin. Invest.* **87,** 1108.
51. Song, X.-Y., Gu, M., Jin, W.-W., Klinman, D. M., and Wahl, S. M. (1998) Plasmid DNA encoding transforming growth factor-β1 suppresses chronic disease in a streptococcal cell wall-induced arthritis model. *J. Clin. Invest.* **101,** 2615.
52. Barnett, M. L., Kremer, J. M., St Clair, E. W., Clegg, D. O., Furst, D., Weisman, M., et al. (1998) Treatment of rheumatoid arthritis with oral type II collagen. Results of a multicenter, double-blind, placebo-controlled trial. *Arthritis Rheum.* **41,** 290.
53. Chen, W., Jin, W., Cook, M., Weiner, H. L., and Wahl, S. M. (1998) Oral delivery of group A streptococcal cell walls augments circulating TGF-β and suppresses streptococcal cell wall arthritis. *J. Immunol.* **161,** 6297.
54. Mottonen, M., Isomaki, P., Saario, R., Toivanen, P., Punnonen, J., and Lassila, O. (1998) Interleukin-10 inhibits the capacity of synovial macrophages to function as antigen-presenting cells. *Br. J. Rheumatol.* **37,** 1207.
55. Chen, C. C. and Manning, A. M. (1995) Transcriptional regulation of endothelial cell adhesion molecules: a dominant role for NF-kappa B. *Agents Actions* **47(Suppl.),** 135.
56. Allen, J. B., Wong, H. L., Costa, G. L., Bienkowski, M. J., and Wahl, S. M. (1993) Suppression of monocyte function and differential regulation of IL-1 and IL-1ra by IL-4 contribute to resolution of experimental arthritis. *J. Immunol.* **151,** 4344.

57. Wong, H. L., Lotze, M. T., Wahl, L. M., and Wahl, S. M. (1992) Administration of recombinant IL-4 to humans regulates gene expression, phenotype, and function in circulating monocytes. *J. Immunol.* **148,** 2118.
58. Isomaki, P., Luukkainen, R., Toivanen, P., and Punnonen, J. (1996) The presence of interleukin-13 in rheumatoid synovium and its antiinflammatory effects on synovial fluid macrophages from patients with rheumatoid arthritis. *Arthritis Rheum.* **39,** 1693.
59. Mangan, D. F., Robertson, B., and Wahl, S. M. (1992) IL-4 enhances programmed cell death (apoptosis) in stimulated human monocytes. *J. Immunol.* **148,** 1812.
60. Kuhn, R., Lohler, J., Rennick, D., Rajewsky, K., and Muller, W. (1993) Interleukin-10-deficient mice develop chronic enterocolitis. *Cell* **75,** 263.
61. Walmsley, M., Katsikis, P. D., Abney, E., Parry, S., Williams, R. O., Maini, R. N., et al. (1996) Interleukin-10 inhibition of the progression of established collagen-induced arthritis. *Arthritis Rheum.* **39,** 495.
62. Joosten, L. A., Lubberts, E., Durez, P., Helsen, M. M., Jacobs, M. J., Goldman, M., et al. (1997) Role of interleukin-4 and interleukin-10 in murine collagen-induced arthritis. Protective effect of interleukin-4 and interleukin-10 treatment on cartilage destruction. *Arthritis Rheum.* **40,** 249.
63. Kasama, T., Strieter, R. M., Lukacs, N. W., Lincoln, P. M., Burdick, M. D., and Kunkel, S. L. (1995) Interleukin-10 expression and chemokine regulation during the evolution of murine type II collagen-induced arthritis. *J. Clin. Invest.* **95,** 2868.
64. Lubberts, E., Joosten, L. A., Helsen, M. M., and van den Berg, W. B. (1998) Regulatory role of interleukin 10 in joint inflammation and cartilage destruction in murine streptococcal cell wall (SCW) arthritis. More therapeutic benefit with IL-4/IL-10 combination therapy than with IL-10 treatment alone. *Cytokine* **10,** 361.

15

Polymorphonuclear Cells

Michael H. Pillinger, Pamela B. Rosenthal, and Bruce N. Cronstein

1. Introduction

The presence of neutrophils (polymorphonuclear leukocytes [PMNs]) within extravascular tissues is a hallmark of acute inflammation. Although Metchnikoff proposed in the nineteenth century that phagocytic neutrophils might release substances capable of injuring tissues, it was not until the mid-twentieth-century that empirical evidence was obtained in support of Metchnikoff's hypothesis. It is now clear from experimental models that neutrophils play a critical role in immune-mediated tissue injury. For instance, depletion of neutrophils reverses tissue injury in the Arthus model of immune-complex-mediated vascular injury, despite the ongoing deposition of immune complexes and complement in vessel walls. Other experimental models in which neutrophils play an active role in the induction of tissue injury include the necrotizing arteritis of serum sickness in rabbits, prolonged proteinuria associated with acute nephrotoxic vasculitis in rats, and the reverse passive Arthus reaction. These studies all indicate that neutrophils are important mediators of the inflammatory tissue injury observed in the rheumatic diseases.

2. Neutrophil Development

Polymorphonuclear leukocytes are terminally differentiated, postmitotic, phagocytic blood cells that form the first line of host defense against microorganisms and mediate the elimination of debris at sites of injury. Three classes of circulating polymorphonuclear leukocyte—the neutrophil, eosinophil, and basophil lines—are easily distinguishable in blood by the staining characteristics of their cytoplasmic granules. The presence of these granules, although different in each line, has led to the alternative term "granulocyte" to describe these cells. By far the most abundant leukocyte in the peripheral circulation is the neutrophil (usually more than 95% of all granulocytes). Indeed, approx 60% of the hematopoietic capacity of the normal bone marrow is dedicated to the production of an enormous number of neutrophils, approx 10^{11} cells per day. Moreover, this number can be greatly increased during conditions of stress, including infection or acute injury.

Neutrophils are derived from myeloid stem cells that populate the bone marrow (1). The myeloblast is the precursor for all polymorphonuclear leukocyte lines. Myeloblasts may then differentiate into neutrophilic promyelocytes, the first committed cell

From: *Current Molecular Medicine: Principles of Molecular Rheumatology*
Edited by: G. C. Tsokos © Humana Press Inc., Totowa, NJ

in the generation of neutrophils, followed, sequentially, by differentiation into neutrophil myelocytes, metamyelocytes, band cells, and, ultimately, mature neutrophils. These differentiation steps take place under the regulation of a variety of cytokines and growth factors, the best characterized of which are granulocyte colony-stimulating factor (G-CSF) and granulocyte/monocyte colony-stimulating factor (GM-CSF). The recent availability of recombinant G-CSF and GM-CSF for clinical use has contributed to a marked decline in the morbidity and mortality associated with chemotherapy-induced leukopenia.

From the myelocyte stage on, neutrophils lose the capacity for further mitosis. The mitotic and postmitotic stages of neutrophil differentiation in the bone marrow last approximately 7 d. However, once they have been released into the circulation, neutrophils have a half-life of approximately 6 h. Senescent neutrophils, like most other cell types, undergo a process of programmed cell death (apoptosis) and are removed from the circulation by the reticuloendothelial system. The half-life of the neutrophils that emigrate from the vasculature into the tissues is, at present, unknown.

In addition to their granules, neutrophils are easily recognized on the basis of their most prominent feature, the multilobed nucleus containing condensed heterochromatin. Neutrophil nuclei tend to have a higher number of lobes than those of other polymorphonuclear leukocytes, typically three to five. Relative to monocytic leukocytes, mature neutrophils do not synthesize a great quantity of proteins, a finding consistent with their condensed chromatin, lack of nucleoli, and relative dearth of endoplasmic reticulum. Neutrophils do synthesize some gene products, however, including interleukin-1α, interleukin-1β, interleukin-8, tumor necrosis factor-α, G-CSF, GM-CSF, c-Raf-1, complement receptor-1, CD11a, receptors for the immunoglobulin constant region (FcγR), actin, and class I major histocompatibility (MHC) molecules.

Within the cytoplasm, the most prominent histologic feature of the neutrophil is its large number of granules. These granules contain a broad spectrum of antimicrobial enzymes and peptides critical for host defense. In addition, their membranes contain a pool of easily mobilized surface proteins that regulate the inflammatory response. Based on morphology and histochemical staining, there are two major, distinct types of granules, designated azurophilic and specific, although using more sensitive techniques, at least two other granule types can be appreciated, gelatinase granules and secretory vesicles. Each of these granules contains a different complement of bactericidal proteins, proteolytic enzymes, and other bioactive molecules. In contrast to the other granules, the secretory vesicles appear to be primarily a reservoir of membrane-associated proteins as opposed to soluble proteins *(2)*.

Neutrophils are motile cells that move both in a directed fashion (chemotaxis) and randomly (chemokinesis). Once they have arrived at their destination, neutrophils phagocytose suitable particles. Both movement and phagocytosis depend on an intact cytoskeleton which is composed, in part, of actin microfilaments and associated proteins. A dense meshwork of actin filaments forms in the subplasmalemmal region of the leading edge (lamellipodium) of neutrophils undergoing chemotaxis. The cytoplasmic domains of integrins (*see* Subheading 3.) serve as organizing centers for the actin microfilaments and actin-associated proteins (myosin, ATPase, etc.) which generate motile force as well as help to invaginate the plasma membrane at the site of contact with phagocytic particles *(3)*.

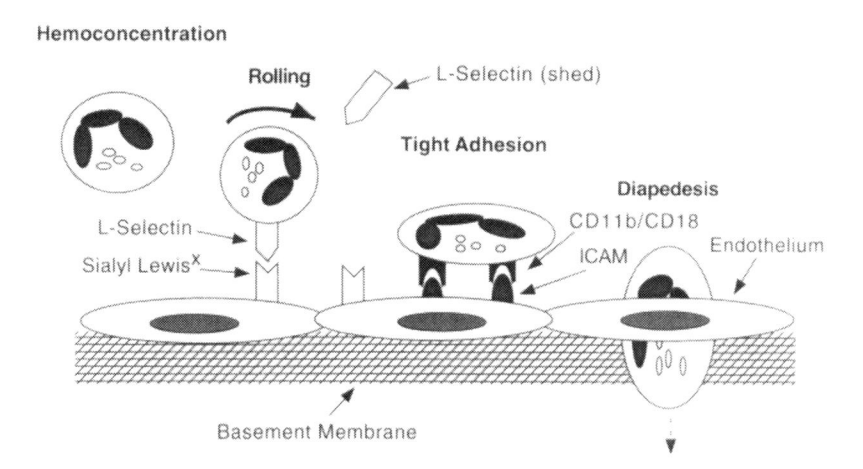

Fig. 1. Neutrophil adhesion to endothelium. Shown at the left of the figure, weak, selectin-dependent neutrophil adhesion to endothelium (rolling) is preceded by margination as a consequence of hemoconcentration. In response to stimuli, additional adhesion molecules (CD11b/CD18 on neutrophils, ICAM on endothelial cells) are activated and/or upregulated, resulting in tight adhesion. Diapedesis of the neutrophil through the endothelium in the direction of a chemoattractant gradient then follows.

In addition to microfilaments, neutrophil cytoskeleton is composed of microtubules. The microtubules, as in other cells, are composed of polymers of tubulin and exist in a dynamic state of assembly and disassembly. Although the assembly and disassembly of microtubules is highly regulated in intact cells, it is also susceptible to disruption with a variety of therapeutic agents, most notably colchicine and vinblastine. Results of studies with agents that disrupt microtubules indicate that microtubules are important for degranulation and fusion of granules with phagolysosomes.

3. Neutrophil Function

3.1. Adhesion, Diapedesis, and Chemotaxis

Neutrophils circulate within the vasculature and must be recruited to infected or inflamed sites. The process by which neutrophils are recruited to inflamed sites has been the subject of a great deal of attention and many of the molecules involved have been identified. Both the neutrophil and the vascular endothelium lining the microvessels play active roles in the process of recruitment.

Neutrophil recruitment is characterized by four different stages. In the first stage, margination, hemoconcentration in the microvasculature at the site of inflammation permits neutrophils to come into closer and more frequent contact with the vascular wall. In the second stage of neutrophil recruitment, the neutrophils adhere loosely to the vascular endothelium and roll along the vessel wall. If sufficiently stimulated, the neutrophils will then spread and adhere more tightly to the vascular wall. Eventually, the neutrophils will find their way out of the vasculature (diapedesis) and follow a trail of chemoattractants to the inflamed or infected site (Fig. 1).

Three families of molecules mediate the adhesive interactions involved in recruitment of neutrophils to an inflamed site. The integrins are a large family of heterodimeric (composed of an a and a b chain) proteins expressed on leukocytes and other cells. One subfamily of integrins, the β2-integrins, is expressed exclusively on neutrophils and other cells of myeloid origin and is particularly important in the recruitment of leukocytes to inflamed sites. The three members of the β2-integrin family share a common β chain (CD18) but have distinct α chains known generally by their cluster designation (CD11a,b,c). The primary integrin adhesion molecules on the neutrophil is CD11b/CD18, which mediates tight neutrophil adhesion to endothelium and is also a receptor for C3bi, a complement activation product. The β2-integrins bind to members of the second class of proteins involved in neutrophil adhesion, the intercellular adhesion molecules (ICAMs). ICAMs are members of the immunoglobulin superfamily of molecules and several of these molecules are expressed on endothelial cells (ICAM-1 and ICAM-2), particularly in response to inflammatory cytokines. The third family of adhesion molecules involved in neutrophil recruitment is the selectins. There are three known members of this group: L-selectin (on neutrophils, T-cells, and monocytes), E-selectin (expressed exclusively on stimulated endothelial cells), and P-selectin (on stimulated platelets and endothelial cells). Selectins bind to specific carbohydrate moieties of glycoproteins expressed on the surface of endothelial cells or neutrophils. In contrast to integrin/ICAM associations, selectins mediate a looser, more easily reversible interaction between neutrophils and endothelial cells (rolling). Thus, the adhesive interactions between neutrophils and the vascular endothelium are mediated initially by selectin-glycoprotein interactions (rolling), followed by β2-integrin/ICAM-1,2-mediated adhesion (tight binding). In addition, the β2-integrins are important for diapedesis and must act to guide the neutrophil into the extravascular space.

3.2. Phagocytosis and Degranulation

Upon reaching a target, the neutrophil must phagocytose and destroy it. Neutrophils are relatively poor at attacking naked bacteria. In most instances, however, bacteria within the body are prepared for neutrophil attack by undergoing coating with immunoglobulins and complement—a process known as opsonization. Interaction of opsonizing immunoglobulins and c3b or c3bi complement fragments with their respective receptors on the neutrophil surface results, not only in bacterial adhesion but also in activation of neutrophil programs for phagocytosis. Recent studies by Caron and Hall suggest that two distinct processes in phagocytosis—extension of filopodia around the opsonized particle and invagination of the cell membrane at the point of particle contact—are stimulated by engagement of immunoglobulin and c3bi receptors, respectively, and regulated by distinct signaling pathways *(4)*.

Degranulation is, technically speaking, the process of stimulated depletion of neutrophil granules. In practice, degranulation may be thought of as two separate processes. In the first, neutrophil phagocytosis of a bacterium results in the fusion of neutrophil granules with the nascent lysosome to form a mature phagolysosome. This process permits the delivery of proteinases and antibacterial proteins to their site of action, including elastase, collagenase, the defensins, and bacterial permeability-inducing protein (BPI) *(5)*. Several of these proteins are maintained within their constituent granules in a latent state and undergo activation only within the phagolysosome. For instance, neutrophil collagenase resides in the specific granules in an inactive form. Fusion of these granules with the phagolysosome brings procollagenase into proximity

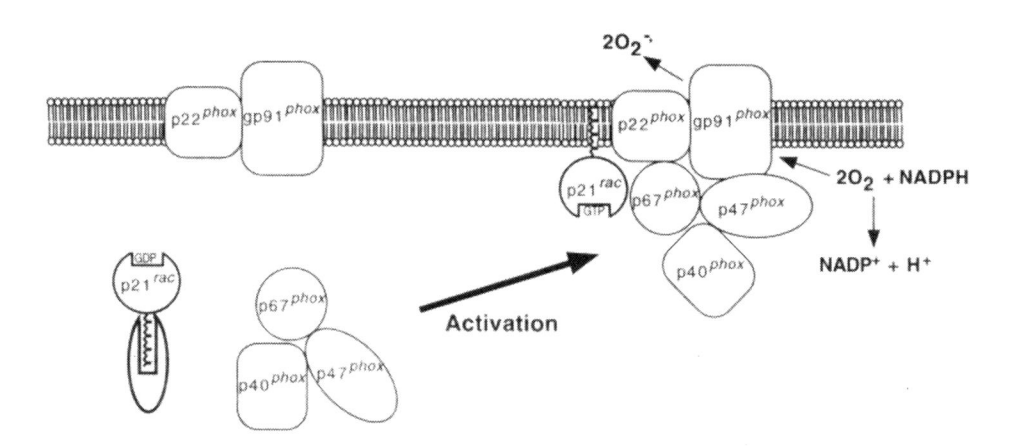

Fig. 2. Assembly of the neutrophil NADPH oxidase system. Stimulation of the neutrophil by chemoattractants results in the translocation of four components (p47^{phox}, p67^{phox}, p40^{phox}, and p21^{rac}) to the neutrophil membrane where the complete oxidase system is assembled, resulting in the generation of O_2^-. Prior to activation and translocation, p21^{rac} is maintained in a soluble form by a chaperon molecule, GDI (unlabeled on the drawing), which sheaths the p21^{rac} hydrophobic tail.

of myeloperoxidase from azurophilic granules, whose products (see Subheading 3.3.) can then mediate collagenase activation. Thus, potentially autodestructive proteins are maintained within the self-protective membranes of granules and, moreover, may be maintained in an inactive state until needed.

A second aspect of degranulation is the fusion of granules with the neutrophil plasma membrane. In addition to soluble molecules, neutrophil granules contain membrane-associated proteins, many with functions on the cell surface. Activation of neutrophils with appropriate stimuli results in the preferential movement of some classes of granules—particularly secretory vesicles—to the plasma membrane, thus resulting in rapid, protein synthesis-independent upregulaton of a number of proteins, as well as an expansion of neutrophil surface area.

3.3. Generation of Toxic Oxygen Radicals

One of the key mechanisms through which neutrophils damage or destroy microorganisms is via the generation of superoxide anion (O_2^-) (Fig. 2). Because of the potential for damage to the cell itself, this process is tightly regulated and only activated in response to appropriate signals. Studies in intact neutrophils, as well as in reconstituted systems consisting of isolated neutrophil cytosolic and membrane components, have revealed the basic system required for superoxide generation. The generating apparatus appears to consist of five proteins: two constitutively associated, membrane-based proteins (gp190^{phox} and p20^{phox}) which collectively make up the electron transport molecule cytochrome b$_{558}$, and three cytosolic proteins (p47^{phox}, p67^{phox}, and p21^{rac}), whose roles appear to be regulatory. A sixth component, p40^{phox}, has recently been described, whose role is not entirely clear. Appropriate stimulation of the neutrophil results in translocation of p47^{phox}, p67^{phox}, and p21^{rac} to the membrane of the phagocytic vacuole and association with the cytochrome b$_{558}$. This complex then employs NADPH as an electron donor to oxidize molecular oxygen to its radical form (6).

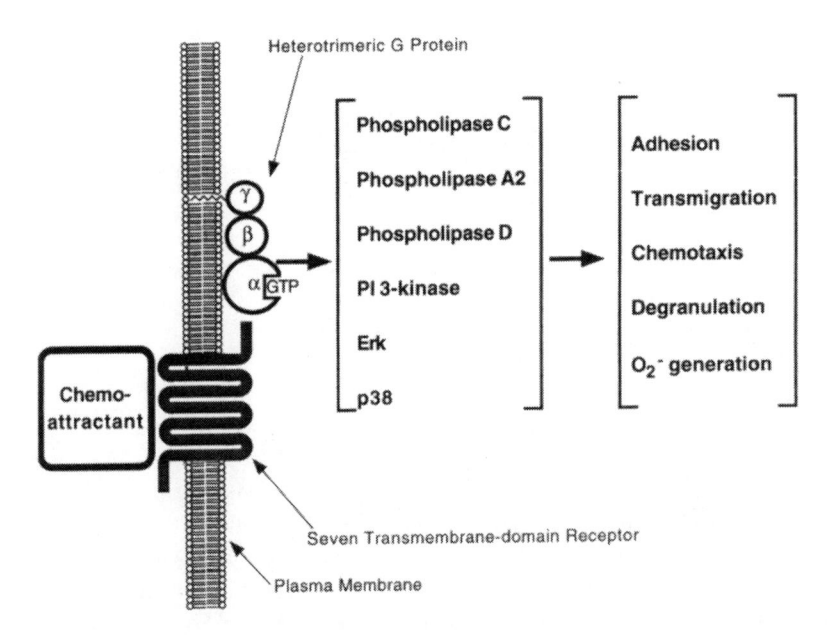

Fig. 3. Signal transduction pathways in human neutrophils. Engagement of a seven-transmembrane domain receptor by a chemoattractant molecule results in GTP-binding and activation of a heterotrimeric GTP-binding protein, followed by the activation of multiple signal transduction pathways and the stimulation of a variety of neutrophil functions. See text for details.

Although superoxide anion is potentially toxic, other forms of oxygen metabolites may be even more toxic to foreign organisms, and the neutrophil possesses the capacity to generate these molecules through the metabolism of superoxide anion. In particular, neutrophil-specific granules contain an enzyme known as myeloperoxidase. In addition to being the molecule responsible for the green color of neutrophil aggregates (i.e., pus), myeloperoxidase has the capacity to catalyze the conversion of hydrogen peroxide (spontaneously generated from O_2^-) to oxidized halides such as HOCl. It is these products that are primarily responsible for the toxic effects of superoxide generation. Whereas the superoxide generating cytochrome b_{558} is localized largely to the specific granule membrane, myeloperoxidase is found exclusively in the matrix of azurophilic granules. Segregation of these proteins thus assures that HOCl will not be produced unless and until the NADPH oxidase is assembled, and specific and azurophilic granules fuse together in the mature phagolysosome *(7)*.

3.4. Signal Transduction

The basic neutrophil functions described (adhesion and transmigration, phagocytosis and degranulation, and the generation of toxic oxygen radicals) all depend on the ability of neutrophils to receive external signals, process them internally, and produce directed, appropriate responses (Fig. 3). Collectively, these processes are referred to as signal transduction *(8)*. In virtually all cases, signal transduction begins when a cytokine or other soluble ligand engages a specific receptor on the surface of the neutrophil. The best studied ligand/receptor pairs in neutrophils include those for chemoattractants such as formylmethionyl-leucyl-phenylalanine (FMLP), the complement split product C5a, interleukin-8, and leukotriene B_4 (LTB_4). These four ligands are from different molecular families, but all possess the ability to stimulate most if not all of the neutrophil activities described earlier. Interestingly, these ligands demonstrate different potencies for different neutrophil functions, suggesting that specificity may exist between agents.

Other receptors observed on neutrophils include those for immunoglobulins and complement C3 components, as well as those for eicosanoids such as arachidonic acid and 5-hydroxyeicosatetraenoic acid (5-HETE). A number of other ligand/receptor pairs have been identified that do not themselves activate neutrophils but potentiate neutrophil responses to the stimuli described earlier. These so-called priming agents include GM-CSF (when administered to mature PMNs) and TNF-α. Interestingly insulin has also been shown to have a priming effect on neutrophils, suggesting one possible explanation for altered neutrophil function in patients with diabetes mellitus.

Receptors on neutrophils, like those on other cells, fall into several distinct classes. Neutrophil chemoattractant receptors share a common basic structure composed of a single protein chain snaking back and forth across the plasma membrane a total of seven times and are therefore referred to as seven-transmembrane domain receptors, or more succinctly, as serpentine seven receptors. Because serpentine seven receptors effect their functions through heterotrimeric, GTP-binding proteins (also known as G proteins), they are alternatively referred to as G-protein-linked receptors or G-protein-coupled receptors. G proteins consist of three subunits designated α, β, and γ. Whereas the γ-subunit possesses a lipid tail that anchors the complex to the cytoplasmic face of the plasma membrane, the α-subunit contains a guanine nucleotide binding pocket that, in the resting state, is occupied by a molecule of GDP. Engagement of the appropriate serpentine seven receptor results in discharge of GDP from the binding pocket, which is then replaced with GTP from the cytosolic pool. This GTP-binding step causes the dissociation of the γ-subunit from the α/β complex, with each of the two components activated and free to stimulate downstream effects.

Until very recently, the consequences of neutrophil chemoattractant receptor activation were understood to consist of a limited number of responses relating to the generation of intracellular lipids. These "classical" responses included the activation of phospholipase C, which cleaves neutrophil membrane lipids to generate diacylglycerol and inositol tris-phosphate (IP_3). Diacylglycerol then directly activates protein kinase C, a phosphorylating enzyme whose significance is confirmed by the fact that synthetic agents that activate PKC possess the ability to activate a variety of neutrophil responses. IP_3, on the other hand, stimulates the influx of calcium ions, another critical signaling event. In addition to phospholipase C, phospholipase A_2 may also be activated, catalyzing the release of arachidonic acid from the plasma membrane, which may serve as a substrate for the generation of leukotriene B_4 (LTB_4), which can further propagate the inflammatory response. Recent studies have also demonstrated the importance of phospholipase D to neutrophil activation.

In addition to the classical neutrophil signals, recent studies have documented the importance of kinase cascades in neutrophil activation. Kinase cascades consist of a series of enzymes that successively phosphorylate and activate each other, resulting in one or more effector function. One such cascade whose importance to neutrophil function is coming to be appreciated is the Erk (for Extracellular signal-Regulated Kinase) pathway. In the classical model of Erk signaling, engagement of a growth factor receptor on mitotic cells activates a cascade that phosphorylates and activates Erk, which then translocates to the nucleus to regulate cell division and differentiation. Although neutrophils are postmitotic and terminally differentiated, engagement of chemoattractant receptors results in the very rapid activation of Erk, in a manner that appears to be critical for some aspects of neutrophil activation (9). Other kinases in the same family as Erk also appear to undergo stimulation in neutrophils, including p38, a kinase implicated in cellular responses to stress. In addition, the enzyme phosphoinositol 3-kinase (PI 3-K), which phosphorylates small lipid molecules, has been shown to be activated in stimulated neutrophils, and studies with specific inhibitors of PI 3-K have implicated this kinase as critical to the stimulation of neutrophil adhesion, degranulation and superoxide anion generation.

The mechanisms through which neutrophil intracellular signals result in phenotypic responses remain incompletely elucidated. As noted earlier, neutrophil adhesion is dependent on the presence of a variety of transmembrane adhesion molecules on the neutrophil surface. Whereas selectins on the neutrophil surface are constitutively "sticky," the neutrophil integrin CD11b/CD18 (CR3) appears to remain in a nonadherent state under resting conditions. Stimulation of neutrophils with agents such as FMLP result in the activation of CD11b/CD18 (inside-out signaling). Although the precise mechanisms for this activation are unknown, some data support a requirement for a phosphorylation event in the CD11b/CD18 activating process. Similarly, a number of authors have observed that one or more components of the NADPH oxidase undergo phosphorylation in the context of oxidase assembly, again implicating kinases in the output stages of neutrophil activation. However, it is likely that other signaling mechanisms—protein complex formations, protein/lipid interactions, and protein posttranslational modifications—also play a role in linking intracellular signals to specific neutrophil end outputs.

4. Neutrophils and Rheumatic Diseases

Neutrophils play a central role in a number of rheumatic diseases. Neutrophils flood the joint space in crystal arthritides as well as autoimmune arthropathies such as rheumatoid arthritis and seronegative arthritides (Reiter's syndrome, reactive arthritis, psoriatic arthritis, and ankylosing spondylitis). Neutrophils are typically less prevalent—although not necessarily less important—in the joints of patients with lupus and postinfectious, immune-complex-mediated arthritides such as rheumatic fever. In addition, neutrophils play a critical role in a number of vasculitides. In addition to the presence of neutrophils in vessel walls, some vasculitides are characterized by the presence of antibodies directed at neutrophil cytoplasm (antineutrophil cytoplasmic antibodies, or ANCA).

4.1. Gout

Gout is a disease of monosodium urate metabolism and neutrophil-mediated inflammation. Urate crystals, formed as a consequence of chronic hyperuricemia, are the inflammatory provocateurs. Urate crystals fix a variety of plasma proteins, among them complement and IgG, which results in the production of chemoattractants and the entry of neutrophils into the synovial space. Synovial macrophages exposed to urate crystals also produce neutrophil chemoattractants, as well as cytokines that upregulate the adhesiveness of vascular endothelium for neutrophils. In addition, monosodium urate crystals stimulate the neutrophil formation of 5-lipoxygenase products such as LTB_4, attracting additional neutrophils into the joint. Moreover, activation of neutrophils by urate crystals, as well as lysis of neutrophils that have phagocytosed crystals, results in the release of neutrophil proteases and generation of O_2^-, with potential for tissue damage. The inflammatory response in gout is sufficiently boisterous as to cause not only local pain and swelling but also systemic manifestations such as fever (attributable to IL-1 production), elevated sedimentation rate, and elevated peripheral white blood cell counts. Synovial fluid neutrophil counts may reach as high as 100,000 cells/mm^3, a level rarely seen in other rheumatic diseases but frequently present in septic joints. Accordingly, care must be taken in distinguishing the gouty from infected joint.

4.2. Rheumatoid Arthritis

Rheumatoid arthritis is typified, in part, by the presence of synovial pannus, an exuberant overgrowth of the normal synovial lining. In addition to hypertrophic, fibroblastlike synoviocytes, and synovial macrophages, infiltrative T-cells and rheumatoid factor-producing B cells are also found in profusion in the pannus tissue. Few neutrophils are found in pannus, but these have been localized to the pannus–cartilage junction, suggesting they may play a role in the marginal erosion of joints. In contrast, the synovial space is typically distended with fluid containing large accumulations of neutrophils *(10)*. Although the numbers of neutrophils in the rheumatoid joint are lower than those in gout, they may still occasionally approach 100,000 cells/mm^3. The inflammatory signals that draw neutrophils into a rheumatoid joint have been studied intensely. Rheumatoid macrophages produce high concentrations of various interleukins (IL-1, IL-6, IL-8) as well as TNF-α and TGF-β. Moreover, the formation of immune complexes containing rheumatoid factor results in complement activation and liberation of the potent chemoattractant C5a. The combined effect of cytokines such as Il-1 and TNF-α (which upregulate adhesion molecules on vascular endothelium) and chemoattractants such as C5a, Il-8, and TGF-β results in increased adhesion of bloodstream neutrophils to vessel walls, and their transmigration out of the circulation and into the joint. Neutrophil production of cytokines (particularly Il-1 and Il-6), although modest on a per-cell basis, may itself be important for the propagation of inflammation given the large numbers of neutrophils present in the joint.

Although the ability of joint fluid neutrophils to directly damage cartilage has never been verified in vivo, numerous in vitro studies support the hypothesis that the neutrophil's destructive capacity, acting upon cartilage, is largely responsible for the symmetrical joint space narrowing that is characteristic of RA. Neutrophil-mediated cartilage destruction may occur when activated neutrophils discharge their destructive enzymes and reactive oxygen radicals directly into the synovial fluid, during either immune-complex consumption (frustrated phagocytosis) or cell death. Such a process is likely to account for the degradation of hyaluronic acid within the joint with accompanying lack of joint fluid viscosity. However, synovial fluid is biologically active and contains both antiproteinases and the capacity to buffer the highly reactive oxygen radicals generated by the NADPH system, and a number of authors have expressed skepticism over the ability of neutrophil toxic mediators released into the joint fluid to damage cartilage. In response to these objections, topologic models of neutrophil-mediated joint destruction have been proposed. One such model emphasizes the importance of rheumatoid-factor-containing immune complexes embedded in the superficial layers of the cartilage. Neutrophils attracted to these complexes via C5a may engage them through interaction with immunoglobulin receptors. As a result, neutrophils attempting to phagocytose a surface much larger than themselves create a closed space into which they degranulate (frustrated phagocytosis). Neutrophil enzymes and oxygen radicals may then act in a harmful manner without the counterregulatory interference of the synovial fluid proteins.

4.3. Vasculitis

The vasculitides are a heterogeneous group of diseases, many of which are defined or characterized by the presence of neutrophils in the vascular inflammatory infiltrate. In some vasculitides (e.g., polyarteritis nodosa, isolated cutaneous vasculitis, Henoch–Schonlein purpura, and essential cryoglobulinemia), immune-complex deposition in blood vessel walls may be responsible for the initiation of the inflammatory cascades that result in tissue destruction. The occasional association of hepatitis virus infection with several of these conditions suggests that exposure to viral or other antigens may lead to immune-complex formation. Subsequently, activation of the complement cascade as well as the elaboration of inflammatory cytokines may result in neutrophil accumulation and tissue destruction.

The presence of antibodies directed at neutrophil cytosol (antineutrophil cytosolic antibodies, or ANCA) is a hallmark of several vasculitic diseases, including Wegener's granulomatosis, Churg–Strauss syndrome, and microscopic polyarteritis. Antineutrophil antibodies were first identified by van der Woude et al. *(11)* and were originally associated with a clinical syndrome of pulmonary infiltrates and glomerulonephritis. Ultimately, the antibodies were further classified into cytoplasmic (cANCA) and perinuclear (pANCA) types depending on their binding patterns to ethanol-fixed neutrophils. It has subsequently been appreciated that both classes of antibody bind to proteins contained within azurophilic granules and that their redistribution in indirect immunofluorescence assays is an artifact of fixation. Whereas cANCA is directed against proteinase 3, pANCA reacts primarily with myeloperoxidase, but also with a variety of other neutrophil antigens including elastase and lysozyme. The presence of cANCA, in particular, is highly associated with Wegener's granulomatosis: In the clinical setting of pulmonary and renal disease, cANCA may be greater than 90% sensitive and specific for the diagnosis of Wegener's.

Whether ANCAs play a pathophysiologic role in the genesis of these vasculitides, or are merely epiphenomena, remains uncertain. However, models have been developed to explain a possible pathophysiologic role. In one such scenario, proteinase 3 and/or myeloperoxidase are released to the cell surface during neutrophil stimulation and adhere there. They then may interact with the variable region of the circulating ANCAs, bringing the ANCA constant domain (Fc portion) into proximity with Fcγ receptors on the neutrophil surface. Engagement of Fcγ receptors results in full-blown activation and degranulation of the neutrophil, releasing neutrophil destructive mediators and chemoattractants. In contrast to RA, where neutrophils may bind directly to cartilage, in the vasculitides, neutrophils are primarily in close approximation to the vascular endothelial surface (upregulated integrin activation and ICAM expression in the context of the proinflammatory milieu), in a position to directly damage the vasculature.

5. Effects of Antirheumatic Drugs on Neutrophil Function

Virtually all of the antirheumatic agents currently in use have pleiotropic effects, including direct or indirect effects on neutrophil function.

5.1. Nonsteroidal Anti-Inflammatory Drugs

Salicylates are among the oldest antirheumatic drugs, having been employed as pharmaceuticals at least since the eighteenth century. The past few decades have seen an explosion in the use of non-salicylate-based, nonsteroidal anti-inflammatory drugs (NSAIDs). Nonetheless, it was not until the 1970s that Vane proposed that aspirin and other NSAIDs act via inhibition of the cyclooxygenase (COX) pathway and resultant blockade of prostaglandin synthesis. Interestingly, the original NSAID—sodium salicylate—is a potent anti-inflammatory but a poor COX inhibitor, suggesting that not all effects of NSAIDs may be the result of COX inhibition. NSAIDs have pleiotropic effects on neutrophils, including (1) inhibition of homotypic neutrophil aggregation and heterotypic neutrophil/endothelial cell adhesion, (2) inhibition of neutrophil O_2^- generation, (3) inhibition of neutrophil G-protein activation, and (4) alterations in neutrophil plasma membrane viscosity. Recently, our laboratory has documented the capacity of salicylates to inhibit activation of the kinase Erk in stimulated neutrophils. The ability of NSAIDs to globally inhibit COX comes at a cost, as COX activity and prostaglandin production is required not only for inflammation but also for the maintenance of gastric mucosal integrity, platelet function, and regulation of renal perfusion; thus, NSAIDs may cause gastritis, ulcers, and platelet and renal dysfunction. The recent discovery of two distinct classes of COXs (COXII, responsible for most phases of inflammation, and COXI, responsible for the homeostatic production of prostaglandins) has led to the development of selective COXII inhibitors, which appear to have efficacy similar to traditional NSAIDs with markedly reduced toxicity *(12)*.

5.2. Glucocorticoids

Glucocorticoids are broadly acting and have primary effects on neutrophils as well as on endothelial cells. Glucocorticoids decrease neutrophil phagocytic activity, phospholipase A_2 activity, and prostaglandin and leukotriene generation. Through their effects on gene transcription they markedly diminish endothelial cell adhesion molecule expression, resulting in decreased transmigration of neutrophils into sites of inflammation. Virtually all pro-inflammatory cytokines are downregulated by corticosteroids, including IL-1 production by neutrophils and other cells; the mechanism for inhibition of cytokine production appears to be related to the ability of glucocorticoids to downregulate the activity of nuclear factor kappa B (NFκB), a transcriptional regulatory molecule of importance to inflammatory responses. In addition, glucocorticoids promote the production of lipocortin, a potent endogenous antiinflammatory compound.

5.3. Methotrexate

For nearly a decade methotrexate has been the drug of choice for treating aggressive rheumatoid arthritis and other rheumatic diseases. Although its mechanism of action has been presumed to be via folate antagonism and an antiproliferative effect, the ability of low doses of methotrexate to block inflammation without lowering white blood cell counts, as well as the ability of folate supplementation to limit the side effects but not the efficacy of methotrexate, suggest that other mechanisms may be pertinent. Cronstein has proposed that a major mechanism of methotrexate action is through the promotion of release of adenosine, a potent anti-inflammatory molecule. Adenosine effects on neutrophils include inhibition of O_2^- generation and adhesion. In contrast, methotrexate itself has no direct effects on neutrophils, but treatment of patients with this agent results in downregulation of neutrophil function. In addition, methotrexate-induced adenosine release had been shown to inhibit the accumulation of neutrophils at sites of tissue injury. Interestingly, sulfasalazine may also act, at least in part, via an ability to promote the release of adenosine *(13)*.

5.4. Colchicine

Colchicine is one of the oldest anti-inflammatory drugs still in use today. Colchicine is commonly used to prevent acute gout attacks and, less commonly, to treat acute attacks of gout as well as dermal vasculitis. The mechanism of colchicine action relates primarily to its ability to interfere with microtubules. Very high concentrations of colchicine (approaching or equivalent to those used to treat acute gouty attacks) prevent neutrophil degranulation and release of chemoattractants. More recently, it has been appreciated that very low concentrations of colchicine interfere with E-selectin-mediated recruitment of neutrophils, an action that may explain the utility of lower-dose colchicine in preventing acute gouty attacks *(14)*.

6. Congenital Disorders of Neutrophil Function

Disorders of neutrophils, both inherited and acquired, result in disordered inflammation and impaired host defense *(15,16)*.

6.1. Neutropenias

A spectrum of inborn diseases are characterized by decreased neutrophil production, and patients with neutrophil counts below 500 cells/μL (absolute neutropenia) are at risk for life-threatening bacterial and fungal infections. *Severe congenital neutropenia* is a marrow-related defect in which the peripheral neutrophil count is chronically low, below 200 cells/μL. In contrast, *cyclic neutropenia* is a hereditary condition characterized by 21-d oscillations in the level of neutrophils. Congenital neutropenias typically present in childhood with recurrent episodes of fever, mucosal ulcerations, and occasional life-threatening infections. The diagnosis is made on the basis of repeated complete blood counts, bone marrow biopsy, and the absence of inciting factors. Despite aggressive therapy with antibiotic, prognosis has been poor. Recently, however, treatment with G-CSF has had a major impact on prognosis in these illnesses.

6.2. NADPH Oxidase Defects: Chronic Granulomatous Disease of Childhood

In the early 1960s, a group of children with recurrent life-threatening infections in association with exuberant granuloma formation were recognized and their syndrome given the name chronic granulomatous disease (CGD). Most patients present before the age of 2 yr. Common presentations include recurrent enlargement of the lymph nodes of the neck and recurrent infection (especially abscesses of skin, lung, and mucous membranes) with catalase-producing organisms such as *Staph. aureus*, *Burkholderia cepacia*, and *Serratia marsescens*, as well as fungi. CGD is a rare disease with an incidence rate of approximately 1 in 250,000.

Chronic granulomatous disease has both X-linked and autosomal recessive patterns of inheritance. Intensive study has revealed that CGD results from the failure of neutrophils and other phagocytes to produce O_2^-. Further study revealed that CGD is actually a heterogeneous group of diseases, each characterized by the deficiency of a single component of the NADPH oxidase. A defect in the $gp91^{phox}$ gene (localized to the X chromosome) is responsible for over 60% of the cases of CGD. The next most common mutation is in the $p47^{phox}$ gene located on chromosome 7 and is responsible for the majority of autosomal recessive cases. $p67^{phox}$ and $p22^{phox}$ gene mutations are each responsible for 5% of cases, but no case has been observed associated with $p21^{rac}$ deficiency. Therapy for CGD includes prophylaxis with trimethoprim/sulfamethoxizole, intensive supportive care with intravenous antibiotics, and granulocyte transfusions when a patient is infected. Recently, interferon-γ therapy has been utilized, with a major impact on morbidity and mortality.

6.3. Granule Abnormalities: Chediak–Higashi Syndrome

A number of rare congenital abnormalities of neutrophil granule formation have been identified, the best studied of which is Chediak–Higashi syndrome. Chediak–Higashi syndrome is an autosomal recessive disorder characterized by abnormal intracellular membrane dynamics in a variety of cell types. Neutrophils are affected, with the result that abnormally large intracellular granules are formed that are easily seen by light microscopy. These represent the fusion of azurophilic granules with each other, or with specific granules. Neutrophil myelopoiesis and function are affected, resulting in a mild neutropenia as well as impaired chemotaxis, degranulation and antibody-mediated bacterial killing.

Clinical manifestations of Chediak–Higashi syndrome include partial occulo-cutaneous albinism, photophobia, nystagmus, peripheral neuropathy, and a prolonged bleeding time. As in other neutrophil abnormalities, recurrent bacterial infections of the skin, lungs, and mucous membranes may be common and severe, and many patients die in childhood as a consequence of infection. Those who survive often go on to an accelerated lymphohistiocytic, lymphoma-like phase of the disease, which often culminates on death. The gene responsible for Chediak–Higashi syndrome has been isolated to chromosome 1 and is named *Lyst*, but its function is unknown. For the moment, therapy is largely supportive, although HLA-matched sibling donor one-marrow transplants have restored normal hematopoiesis and immune function in select cases.

6.4. Adhesion Deficiencies

Leukocyte adhesion deficiency type I and II (LAD I and LAD II) are rare autosomal recessive entities that result in impaired healing of the umbilicus in neonates and recurrent abscesses. As the major defect in both LADs is the inability of leukocytes to adhere to the endothelium and emigrate from the vasculature, these conditions are characterized in part by marked neutrophilia with peripheral white blood cell counts from 15,000–60,000/mm³.

Patients with LAD I demonstrate a deficiency in production of common integrin β chain, CD 18. Neutrophils are unable to adhere tightly to, and diapedese through, the vascular endothelium. Severe LAD I manifests early in life with delayed umbilical stump separation with associated infection (omphalitis). Subsequent infections include destructive periodontitis, recurrent otitis media, pharyngitis, cutaneous abscesses, and cellulitis. In the absence of acute inflammation infections often spread before coming to attention, and patients often die before the age of 5 yr. Patients with a moderate form of the disease express reduced quantities of β2-integrins and are more likely to survive into adolescence. Therapy consists of aggressive antibiosis and, occasionally, bone marrow transplantation.

Leukocyte adhesion deficiency type II is characterized by a defect in the generation of the protein-linked sugars (such as sialyl–Lewis) that are the counterligands for selectins. Patients with LAD II have a defect in neutrophil loose adherence to, and rolling along, vascular endothelium. Like LAD I, LAD II is characterized by recurrent pulmonary, periodontal, and cutaneous infections. In addition, patients with LAD II manifest short stature, learning disabilities, distinctive facies, and the Bombay blood phenotype. The underlying molecular defect is unknown but may relate to errors in fructose metabolism.

6.5. Acquired Deficiencies of Neutrophil Function

In addition to inborn errors, neutrophils acquire functional disorders under a variety of clinical circumstances. Aging and diabetes are both known to be associated with an increased risk of infection. In each case, studies on neutrophils have revealed defects in adhesive behavior and/or oxidative metabolism. In studies by Cronstein and Perskin, neutrophils from elderly patients were found to have a decrease in membrane viscosity, which correlated with decreased adherence to collagen, a component of the extracellular matrix, as well as a decrease in oxygen radical generation when appropriately challenged. Others have found that PMN of the elderly are more inclined to undergo apoptosis even when presented with counterapoptotic signals such as GM-CSF. The neutrophils of diabetics are also known to have impaired adhesive behavior in response to stimuli as well as impaired phagocytosis and a decreased oxidative burst. These acquired defects may contribute to the increased susceptibility to infection found in diabetics and the elderly.

References

1. Bainton, D. F. (1992) Developmental biology of neutrophils and eosinophils, in *Inflammation: Basic Principles and Clinical Correlates*, 2nd ed. (Gallin, J., Goldstein, I. M., and Snyderman, R., eds.) Raven, New York, pp. 303–324.
2. Borregaard, N., Lollike, K., Kjeldsen, L., Sengelov, H., Bastholm, L., Nielsen, M. H., et al. (1993) Human neutrophil granules and secretory vesicles. *Eur. J. Hematol.* **51,** 187–198.
3. Hallett, M. B. (1997) Controlling the molecular motor of neutrophil chemotaxis. *BioEssays* **19,** 615–621.
4. Caron, E. and Hall, A. (1998) Identification of two distinct mechanisms of phagocytosis controlled by different Rho GTPases. *Science* **282,** 1717–1721.
5. Weiss, J. (1994) Leukocyte-derived antimicrobial proteins. *Curr. Opin. Hematol.* **1,** 78–84.
6. DeLeo, F. R. and Quinn, M. T. (1996) Assembly of the phagocyte NADPH oxidase: molecular interaction of oxidase proteins. *J. Leukoc. Biol.* **60,** 677–691.

7. Weiss, S. J. (1989) Tissue destruction by neutrophils. *N. Eng. J. Med.* **320**, 365–376.
8. Bokoch, G. M. (1995) Chemoattractant signaling and leukocyte activation. *Blood* **86**, 1649–1660.
9. Pillinger, M. H., Feoktistov, A. S., Capodici, C., Solitar, B., Levy, J., Oei, T. T., et al. (1996) Mitogen-activated protein kinase in neutrophils and enucleate neutrophil cytoplasts: evidence for regulation of cell-cell adhesion. *J. Biol. Chem.* **271**, 12,049–12,056.
10. Kishimoto, T., Taga, T., and Akira, S. (1994) Cytokine signal transduction. [Review]. *Cell* **76**, 253–262.
11. van der Woude, F. J., Rasmussen, N., Lobatto, S., Wiik, A., Permin, H., van Es, L. A., et al. (1985) Autoantibodies against neutrophils and monocytes: tool for diagnosis and marker of disease activity in Wegener's granulomatosis. *Lancet* **1**, 425–429.
12. Amin, A. R., Attur, M. G., Pillinger, M., and Abramson, S. B. (1999) The pleiotropic functions of aspirin: mechanisms of action. *Cell Mol. Life Sci.* **56**, 305–312.
13. Cronstein, B. N. (1997) The mechanism of action of methotrexate. *Rheum. Dis. Clin. North. Am.* **23**, 739–755.
14. Molad, Y., Cronstein, B. N., and Malawista, S. E. (1999) Colchicine, in *Gout, Hyperuricemia and Other Crystal-Associated Arthropathies* (Smyth, C. J. and Holers, V. M., eds.,) Marcel Dekker, New York.
15. Holland, S. M. and Gallin, J. I. (1998) Evaluation of the patient with recurrent bacterial infections. *Annu. Rev. Med.* **49**, 185–199.
16. Mills, E. L. and Noya, F. J. D. (1993) Congenital neutrophil deficiencies, in *The Neutrophil* (Abramson, J. S. and Wheeler, J. G., eds.), IRL/Oxford University Press, Oxford, pp. 183–227.

16
Synoviocytes

David E. Yocum

1. Normal Characteristics

Normal synovium is made up of two distinct layers, the synovial lining intima, which is in direct contact with the joint space, and the subsynovium or sublining *(1,2)*. The sublining is relatively acellular, containing blood vessels, fat cells, and fibroblasts.

There are two types of synoviocytes that predominate in the normal synovial lining or intima, the type A and type B synoviocyte. The type A synoviocytes resemble tissue macrophages, whereas the type B resemble fibroblasts. About one-third of the cells in the lining are type A and two-thirds are type B. It appears that the type A cells are of bone marrow origin and the type B cells of mesencymal origin, locally derived *(2,3)*. The major function of the synoviocytes in the normal joint is to provide the joint cavity with lubricant molecules such as glycosaminoglycans, as well as oxygen and nutritive plasma proteins. However, it is clear that these two morphologically distinct cell types have different biologic and molecular functions, both in health and disease.

The type A synoviocytes, which express macrophage markers, not only remove debris from the joint cavity but also have antigen-processing functions *(1,2)*. These cells show high activity for nonspecific esterase and express major histocompatibility complex (MHC) class II antigens, Fc receptors, as well as estrogen and androgen receptors. Resembling tissue macrophages, these cells also possess a prominent Golgi apparatus and abundant digestive vacuoles. A distinct subgroup of the type A synoviocyte is the CD14/CD33 positive group, also called dendritic cells. Characteristics of these cells include antigen presentation to T-cells as well as the ability to produce prostaglandin.

The type B cells have a bipolar fibroblastlike morphology, prominent rough endoplasmic reticulum and regular ribosomal assays *(1,2)*. One of the major functions of the type B synoviocyte in the normal joint is the production of hylauronan for joint lubrication as well as the synthesis of matrix components, including collagen. They show intense activity for the enzyme uridine diphospho-glucose dehydrogenase as well as a variety of other enzymes, capable of degrading cartilage and bone. Although the type B synoviocytes lack MHC II markers, they do express a number of other cell-surface-related molecules, including vascular cell adhesion molecule-1 (VCAM-1) and complement decay-accelerating factor *(4)*. The type B cells are capable of interacting with the type A cell by signal reception and mediation via cytokines and growth factors.

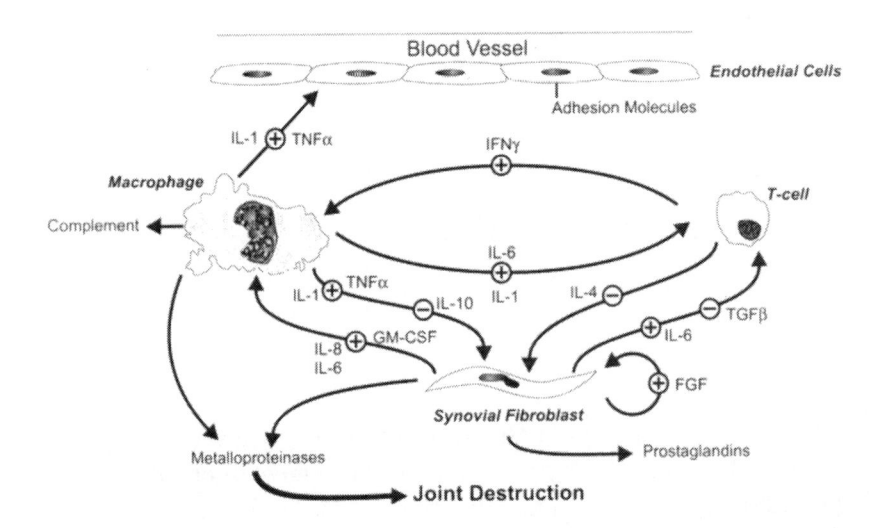

Fig. 1. Pathogenesis of tissue degradation in rheumatoid arthritis.

The characteristics of the two types of intimal synoviocytes implicate them not only in the healthy function of the joint but also the abnormal activities that occur during inflammatory diseases such as rheumatoid arthritis (RA). The mechanisms by which this appears to occur will be discussed in depth.

2. Pathophysiology of Rheumatoid Arthritis

To address the abnormal events that occur in an inflammatory arthritic situation, one must consider the sequence of events in the inflammatory cascade. This includes antigen presentation, adhesion molecule expression, oncogene expression, cytokine and growth factor generation, synovial proliferation, and tissue degradation. Each of these will be dealt with in the context of the cells and molecular mechanisms involved, using RA as a model (Fig. 1). In RA, oncogene expression is also an important part of the synovial proliferation and tissue degradation that occurs, especially in the established phase.

2.1. Antigen Presentation

The primary antigen-presenting cells in the synovium are the synovial macrophage (type A synoviocyte) and the dendritic cell. Although no specific antigens, either exogenous or of synovial origin, have been identified, it is likely that such exists and represents the initiating factor in diseases such as RA. Suspected arthrotropic agents include infectious agents such as a retrovirus, spirochetes, chlamydia, or mycobacterium *(1)*. It is also possible that it results from chronic inflammation induced by a product of one of these agents.

The association of rheumatoid factor with more aggressive disease suggests that immune complexes play an important role *(5)*. In addition, human leukocyte antigen (HLA)-DR expression is very high on the synovial macrophages and dendritic cells suggesting that active antigen presentation is ongoing. In fact, early RA synovium demonstrates areas similar to those seen in lymphoid follicles of lymph nodes *(3)*. However, the major lymphocyte population involving the area is of the T helper subset or CD4$^+$ cell with a paucity of the T suppression or CD8$^+$ cell *(6)*. This latter finding supports ongoing antigen stimulation.

Dendritic cells are potent antigen-presenting cells that express large amounts of MHC class II antigens (HLA-DQ), but lack macrophage antigens such as CD14 and Fc receptors *(3)*. These cells are found in high numbers in the synovial fluid (15% vs 1% in peripheral blood) of patients with RA, suggesting ongoing antigen challenge. In chronic RA, over 70% of patients demonstrate few lymphocytes and have heavy infiltration of macrophages, which are also HLA-DR positive *(6)*.

2.2. Adhesion Molecules

Adhesion molecules mediate cellular interaction. Although discussed largely in the context of T-cells and endothelial cells, there is recent data on adhesion molecule expression on synoviocytes. Large amounts of VCAM-1 are found in the lining layer, primarily on synovial fibroblasts in rheumatoid and, to a lesser degree, osteoarthritic synovium. VCAM-1 is important in the binding of T-lymphocytes via the very late activation antigen-4 (VLA-4) and it probably aids in the binding of the synovial fibroblasts to cartilage and bone *(3,4)*. Whereas normal synovial fibroblasts express low levels of ICAM-1, cytokines such as interferon-γ (IFN-γ), tumor necrosis factor-α (TNF-α), and interleukin-1 (IL-1) greatly enhance its expression. In addition, VCAM-1 expressing cells are strongly associated with B-lymphocytes. In fact, synovial fibroblasts are superior to all other fibroblasts in the promotion of B-cell survival and terminal differentiation into plasma cells *(7)*. This suggests that the VCAM-1 expressing fibroblasts may play an important role in sustaining the ectopic lymphoid tissue seen in RA.

Synovial macrophages express high levels of intercellular adhesion molecule-1 (ICAM-1), which binds to the lymphocyte function-associated antigen-1 (LFA-1), which is expressed on normal as well as RA synoviocytes *(2,4)*. In RA, they also express elevated levels of LFA-3, but not VCAM-1. TNF-α and IL-1 enhance the expression of LFA-1, VCAM-1, and ICAM-1, whereas IFN-γ further enhances ICAM-1. Another adhesion molecule, ICAM-3, whose counterreceptor is also LFA-1, is also present on synovial macrophages. However, its function is presently not known.

Finally, CD31, a member of the immunoglobulin supergene family, is also present on both synovial macrophages and fibroblasts and appears to serve an adhesive role in RA synovium *(8)*. Overall, the adhesion molecules not only play important roles in cellular interactions, but probably play critical roles in the adhesion of pannus to cartilage and bone, as well as the production and release of metalloproteinases, which destroy the latter tissues. Both synovial macrophages and fibroblasts produce these matrix-degrading enzymes. Recent therapeutic development in RA is targeting adhesion molecules and the metalloproteinases to suppress inflammation and tissue destruction.

2.3. Cytokine and Growth Factor Production

Whereas T-cells are felt to play an important role in the pathogenesis of RA, T-cell cytokines are noticeably absent from established RA tissue and synovial fluids *(3)*. Both synovial fibroblasts and macrophages are capable of producing and responding to a variety of growth factors and cytokines. The major cytokines measured in established RA synovium are IL-1, IL-6, and TNF-α, which are produced primarily by cells of the macrophage lineage *(3)*.

Both IL-1 and TNF-α are arthritogenic in animals and have been implicated in the pathogenesis of RA. Injections of either result in transient synovitis and IL-1 injected systemically can act as an adjuvant in antigen-induced arthritis in animals *(3)*.

Large amounts of IL-1 and TNF-α can be measured in RA synovial fluid and synvovial tissue explants *(3,9)*. Localization techniques using immunoperoxidase staining or in vitro hybridization demonstrates that about 40% of the cells of the lining stain positive for these cytokines as compared to only 10–15% of the sublining. Double-staining techniques demonstrate the cells expressing macrophage markers are the predominate producing cell for both cytokines.

Both TNF-α and IL-1 are potent stimulators of synovial fibroblast proliferation, adhesion molecule expression, and matrix-degrading enzyme production *(3)*. In fact, both usually are synergistic in their actions, and IL-1 can act as an autocrine growth factor for synoviocytes. It appears that IL-1 is responsible for the destructive component of RA, and TNF-α is more important for the proliferative and inflammatory phase. This information comes as a result of animal model work. So far, trials using antagonists for each IL-1 (i.e., IL1-ra) and TNF-a (soluble TNF-a receptor) support this concept *(10,11)*. Trials combining both antagonists will be interesting.

Unlike IL-1 and TNF-α, IL-6 is produced predominately by synovial fibroblasts *(3)*. Its role appears to be as a B cell stimulator, probably contributing to local antibody and rheumatoid factor production. With levels of IL-6 elevated in both the joint and serum of RA patients, it probably plays an important role in stimulating acute-phase reactants (i.e., c-reactive protein) from the liver.

Granulocyte-macrophage colony-stimulating factor (GM-CSF) is found in RA synovial fluid, and although produced primarily by macrophages, it can also be produced by synovial fibroblasts stimulated by IL-1 and TNF-α *(3)*. GM-CSF appears to be important in the induced expression of MHC class II antigens on macrophages as well as the enhanced release and secretion of IL-1 and TNF-α.

There are a variety of other cytokines and chemokines found elevated in the synovial fluid and serum of RA patients. Most of these are produced by macrophages and activated synovial fibroblasts. Although most are regulated by TNF-α, IL-1, IFN-γ, IL-4, and IL-8, their exact role in the pathophysiology of RA is not clear.

In addition to the variety of cytokines, researchers have found that there are a variety of growth factors in RA synovium *(1,3)*. Although the distinction between growth factors and cytokines has significant overlap, one should think of growth factors as predominately inducers of cell growth with little pro-inflammatory characteristics. The growth factor, PDGF, is produced by synovial macrophages and has been shown to be a major stimulator of synovial fibroblast proliferation. PDGF can also stimulate oncogene-triggered transformation, a feature of RA tissue.

Synovial fibroblasts produce and react to fibroblast growth factor (FGF), an autocrine growth factor *(3)*. In addition to stimulating fibroblast proliferation, FGF can also act as an angiogenesis factor, thus stimulating blood vessel growth in RA. Epidermal growth factor (EGF) is also found in RA synovium, but its role is less clear. Vascular EGF (VEGF) is also found increased in RA synovial tissue and also plays an important role in the angiogenesis seen in RA.

The role of transforming growth factor-β (TGF-β) is controversial *(3)*. Whereas it can induce synovial lining proliferation, it also induces the production of collagen by synovial fibroblasts and at certain concentrations is anti-inflammatory. As to this latter role, TGF-β can downregulate IL-1 production and is a potent inhibitor of T-cell proliferation and cytokine production.

2.4. Proliferation and Oncogene Expression

Fassbender originally described the transformed appearance of synovial cells seen in RA *(12)*. Other researchers have further characterized these transformed features of the RA synovial fibroblast, even demonstrating the ability for tumorlike growth in nude (T-cell-deficient) mice *(13)*. Some of these cells described as pannocytes demonstrate paracrine growth characteristics and the capability to adhere to cartilage and bone (*see* Subheading 2.2.) *(14)*. In another model, Rendt et al. found that synovium extracted from rheumatoid joints could survive for up a year when implanted into severe combined immunodeficient (SCID) mice *(15)*. Rheumatoid synoviocytes also demonstrate other characteristics of transformed cells, including defective apoptosis and excessive growth factor and matrix-degrading enzyme production *(1,3)*.

Research from several labs suggest that the abnormal growth and function of rheumatoid synoviocytes is being regulated by a group of genes, called oncogenes, that are involved in the regulation of the cell cycle *(1,3)*. For example, PDGF-B/c-sis is a growth factor overexpressed in rheumatoid synovium. Lafyatis et al. found that it stimulated anchorage-independent growth of synoviocytes, similar to that seen with rheumatoid synoviocytes *(16)*. Other genes, such as egr-1 (an early response gene) are significantly upregulated in RA synovial fibroblasts *(3)*. Egr-1 regulates the expression of other oncogenes such as sis and ras, which are also overexpressed in RA. As an early response gene, egr-1 may be responsible for initial events in early RA.

Normally, there is an important balance between proliferation and cell death (apoptosis) in any normal cell, including synovial fibroblasts. In the transformed-appearing synoviocytes seen in RA, less than 3% are undergoing apoptosis *(1,17)*. In RA synovium, synovial-lining cells attaching to and invading cartilage express the oncogene Bcl-2 that is a potent inhibitor of apoptosis. Meanwhile, the oncogene associated with apoptosis, ras is seen only in cells near terminal vessels. These data strongly suggest that the abnormal growth characteristics seen in RA synovial fibroblasts is not the result of rapid proliferation, but to the lack of apoptosis.

Placed in an assay to examine the invasiveness of malignant melanoma cells isolated from patients, RA synovial fibroblasts are able to rapidly digest a collagen type II matrix and migrate to an adjacent chamber *(18)*. This characteristic appears linked to integrin expression and overproduction of matrix-degrading enzymes. Expression of this function correlated with the clinical course of the patients from which the synovial tissue was original obtained.

2.5. Matrix-Degrading Enzymes

In patients with aggressive RA, cartilage and bone destruction are prominent, occurring early in the course of disease, causing disability often within 5 yr of the onset. Metalloproteinases represent a family of enzymes responsible for tissue destruction and remodeling. They appear to play an important role in RA.

Stromelysin, a metalloproteinase responsible for digesting interstitial collagen, cleaves proteoglycans, laminin, and fibronectin *(3)*. In addition, it can activate latent collagenase. Stromelysin frequently appears early in the genesis of inflammatory arthritis and can be found in the lining and sublining of RA synovium. Interestingly, stromelysin gene expression occurs predominately in only the lining. Although produced in only small amounts by resting synovial fibroblasts, gene expression is rapidly upregulated after exposure to cytokines such as IL-1 and TNF-α.

Similar to stromelysin, another metalloproteinase collagenase is produced in large amounts by RA synovial lining cells (3). Collagenase digests native triple helical collagenase, and in combination with stromelysin, it is capable of degrading nearly all important structural proteins within the joint. Recently, a study examining early (1–3 mo) RA synovitis found metalloproteinase gene expression already upregulated. Interestingly, methotrexate suppresses the gene expression for collagenase but not stromelysin. This may explain its apparent ability to partially suppress erosions in clinical RA trials. IL-4 appears capable of inhibiting both collagenase and stromelysin.

The upregulation of matrix-degrading enzymes in the rheumatoid joint appears linked to the activation of oncogenes that regulate cell cycle. For example, Trabandt et al. demonstrated that the expression of collagenase and the cathepsins B and L in human RA synoviocytes is associated with the proliferation-associated oncogenes ras and myc (19). Another oncogene, c-fos, is also activated in RA synovial fibroblasts (1). One of its major functions is the activation of matrix-degrading molecules such as collagenase and stromelysin. It is likely that growth factors such as PDGF mediate the transcription of c-fos gene products, which trigger the expression of the matrix-degrading enzymes through the AP-1 promoter (3). Therapeutically, RA treatments such as steroids and gold can interfere with AP-1, which may explain their effects at slowing joint destruction.

3. Conclusions

Synoviocytes play critical roles in both the normal and diseased joint. Whereas the synovial macrophage appears important in many of the initiating inflammatory events in RA, the synvovial fibroblast appears important in the perpetration of the disease. Both cells produces a variety of cytokines, growth factors, and matrix-degrading enzymes that result in joint destruction. Much of this aberrant behavior is under control of oncogene expression. Only through a variety of treatments, probably in combination, targeting different elements of the process can this behavior be controlled.

References

1. Müller-Ladner, V., Gay, R. E., and Gay, S. (1997) Structure and function of synoviocytes, in *Arthritis and Allied Conditions. A Textbook of Rheumatology* (Koopman, W., ed.), Williams and Wilkins, pp. 243–254.
2. Edwards, J. C. W. (1998) The synovium, in *Rheumatology* (Klippel, J. H. and Dieppe, P. A., eds.), Mosby, London, pp. 6.1–6.8.
3. Firestein, G. S. (1998) Rheumatoid synovitis and pannus, in *Rheumatology* (Klippel, J. H. and Dieppe, P. A., eds.), Mosby, London, pp. 13.1–13.24.
4. Mojcik, C. F. and Shevach, E. M. (1997) Adhesion molecules: a rheumatologic perspective. [Review]. *Arthritis Rheum.* **40,** 991–1004.
5. Van Zeben, D., Hazes, J. M., Zwinderman, A. H., et al. (1993) Factors predicting outcome of rheumatoid arthritis results of a follow-up study. *J. Rheumatol.* **20,** 1288–1296.
6. Mulene, D. G., Wahl, S. M., Tsokos, M., et al. (1984) Immune function in severe, active rheumatoid arthritis: a relationship between peripheral blood mononuclear cell proliferation

to soluble antigens and synovial tissue immunohistologic characteristics. *J. Clin. Invest.* **74,** 1173–1185.

7. Dechanet, J., Merville, P., Durand, I., et al. (1995) The ability of synoviocytes to support terminal differentiation of activated B cells may explain plasma cell accumulation in rheumatoid synovium. *J. Clin. Invest.* **95,** 456–463.
8. Johnson, B. A., Haines, G. K., Harlow, L. A., and Koch, A. E. (1993) Adhesion molecule expression in human synovial tissue. *Arthritis Rheum.* **36,** 137–146.
9. Yocum, D. E., Esparza, L., Dubry, S., et al. (1989) Characteristics of tumor necrosis factor production in rheumatoid arthritis. *Cell. Immunol.* **122,** 131–145.
10. Elliott, M. J., Maini, R. N., Feldmann, M., et al. (1994) Randomized double-blind comparison of chimeric monoclonal antibody to tumor necrosis factor alpha (cAZ) versus placebo in rheumatoid arthritis. *Lancet* **344,** 1105–1110.
11. Brennan, F. M., Butler, D. M., Maini, R. N., and Feldmann, M. (1995) Modulation of proinflammatory cytokine release in rheumatoid synovial membrane cell cultures with an anti-TNF-alpha monoclonal antibody: comparison with blockade of IL-1 using the recombinant IL-1 receptor antagonist. *Arthritis Rheum.* **38,** S400.
12. Fassbender, H. G. (1983) Histomorphologic basis of articular cartilage destruction in rheumatoid arthritis. *Cell Related Res.* **3,** 141–155.
13. Geiler, T., Kriegsmann, J., Keyszer, G., et al. (1994) A new model for rheumatoid arthritis generated by engraftment of rheumatoid synovial tissue and normal human cartilage into SCID mice. *Arthritis Rheum.* **37,** 1664–1671.
14. Zvaifler, N. J. and Firestein, G. S. (1994) Pannus and pannocytes. Alternative models of joint destruction in rheumatoid arthritis. *Arthritis Rheum.* **37,** 783–789.
15. Rendt, K. E., Barry, T. S., Jones, D. M., et al. (1993) Engraftment of human synovium into severe combined immune deficient (SCID) mice: migration of human peripheral blood T-cells to engrafted human synovium and to mouse lymph nodes. *J. Immunol.* **151,** 7324–7336.
16. Lafyatis, R., Remmers, E. F., Roberts, A. B., et al. (1989) Anchorage independent growth regulation of synoviocytes from arthritis and normal joints stimulation by exogenous platelet-derived growth factor and inhibition by transforming growth factor-beta and retinoids. *J. Clin. Invest.* **83,** 1267–1276.
17. Müller-Ladner, V., Kriegsmann, J., Gay, R. E., et al. (1994) Upregulation of bcl-2 and fas mRNA in synovium of patients with rheumatoid arthritis (RA). *Arthritis Rheum.* **37,** S163.
18. Frye, C. A., Tuan, R., Yocum, D. E., and Hendrix, M. J. C. (1993) An *in vitro* model for studying mechanisms underlying cartilage destruction associated with rheumatoid arthritis. *Arthritis Rheum.* **36,** S174.
19. Trabandt, A., Aicher, W. K., Gay, R. E., et al. (1990) Expression of the collagenolytic and ras-induced cysteine protease cathepsin L and proliferation-associated oncogenes in synovial cells of MRL/l mice and patients with rheumatoid arthritis. *Matrix* **10,** 349–361.

17
Chondrocytes

Tariq M. Haqqi, Donald D. Anthony, and Charles J. Malemud

1. Articular Cartilage Development
1.1. Synovial Joint Morphogenesis

The basic role of articular cartilage is to serve as a cap on top of skeletal long bones of synovial joints. Articular cartilage is crucial to the normal function of synovial joints because it enables articulating surfaces to transmit high loads while maintaining contact stresses at low levels. In addition, articular cartilage functions to allow articulating surfaces to resist compressive force with low frictional resistance.

The development of synovial joints require spatial and temporal events involving chondrocyte proliferation modulated by extrinsic morphogenetic factors transduced via the extracellular matrix (ECM). The result of these events is the specialized divisions of articular cartilage. After form is established during embryogenesis, changes in form and ECM composition proceed more slowly. Nonetheless, constant remodeling of cartilage and subchondral bone occurs during the lifetime of the synovial joint (for a review, *see* ref. *1*).

Adult articular cartilage has been described as a composite tissue with variable topographical distributions of ECM. Tissue subdivisions have been defined as superficial, middle, deep, and calcified, based on the morphology of the chondrocytes, collagen fiber orientation, and the types and distribution of sulfated proteoglycans and accessory proteins found within the ECM (for a review, *see* ref. *2*). Biochemical studies have defined subdivisions of articular cartilage based on ECM composition. The cells of articular cartilage (chondrocytes) are responsible for the biosynthesis of ECM proteins and their transport into the space occupied by the ECM. ECM proteins possess the structural capacity to self-assemble. What has been clarified recently is that the cellular signals required to initiate and stabilize the chondrogenic phenotype are produced during cartilage development. Once the cartilage form and shape are stabilized, some cellular signals once required during joint morphogenesis are no longer needed or required to maintain cartilage homeostasis. A recent tenet of synovial joint degeneration (as is commonly found in osteoarthritis or rheumatoid arthritis) holds that cellular signals, which are normally repressed, become derepressed and result in significant alterations in the cartilage ECM.

1.2. Chondrocyte Transactivating Proteins: Regulation of Phenotype

The establishment and maintenance of the chondrogenic phenotype is still poorly understood at the molecular level. Articular cartilage ECM proteins have long been

From: *Current Molecular Medicine: Principles of Molecular Rheumatology*
Edited by: G. C. Tsokos © Humana Press Inc., Totowa, NJ

considered to be signature macromolecules that define the differentiated state of the tissue. Thus, ECM macromolecules, namely type II collagen, type IX collagen, and type XI collagen, together with the large proteoglycan, aggrecan, are genetic markers and define the chondrogenic phenotype of articular cartilage (for a review, *see* ref. *3*). There remains controversy as to whether "normal" articular cartilage synthesizes and deposits type X collagen into the ECM. Type X collagen has been localized to the calcified region of canine articular cartilage. Type X collagen has been found in both osteoarthritic articular cartilage and the osteochondrophytic spurs that accompany the remodeling of the synovial joint as part of the osteoarthritic process. Type X collagen is an important prerequisitory macromolecule in the growth plate cartilage transition to ossifying bone. In that respect, type X collagen gene expression has largely been confined to the hypertrophic chondrocytes of the growth plate *(4)*. Skeletal abnormalities and other malformations such as the Schmid epiphyseal dysplasia have been shown to result as a consequence of mutations in the type X collagen gene *(5)*.

Recent studies have begun to shed some light on the molecular events underlying the development of the chondrogenic phenotype of articular cartilage. For example, SOX9 is a member of a large family of proteins that possess a DNA-binding domain with greater than 50% similarity to that of the sex-determining region Y (SRY), the testicular-determining gene in mammals. The DNA-binding domain is synthesized by a variant of the HMG (high-mobility group) proteins, which were first identified as a component of chromatin. SOX9 was shown to be an activator of the chondrocyte-specific enhancer of the type II collagen promoter derived from chondrocytes (for a review, *see* ref. *6*). Thus, SOX9 and type II collagen are co-expressed in cells of the murine chondrocytic lineage Furthermore, SOX9 expression in ectopic sites upregulates the type II procollagen gene, and additional studies support the view that SOX9 directly induces the chondrogenic phenotype. Furthermore, a mutation in SOX9 results in campomelic dwarfism in which cartilaginous structures are affected *(7)*.

Type II collagen essentially fails to turnover in adult cartilage. Does that mean that chondrocytes of adult articular cartilage do not require expression of SOX9, but after injury when small cartilage lesions ensue, SOX9 upregulation is required for normal repair? Activation of type II collagen synthesis accompanies the osteoarthritic process *(8)* and the repair of superficial cartilage lesions will ultimately require chondrocyte synthesis and deposition of type II collagen into the repair site *(9)*. It will now be important to determine whether upregulation of SOX9 gene expression accompanies these events. Furthermore, it will be necessary to define precisely those molecular or physicochemical events that may be occurring upstream of SOX9 that could modulate SOX9 expression. For example, compressive force was shown to upregulate SOX9 expression in mouse embryonic limb bud mesenchymal cells *(10)*, which was accompanied by increased synthesis of type II collagen and aggrecan and inhibition of interleukin-1 (IL-1) (*see also* Chapter 11).

Molecules such as Indian hedgehog (Ihh), parathyroid-related peptide (PTHp), and its receptor, PTH/PTHrp, have been shown to regulate the differentiation of hypertrophic chondrocytes. Thus, PTH/PTHrp may need to be suppressed to prevent the derepression of the type X collagen gene in articular cartilage (for a review, *see* ref. *11*). It is interesting to note that immunohistochemical staining for PTHp was found in human femoral head cartilage from patients with osteoarthritis and rheumatoid arthritis, but not in control specimens *(12)*.

The protooncogene c-fos was shown to inhibit proteoglycan biosynthesis in transfected HCS 2/8 cells, a cell line with chondrocytic differentiation markers. Macroscopic effects on chick limb bud development were seen when ectopic expression of *fos* was induced by the microinjecting replication-competent retrovirus into the presumptive leg field of stage 10 embryos. This suggests that chondrocytes are a specific target for c-fos expression and c-fos could be responsible for inhibiting chondrocyte differentiation *(13,14)*.

2. Biosynthesis and Integration of Cartilage ECM

2.1. Intracellular Events

The biosynthesis of cartilage ECM proteins occurs typically in the endoplasmic reticulum. What defines the biosynthesis of these ECM proteins is the significant posttranslational events that modify the structure of ECM proteins and that enable them to perform their function.

2.1.1. Proteoglycans

Proteoglycans are large ECM proteins that possess a protein core to which polymers of the glycosaminoglycans (GAG) chondroitin sulfate, dermatan sulfate, keratan sulfate, and miscellaneous N- or O-linked oligosaccharides are covalently associated (for a review, *see* ref. *15*).

2.1.2. The Chondroitin Sulfate Proteoglycans

Intracellular biosynthesis resulting in the formation of chondroitin sulfate proteoglycans is initiated in the endoplasmic reticulum where the core protein is synthesized and where xylosyl transferase catalyzes the attachment of a xylose–ester linkage region glucuronic acid–galactose–galactose–xylose, a prerequisite for the covalent attachment of GAGs. GAG polymerization occurs in the Golgi complex. The size of the individual GAG polymers ($[1–2] \times 10^5$ Dalton) is, in all likelihood, regulated by the activity of galactosyl and glucosyl transferases and the topology of the Golgi cis–trans membrane. The final step in the completion of a GAG polymer is sulfation. Sulfation was shown to be a crucial step not only in the completion of GAGs but also to the function of proteoglycans. The principal source of sulfur in this pathway is free SO_4^{2-} which is transported into the cytoplasm by transmembrane symporter or antiporter molecules. In the cytoplasm, sulfur is activated using ATP and sulfate as substrates and the action of ATP sulfurylase, which catalyzes the synthesis of adenosine 5'-phosphosulfate (APS). A phosphokinase adds phosphorus to APS to create PAPS, which is the universal donor molecule for the addition of sulfate to chondroitin. Direct evidence linking the addition of sulfate to GAG polymers as important in ECM and cartilage function was revealed when specific genetic abnormalities were defined as stemming from mutations in either the sulfate transporter or the ATP sulfurylase–ATP kinase complex giving rise to the abnormal cartilage ECM seen in the brachymorphic mouse or human spondylometaphyseal dysplasia (for a review, *see* ref. *16*).

2.1.3. Aggregating Chondroitin-Sulfate-Containing Proteoglycans (Aggrecan and Versican)

The largest of the cartilage proteoglycans is aggrecan. Aggrecan is hydrodynamically large (average molecular mass, 3 MDa) consisting of both chondroitin-4 and/or

6-sulfate and keratan sulfate covalently attached to a core protein (molecular mass, 2.5×10^5 Dalton) in various structural domains (for a review, see ref. *15*). There are three globular domains devoid of GAG. Globular domain 1 (G1) is located at the N-terminus of the core protein and provides the structural foundation for the formation of noncovalent aggrecan–hyaluronan interactions. This interaction is stabilized by another glycoprotein, link protein, that shares structural homology with the G1 domain. Globular domain 2 (G2) is located near the N-terminus and is separated from the G1 domain by a linear interglobular domain or IGD. The G2 domain cannot interact with hyaluronan. Otherwise, its function is unknown. A large heavily GAG-substituted region extends from the G2 domain to the G3 globular region located at the C-terminus of the core protein. The G3 region contains sequence homologous to epidermal growth factor, complement regulatory proteins, and a lectinlike structure. Approximately one-half of the aggrecans in cartilage ECM lack the G3 domain, suggesting that it is proteolytically cleaved as a part of aggrecan turnover. When the G3 domain is present, it could serve to stabilize the network of ECM proteins.

Aggrecan–hyaluronan interactions provide a way for integrating aggrecan into the ECM and also inhibits aggrecan diffusion from the ECM. Newly synthesized aggrecan exhibits low affinity for binding hyaluronan. Gradually, aggrecan structural modifications occurring in the G1 domain improve aggrecan–hyaluronan interaction. This G1 "maturation" event presumably ensures that maximal aggrecan–hyaluronan interactions occur in the ECM. The many chondroitin sulfate chains covalently attached to the aggrecan core protein attract water, which provides a physiochemical explanation for the ability of articular cartilage to resist high compressive loads. The role played by keratan sulfate and the N- or O-linked oligosaccharides in this mechanism is not known. Keratan sulfate polymers are synthesized on asialo branches of O-linked oligosaccharides. No structural cartilage defect has been detected in rat cartilage, which contain a consensus sequence required for substitution with keratan sulfate, but contains no keratan sulfate (for a review, see ref. *15*).

Versican is a chondroitin sulfate proteoglycan with hyaluronan-binding capacity that does not contain keratan sulfate. Versican mRNA is expressed by chondrocytes *(17)* and abnormal amounts of versican have been found in osteoarthritic cartilage *(18)*.

2.1.4. Proteins/Proteoglycans with Leucine-Rich Repeats

Articular cartilage ECM contains small proteoglycans in addition to the large aggregating proteoglycans. In cartilage, this family of proteoglycans contain leucine-repeat sequences in the core protein and include decorin, biglycan, fibromodulin, and lumican (for a review, see ref. *19*). Decorin and biglycan contain one and two chondroitin sulfate/dermatan sulfate chains, respectively. Fibromodulin and lumican usually contain one to two keratan sulfate chains per core protein, and in addition, fibromodulin contains two tyrosine sulfate residues in the N-terminal domain of the molecule. Unlike the aggregating large proteoglycans that interact with hyaluronan, this family of proteoglycans interacts directly with collagen. There appears to be some specificity to the collagen binding. For example, decorin and fibromodulin were shown to bind to types I and II collagen, whereas biglycan bound only to type VI collagen. One potential consequence for the direct binding of this proteoglycan family to collagen is that these proteoglycans play a role in limiting collagen fiber diameter. Furthermore, the GAG side chains may serve to bridge the gap between other ECM molecules subserving type II collagen to stabilize the ECM and augment the mechanical qualities of cartilage.

2.1.5. The Collagens of Articular Cartilage

Chondrocytes synthesize several collagen isotypes that, after extensive posttranslational modification, are transported into the ECM. These posttranslational modifications that occur in the Golgi complex include hydroxylation of prolyl and lysyl residues and glycosylation of lysyl residues subsequent to its hydroxylation. Additional intracellular events are required prior to procollagen transport into the ECM. These include proteolytic cleavage of the procollagen peptides located proximal to the triple helical domain at both the C- and N-terminus prior to transport of collagen into the ECM. The formation of collagen fibers in the cartilage ECM is dependent on these posttranslational modifications, as defects in prolyl hydroxylation or in procollagen peptidases results in accumulation of procollagen intracellularly or abnormal and highly fragile collagen fibers. Lysyl oxidase is required for intramolecular and intermolecular cross-link formation (for a review, *see* ref. *20*).

The structure of collagen genes and the regulation of collagen gene expression in articular cartilage has been elucidated and several characteristics of the regulatory sequences of procollagen genes have been described (for a review, *see* ref. *21*). The most abundant of the cartilage collagen isotypes is type II collagen, which comprises over 90% of the cartilage ECM collagen. Other collagen isotypes present in smaller amounts in cartilage include type VI, type IX, and type XI collagens. Despite their lack of abundance in articular cartilage, these so-called "minor" collagens are strategically located in cartilage ECM and may, in fact, play important roles in the maintenance of cartilage homeostasis. For example, type VI collagen is primarily located in the territorial ECM surrounding chondrocytes. Changes in the abundance of type VI collagen have been seen in human osteoarthritic cartilage and experimental osteoarthritic canine cartilage. Types IX and XI collagens interact with type II collagen fibers to form hybrid collagen fibers. This relationship of types IX and XI collagen with type II collagen may serve to stabilize the collagen fibers of the cartilage ECM as well as to provide spatial orientation with respect to the collagen fibers themselves. Chondrocytes are also capable of expressing the genes for the type I and type III collagen isotypes, which may play a particularly important role in osteoarthritis as well as serving as markers for phenotypic modulation *(22)*.

2.1.6. Modulation of Collagen Gene Expression

Type II collagen fibers provide the structural mechanism for the tensile strength of articular cartilage. Single-amino-acid-substitution mutations in the type II procollagen gene have been found in association with several disorders of articular cartilage, including an early-onset form of osteoarthritis and spondyloepiphyseal dysplasia (for a review, *see* ref. *23*). Thus, the stability of type II collagen engendered by the correct amino acid sequence appears to be a requirement for normal ECM structure, and alterations in the type II collagen structure compromises the normal resistance of articular cartilage to precocious degeneration. The significance of the "derepression" of type X collagen gene expression and the deposition of type X collagen into the osteoarthritic cartilage and osteochondrophytic spur ECM is still unknown. The deposition of type X collagen into articular cartilage ECM might serve as a prerequisite for ossification similar to that seen prior to mineralization of the growth plate. Calcification of articular cartilage would undoubtedly alter the function of articular cartilage and could, in combination with abnormal mechanics, be responsible for the fissuring and fragmentation of cartilage frequently observed during the osteoarthritic process.

2.1.7. Cartilage ECM Accessory Proteins

Articular cartilage ECM contains many accessory proteins, including cartilage oligomeric matrix protein (COMP), fibronectin, matrix gla-protein, chondrocalcin, and GP-39 (for a review, see ref. *19*). The function of COMP and matrix gla-protein have not been elucidated. COMP bears structural similarity to thrombospondin. Fibronectin interacts with other ECM proteins to form an intrafibrillar network in the ECM. Chondrocalcin was identified as the C-terminal propeptide of type II collagen that remains in the ECM after cleavage from the procollagen molecule. Although chondrocalcin binds to hydroxyapatite in mineralizing cartilages, its role in normal articular cartilage has not been elucidated. GP-39 (molecular mass, 39 kDa) is preferentially expressed in the superficial region of articular cartilage and in synovial membrane. The function of GP-39 in cartilage has not been determined, but recent studies have suggested that GP-39 may serve as an autoantigen in rheumatoid arthritis (*see* Subheading 4.).

3. Role of Chondrocytes in Degenerative Joint Disease

3.1. Osteoarthritis as a Process of Imbalance in Chondrocyte Anabolic/Catabolic Pathways and Concomitant Systemic Disturbances

Cartilage homeostasis is maintained by the proper balance between anabolic pathways, resulting in the biosynthesis of ECM proteins and catabolic pathways resulting in ECM protein turnover. Several studies have shown that cartilage proteoglycans and collagen are long-lived. When ECM protein turnover is required, *de novo* ECM protein gene transcription must occur. If the rate of ECM protein turnover and/or degradation exceeds the rate of compensatory ECM protein biosynthesis, the ECM may become seriously compromised and no longer retain its function. Recent studies have established that in degenerative joint diseases such as osteoarthritis, there occurs a metabolic imbalance between anabolic and catabolic pathways, driven, in part, by systemic disturbances (for a review, *see* ref. *24*).

3.1.1. In Vitro Studies of Chondrocyte ECM Gene Expression

Maintenance of human cartilage as organ-cultures demonstrates that chondrocytes synthesize ECM proteins, which are quite similar to the ECM proteins found in the tissue (for a review, *see* ref. *3*). Long-term culture of human cartilage demonstrated changes typical of aging and osteoarthritis with an increased amount of keratan sulfate in the proteoglycans of large hydrodynamic size. A comparison of proteoglycans synthesized by human osteoarthritic femoral head cartilage types (i.e., discolored, fibrillated) showed patterns of proteoglycan synthesis indicative of a continuum of change as a function of joint topography and disease severity. These results were confirmed by histological studies that indicated distinct patterns of newly synthesized proteoglycans and histochemical tissue type in resident osteoarthritic cartilage. Taken together, the evidence suggests that chondrocytes of osteoarthritic cartilage are capable of compensatory proteoglycan biosynthesis. Additional studies, however, indicated that the profile of newly synthesized chondrocyte proteoglycan core proteins derived from human osteoarthritic cartilage differed from the proteoglycan core proteins synthesized by age-matched nonarthritic cartilage. The fundamental differences were the synthesis of a single, large, proteoglycan core protein that contained both chondroitin sulfate and keratan sulfate in the osteoarthritic chondrocytes vis-à-vis three large proteoglycan core proteins synthesized by age-matched, nonarthritic chondrocytes. An apparent increase in the biosynthesis of the small proteoglycans at the expense of the large proteoglycans was also seen. An increase in mRNA of the small proteoglycans decorin, biglycan, and fibromodulin was seen in experimental canine osteoarthritic cartilage *(25)*. Methods employing monoclonal antibodies to study the small proteoglycan content of human osteoarthritic cartilage *(26)* have not sustained the biosynthesis studies. An increase in the biosynthesis of small proteoglycans, without a concomitant increase in small proteoglycan content, may be explained on the basis of increased proteoglycan degradation in osteoarthritic cartilage. Indeed, proteoglycan fragments generated from the small proteoglycans have been found in osteoarthritic cartilage. The newly synthesized proteoglycans produced in human osteoarthritic cartilage explants were as susceptible to proteolytic degradation as the endogenous cartilage proteoglycan population.

Whereas proteoglycan synthesis may be altered in osteoarthritic human cartilage, osteoarthritic chondrocytes in culture continue to express types II, IX, and XI collagen genes. Immunohistochemical studies have confirmed that collagen synthesis is activated in osteoarthritic cartilage *(8)*, so that any failure to incorporate collagen into the ECM may result from activation of chondrocyte or synoviocyte collagenases and/or gelatinases, which degrade the newly synthesized collagen, resulting in no net gain of collagen in the ECM.

3.1.2. Matrix Metalloproteinase Gene Expression and ECM Degradation by Chondrocytes in Osteoarthritis

Proteoglycan and collagen fragments have been detected immunochemically in osteoarthritic cartilage, confirming the relevance of proteolysis to the osteoarthritic process *in situ (27)*. The proteinases relevant to this event have been termed matrix metalloproteinases (MMPs) and include stromelysin and collagenases, both of which have been found in osteoarthritic human and animal cartilages and produced by normal and osteoarthritic chondrocytes in culture.

The amount of proteolytic degradation of cartilage ECM appears to depend on several phases of a catabolic pathway, which includes the upregulation of MMPs by cytokines such as IL-1 and tumor necrosis factor-α (TNF-α) produced by chondrocytes and synovial cells (for a review, *see* ref. *28*). Additional cytokines such as IL-6, IL-10, and IL-17 may serve to modulate MMP gene expression and other signaling pathways relevant to the osteoarthritic process such as the induction of nitric oxide (*see* Subheading 3.1.4.).

The activation step in osteoarthritic cartilage required to convert latent MMPs to active enzymes is not without controversy. Several candidate activators (most notably, plasminogen activator and plasmin) have been implicated in the process. Normally, levels of activated MMPs required for normal ECM protein turnover are controlled by the endogenous tissue inhibitor of metalloproteinase (TIMP), but in osteoarthritic cartilage, much more activated MMPs are found than can be inhibited by cartilage TIMP (for a review, *see* ref. *28*). Thus, a metabolic pathway imbalance ensues. This pathway imbalance could be initiated by tissue injury subsequent to trauma, by mechanical forces acting on subtle dysplasias not readily detected by x-ray, by a genetic predisposition that has resulted in an inadequate ECM, or by unknown causes. The cartilage response is characterized by activation of chondrocyte MMP gene transcription, conversion of latent to active chondrocyte MMPs, and degradation of both newly synthesized and endogenous chondrocyte ECM proteins. This process cannot be overcome by chondrocyte ECM protein compensatory biosynthesis.

Processes occurring locally in the joint may be further compromised by the inability of growth factors, such as insulin-like growth factor I (IGF-1) to adequately stimulate chondrocyte proteoglycan synthesis. The serum of patients with osteoarthritis contains significantly less IGF-1 than age-matched controls *(29)*. These results suggest that, in addition to a metabolic pathway imbalance in the joint, systemic disturbances as exemplified by perturbations in the growth hormone/IGF-1 axis may also participate in the process of progressive cartilage destruction in osteoarthritis *(30)*.

3.1.3. Characteristics of Chondrocyte-Mediated ECM Protein Degradation in Osteoarthritis: Emergence of Predominating Signal Pathways in Human Cartilage

A major cleavage site for chondrocyte metalloproteinases reactive with cartilage ECM is the IGD of aggrecan. Stromelysin (MMP-3) and an enzyme activity, termed aggrecanase, have been implicated in this process. The activities of these enzymes are separable and clearly delineated N-terminal sequences, indicating that at least two enzymes participate (perhaps sequentially) in the degradation of aggrecan. Other enzymes, including Cathepsin G, were shown to also cleave aggrecan in the IGD domain. The chondroitin-sulfate-rich domain spanning the aggrecan core protein from G2 to the G3 domain may also be degraded. The ultimate effect of these proteolytic cleavage events is the production of proteoglycan fragments capable of diffusing from cartilage (for a review, *see* ref. *31*). This event compromises cartilage function, and ECM protein fragments derived from both large and small proteoglycans are retained in synovial fluid, where the fragments serve a markers for cartilage degradation. These proteoglycan fragments may also serve to activate synovial cells that perpetuates the cycle of cartilage destruction.

The complexity of these enzyme activities on aggrecan has made it difficult to design any one inhibitor that might be useful in the treatment of osteoarthritis. For example, aggrecanase may be similar in structure to neutrophil collagenase (MMP-8), but this is controversial and stromelysin may also be critical to normal chondrocyte-mediated turnover of cartilage ECM.

Whereas type II collagen is slowly degraded by mammalian collagenase (MMP-1), a collagenase (collagenase-3) with strong activity against type II collagen was described in cultured chondrocytes, but not synovial cells *(32)*. Stromelysin also degrades types IX and type XI collagens, which may further destabilize the type II collagen-rich cartilage fibers.

3.1.4. Chondrocyte Signaling Pathways Relevant to Cartilage Degradation: Induction of Nitric Oxide

The production of nitric oxide (NO) mediated by the inducible nitric oxide synthase (iNOS) occurs in chondrocytes exposed to IL-1. NO synthesis is accompanied by concomitant apoptosis (programmed cell death) in human cartilage. Apoptotic chondrocytes have been linked to areas of cartilage degradation in human osteoarthritis *(33)*. Taken together, the current view is that several signaling pathways converge to cause upregulation of metalloproteinase gene expression, induction of nitric oxide, and apoptosis, all of which are hallmarks of osteoarthritic pathology *(34)*.

4. Activation of Fibroblasts and Chondrocytes in Rheumatoid Arthritis

Current models accounting for synovial tissue inflammation and cartilage and bone destruction in rheumatoid arthritis involve complex cell–cell interactions (for a review, *see* ref. *35*). Strong evidence exists for the involvement of the monocyte/macrophage lineage in the effector arm of inflammation and tissue destruction. In addition, evidence exists for the involvement of potential antigen-presenting cells, namely monocytes/macrophages, B-cells, fibroblasts, and chondrocytes, in initiating or perpetuating the inflammatory state. T-cells may play an important role in this process by activating the resident synovial macrophage. Several mechanisms for initial T-cell activation have been proposed (for a review, *see* ref. *36*). Alternatively, some data suggest that the monocyte/macrophage may, in and of itself, become activated in a T-cell-independent fashion. Once the T-cell is activated, the monocyte/macrophage may, in turn, activate synovial fibroblasts and chondrocytes via elaboration of TNF-α, IL-1, or platelet-derived growth factor (PDGF). Activated fibroblasts, chondrocytes and macrophages are capable of synthesizing tissue-destructive enzymes (*see* Subheading 3.). which result in cartilage and bone invasion. Many other paracrine and autocrine factors are capable of maintaining a chronic state of inflammation *(34)*. Additionally, a proposed contribution to chronic destructive synovitis is a defect in apoptosis that results in decreased inflammatory cell death *(37)*.

References

1. Urist, M. K. (1983) The origin of cartilage: investigations in quest of chondrogenic DNA, in *Cartilage, Vol. 2, Development, Differentiation and Growth* (Hall, B. K., ed.), Academic, New York, pp. 1–85.
2. Malemud, C. J. and Shuckett, R. (1987) Impact-loading and lower extremity disease, in *Clinical Concepts in Regional Musculoskeletal Illness* (Hadler, N. M, ed.), Grune & Stratton, Orlando, FL, pp. 109–135.
3. Malemud, C. J. and Hering, T. M. (1992) Regulation of chondrocytes in osteoarthrosis, in *Biological Regulation of the Chondrocytes* (Adolphe, M., ed.), CRC, Boca Raton, FL, pp. 295–319.
4. LuValle, P., Iwamoto, M., Fanning, P., Pacifici, M., and Olsen, B. R. (1993) Multiple negative elements in a gene codes for an extracellular matrix protein, collagen X, restrict expression to the hypertrophic chondrocytes. *J. Cell Biol.* **121,** 1173–1179.
5. Warman, M. L., Abbott, M., Apte, S. S., Hefferon, T., McIntosh, I., Cohn, D. H., et al. (1993) A type X collagen mutation causes Schmid metaphyseal chondrodysplasia. *Nature Genet.* **5,** 79–82.
6. Lefebvre, V. and de Crombrugghe, B. (1997/1998) Toward understanding SOX9 function in chondrocyte differentiation. *Matrix Biol.* **16,** 529–540.
7. Foster, J. W., Dominguez-Steglich, M. A., Guioli, S., Kwok, C., Weller, P. A., Stevanovic, M., et al. (1994) Campomelic dysplasia and autosomal sex reversal caused by mutations in an SRY-related gene. *Nature* **372,** 525–530.

8. Aigner, T., Stöß, H., Weseloh, G., Zeiler, G., and von der Mark, K. (1992) Activation of collagen type II expression in osteoarthritic and rheumatoid cartilage. *Vichows Arch. B Cell. Pathol.* **62,** 337–345.
9. Caplan, A. I., Elyaderani, M., Mochizuki, Y., Wakitani, S., and Goldberg, V. M. (1997) Principles of cartilage repair and regeneration. *Clin. Orthop. Rel. Res.* **342,** 254–269.
10. Takahashi, I., Nuckolis, G. H., Takahashi, K., Tanaka, O., Semba, I., Dashner, R., et al. (1998) Compressive force promotes Sox9, type II collagen and aggrecan and inhibits IL-1β expression resulting in chondrogenesis in mouse embryonic limb bud mesenchymal cells. *J. Cell Sci.* **111,** 2067–2076.
11. Tabin, C. J. and McMahon, A. P. (1997) Recent advances in Hedgehog signalling. *Trends Cell Biol.* **7,** 442–446.
12. Okano, K., Tsukazaki, T., Ohtsuru, A., Osaki, M., Yonekura, A., Iwasaki, K., et al. (1997) Expression of parathyroid hormone-related peptide in human osteoarthritis. *J. Orthop. Res.* **15,** 175–180.
13. Tsuji, M., Funahashi, S-i., Takigawa, M., Seiki, M., Fujii, K., and Yoshida, T. (1996) Expression of c-fos inhibits proteoglycans synthesis in transfected chondrocyte. *FEBS Lett.* **381,** 222–226.
14. Watanabe, H., Saitoh, K., Kameda, T., Murakami, M., Niikura, Y., Okazaki, S., et al. (1997) Chondrocytes as a specific target of ectopic Fos expression in early development. *Proc. Natl. Acad. Sci. USA* **94,** 3994–3999.
15. Vertel, B. M. (1995) The ins and outs of aggrecan. *Trends Cell Biol.* **5,** 458–464.
16. Faiyaz ul Haque, M., King, L. M., Krakow, D., Cantor, R. M., Rusiniak, M. E., Swank, R. T., et al. (1998) Mutations in orthologous genes in human spondylometaphyseal dysplasia and the brachymorphic mouse. *Nature Genet.* **20,** 157–162.
17. Melching, L. I., Cs-Szabo, G., and Roughley, P. J. (1997) Analysis of proteoglycan messages in human articular cartilage by a competitive PCR technique. *Matrix Biol.* **16,** 1–11.
18. Nishida, Y., Shinomura, T., Iwata, H., Miura, T., and Kimata, K. (1994) Abnormal occurrence of a large chondroitin-sulfate proteoglycan, PG-M/versican in osteoarthritic cartilage. *Osteoarthritis Cart.* **2,** 43–49.
19. Heinegård, D., Lorenzo, P., and Sommarin, Y. (1995) Articular cartilage matrix proteins, in *Osteoarthritic Disorders* (Kuettner, K. E. and Goldberg, V. M., eds.), American Academy of Orthopaedic Surgeons, Rosemont, IL, pp. 229–237.
20. Linsenmayer, T. F. (1981) Collagen, in *Cell Biology of Extracellular Matrix* (Hay, E. D., ed.), Plenum, New York, pp. 1–37.
21. Sandell, L. J. (1995) Molecular biology of collagens in normal and osteoarthritic cartilage, in *Osteoarthritic Disorders* (Kuettner, K. E. and Goldberg, V. M., eds.), American Academy of Orthopaedics Surgeons, Rosemont, IL, pp. 131–146.
22. Aigner, T., Bertling, W., Stöss H., Weseloh, G., and von der Mark, K. (1993) Independent expression of fibril-forming collagens I, II and III in chondrocytes of human osteoarthritic cartilage. *J. Clin. Invest.* **91,** 829–837.
23. Kuivaniemi, H., Tromp, G., and Prockop, D. J. (1991) Mutations in collagen genes: causes of rare and some common diseases in man. *FASEB J.* **5,** 2052–2060.
24. Poole, A. R. (1995) Imbalances of anabolism and catabolism of cartilage matrix components in osteoarthritis, in *Osteoarthritic Disorders* (Kuettner, K. E. and Goldberg, V. M., eds.), American Academy of Orthopaedic Surgeons, Rosemont, IL, pp. 247–260.
25. Dourado, G. S., Adams, M. E., Matyas, J. R., and Huang, D. (1996) Expression of biglycan, decorin and fibromodulin in the hypertrophic phase of experimental osteoarthritis. *Osteoarthritis Cart.* **4,** 187–196.
26. Poole, A. R., Rosenberg, L. C., Reiner, A., Ionescu, M. Bogoch, E., and Roughley, P. J. (1996) Contents and distribution of the proteoglycans decorin and biglycan in normal and osteoarthritic human articular cartilage. *J. Orthop. Res.* **14,** 681–689.

27. Rizkalla, G., Reiner, A., Bogoch, E., and Poole, A. R. (1992) Studies of the articular cartilage proteoglycan aggrecan in health and disease. Evidence for molecular heterogeneity and extensive molecular change in disease. *J. Clin. Invest.* **90,** 2268–2277.
28. Woessner, J. F., Jr. (1995) Imbalance of proteinases and their inhibitors in osteoarthritis, in *Osteoarthritic Disorders* (Kuettner, K. E. and Goldberg, V. M., eds.), American Academy of Orthopaedic Surgeons, Rosemont, IL, pp. 281–290.
29. Denko, C. W., Boja, B., and Moskowitz, R. W. (1990) Growth promoting peptides in osteoarthritis: insulin, insulin-like growth factor, growth hormone. *J. Rheumatol.* **17,** 1217–1221.
30. Denko, C. W. and Malemud, C. J. (1999) Metabolic disturbances and synovial joint responses in osteoarthritis. *Front. Biosci.* **4,** D686–D693.
31. Rizkalla, G., Reiner, A., Bogoch, E., and Poole, A. R. (1992) Studies of the articular cartilage proteoglycan aggrecan in health and disease. Evidence for molecular heterogeneity and extensive molecular change in disease. *J. Clin. Invest.* **90,** 2268–2277.
32. Reboul, P., Pelletier, J.-P., Tardif, G., Cloutier, J.-M., and Martel-Pelletier, J. (1996) The new collagenase, collagenase-3, is expressed and synthesized by human chondrocytes but not by synoviocytes. *J. Clin. Invest.* **97,** 2011–2019.
33. Hashimoto, S., Ochs, R. L., Komiya, S., and Lotz, M. (1998) Linkage of chondrocyte apoptosis and cartilage degradation in human osteoarthritis. *Arthritis Rheum.* **41,** 1632–1638.
34. Blanco, F.J., Ochs, R. L., Schwarz, H., and Lotz, M. (1995) Chondrocyte apoptosis induced by nitric oxide. *Am. J. Pathol.* **146,** 75–85.
35. Burmester, G. R., Stuhlmuller, B., Keyser, G., and Kinne, R. W. (1997) Mononuclear phagocytes and rheumatoid synovitis: mastermind or workhorse in arthritis. *Arthritis Rheum.* **40,** 5–18.
36. Goronzy, J. J. and Weyland, C. M. (1995) T cells in rheumatoid arthritis. *Rheum. Dis. Clin. North Amer.* **21,** 655–674.
37. Nishioka, K., Hasunuma, T., Kato, T., Sumida, T., and Kobata, T. (1998) Apoptosis in rheumatoid arthritis: a novel pathway in the regulation of synovial tissue. *Arthritis Rheum.* **41,** 1–9.

18

Osteoblasts and Osteoclasts

Stavros C. Manolagas

1. Introduction

The skeleton is a highly specialized and dynamic organ that undergoes continuous regeneration. Its functions are to maintain the shape of the body, protect vital organs, serve as a scaffold for the muscles, allowing their contractions to be translated into bodily movements, resist mechanical load during locomotion and weight bearing, and provide a reservoir of calcium, magnesium, bicarbonate, and phosphate. The skeleton consists of highly specialized cells, mineralized and unmineralized connective tissue matrix, and spaces that include the bone marrow cavity, vascular canals, canaliculi, and lacunae. During development and growth, the skeleton is sculpted in order to achieve its shape and size by the removal of bone from one site and deposition at a different one; this process is called modeling. Once the skeleton has reached maturity, regeneration continues in the form of a periodic replacement of old bone with new at the same location *(1)*. This process is called remodeling. Removal of bone is the task of osteoclasts. The cells responsible for new bone formation are osteoblasts.

Remodeling is carried out not by individual osteoclasts and osteoblasts, but rather by temporary anatomical structures, termed basic multicellular units (BMUs), comprised of teams of osteoclasts in the front and osteoblasts in the rear (Fig. 1). In cortical bone, the BMUs tunnel through the tissue, whereas in cancellous bone, the BMUs move across the trabecular surface, forming a trench. In any established BMU, bone resorption and formation are happening at the same time; formation begins to occur while resorption advances. New osteoblasts assemble only at sites where osteoclasts have recently been active—a phenomenon referred to as coupling. Although, during modeling, one cannot distinguish anatomical units analogous to BMU *per se*, sculpting of the growing skeleton requires spatial and temporal orchestration of the display of osteoblasts and osteoclasts, albeit with different rules and coordinates than those operating in the BMU of the remodeling skeleton.

2. Origin and Differentiation of Osteoblasts and Osteoclasts

Both osteoblasts and osteoclasts are derived from precursors originating in the bone marrow. The precursors of osteoblasts are multipotent mesenchymal stem cells, which also give rise to bone marrow stromal cells, chondrocytes, muscle cells, and adipocytes *(2)*. The existence of multipotent mesenchymal stem cells had been suspected, long

From: *Current Molecular Medicine: Principles of Molecular Rheumatology*
Edited by: G. C. Tsokos © Humana Press Inc., Totowa, NJ

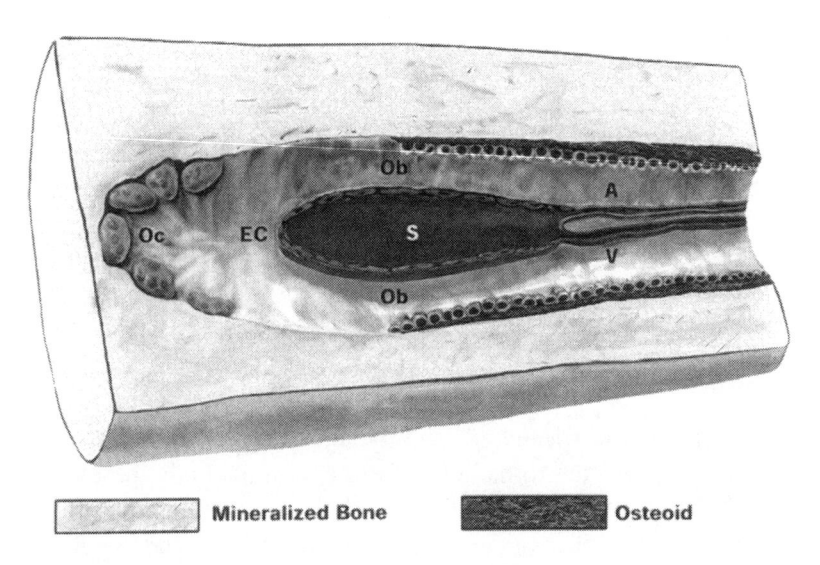

Fig. 1. Schematic of cortical BMU in normal human iliac bone. The structure is traveling from right to left at about 25 μm/d, excavating a tunnel. The cavity in the bone is approximately 500 μm long and 200 μm in maximum width. The space between the cells lining the cavity and the central blood vessel is filled with a loose connective tissue stroma. Oc, osteoclasts; EC, endothelial cells; Ob, osteoblasts; S, sinusoid; A, arteriole; and V, venule. The latter structures have been demonstrated in cross-sections of Haversian canals, but their three-dimensional relationship to the sinusoid within the BMU is conjectural. The sinusoid maintains the same distance behind the cutting cone of osteoclasts for many months, but its manner of growth is unknown. The circulating mononuclear osteoclast precursors pass through the wall of the sinusoid by diapedesis and travel for about 150 μm through the stroma to join the team of osteoclasts of [From A. M. Parfitt, *Bone* **23,** 491–494 (1998), reproduced with the permission.]

before these cells could be cultured, based on the evidence that fibroblastic colonies formed in cultures of adherent bone marrow cells can differentiate, under the appropriate stimuli, into each of the above-mentioned cells; these progenitors were named colony-forming-unit fibroblasts (CFU-F). The subset of cells within the CFU-F that can form a mineralized bone nodule in vitro in the presence of β-glycerophosphate have been termed CFU osteoblast (CFU-OB) *(3)*.

The precursors of osteoclasts are hematopoietic cells of the monocyte/macrophage lineage. Specifically, osteoclasts arise in vitro from the colony-forming-unit granulocyte/macrophage (CFU-GM) *(4)*. Osteoclast development cannot be accomplished unless cells derived from the CFU-F colonies are present to provide essential support. The precise stage of differentiation of the mesenchymal cells that support osteoclast development remains unknown. In vitro studies suggest that these cells are closely related to the osteoblast lineage. Nonetheless, it is unlikely that they are fully differentiated matrix-synthesizing osteoblasts. Instead, the cells that support osteoclast development seem to represent an earlier stage of the progeny of the CFU-F. For convenience, the cells that support osteoclast development have been designated as stromal/osteoblastic cells to indicate their similarities to both bone marrow stromal cells and osteoblasts. The mechanistic basis of the dependency of osteoclastogenesis on mesenchymal cells has been recently established by the discovery of two membrane-bound cytokine-like molecules: the receptor activator of NFκB (RANK) and the RANK ligand *(5)*. RANK is expressed in the hematopoietic osteoclast progenitors; whereas RANK ligand is expressed in committed preosteoblastic cells. Other names used for RANK are osteoprotegerin ligand and TRANCE. The RANK ligand recognizes RANK and binds to it with high affinity. This interaction is essential and, together with M-CSF, sufficient for osteoclastogenesis. Osteoprotegerin is another protein related to the tumor necrosis factor (TNF) receptor *(6)*. However, unlike RANK and RANK ligand, osteoprotegerin occurs in a soluble form. Osteoprotegerin can block the RANK ligand–RANK interaction and, as a consequence, is a potent antiresorptive factor that inhibits osteoclast development as well as activity.

Under certain conditions, fibroblastic stromal cells may become fatty. The replacement of fibroblastic stromal cells by large adipocytes reduces the space available for hematopoiesis. In these conditions, the marrow appears yellow, as there is less red cell production. Osteoblast differentiation has a reciprocal relationship with adipocyte differentiation. Specifically, increased bone marrow adipocyte differentiation occurs at the expense of osteoblastogenesis in age-related osteoporosis in animals and humans. This situation may also apply to the case of glucocorticoid excess, as prednisolone administration to mice suppresses osteoblast formation while it increases adipocyte differentiation in the marrow *(7,8)*.

Not only do fibroblastic stromal cells of the hematopoietic marrow support osteoclast development and are close relatives of the bone-forming osteoblast, but osteoblasts also seem to be involved in hematopoiesis. Indeed, like adipocytes and fibroblastic stromal cells of the bone marrow, osteoblast-like cells exhibit the ability to provide microenvironmental support for the development of macrophages and neutrophils, because they are a rich source of G-CSF. Thus, hematopoiesis and bone remodeling are highly interdependent in spite of the fact that these processes ultimately carry out distinct functions.

3. Control of Osteoblast and Osteoclast Development and Differentiation

The development and differentiation of osteoblasts and osteoclasts is controlled by growth factors and cytokines produced in the bone marrow microenvironment as well as adhesion molecules that mediate cell–cell and cell–matrix interactions. Several systemic hormones as well as mechanical signals also exert potent modulation of osteoclast and osteoblast development and differentiation. Although many details remain to be established about the operation of this network, a few themes have emerged *(9)*. First, several of the growth factors and cytokines control each other's production in a cascade fashion and, in some instances, form negative feedback loops. Second, there is extensive functional redundancy among them. Third, some of the same factors are capable of influencing the differentiation of both osteoblasts and osteoclasts. Fourth, agents arising from the circulation (i.e., endocrine hormones) influence the process of osteoblast and osteoclast formation via their ability to control the production and/or action of local mediators. Moreover, mesenchymal cell differentiation toward the osteoblast phenotype and osteoclastogenesis are inseparably linked, as both are stimulated by the same factors, proceed simultaneously, and the former event is a prerequisite for the latter. This tight association between osteoblast and osteoclast production is the means of assuring the balance between bone formation and resorption under normal conditions.

3.1. Growth Factors

Members of the tumor growth factor-β (TGF-β) super family, platelet-derived growth factor (PDGF), insulin-like growth factors (IGFs), and members of the fibroblast growth factor (FGF) family can all stimulate osteoblast differentiation *(10)*. Some of these factors are produced by mesenchymal cells and act in an autocrine fashion. Others, particularly IGFs and TGF-β, are derived from the bone matrix and are released in an active form during the resorption of bone by osteoclasts. TGF-β, PDGF, FGF, and IGFs are able to influence the replication and differentiation of committed osteoblast progenitors toward the osteoblastic lineage. However, TGF-β, IGF-1, or FGF alone cannot induce osteoblast differentiation from uncommitted progenitor cells.

Bone morphogenetic proteins (BMPs), which are members of the TGF-β family, are unique in their ability to initiate osteoblastogenesis, as they are able to initiate osteoblast differentiation from uncommitted progenitors in vitro as well as in vivo *(11)*. BMPs have been long known as the factors responsible for skeletal development during embryonic life and fracture healing. More recently, it has become apparent that BMPs and, in particular, BMP-2 and BMP-4 also initiate the commitment of pluripotent mesenchymal precursors of the adult bone marrow to the osteoblastic lineage *(12)*. BMPs stimulate the transcription of the gene-encoding Osf2/Cbfa1—an osteoblast transcription factor *(13)*. In turn, Osf2/Cbfa1 activates the genes for osteoblast-specific genes such as osteopontin, bone sialoprotein, type I collagen, and osteocalcin. Lack of Osf-2 prevents osteoblast development and also leads to a paucity of osteoclasts. Based on evidence that the RANK ligand gene promoter contains two functional Cbfa1 sites, it is likely that a BMP→Cbfa1→RANK ligand gene expression cascade in cells of the bone marrow stromal/osteoblastic lineage constitutes the molecular basis of the linkage between osteoblastogenesis and osteoclastogenesis, with BMPs providing the tonic baseline control of both processes—and thereby the rate of bone remodeling—upon which other inputs (e.g., biomechanical, hormonal, etc.) operate.

Besides growth factors, bone cells produce proteins that modulate the activity of growth factors either by binding to them and thereby preventing interaction with their receptors, by competing for the same receptors, or by promoting the activity of a particular factor. For example, osteoblasts produce several IGF-binding proteins (IGFBP). Of these, IGFBP-4 binds to IGF and blocks its action, whereas IGFBP-5 promotes the stimulatory effects of IGF on osteoblasts. During the last few years, several proteins able to antagonize BMP action have also been discovered. Of them, noggin and chordin, were initially found in the Spemann organizer of the Xenopus embryo and shown to be essential for neuronal development. Their localization is strictly limited to the dorsal region of the Xenopus embryo, whereas BMPs were localized in the ventral region. More important, noggin and chordin are strong inhibitors of BMP actions and vice versa, as injection of noggin or chordin to the ventral region or injection of BMP to the dorsal region prevented further development. Noggin and chordin inhibit the action of BMPs by binding directly and with high affinity with the latter proteins. Such binding is highly specific for BMP-2 and BMP-4, as noggin binds BMP-7 with very low affinity and does not bind TGF-β or IGF-1. The addition of human recombinant noggin to bone marrow cell cultures from normal adult mice inhibits not only osteoblast formation but also osteoclast formation; these effects can be reversed by exogenous BMP-2 *(12)*. Consistent with this evidence, BMP-2, BMP-4 and BMP-2/4 receptor transcripts and proteins are found in bone marrow cultures, bone-marrow-derived stromal/osteoblastic cell lines, as well as in murine adult whole bone. Noggin expression has also been documented in all these cell preparations. These findings indicate that BMP-2 and BMp-4 are expressed in the bone marrow in postnatal life and serve to maintain the continuous supply of osteoblasts and osteoclasts and that, in fact, BMP-2/4-induced commitment to the osteoblastic lineage is a prerequisite for osteoclast development. Hence, BMPs (in balance with noggin and possibly other antagonists) may provide the tonic baseline control of the rate of bone remodeling upon which other inputs (e.g., hormonal, biomechanical, etc.) operate. Fetuin (also known as a2-HS glycoprotein or pp63) is another protein able to antagonize BMP actions. Fetuin is a member of the sialoprotein family and is produced in the liver, kidney, lung, and brain, and its levels in serum are very high at the fetal stage, but decrease after birth.

Not only are there cascades of growth factor action and functional redundancy, but there also exists an extensive combinatorial overlap and commonality in their receptors, and therefore their signal transduction pathways. For example, the receptors that mediate the effects of the TGF-β superfamily that includes the BMPs are serine/threonine receptor kinases, which are composed of two subunits, called type I and type II. Each subunit exists in various isoforms and each ligand (i.e., BMP-2 or TGF-β) recognizes different constellations of type I and type II subunits (14).

3.2. Cytokines

Because the early stages of hematopoiesis and osteoclastogenesis proceed along identical pathways, it is not surprising that a large group of cytokines and colony-stimulating factors that are involved in hematopoiesis also affect osteoclast development (15). This group includes the interleukins IL-1, IL-3, IL-6, and IL-11, leukemia inhibitory factor (LIF), oncostatin M (OSM), ciliary neurotropic factor (CNTF), tumor necrosis factor (TNF), GM-CSF, and M-CSF. The importance of M-CSF for osteoclastogenesis has been well established by demonstrating that a mutation of the M-CSF gene causes osteopetrosis. Osteoblasts isolated from adult human trabecular bone, neonatal murine calvaria cells, or osteoblastic cell lines are capable of producing IL-1 and TNF constitutively or in response to stimulation by lipopolysaccharide or other cytokines. Despite the very low level of production of TNF in the bone microenvironment, this particular cytokine may serve as an important amplifier for the effects of other local cytokines and systemic hormones that stimulate osteoclast development. As opposed to the above-mentioned cytokines that stimulate osteoclast development, IL-4, IL-10, IL-18, and interferon-γ (IFN-γ) inhibit osteoclast development. In the case of IL-18, the effect is mediated through GM-CSF.

Interleukin-6 is produced at high levels by cells of the stromal/osteoblastic lineage in response to stimulation by a variety of growth factors and other cytokines such as TGF-β, PDGF, IL-1, and TNF. Alone or in concert with other agents, IL-6 stimulates osteoclastogenesis and promotes bone resorption. Along with IL-3, IL-6 stimulates CFU-GM development and the formation of osteoclast precursors from this colony type. IL-6 stimulates osteoclast formation and bone resorption in fetal mouse bone in vitro and, in combination with parathyroid hormone-related protein (PTHrP), stimulates bone resorption in vivo. The cells that mediate the actions of the IL-6 type cytokines on osteoclast formation appear to be the stromal/osteoblastic cells, as stimulation of gp80 expression on these cells by pretreatment with dexamethasone allows them to support osteoclast formation in response to IL-6 alone. These findings indicate that the osteoclastogenic property of IL-6 depends not only on its ability to act directly on hematopoietic osteoclast progenitors but also on the activation of gp130 signaling in the stromal/osteoblastic cells that provide essential support for osteoclast formation. Despite the effects of IL-6 on osteoclastogenesis in experimental in vitro systems, IL-6 is not required for osteoclastogenesis in vivo under normal physiologic conditions. In fact, osteoclast formation is unaffected in sex-steroid-replete mice treated with a neutralizing anti-IL-6 antibody or in IL-6 deficient mice. The expression of the gp80 subunit of the IL-6 receptor in bone is a limiting factor for the effects of the cytokine. In agreement with the notion that IL-6 attains its importance for bone metabolism in pathologic states where there is increased IL-6 production in combination with increased sensitivity to the effects of IL-6, increased IL-6 receptor production has been documented in several disease states *(15)*.

Interleukin-6-type cytokines are capable of influencing the differentiation of osteoblasts as well *(16)*. Thus, receptors for these cytokines are expressed on a variety of stromal/osteoblastic cells and ligand binding induces progression toward a more mature osteoblast phenotype characterized by increased alkaline phosphatase and osteocalcin expression, and a concomitant decrease in proliferation. Moreover, IL-6-type cytokines stimulate the development of osteoblasts from noncommitted embryonic fibroblasts obtained from 12-d-old murine fetuses. Consistent with the in vitro evidence, several in vivo studies have demonstrated increased bone formation in transgenic mice overexpressing OSM or LIF. The ability of IL-6 type cytokines to stimulate both osteoclast and osteoblast development is consistent with the contention that they can increase the rate of bone remodeling.

Tumor growth factor-β is another example of a factor affecting both bone formation and bone resorption *(10)*. Thus, in addition to its ability to stimulate osteoblast differentiation, TGF-β increases bone resorption by stimulating osteoclasts formation. Injection of TGF-β into the subcutaneous tissue that overlies the calvaria of adult mice causes increased bone resorption accompanied by the development of unusually large osteoclasts, as well as increased bone formation. The effects of TGF-β might be mediated by other cytokines involved in osteoclastogenesis, as TGF-β can stimulate their production. Mice lacking the TGF-β1 gene because of targeted disruption exhibit excessive production of inflammatory cells suggesting that this growth factor normally operates to suppress hematopoiesis.

3.3. Systemic Hormones

The two major hormones of the calcium homeostatic system, namely PTH and 1,25-dihydroxyvitamin D_3 [$1,25(OH)_2D_3$], are potent stimulators of osteoclast formation *(4)*. The ability of these hormones to stimulate osteoclast development and to regulate calcium absorption and excretion from the intestine and kidney, respectively, are the key elements of extracellular calcium homeostasis. Calcitonin, the third of the classical bone-regulating hormones, inhibits osteoclast development and activity and promotes osteoclast apoptosis. Although the antiresorptive properties of calcitonin have been exploited in the management of bone diseases with increased resorption, the role of this hormone in bone physiology in humans, if any, remains questionable. PTH,

PTH-related peptide, and 1,25(OH)$_2$D$_3$ stimulate the production of IL-6 and IL-11 by stromal/osteoblastic cells. Moreover, PTH, PTHrP, 1,25(OH)$_2$D$_3$, IL-6, IL-11, as well as IL-1 induce the expression of the RANK ligand in stromal/osteoblastic cells.

Several other hormones, including estrogen, androgen, glucocorticoids, and thyroxin, exert potent regulatory influences on the development of osteoclasts and osteoblasts by regulating the production and/or action of several cytokines, such as IL-6. Importantly, changes in the production and/or action of cytokines are crucial pathogenetic mechanisms of the adverse affects of decreased (estrogen, androgen) or increased (glucocorticoids, thyroxin) hormonal levels on bone homeostasis *(15)*.

3.4. Adhesion Molecules

Besides autocrine, paracrine, and endocrine signals, cell–cell and cell–matrix interactions are also required for the development of osteoclasts and osteoblasts. Such interactions are mediated by proteins expressed on the surface of these cells and are responsible for contact between osteoclast precursors with stromal/osteoblastic cells and facilitation of the action of paracrine factors anchored to the surface of cells that are required for bone cell development. An example of the latter is M-CSF, which can exert its action while anchored to the cell membrane of osteoblastic cells. Adhesion molecules are also involved in the migration of osteoblast and osteoclast progenitors from the bone marrow to sites of bone remodeling as well as the cellular polarization of osteoclasts and the initiation and cessation of osteoclastic bone resorption. The list of adhesion molecules involved in bone cell development and function includes the integrins, the intercellular adhesion molecules, selectins, cadherins, leucine-rich glycoproteins, mucins, and CD36 and CD44 molecules. Each of these proteins recognizes distinct ligands. For example, integrins recognize a specific amino acid sequence (RGD) present in collagen, fibronectin, osteopontin, thrombospondin, bone sialoprotein, and vitronectin.

4. Function of the Differentiated Osteoblast

The fully differentiated osteoblasts produce and secrete proteins that constitute the bone matrix *(17)*. The collagenous matrix is subsequently mineralized under the control of the same cells. Osteoblasts engaged in bone formation are polarized cuboidal mononuclear cells with an average diameter of 10–15 μm. Bone-forming osteoblasts contain a well-developed secretory apparatus of rough endoplasmic reticulum and Golgi complexes oriented toward the bone surface (Fig. 2).

A major product of the bone-forming osteoblast is type I collagen. This polymeric protein is initially secreted in the form of a precursor, which contains peptide extensions at both the amino terminal and carboxyl ends of the molecule. The propeptides are proteolytically removed at the time of exocytosis. Further extracellular processing results in mature three-chained type I collagen molecules, which then assemble themselves into a collagen fibril. Individual collagen molecules become interconnected by the formation of pyridinoline crosslinks, which are unique to bone. Bone-forming osteoblasts synthesize a number of other proteins that are incorporated into the bone matrix, including osteocalcin and osteonectin, which constitute 40–50% of the noncollagenous proteins of bone *(17)*. The precise function of these proteins remains unknown. Other osteoblast-derived proteins include glycosaminoglycans, which are

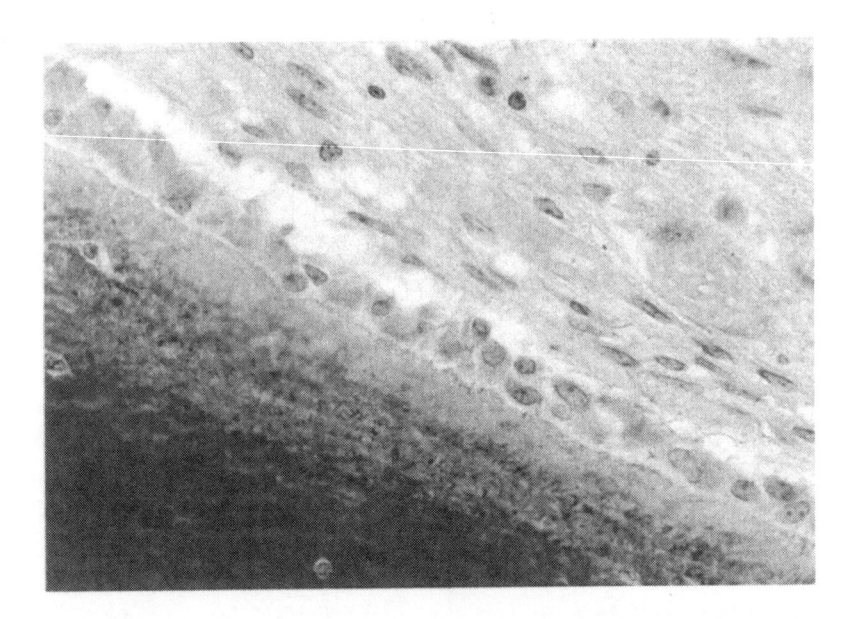

Fig. 2. Histology of the osteoblast. Plump, cuboidal osteoblasts are lining a partly mineralized layer, or seam, of osteoid in a patient with an increased rate of bone formation. Note the perinuclear halo of the prominent Golgi apparatus. Osteoblasts have a volume ranging from about 900 to 1200 m^3. Mineralized bone is black, osteoid is grey; modified Masson stain; ×250. (Courtesy of Dr. Robert S. Weinstein.)

attached to one of two small core proteins: PG-I (or biglycan) and decorin; the later has been implicated in the regulation of collagen fibrillogenesis. A number of other minor proteins such as osteopontin, bone sialoprotein, fibronectin, vitronectin, and thrombospondin serve as attachment factors that interact with integrins.

Osteoblasts express relatively high amounts of alkaline phosphatase, which is anchored to the external surface of the plasma membrane. Some alkaline phosphatase is released from the surface of the osteoblast and reaches the circulation, accounting for approximately one-half of the total alkaline phosphatase activity present in adult serum. For a long time, alkaline phosphatase has been thought to play a role in bone mineralization. Consistent with this, deficiency of alkaline phosphatase due to genetic defects leads to hypophosphatasia, a condition characterized by defective bone mineralization *(18)*. However, the precise mechanism of mineralization and the exact role of alkaline phosphatase in this process remains unclear. In any event, mineralization is the result of deposition of hydroxyapatite crystals in the collagenous matrix. This process lags behind matrix production and, in remodeling sites in the adult bone, occurs at a distance of 8–10 μm from the osteoblast. Matrix synthesis determines the volume of bone but not its density. Mineralization of the matrix under the control of osteoblasts increases the density of bone by displacing water, but does not alter its volume. Osteoblasts are thought to regulate the local concentrations of calcium and phosphate in such a way as to promote the formation of hydroxyapatite. In view of the highly ordered, well-aligned, collagen fibrils complexed with the noncollagenous proteins formed by the osteoblast in lamellar bone, it may be that mineralization proceeds in association with, and perhaps governed by, the heteropolymeric matrix fibrils themselves.

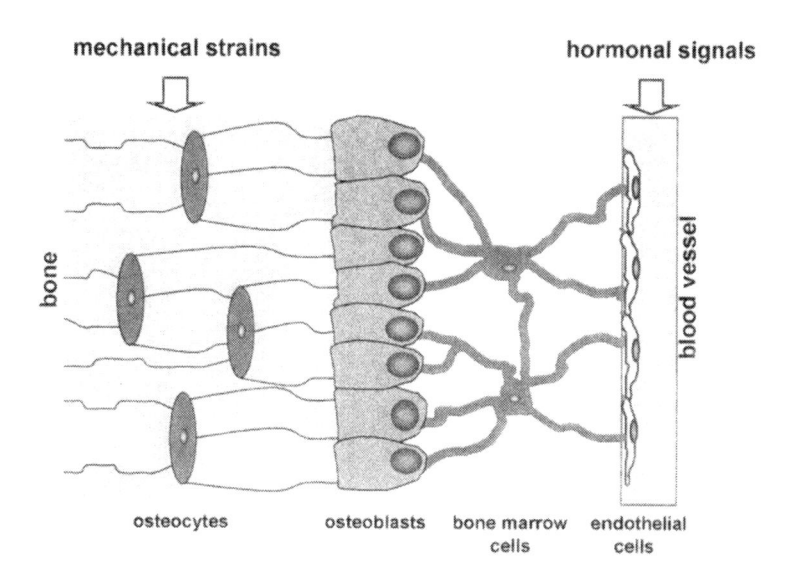

Fig. 3. Functional syncytium comprising osteocytes, osteoblasts, bone marrow stromal cells, and endothelial cells. (From Plotkin et al., *J. Clin. Invest.* **104**, 1363–1374, 1999, with permission from the authors.)

4.1. Osteocytes

Some osteoblasts are eventually buried within lacunae of mineralized matrix. These cells are termed osteocytes and are characterized by a striking stellate morphology, reminiscent of the dendritic network of the nervous system *(19)*. Osteocytes are the most abundant cell types in bone: There are 10 times as many osteocytes as osteoblasts. Osteocytes are regularly spaced throughout the mineralized matrix and communicate with each other and with cells on the bone surface via multiple extensions of their plasma that run along the canaliculi; osteoblasts, in turn, communicate with cells of the bone marrow stroma, which extend cellular projections onto endothelial cells inside the sinusoids. Thus, a syncytium extends from the entombed osteocytes all the way to the vessel wall (Fig. 3). As a consequence, the strategic location of osteocytes makes them excellent candidates for mechanosensory cells able to detect the need for bone augmentation or reduction during functional adaptation of the skeleton and the need for repair of microdamage, and, in both cases, to transmit signals leading to the appropriate response. Osteocytes evidently sense changes in interstitial fluid flow through canaliculi produced by mechanical forces and detect changes in the levels of hormones such as estrogen and glucocorticoids that influence their survival and that circulate in the same fluid. Disruption of the osteocyte network is likely to increase bone fragility.

4.2. Lining Cells

The surface of normal quiescent bone (i.e., bone that is not undergoing remodeling) is covered by a 1- to 2-µm-thick layer of unmineralized collagen matrix on top of which there is a layer of flat and elongated cells. These cells are called lining cells and are descendents of osteoblasts *(1)*. Conversion of osteoblasts to lining cells represents one of the three fates of osteoblasts that have completed their bone-forming function, the other two being entombment into the matrix as osteocytes and apoptosis. Osteo-

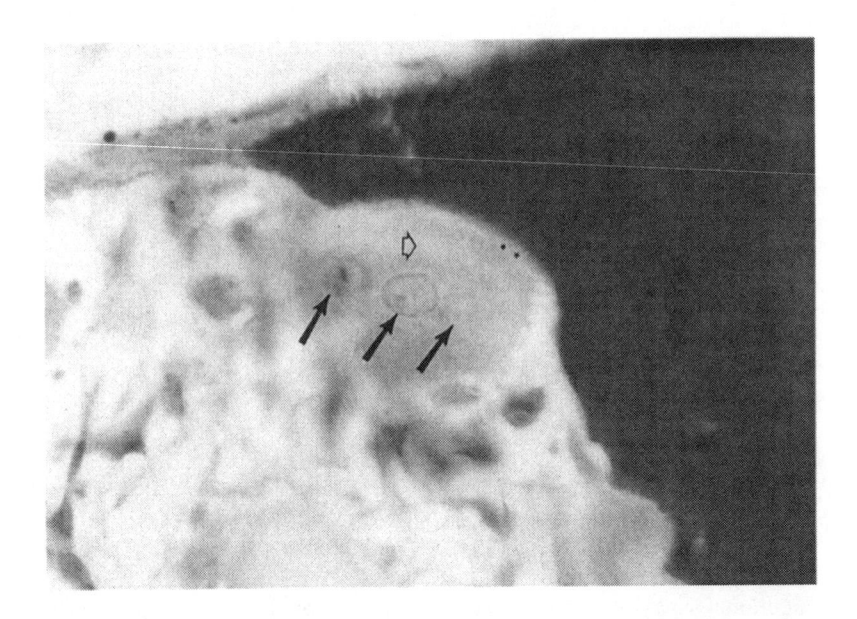

Fig. 4. Histology of the osteoclast. A large multinucleated osteoclast. Three nuclei (black arrows), each with a prominent nucleolus, are polarized to the area opposite to the bone interface. The clear zone (open arrow head) and the ruffled border (small stars) are adjacent to the site of active resorption of mineralized bone (dark area in the right half of this picture). Modified Masson stain, ×250. (Courtesy of Dr. Robert S. Weinstein.)

clasts cannot attach to the unmineralized collagenous layer that covers the surface of normal bone. Therefore, other cells, perhaps the lining cells, secrete collagenase, which removes this matrix before osteoclasts can attach to bone.

5. Function of the Differentiated Osteoclast

Osteoclasts are usually large (50–100 µm in diameter) multinucleated cells with abundant mitochondria, numerous lysosomes, and free ribosomes (Fig. 4). The most remarkable morphologic feature of osteoclasts is the ruffled border, a complex system of finger-shaped, flat-plate-shaped projections of the membrane, the function of which is to mediate the resorption of the calcified bone matrix. This structure is completely surrounded by another specialized area, called the clear zone. The cytoplasm in the clear zone area has a uniform appearance and contains bundles of actinlike filaments. The clear zone delineates the area of attachment of the osteoclast to the bone surface and seals off a distinct area of the bone surface that lies immediately underneath the osteoclast and that eventually will be excavated. The ability of the clear zone to seal off this area of bone surface allows the formation of a microenvironment suitable for the operation of the resorptive apparatus *(4)*.

The mineral component of the matrix is dissolved in the acidic environment of the resorption site, which is created by the action of an ATP-driven proton pump (the so-called vaculoar H+-ATPase) located in the ruffled border membrane. The protein components of the matrix, mainly collagen, are degraded by matrix metalloproteinases and cathepsins O, K, B, and L secreted by the osteoclast into the area of bone resorption. The degraded bone matrix components are endocytosed along the ruffled border within the resorption lacunae and then transcytosed to the membrane area opposite the bone, where they are released. Another feature of osteoclasts is the presence of high amounts of the phosphohydrolase enzyme, tartrate-resistant acid phosphatase. In fact, this feature is frequently used for the detection of osteoclasts in bone specimens. In contrast to the role of the lysosomal proteolytic enzymes, little is known about the role of TRAPase in osteoclastic bone resorption.

Osteoclasts bear on their surface several antigens that are also present on hematopoietic cells. These include CD54, the cellular ligand for certain integrin proteins, CD45, the common leukocyte antigen, and the CD49b and CD29 antigens that constitute the collagen receptor. In addition, osteoclasts express CD9 (function unknown), CD13, which is the aminopeptidase N that regulates the tissue half-life of small peptides in the case of inflammatory cells, CD71, the transferrin receptor that may be related to the presence of high levels of the iron-containing TRAPase present in osteoclasts, and CD51 and CD61, which constitute the vitronectin receptor responsible for mediating the attachment of osteoclasts to the bone surface.

6. Death of Osteoclasts and Osteoblasts

The average life-span of human osteoclasts is about 2 wk, whereas the average life-span of osteoblasts is 3 mo. After osteoclasts have eroded to a particular distance, either from the central axis in cortical bone or to a particular depth from the surface in cancellous bone, they die by apoptosis and are quickly removed by phagocytes (20). The majority (65%) of the osteoblasts that originally assembled at the remodeling site also die by apoptosis (21). The remaining are converted to lining cells that cover quiescent bone surfaces or are entombed within the mineralized matrix as osteocytes. The life-span of the BMU is 6–9 mo; much longer than the life-span of its executive cells. Therefore, a continuous supply of new osteoclasts and osteoblasts from their respective progenitors in the bone marrow is essential for the origination of BMUs and their progression on the bone surface. Consequently, the balance between the supply of new cells and their life-span (reflecting the timing of their death by apoptosis) are key determinants of the number of either cell type in the BMU and the work performed by each type of cell, hence critical for the maintenance of bone homeostasis. The frequency of osteoblast apoptosis in vivo is such that changes in its timing and extent could have a significant impact in the number of osteoblasts present at the site of bone formation (22).

Osteocyte apoptosis could be of importance to the origination and/or progression of the BMU. Targeting of osteoclast precursors to a specific location on bone depends on a "homing" signal given by lining cells. Lining cells are instructed to do so by osteocytes—the only bone cells that can sense the need for remodeling at a specific time and place. This and the evidence that antiresorptive agents such as bisphosphonates, calcitonin, and estrogen affect osteoclasts not only directly but also indirectly via effects on osteoblastic cells indicates that prolongation of the life-span of osteocytes (and osteoblastic cells in general) may contribute to the reduction in the frequency of origination and/or premature termination of BMU progression that characterize the decrease in bone resorption induced by such agents. Prolongation of the bone-forming function of osteoblasts and preservation of the mechanosensory function of osteocytes by pharmacotherapeutic agents like bisphosphonates, calcitonin, and estrogen may contribute to the efficacy of these drugs in the management of disease states because of the loss of bone. The former may lead to a slow increase in trabecular thickness and the latter may contribute to their antifracture efficacy.

References

1. Parfitt. A. M. (1994) Osteonal and hemi-osteonal remodeling: the spatial and temporal framework for signal traffic in adult human bone. *J. Cell Biochem.* **55,** 273–286.
2. Pittenger, M. F., Mackay, A. M., Beck, S. C., Jaiswal, R. K., Douglas, R., Mosca, J. D., et al. (1999) Multilineage potential of adult human mesenchymal stem cells. *Science* **284,** 143–147.
3. Triffitt, J. T. (1996) The stem cell of the osteoblast, in *Principles of Bone Biology* (Bilezikian, J. P., Raisz, L. G., and Rodan, G. A., eds.), Academic, San Diego, pp. 39–50.
4. Roodman, G. D. (1996) Advances in bone biology: the osteoclast. *Endocr. Rev.* **17,** 308–332.
5. Lacey, D. L., Timms, E., Tan, H. L., Kelley, M. J., Dunstan, C. R., Burgess, T., et al. (1998) Osteoprotegerin ligand is a cytokine that regulates osteoclast differentiation and activation. *Cell* **93,** 165–176.
6. Simonet, W. S., Lacey, D. L., Dunstan, C. R., Kelley, M., Chang, M. S., Luthy, R., et al. (1997) Osteoprotegerin: a novel secreted protein involved in the regulation of bone density. *Cell* **89,** 309–319.
7. Kajkenova, O., Lecka-Czernik, B., Gubrij, I., Hauser, S. P., Takahashi, K., Parfitt, A. M., et al. (1997) Increase adipogenesis and myelopoiesis in the bone marrow of SAMP6, a murine model of defective osteoblastogenesis and low turnover osteopenia. *J. Bone Miner. Res.* **12,** 1772–1779.
8. Lecka-Cznernik, B., Gubrij, I., Moerman, E. A., Kajkenova, O., Lipschitz, D. A., Manolagas, S. C., et al. (1999) Inhibition of Osf2/Cbfa1 expression and terminal osteoblast differentiation by PPAR-gamma 2. *J. Cell Biochem.* **74,** 357–371.
9. Manolagas, S. C. and Jilka, R. L. (1995) Bone marrow, cytokines, and bone remodeling—emerging insights into the pathophysiology of osteoporosis. *N. Engl. J. Med.* **332,** 305–311.
10. Bonewald, L. F. and Dallas, S. L. (1994) Role of active and latent transforming growth factor β in bone formation. *J. Cell Biochem.* **55,** 350–357.
11. Rosen, V., Cox, K., and Hattersley, G. (1996) Bone morphogenetic proteins, in *Principles of Bone Biology* (Bilezikian, J. P., Raisz, L. G., and Rodan, G. A., eds.), Academic, San Diego, pp. 661–671.
12. Abe, E., Yamamoto, M., Taguchi, Y., Lecka-Czernik, B., O'Brien, C. A., Economides, A. N., Stahl, N., et al. (2000) Essential requirement of BMPs2/4 for both osteoblast and osteoclast formation in murine bone marrow cultures from adult mice: Antagonism by noggin. *J. Bone Miner. Res.* **15,** 663–673.
13. Ducy, P., Zhang, R., Geoffroy, V., Ridall, A. L., and Karsenty, G. (1997) Osf2/Cbfa1: a transcriptional activator of osteoblast differentiation. *Cell* **89,** 747–754.
14. Massagué, J. (1996) TGFβ signaling: receptors, transducers, and mad proteins. *Cell* **85,** 947–950.
15. Manolagas, S. C., Jilka, R. L., Bellido, T., O'Brien, C. A., and Parfitt, A. M. (1996) Interleukin-6-type cytokines and their receptors, in *Principles of Bone Biology* (Bilezikian, J. P., Raisz, L. G., and Rodan, G. A., eds.), Academic, San Diego, pp. 701–713.
16. Taguchi, Y., Yamate, T., Lin, S.-C., DeTogni, P., Nakayama, N., Abe, E., et al. (1998) Glycoprotein 130 activation stimulates murine embryonic fibroblast differentiation exclusively toward the osteoblastic lineage. *Proc. Assoc. Am. Physicians* **110,** 559–574.
17. Robey, P. G. and Bosky, A. L. (1995) The biochemistry of bone, in *Osteoporosis* (Marcus, R., Feldman, D., Bilezikian, J. P., and Kelsey, J., eds.), Academic, New York, pp. 95–183.
18. Whyte, M. P. (1994) Hypophosphatasia and the role of alkaline phosphatase in skeletal mineralization. *Endocr. Rev.* **15,** 439–461.

19. Nijweide, P. J., Burger, E. H., Klein Nulend, J., and Van der Plas, A. (1996) The osteocyte, in *Principles of Bone Biology* (Bilezikian, J. P., Raisz, L. G., and Rodan, G. A., eds.), Academic, San Diego, pp. 115–126.
20. Hughes, D. E., Dai, A., Tiffee, J. C., Li, H. H., Mundy, G. R., and Boyce, B. F. (1996) Estrogen promotes apoptosis of murine osteoclasts mediated by TGF-β. *Nature Med.* **2,** 1132–1136.
21. Jilka, R. L., Weinstein, R. S., Bellido, T., Parfitt, A. M., and Manolagas, S. C. (1998) Osteoblast programmed cell death (apoptosis): modulation by growth factors and cytokines. *J. Bone Miner. Res.* **13,** 793–802.
22. Weinstein, R. S., Jilka, R. L., Parfitt, A. M., and Manolagas, S. C. (1998) Inhibition of osteoblastogenesis and promotion of apoptosis of osteoblasts and osteocytes by glucocorticoids: potential mechanisms of their deleterious effects on bone. *J. Clin. Invest.* **102,** 274–282.

19
Animal Models

Thomas J. Lang and Charles S. Via

Animal models have been of enormous value in studying immune-mediated rheumatic diseases such as systemic lupus erythematosus (SLE) and rheumatoid arthritis (RA). Studies employing human patients are complicated by such factors as (1) variability in disease expression among patients, (2) difficulty in accurately staging disease activity, particularly for SLE patients, complicating between-patient comparisons, and (3) the effect of medications, many of which are immunosuppressive. Inasmuch as human patients exhibit considerable heterogeneity, animal models may not perfectly mimic human disease. Nevertheless, they allow insight into immune mechanisms that may be operative in a subset of patients. Murine models of human conditions also allow the testing of potential therapeutic agents in vivo to fully characterize beneficial and untoward effects prior to use in humans.

1. Animal Models of Inflammatory Arthritis

1.1. Bacterial Cell-Wall Arthritis

Bacteria have been implicated as causative agents in inflammatory forms of arthritis such as reactive arthritis, rheumatic fever, and poststreptococcal arthritis. These arthritides are not necessarily caused by the persistence of live bacteria in the joint, but rather by a pathogenic inflammatory response against bacterial antigens that persist in the joint. The rat streptococcal cell-wall-induced (SCW) model of arthritis occurs through such a mechanism.

The intraperitoneal injection of cell walls from a number of bacteria, of which SCW are the most extensively studied, results in a biphasic inflammatory polyarthritis *(1)*. After the initial intraperitoneal injection of SCW, there is an acute inflammatory arthritis lasting 1–2 wk, affecting primarily the distal joints, followed by a chronic inflammatory arthritis persisting for months with gradual resolution.

The initial joint pathology is characterized by a polymorphonuclear leukocytic exudate into the synovium and joint space *(2)*. After disease induction, cell-wall fragments can be detected in synovial monocytes, as well as in the liver, spleen, and lymph nodes *(2)*. SCW antigens may persist throughout the course of disease *(2)*. Neutrophil migration to the synovium is dependent on the upregulation of adhesion molecules in the synovial endothelium and on the expression of chemokines such as macrophage inhibitory protein-2 (MIP-2) *(3)*. Once the acute response subsides, the synovium enters a chronic inflammatory phase, which is dependent on mononuclear cells *(1)* and is characterized by synovial proliferation with periarticular bone and cartilage destruction *(4)*. The role of lymphocytes, particularly T-cells, in SCW-induced arthritis is particularly important in the chronic phase of the arthritis. Athymic nude mice treated with SCW will only develop the acute arthritis, but not the chronic phase of arthritis *(5)*. The chronic phase of the disease can also be prevented by treatment with either antilymphocyte serum or by T-cell depletion *(6,7)*, although arthritis still occurs.

A number of potential therapeutic targets have been defined in the SCW model. Anti-interleukin-1 (IL-1) and anti-tumor necrosis factor-α (TNF-α) monoclonal antibody (mAb) when given at the time of disease induction can prevent arthritis development *(3)*. Anti-transforming growth factor-β (TGF-β) mAb has been noted to prevent both the acute and chronic phases of arthritis when given intra-articularly or delivered systemically by an expression vector *(8,9)*. The use of anti-IL-4 mAb has been found to prevent disease possibly by inhibiting IL-4-dependent production of mononuclear chemoattractants such as monocyte chemoattractant protein 1 (MCP-1) *(10)*.

1.2. Adjuvant-Induced Arthritis

Similar to the SCW model, adjuvant-induced inflammatory arthritis depends on the immune recognition of bacterial antigens, which, in this case, are derived from mycobacteria. Arthritis is induced in susceptible inbred rat strains by a single intradermal injection of complete Freund's adjuvant, which contains killed mycobacterium tuberculosis. Within 9–12 d, acute periarticular inflammation develops in the distal joints characterized by a synovial mononuclear cell infiltrate *(4)*. The acute phase is followed by a chronic arthritis characterized by synovial hyperplasia and destruction of periarticular bone and cartilage similar to that seen in RA. There is also new bone formation in the periosteum analogous to that seen in spondyloarthritis. The joint disease eventually progresses to bony ankylosis. Animals may also develop extra-articular disease such as tendinitis, keratitis, uveitis, and urethritis.

Lymphocytes are critical to disease pathogenesis because nude mice, which lack T-cells, are resistant to disease induction *(11)*. In addition, the mycobacterial antigen heat-shock protein 65 (hsp65) plays a critical role. Although hsp65 does not induce arthritis when given alone or in adjuvant, it does induce resistance to arthritis *(12)*. However, Hsp65-specific T-cell clones have been identified that are arthritogenic when injected into naive recipients *(13)*. An Hsp65-specific cell line, A2b, can also recognize normal cartilage antigens and is arthritogenic when transferred into naive animals *(14)*, suggesting that adjuvant arthritis may be a model of molecular mimicry, whereby an immune response directed against a foreign antigen also recognizes a self antigen and induces disease.

Effective therapeutic interventions in adjuvant-induced arthritis have included anti-CD4 mAb treatment and deletion of CD4+ T-cells *(15)*. The frequency of disease can also be reduced by tolerizing rats with collagen *(16)* or synthetic Hsp65 *(12)*. Oral administration of mycobacteria is not effective in preventing disease *(16)*.

1.3. Type II Collagen-Induced Arthritis

Since cell-mediated and humoral immunity against collagen has been noted in RA, SLE, scleroderma, and other connective tissue diseases, collagen has been studied as a potential autoantigen in animal models of autoimmunity *(17)*. Unlike the previous two models, the native (nondenatured) type II collagen (CII) model of arthritis involves the induction of a pathologic immune response to a normal component of cartilage. It should be noted that disease is most effectively induced with collagen from a species different from the recipient (heterologous).

Induction of disease in this model is achieved by injecting native CII or specific purified peptide fragments of CII intradermally in either incomplete or complete Freund's adjuvant in susceptible rat or mouse strains *(17)*. A severe polyarthritis involving the distal joints develops within 2–3 wk in rats and 2–8 wk in mice, which is characterized by synovial pannus formation and erosion of periarticular bone and cartilage. The disease course is monophasic with a gradual resolution of inflammation resulting in joint ankylosis. The pattern of joint involvement and histologic changes are similar to RA; however, the monophasic course and lack of rheumatoid factor distinguish the model from RA. A notable extra-articular manifestation is the development of polychondritis-like lesions of the ear cartilage.

As in humans with RA, disease susceptibility of rats and mice is associated with major histocompatibility complex (MHC) molecules. The specific MHC allele that confers susceptibility is dependent on the species of CII used. Only mice with the $H-2^q$ haplotype are susceptible to chicken CII *(18)*, whereas $H-2^r$ mice are susceptible to bovine or pig CII *(19)*. Expression of the human HLA-DR1 molecule (an allele linked to RA in humans) in transgenic mice results in the induction of arthritis when human CII is used, suggesting that RA can be induced by human CII when presented by the appropriate MHC molecules *(20,21)*.

Humoral immunity in the form of anti-cartilage antibodies is the causative agent of the pathology in this model *(18)* because arthritis can be produced in naive animals by the transfer of serum from animals with CII-induced arthritis *(19)*. Abrogation of disease with anti-CD4 treatment *(17)* likely reflects the requirement for T-cell help to CII-specific B-cells in order to produce arthritogenic antibodies. Cytokines, particularly IL-1 and TNF-α, also play a role in disease pathogenesis, as anti-IL-1 monoclonal antibody and soluble IL-1 receptor antagonist both reduce disease severity *(17)*, whereas rTNF-α administration can exacerbate arthritis. Neutralization of TNF-α is not as effective as the neutralization of IL-1 in reducing disease manifestations. Endogenous IL-4 and IL-10 may play a downregulatory role as neutralization of these cytokines in vivo results in more severe arthritis *(17)*, whereas administration of rIL-4 or rIL-10 reduces the severity of joint destruction.

The administration of oral collagen to induce tolerance results in reduced T-cell responses to CII, reduced antibody production to CII, and reduced frequency of arthritis *(17)*. An hypothesized mechanism for this effect is that the T-cell response is shifted to one dominated by Th2 cytokines such as IL-4 and IL-10. If animals are tolerized by CII they are observed to produce more IL-4 and IL-10 than nontolerized animals with CII-induced arthritis *(17)*. Arthritis can also be prevented by antibody depletion of T-cells bearing T-cell receptors prominent in CII-induced arthritis such as Vβ6 and Vβ8 *(17)*. These results support a similar approach for treating human inflammatory arthritis where the dominant T-cell receptor types can be identified.

1.4. Proteoglycan-Induced Arthritis

In this model, a normal component of cartilage can induce an inflammatory arthritis. Proteoglycan in either complete or incomplete Freund's adjuvant is injected weekly for 4 wk into susceptible mouse strains and joint swelling develops by the fourth week. A chronic polyarthritis ensues with periarticular joint destruction of both peripheral and axial joints. B- and T-cells appear critical in disease pathogenesis because disease can be transferred to naive animals with B- and T-cells already sensitized to proteoglycans. Depletion of either B- or T-cells prevents the development of disease *(22)*. Depletion of CD4+ T-cells alone completely prevents disease *(23)*, whereas depletion of CD8+ T-cells alone accentuates disease suggesting a regulatory role for CD8+ T-cells.

2. Animal Models of Spondyloarthritis

2.1. Ank/Ank Mice

Spontaneous murine progressive ankylosis was first described by Sweet and Green in 1981 *(20)* and resembles human spondyloarthropathies. Animals homozygous for the autosomal recessive mutation *(ank/ank)* develop early-onset progressive joint ankylosis in the spine and peripheral joints with eventual loss of mobility and death within 6 mo. Originally, the pathology was felt to reflect solely excessive tissue calcification; however, subsequent studies in young mice demonstrated synovial inflammation with both polymorphonuclear and mononuclear cell infiltrates *(21)*. As the disease progresses, there is synovial proliferation, cartilage erosion, bony proliferation, and eventual ankylosis. The prominent inflammatory component leading to ankylosis resembles that seen in human spondyloarthritis. Radiographic studies demonstrate that ankylosis progresses from distal to proximal joints and is associated with vertebral syndesmophytes and the classic "bamboo" spine typical of ankylosing spondylitis *(24)*. Animals do not develop evidence of ocular inflammation *(25)*.

2.2. HLA-B27 Transgenic Rat Model

In humans, HLA-B27 is closely linked to spondyloarthritis. Similarly, transgenic rats expressing HLA-B27 develop a spontaneous systemic inflammatory disease with spondyloarthritis *(26)*. Initially, animals develop a diarrheal illness with a mononuclear infiltrate in the colon and small bowel *(27)*, followed several weeks later by a peripheral arthritis with histologic evidence of enthesopathy progressing to fibrosis and ankylosis *(26,28)*. Animals also develop testicular inflammation *(28)* and rarely anterior uveitis *(29)*. Skin changes include nail dystrophy, psoriasiform skin lesions, and folliculitis *(26,30)*. Intestinal flora play a critical role in this model, as germ-free animals do not develop gut inflammation or arthritis *(31)*; however, reconstitution of normal gut flora results in typical disease *(31,32)*.

Disease can be transferred to normal nontransgenic rats by bone marrow and spleen cells from transgenic rats but not by spleen cells alone *(33)*. T-Cells are critical to disease development, as athymic HLA-B27 rats do not develop disease unless T-cells from euthymic HLA-B27 rats are transferred *(34)*. The requirement for bone marrow cells in development of disease suggests that cells derived from bone marrow precursors are important in disease. Because T-cell-depleted bone marrow can still induce disease in nontransgenic animals, it is hypothesized that antigen-presenting cells expressing HLA-B27 derived from bone marrow precursors are critical.

3. Animal Models of Lupus
3.1. Spontaneous Lupus
3.1.1. New Zealand Black and New Zealand Black/New Zealand White F1

New Zealand Black (NZB) mice are an inbred strain that develop an autoimmune hemolytic anemia, thymic atrophy, and late-onset immune-complex glomerulonephritis. Mice produce autoantibodies against erythrocytes and DNA primarily of the IgM isotype *(35)*.

The first generation offspring of a cross between NZB mice (H-2^z) with New Zealand White (NZW) (H-2^d) mice, (NZB/W)F1 (H-2 $^{z/d}$) develop a lupus-like phenotype characterized by a severe immune-complex glomerulonephritis *(35)*. Female NZB/W as compared to male NZB/W are affected at an earlier age and more severely than male animals. Renal disease, initially manifested by proteinuria, occurs by 5 mo of age in females. The average life-span is approximately 8 mo in females and 13 mo in male NZB/W mice. Estrogens have been shown to be critical in the development of the more severe female phenotype by as yet unknown mechanisms *(35)*.

Renal disease is characterized by immune complex and C3 deposition in the glomeruli. The deposited antibody is a high-affinity IgG anti-dsDNA antibody complexed to nuclear antigens. Compared to NZB mice, NZB/W mice have higher titer anti-dsDNA antibody, with a greater proportion being IgG1 and IgG2.

The production of IgG anti-DNA in NZB/W mice, as opposed to primarily IgM anti-DNA in NZB mice, suggests a role for cytokine producing T-cells, which promote B-cell class switching from IgM to IgG. Supporting the role of T-cells is the observation that treatment of NZB/W mice with anti-CD4 mAb prevents autoantibody production and disease progression. However, B-cells may also be abnormal independent of T-cells. In both the NZB and NZB/W mouse, B-cells spontaneously proliferate and produce antibody in vitro and are hyperresponsive to T-cell-derived stimuli. In vivo, NZB/W B cells are activated and hypersecretory as early as 1 mo of age *(35,36)*.

Regarding the role of cytokines, neutralization of interferon-γ (IFN-γ), a Th1 cytokine, or IL-6 or IL-10, both Th2 cytokines, reduces disease severity *(37,38)*. Neutralization of IL-4 or IL-12, cytokines important in Th2 and Th1 cell development, respectively, prevents the development of IgG autoantibody, but only neutralization of IL-4 prevents nephritis *(39)*, implying that this cytokine has a key pathogenic role. Surprisingly, neutralization of both IL-4 and IL-12 simultaneously did not alter the disease. A mechanism for the prevention of disease by anti-IL-4 treatment may relate to increased TNF-α production, which has been shown to reduce disease severity when administered to NZB/W mice *(40)*.

Although maximal disease susceptibility is correlated with the heterozygous H-2$^{d/z}$ genotype, genetic loci on chromosomes 1, 4, 7, 10, and 13 have also been associated with disease development, emphasizing the contribution of multiple genes *(41)*.

3.1.2. MRL/lpr/lpr

Mice homozygous for the lymphoproliferative mutation *(lpr)* possess a functional defect in the membrane protein Fas, a member of the TNF family that mediates apoptosis when engaged by Fas ligand (FasL) expressed on the surface of another cell such as a CD8+ cytotoxic T-cell. Wild-type MRL/+ mice spontaneously produce anti-dsDNA antibodies and develop a mild immune-complex glomerulonephritis late in life. When the *lpr* mutation is bred onto the MRL background, MRL/*lpr*/*lpr* mice develop severe lymphadenopathy because of the accumulation of a double-negative CD4-CD8-Thy1+B220+ population (DN) of cells and an accelerated and more severe autoimmune disease compared to MRL/+ mice *(35)*. Disease in MRL/*lpr* mice is characterized by a proliferative nephritis, a vasculitis involving primarily the renal and coronary arteries, and a rheumatoid factor positive arthritis. Thus, the MRL/+ mouse contributes a predisposition to autoimmunity; however, the *lpr* mutation enhances and accelerates autoimmunity on the MRL/+ background.

MRL/*lpr*/*lpr* mouse develops serologic abnormalities typical of lupus, including hypergammaglobulinemia, high-titer anti-dsDNA antibody, anti-Smith antibody, hypocomplementemia, and rheumatoid factor. B-Cells exhibit polyclonal activation early in life *(35)*.

T-Cells are critical in this model because neonatal thymectomy prevents autoimmunity in MRL/*lpr*/*lpr* mice *(42)*. Additionally, chronic treatment with anti-CD4 mAb reduces autoimmune disease and lymphoproliferation *(43)*. Other studies using MHC class II-deficient MRL/*lpr*/*lpr* mice, which lack CD4+ T-cells, have found a similar reduction in autoimmune disease but no change in the degree of lymphoproliferation *(44)*. However, with long observation periods (i.e., 8–9 mo, there is eventual development of glomerulonephritis with IgG and C3 deposition. These results suggest that lymphoproliferation is CD4+ T-cell independent, that autoantibody is CD4+ dependent, and that nephritis may result from CD4-dependent and -independent mechanisms.

Normally, the presence of Fas on B- and T-cells allows for the removal of autoreactive or otherwise abnormal cells. Transgenic expression of Fas on only T-cells in MRL/*lpr*/*lpr* mice prevents the proliferation of T-cells, including the CD4–CD8–Thy1+B220+ cells, but it does not alter the production of autoantibodies or the incidence and severity of glomerulonephritis *(45)*. These data suggest that autoimmunity is not dependent on the proliferation of CD4–CD8– cells or CD4+ T-cells and that disease susceptibility may reflect an inability to eliminate autoreactive B-cells through fas-dependent mechanisms.

Regarding the role of cytokines, TNF-α, interferon-γ, and IL-1β expression have been noted to be elevated in MRL/*lpr*/*lpr* mice *(46,47)*. TNF-α administered prior to disease onset produces a rapid deterioration in renal function, especially in the presence of colony-stimulating factor-1 (CSF-1), a macrophage-stimulating cytokine that is also elevated in this animal model *(46)*. The role of interferon-γ remains controversial, because its neutralization did not produce any change in disease severity *(48)*, although the use of MRL/*lpr*/*lpr* mice homozygous for a mutation that knocks out the interferon-γ receptor results in reduced disease severity without changing the quantity of double-negative T-cells or adenopathy *(49)*.

3.1.3. BSXB Model

Initial crosses between the C57BL/6J and SB/LE mouse strains resulted in lymphoproliferation. Subsequent strict inbreeding was used to produce the final BXSB strain in which male mice develop an accelerated autoimmune disease starting at approximately 5 mo of age, whereas females are disease free until about 15 mo of age. Males develop a proliferative glomerulonephritis with heavy glomerular deposition of anti-DNA antibody, particularly of the IgG2b isotype. The male predominance is not related to male sex hormones because castrated males develop the same degree of autoimmunity (35).

The genetic loci for disease susceptibility was localized to the Y chromosome and is termed the Y-chromosome-linked autoimmune accelerator or Yaa+ locus *(50)*. The nature of the gene is not known; however, B-cells that carry the Yaa+ gene are able to produce antibodies against self antigens, whereas Yaa− B-cells do not. Both types of B-cells respond equally well to foreign antigen *(51)*.

As noted for NZB/W mice, multiple genes contribute to autoimmune disease in addition to the originally described autoimmune accelerator genes such as *lpr* and Yaa+. The expression of certain MHC alleles also influences disease expression because replacement of the normal H-2^b allele in BXSB mice with the H-2^d allele results in prolonged survival *(52)*. Other genetic loci are also linked to autoimmunity in general and to specific features such as anti-dsDNA antibody production, splenomegaly, and nephritis *(53)*.

The BXSB mouse also serves as a model of antiphospholipid syndrome. Male offspring of male BXSB and female NZW [i.e., (BXSB × NZW)F1] develop thrombocytopenia and early coronary artery disease with infarction correlated with the appearance of antiplatelet and anticardiolipin antibodies *(54,55)*. Genetic studies have identified multiple loci linked to the development of antiplatelet and anticardiolipin antibodies in addition to Yaa+ *(56)*. Several of these loci are in close proximity to the MHC locus, although the genes have not been identified.

3.1.4. Palmerston North Model

Palmerston North (PN) mice spontaneously develop an autoimmune disease characterized by hypergammaglobulinemia, anti-dsDNA antibodies, glomerulonephritis, polyarteritis, and early mortality *(57)*. Female F1 offspring produced by breeding the Palmerston North × NZB develop more severe disease with vasculitis, renal disease, and lymphoma. PN mice express a broad variety of autoantibodies against dsDNA, cardiolipin, erythrocytes, ribonucleoprotein (RNP), Smith antigen, and other phospholipids *(58)*. The IgA isotype is prominent among the anti-DNA antibodies and also among antibodies specific for IgG.

3.2. Induced Lupus

3.2.1. 16/6 Idiotype Administration

Idiotypes define a collection of immunoglobulin heavy- and light-chain variable-region structures that participate in antigen recognition and can be recognized specifically by anti-idiotype antibody. Certain idiotypes are shared among autoantibodies from different SLE patients despite having different antigenic specificities. One such idiotype is termed the 16/6 idiotype. When these antibodies are injected into mice, there is a resultant lupus-like disease. Mice are immunized with anti-DNA antibody of the 16/6 idiotype followed in 3 wk by a repeat injection. These animals subsequently develop high-titer anti-16/6 idiotype, anti-dsDNA, anti-RNP, anti-Ro, anti-La, and anti-Sm antibody. The spectrum of autoantibodies is believed to be the result of the production of anti-anti-16/6 antibodies, which also have the characteristic of binding to autoantigens. Clinically, these mice develop lupus-like disease with prominent immune-complex glomerulonephritis.

CD4+ T-cell depletion prior to, but not after, 16/6 administration inhibits disease *(59)*. CD8+ T-cell depletion before or after immunization increases disease severity, suggesting a regulatory role for CD8+ T-cells *(59)*. IL-1 and TNF-α production are both prominent and correlate with disease activity. IL-2 and IFN-γ are increased 2–4 mo after disease induction. Methotrexate treatment normalizes both IL-1 and TNF-α levels and reduces the frequency and severity of disease *(59)*.

3.2.2. Parent-into-F1 Chronic Graft-Versus-Host Disease

The injection of homozygous parental T-cells into normal unirradiated F1 mice results in either an acute suppressive graft-versus-host disease (GVHD) or a chronic lupus-like autoimmune GVHD. Chronic GVHD is characterized by high serum levels of IgG autoantibodies (antinuclear, anti-double-stranded DNA, antihistone and anti-RBC [red blood cell] antibodies) characteristic of human SLE *(60–62)*. Ig is deposited along the dermal basement membrane *(63)* and immune-complex formation occurs with deposition in the renal glomeruli and death because of renal failure *(63,64)*. Acute GVHD is characterized initially by a reduction in host lymphocytes, demonstrable antihost cytotoxic T-cell activity, and immunodeficiency; however, long-term survivors develop a scleroderma-like disease (*see* Subheading ?.).

Chronic GVHD can be induced by the intravenous injection of CD8+ T-cell-depleted donor T-cells into an F1 mouse differing from the donor at least at the MHC class II loci. Alternatively, the injection of unfractionated splenocytes from DBA/2 mice into (C57Bl/6 × DBA/2)F1 mice will also result in chronic GVHD. The common feature of chronic GVHD induction is the selective activation of donor CD4+ T-cells (and not CD8+ T-cells) following recognition of host alloantigens. If both donor CD4+ and CD8+ T-cells are activated, as would occur with unfractionated splenocytes injected into a fully MHC class I + II disparate F1, acute GVHD results. Chronic GVHD occurring in the DBA-into-F1 model is related to the observation that the anti-F1 precursor cytotoxic lymphocyte (CTL) frequency of DBA/2 mice is approximately 10-fold less than that of mice from the C57Bl/6 background, and as a result, CD8 activation is suboptimal.

The initiation of acute and chronic GVHD has several similarities *(65,66)* characterized by (1) lymphoproliferative changes, with an increase in total spleen cells, host B-cells, and host T-cells and (2) B-cell activation as measured by increased MHC class II expression and autoantibody production. These changes correlate with the engraftment and expansion of donor CD4+ T-cells in both models.

At 1 wk of disease, acute and chronic GVHD begin to diverge. In acute GVHD, significant expansion of donor CD8+ T-cells has occurred and antihost CTL are readily detectable. As a result, host lymphocytes, including autoantibody secreting B-cells are eliminated, serum autoantibody levels are reduced, and the characteristic profound immunodeficiency develops. Interestingly, the surviving B-cells remain activated until their elimination. By contrast, in chronic GVHD, there is no significant expansion of donor CD8+ T-cells, no development of anti-host CTL *(67)*, and, consequently, no reduction in the lymphoproliferation and B-cell stimulation begun earlier. During the first 2 wk of GVHD, both forms of GVHD exhibit an initial (d 1–3) increase in IL-2 production *(65)* followed by increased B-cell-stimulatory cytokines (IL-4 and IL-10) *(66)* beginning at d 4 of GVHD. Importantly, an increase in the Th1 cytokine, IFN-γ, is seen beginning at 5–7 d of disease only for acute GVHD. These data suggest that IFN-γ and donor CD8+ CTL play a major role in mediating acute GVHD and that in their absence, chronic GVHD, and lupus-like autoimmunity ensue. Thus, in this model, lupus-like disease is clearly T-cell driven and results from (1) donor CD4+ T-cell production of Th2 cytokines, which activate autoreactive host B-cells and drive autoantibody production and (2) an absence of donor CD8+ T-cell activation, which would otherwise regulate or eliminate autoreactive B-cells.

4. Animal Models of Vasculitis

Animal models of vasculitis as with other autoimmune diseases fail to mimic all features of a particular human form of vasculitis. Several animal models of vasculitis and what they suggest about human vasculitis are discussed in the following subsections.

4.1. Mercuric-Chloride-Induced Vasculitis

The exposure of Brown Norway Rats to mercuric chloride causes T-cell-dependent polyclonal B-cell activation with the production of multiple autoantibodies, including anti-DNA, anticollagen, and antiglomerular basement membrane antibody *(68)*. Animals also develop multiorgan necrotizing vasculitis of small to medium-sized vessels, particularly in the gastrointestinal tract, similar to that seen in polyarteritis nodosa. Animals produce antimyeloperoxidase (MPO) antibody which is responsible for the p-ANCA pattern in human ANCA-associated vasculitis. These antibodies do not appear pathogenic because transfer of sera to normal Brown Norway rats does not transfer disease.

4.2. Spontaneous Murine Vasculitis

MRL/*lpr/lpr* mice develop a small to medium vessel-necrotizing vasculitis, affecting the kidney and gallbladder primarily. Perivascular infiltrates initially consist of neutrophils, with lymphocytes eventually predominating. Approximately 20% of females are ANCA positive. A second mouse strain, SCG/Kj mice, derived from BXSB × MRL/*lpr/lpr* crosses, spontaneously develop rapidly progressive crescentic glomerulonephritis and necrotizing vasculitis *(69)*. These mice also have antimyeloperoxidase antibody, although, again, there is no evidence that the antibody is pathogenic. Palmerston North mice develop a multiorgan non-necrotizing vasculitis involving the small and medium-size arteries and veins *(70)*.

4.3. Myeloperoxidase Immunization

In contrast to the previous models, immunization of Brown Norway rats myeloperoxidase (MPO) results in pathogenic anti-MPO antibody *(68)*. A necrotizing crescentic glomerulonephritis is observed in the kidneys of anti-MPO antibody-producing animals following renal perfusion with MPO, peroxide, and products of activated neutrophils (i.e., elastase and proteinase 3 among others). IgG and C3 are deposited in the glomerular basement membrane. These experiments demonstrate that antibody–antigen complexes composed of MPO and anti-MPO antibody can induce renal damage.

4.4. Experimental ANCA-Associated Vasculitis

A model of ANCA-associated vasculitis has been developed based on the theory that during a viral or bacterial infection, anti-idiotypic antibody may induce pathology analogous to that seen in the 16/6 idiotype model of lupus *(68)*. Immunization of normal Balb/c mice with purified anti-proteinase-3 IgG antibody, the antibody that produces the c-ANCA pattern, induces an idiotypic antibody response that recognizes proteinase 3 as well as MPO and other undefined endothelial surface antigens. These antibodies can also activate neutrophils. As yet, there is no evidence supporting the role of anti-idiotype antibodies as causative agents in Wegener's granulomatosis or any other ANCA-associated human vasculitis.

5. Animal Models of Scleroderma
5.1. Tight Skin Mouse Model

Two spontaneous models of systemic sclerosis are the tight skin 1 (tsk 1) and the tight skin 2 (tsk 2) mouse. Both are autosomal dominant mutations in which homozygotes die *in utero*. Tsk 1 arose spontaneously, whereas tsk 2 was induced by a chemical mutagenesis. Pathology in the tsk1 mutant is characterized by cutaneous and visceral fibrosis involving the lungs and heart, similar to that seen in systemic sclerosis. Biochemically, there is increased production of $\alpha1(I)$, $\alpha2(I)$, and $\alpha1(III)$ procollagens, as well as type VI collagen *(71)*. Both models develop fibrosis within the first month of life, with progression of disease throughout the shortened life-span of the animal *(72)*. Histologically, the skin shows densely packed connective tissue in the dermis, which in the case of tsk 2 is associated with a mononuclear infiltrate. The increased connective tissue is made up predominantly of collagen with a predominant increase in type I procollagen. The tsk 2 mutation has been localized to chromosome 1, whereas the tsk 1 mutation is mapped to chromosome 2. Tsk 1 is associated with a duplication within the gene for fibrillin, which results in an altered protein product.

Tsk animals produce autoantibodies such as ANA, antitopoisomerase, anti-RNA polymerase, and antimitochondrial antibodies. ANA and antitopoisomerase are prominent in old mice *(73)*. These antibodies do not appear pathogenic because tsk animals without B-cells still develop disease. Tsk 1 animals that lack CD4+ T-cells show reduced dermal fibrosis. Tsk 1 CD4+ T-cells transferred to normal animals, though, do not cause disease. IL-4 has been implicated in disease pathogenesis, because it can stimulate collagen synthesis as well as fibroblast proliferation in normal mice. If anti-IL4 is given to tsk 1 animals starting immediately after birth, mice do not develop dermal fibrosis but still develop lung pathology *(74)*.

5.2. Acute Murine GVHD (Parent-into-F1)

It has been observed that some bone-marrow-transplant recipients, particularly those who developed acute GVHD, develop an autoimmune disorder termed chronic GVHD, which resembles scleroderma and has features of Sjögren's syndrome with interstitial lung disease *(75,76)*. Although this disorder is not identical to human scleroderma, particularly with regard to the autoantibody profile and collagen-deposition patterns, it supports the idea that chimerism or the persistence of allogeneic T-cells in an unirradiated recipient can mediate autoimmune diseases such as scleroderma and Sjögren's syndrome. In murine models, bone marrow transplantation across minor histocompatibility differences in irradiated recipients results in sclerodermatous features such as dermal T-cell infiltration and collagen deposition. Alloreactive T-cell clones that produce cytokines that promote collagen deposition and fibroblast proliferation have been isolated *(77,78)*. Although these murine models mimic bone marrow transplantation from identical donor/recipient pairs and provide an approach to study in vivo conditions that lead to altered collagen deposition, it is not clear that they are models for other aspects of scleroderma.

Sclerodermatous skin lesions also develop following the injection of immunologically competent lymphocytes into tolerant rats. Following an acute dermal infiltration consistent with acute GVHD, surviving rats developed epidermal atrophy, collagenization of the dermis, and disappearance of skin appendages *(79)*. More recently, using the parent-into-F1 model of acute GVHD, it was shown that mice that do not succumb to disease, go on to develop scleroderma-like skin lesions, as well as a chronic progressive polyarthritis (RA-like), Sjögren-like salivary gland lesions, and lesions resembling sclerosing cholangitis. These mice develop positive ANA (100%), anti-dsDNA (50%), antihistone (25%), and low-titer anti-snRNP (35%) antibodies *(80,81)*. Importantly, the scleroderma-like changes require 9–12 mo to develop.

6. Animal Models of Myositis

Prior viral infections, such as influenza and adenovirus, have been associated with the occurrence of myositis in humans. Likewise, animal models of myositis have been developed in which the causative agent is either Coxsackie B, encephalomyocarditis virus, or picornaviruses *(82,83)*. Mice infected with these viruses develop muscle weakness, which is monophasic in character and is associated with elevation of serum muscle enzymes and histologic evidence of muscle inflammation. T-Cells appear important in the development of prolonged weakness because athymic mice infected with Coxsackie B develop only an acute transient episode of myositis followed by full recovery *(84)*.

7. Knockout Mice as Models of Autoimmunity

Mice genetically engineered with mutations rendering specific cytokines inactive provide insight into the role of cytokines in autoimmune disease. Several knockout mice produced in nonautoimmune mouse strains have been noted to develop autoimmune disease. The IL-2 knockout mouse (IL-2$^{-/-}$) develops an ulcerative colitis-like disorder and hemolytic anemia *(85)* associated with a polyclonal expansion of B- and T-cells. Administration of rIL-2 to these mice prevents B- and T-cell expansion and autoimmune manifestations *(85)*. IL-2 is believed to be critical in the development of regulatory T-cells because the transfer of lymphocytes from IL-2-treated IL-2$^{-/-}$ to untreated IL-2$^{-/-}$ prevents disease development.

The TGF-β knockout mice develop autoimmune features of SLE and Sjögren's syndrome. There is a massive infiltration of lymphocytes and monocytes into the lungs, liver, heart, salivary glands, and intestinal tract *(86)* with production of serum autoantibodies to dsDNA, ssDNA, and Sm antigen, with associated glomerular immunoglobulin deposits *(87)*. Similarly, animals in which the C1q gene is knocked out also develop a SLE-like disease with autoantibodies and glomerulonephritis. There is accumulation of apoptotic cells, which may be a source of autoantigen *(88)*.

References

1. Cromartie, J. G., Craddock, J. H., Schwab, S. K., Anderle, C., and Yang, C. (1977) Arthritis in rats after systemic injection of streptococcal cells or cell walls. *J. Exp. Med.* **146**, 1585–1595.

2. Allen, J. B., Malone, D. G., Wahl, S. M., Calandra, G. B., and Wilder, R. L. (1985) Role of the thymus in streptococcal cell wall-induced arthritis and hepatic granuloma formation. *J. Clin. Invest.* **76,** 1042–1056.
3. Schimmer, R. C., Schrier, D. J., Flory, C. M., Dykens, J., Tung, D. K.-L, Jacobson, P. B., et al. (1997) Streptococcal cell wall-induced arthritis: requirements for neutrophils, P-selectin, intercellular adhesion molecule-1, and macrophage-inflammatory protein-2. *J. Immunol.* **159,** 4103–4108.
4. Sokoloff, L. (1984) Animal models of rheumatoid arthritis. *Int. Rev. Exp. Pathol.* **26,** 107–145.
5. Wilder, R. L., Allen, J. B., and Hansen, C. (1987) Thymus-dependent and -independent regulation of Ia antigen expression in situ by cells in synovium of rats with streptococcal cell wall-induced arthritis. Differences in site and intensity of expression in euthymic, athymic, and cyclosporin A-treated LEW and F344 rats. *J. Clin. Invest.* **79,** 1160–1171.
6. Lens, J. W., Van den Berg, W. B., Van de Putte, L. B. A., Berden, J. H. M., and Lems, S. P. M. (1984) Flare-up of antigen-induced arthritis in mice after challenge with intravenous antigen: effects of pre-treatment with cobra venom factor and anti-lymphocyte serum. *Clin. Exp. Immunol.* **57,** 520–527.
7. Van den Broek, M. F., Van Bruggen, M. C. J., Stimpson, S. A., and Severijen, A. J. (1990) Flare-up reaction of streptococcal cell wall induced arthritis in Lewis and F344 rats: the role of T lymphocytes. *Clin. Exp. Immunol.* **79,** 297–303.
8. Wahl, S. M., Allen, J. B., Costa, G. L., Wong, H. L., and Dasch, J. R. (1993) Reversal of acute and chronic synovial inflammation by anti-transforming growth factor beta. *J. Exp. Med.* **177,** 225–230.
9. Song, X.-Y., Gu, M. L., Jin, W.-W., Klinman, D. M., and Wahl, S. M. (1998) Plasmid DNA encoding transforming growth factor-beta1 suppresses chronic disease in a streptococcal cell wall-induced arthritis model. *J. Clin. Invest.* **101,** 2615–2621.
10. Schimmer, R. C., Schrier, D. J., Flory, C. M., Laemont, K. D., Tung, D., Metz, A. L., et al. (1998) Streptococcal cell wall-induced arthritis: requirements for IL-4, IL-10, IFN-gamma, and monocyte chemoattractant protein-1. *J. Immunol.* **160,** 1466–1471.
11. Kohashi, O., Aihara, K., Ozawa, A., Kotani, S., and Azuma, I. (1982) New model of a synthetic adjuvant, *N*-acetylmuramyl-L-alanyl-D-isoglutamine-induced arthritis. *Lab. Invest.* **47,** 27–35.
12. Billingham, M., Carney, S., Butler, R., and Colston, M. (1990) A mycobacterial 65-kD heat shock protein induces antigen-specific suppression of adjuvant arthritis, but is not itself arthritogenic. *J. Exp. Med.* **171,** 339–344.
13. Holoshitz, J., Naparsted, Y., Ben-Nun, A., and Cohen, I. (1983) Lines of T-lymphocyte induce or vaccinate against autoimmune disease. *Science* **217,** 56–58.
14. van Eden, W., Holoshitz, J., and Nevo, A. (1985) Arthritis induced by a T-lymphocyte clone that responds to mycobacterium tuberculosis and to cartilage proteoglycans. *Proc. Natl. Acad. Sci. USA* **82,** 5117–5120.
15. Pelegri, C., Morante, M. P., Castellote, C., Franch, A., and Castell, M. (1996) Treatment with an anti-CD4 monoclonal antibody strongly ameliorates established rat adjuvant arthritis. *Clin. Exp. Immunol.* **103,** 273–278.
16. Zhang, A., Lee, C., Lider, O., and Weiner, H. (1990) Suppression of adjuvant arthritis in Lewis rats by oral administration of type II collagen. *J. Immunol.* **145,** 2489–2493.
17. Myers, L. K., Rosloniec, E. F., Cremer, M. A., and Kang, A. H. (1997) Collagen-induced arthritis, an animal model of autoimmunity. *Life Sci.* **61,** 1861–1878.
18. Stuart, J. M., Tomoda, K., Yoo, T. J., Townes, A. S., and Kang, A. H. (1983) Serum transfer of collagen-induced arthritis. *Arthritis Rheum.* **26,** 1237–1244.
19. Watson, W. C., Brown, P. S., Pitcock, J. A., and Townes, A. S. (1987) Passive transfer studies with type II collagen antibody in B10.D2/old and new line and C57Bl/6 normal and beige (Chediak-Higashi) strains: evidence of important roles for C5 and multiple inflammatory cell types in the development of erosive arthritis. *Arthritis Rheum.* **30,** 460–465.

20. Sweet, H. O. and Green, M. C. (1981) Progressive ankylosis, a new skeletal mutation in the mouse. *J. Heredity* **72**, 87–93.
21. Hakim, F. T., Crawley, R., Brown, K. S., Evans, E. D., Harne, L., and Oppenheim, J. J. (1984) Hereditary joint disorder in progressive ankylosis *(ank/ank)* mice: I. Association of calcium hydroxyapatite deposition with inflammatory arthropathy. *Arthritis Rheum.* **27**, 1411–1420.
22. Mikecz, K., Glant, T. T., Buzas, E., and Poole, A. R. (1990) Proteoglycan-induced polyarthritis and spondylitis adoptively transferred to naive (nonimmunized) BALB/c mice. *Arthritis Rheum.* **33**, 866–876.
23. Banerjee, S., Webber, C., and Poole, A. R. (1992) The induction of arthritis in mice by the cartilage proteoglycan aggrecan: roles of CD4+ and CD8+ T cells. *Cell. Immunol.* **144**, 347–357.
24. Mahowald, M. L., Krug, H., and Taurog, J. (1988) Progressive ankylosis in mice. An animal model of spondyloarthropathy. *Arthritis Rheum.* **31**, 1390–1399.
25. Mahowald, M. H., Krug, H., and Halverson, P. (1989) Progressive ankylosis *(ank/ank)* in mice. An animal model of spondyloarthropathy. II. Light and electron microscopy findings. *J. Rheum.* **16**, 60–66.
26. Hammer, R. E., Maika, S. D., Richardson, J. A., Tang, J.-P., and Taurog, J. (1990) Spontaneous inflammatory disease in transgenic rats expressing HLA-B27 and human beta2-m: an animal model of HLA-B27 associated human disorders. *Cell* **63**, 1099–1112.
27. Aiko, S. and Grisham, M. B. (1995) Spontaneous inflammation and nitric oxide metabolism in HLA-B27 transgenic rats. *Gastroenterology* **109**, 142–150.
28. Taurog, J., Maika, S. D., Simmons, W. A., Breban, M., and Hammer, R. E. (1993) Susceptibility to inflammatory disease in HLA-B27 transgenic rat lines correlates with the level of B27 expression. *J. Immunol.* **150**, 4168–4178.
29. Baggia, S., Lyons, J. L., Angell, E., Barkhuizen, A., Han, Y. B., and Planck, S. R. (1997) A novel model of bacterially induced acute anterior uveitis in rats and lack of effect of HLA-B27 expression. *J. Invest. Med.* **45**, 295–301.
30. Yanagisawa, H., Hammer, R. E., Taurog, J. D., and Richardson, A. (1995) Characterization of psoriasiform and alopecic skin lesions in HLA-B27 transgenic rats. *Am. J. Pathol.* **147**, 955–964.
31. Taurog, J. D., Richardson, J. A., Croft, J. T., Simmons, W. A., Zhou, M., Fernandez-Sueiro, J. L., et al. (1994) The germ free state prevents development of gut and joint inflammatory disease in HLA-B27 transgenic rats. *J. Exp. Med.* **180**, 2359–2364.
32. Rath, H. C., Herfarth, H. H., Ikeda, J. S., Grenther, W. B., Hamm, T. E., Balish, E., et al. (1996) Normal luminal bacteria especially bacteroides species, mediate chronic colonic, gastric, systemic inflammation in HLA-B27/hbeta2m transgenic rats. *J. Clin. Invest.* **98**, 945–953.
33. Breban, M., Hammer, R. E., Richardson, J. A., and Taurog, J. D. (1993) Transfer of the inflammatory disease on HLA-B27 transgenic rats by bone marrow engraftment. *J. Exp. Med.* **178**, 1606–1616.
34. Breban, M., Fernandez-Sueiro, J. L., Simmons, W. A., Hadavand, R., Maika, S. D., Hammer, R. E., et al. (1996) T cells but not thymic exposure to HLA-B27 are required for the inflammatory disease of HLA-B27 transgenic rats. *J. Immunol.* **156**, 794–803.
35. Theofilopoulos, A. N. and Dixon, F. J. (1985) Murine models of systemic lupus erythematosus. *Adv. Immunol.* **37**, 269–390.
36. Theofilpoulos, A. N., Shawler, D. L., Eisenberg, R. A., and Dixon, F. J. (1980) Splenic immunoglobulin secreting cells and their regulation in autoimmune mice. *J. Exp. Med.* **151**, 446–466.
37. Jacob, C. O., Van der Meide, P. H., and McDevitt, H. O. (1987) In vivo treatment of (NZB × NZW)F1 lupus-like nephritis with monoclonal antibody to interferon-gamma. *J. Exp. Med.* **166**, 798–803.
38. Ishida, H., Muchamuel, T., Sakaguchi, S., Andrade, S., Menon, S., and Howard, M. (1994) Continuous administration of anti-interleukin 10 antibodies delays onset of autoimmunity in NZB/W F1 mice. *J. Exp. Med.* **179**, 305–310.

39. Nakajima, A., Hirose, S., Yagita, H., and Okumura, K. (1997) Roles of IL-4 and IL-12 in the development of lupus in NZB/W F1 mice. *J. Immunol.* **158**, 1466–1472.
40. Jacob, C.O. and McDevitt, H.O. (1988) Tumor necrosis factor-α in murine autoimmune "lupus" nephritis. *Nature* **331**, 356–358.
41. Morel, L., Rudofsky, U. H., Longmate, J. A., Schiffenbauer, J., and Wakeland, E. K. (1994) Polygenic control of susceptibility to murine systemic lupus erythematosus. *Immunity* **1**, 219–229.
42. Theofilopoulos, A. N., Balderas, R. S., Shawler, D. L., Lee, S., and Dixon, F. J. (1980) Influence of thymic genotype on the systemic lupus erythematosus-like disease and T cell proliferation of MRL/lpr/lpr mice. *J. Exp. Med.* **153**, 1405–1414.
43. Santoro, T. J., Portanova, J. P., and Kotzin, B. L. (1988) The contribution of L3T4+ T cells to lymphoproliferation and autoantibody production in MRL-lpr/lpr mice. *J. Exp. Med.* **167**, 1713–1718.
44. Chesnutt, M. S., Finck, B. S., Killeen, N., Connolly, M. K., Goodman, H., and Wofsy, D. (1998) Enhanced lymphoproliferation and diminished autoimmunity in CD4-deficient MRL/lpr mice. *Clin. Immunol. Immunopathol.* **87**, 23–32.
45. Fukuyama, H., Adachi, M., Suematsu, S., Miwa, K., Suda, T., Yoshida, N., et al. (1998) Transgenic expression of fas in T cells blocks lymphoproliferation but not autoimmune disease in MRL/lpr mice. *J. Immunol.* **160**, 3805–3811.
46. Boswell, J. M., Yui, M. A., Burt, D. W., and Kelley, V. E. (1988) Increased tumor necrosis factor and IL-1β expression in the kidneys of mice with lupus nephritis. *J. Immunol.* **141**, 3050–3058.
47. Takahashi, S., Fossati, L., Iwamoto, M., Merino, R., Motta, R., Kobayakawa, T., et al. (1996) Imbalance towards Th1 predominance is associated with acceleration of lupus-like autoimmune syndrome in MRL mice. *J. Clin. Invest.* **97**, 1597–1604.
48. Nicoletti, F., Meroni, P., DiMarco, R., Barcellini, W., Borghi, M. O., Gariglio, M., et al. (1992) In vivo treatment with monoclonal antibody to interferon-gamma neither affects the survival nor the incidence of lupus-nephritis in the MRL/*lpr-lpr* mouse. *Immunopharmacology* **24**, 11–20.
49. Haas, C., Ryffel, B., and Hir, M. L. (1997) IFN-g is essential for the development of autoimmune glomerulonephritis in MRL/lpr mice. *J. Immunol.* **158**, 5484–5491.
50. Hudgins, C. C., Steinberg, R. T., Klinman, D. M., Reeves, M. J. P., and Steinberg, A. D. (1985) Studies of consomic mice bearing the Y chromosome of the BXSB mouse. *J. Immunol.* **134**, 3849–3854.
51. Merino, R., Fossati, L., Lacour, M., and Izui, S. (1991) Selective autoantibody production by Yaa+ B cells in autoimmune Yaa+-Yaa− bone marrow chimeric mice. *J. Exp. Med.* **174**, 1023–1029.
52. Merino, R., Iwamoto, M., Gershwin, M. E., and Izui, S. (1994) The Yaa gene abrogates the major histocompatibility complex association of murine lupus in (NZB × BXSB)F1 hybrid mice. *J. Clin. Invest.* **94**, 521–530.
53. Hogarth, M. B., Slingsby, J. H., Allen, P. J., Thompson, E. M., Chandler, P., Davies, K. A., et al. (1998) Multiple lupus susceptibility loci map to chromosome 1 in BXSB mice. *J. Immunol.* **161**, 2753–2761.
54. Hang, L. M., Izui, S., and Dixon, F. (1981) (NZW × BXSB)F1 hybrid: a model of acute lupus and coronary vascular disease with myocardial infarction. *J. Exp. Med.* **154**, 216–221.
55. Oyaizu, N., Yasumizu, R., Miyama-Inaba, M., Nomura, S., Yoshida, H., Miyawaki, S., et al. (1988) (NZW × BXSB) F1 mouse: a new model of idiopathic thrombocytopenic purpura. *J. Exp. Med.* **167**, 2017–2022.
56. Ida, A., Hirose, S., Hamano, Y., Kodera, S., Jiang, Y., Abe, M., et al. (1998) Multigenic control of lupus-associated antiphospholipid syndrome in a model of (NZW × BXSB) F1 mice. *Eur. J. Immunol.* **28**, 2694–2703.
57. Walker, S. E., Gray, R. H., Fulton, M., and Wigley, R. D. (1978) Palmerston North mice: a new animal model of systemic lupus erythematosus. *J. Lab. Clin. Med.* **92**, 932–945.

58. Handwerger, B. S., Storrer, C. E., Wasson, C. S., Movafagh, F., and Reichlin, M. (1999) Further characterization of the autoantibody response of Palmerston North mice. *J. Clin. Immunol.* **19**, 45–57.
59. Dayan, M., Segal, R., and Mozes, E. (1997) Cytokine manipulation by methotrexate treatment in murine experimental systemic lupus erythematosus. *J. Rheum.* **24**, 1075–1082.
60. Van Rappard-Van Der Veen, F. M., Kiessel, U., Poels, L., Schuler, W., Melief, C. J. M., Landegent, J., and Gleichmann, E. (1984) Further evidence against random polyclonal antibody formation in mice with lupus-like graft-vs-host disease. *J. Immunol.* **132**, 1814–1820.
61. Gleichmann, E., van Elven, E. H., and Van Der Veen, P. J. W. (1982) A systemic lupus erythematosus (SLE)-like disease in mice induced by abnormal T-B cell cooperation. Preferential formation of autoantibodies characteristic of SLE. *Eur. J. Immunol.* **12**, 152–160.
62. Portanova, J. P., Claman, H. N., and Kotzin, B. L. (1985) Autoimmunization in murine graft-vs-host disease: I. Selective production of autoantibodies to histones and DNA. *J. Immunol.* **135**, 3850–3858.
63. van Elven, E. H., Agterberg, J., Sadel, S., and Gleichmann, E. (1981) Diseases caused by reactions of T lymphocytes to incompatible structures of the major histocompatibility complex: II. Autoantibodies deposited along the basement membrane of skin and their relationship to immune-complex glomerulonephritis. *J. Immunol.* **126**, 1684–1690.
64. Rolink, A. G., Gleichmann, H., and Gleichmann, E. (1983) Diseases caused by reaction of T lymphocytes to incompatible structures of the major histocompatibility complex: VII. Immune complex glomerulonephritis. *J. Immunol.* **130**, 209–216.
65. Via, C. S. (1991) Kinetics of T cell activation in acute and chronic forms of murine graft-versus-host disease. *J. Immunol.* **146**, 2603–2609.
66. Rus, V., Svetic, A., Nguyen, P., Gause, W., and Via, C. S. (1995) Kinetics of Th1 and Th2 cytokine production during the early course of acute and chronic murine graft-versus-host disease. *J. Immunol.* **155**, 2396–2406.
67. Via, C. S. and Shearer, G. M. (1988) T-cell interactions in autoimmunity: insights from a murine model of graft-versus-host disease. *Immunol. Today* **9**, 207–210.
68. Heeringa, P., Brouwer, E., Tervaert, J. W. C., Weening, J. J., and Kallenberg, C. G. M. (1998) Animal models of anti-neutrophil cytoplasmic antibody associated vasculitis. *Kidney Int.* **53**, 253–263.
69. Kinjoh, K., Kyogoku, M., and Good, R. A. (1993) Genetic selection for crescent formation yields mouse strain with rapidly progressive glomerulonephritis and small vessel vasculitis. *Proc. Natl. Acad. Sci. USA* **90**, 3413–3417.
70. Luzina, I. G., Knitzer, R. H., Atamas, S. P., Gause, W. C., Papadimitriou, J. C., Sztein, M. B., et al. (1999) Vasculitis in the Palmerston North mouse model of lupus. *Arthritis Rheum.* **42**, 561–568.
71. Jimenez, S. A. and Christner, P. J. (1994) Animal models of systemic sclerosis. *Clin. Dermatol.* **12**, 425–436.
72. Christner, P. J., Peters, J., Hawkins, D., Siracusa, L. D., and Jimenez, S. A. (1995) The tight skin 2 mouse. An animal model of scleroderma displaying cutaneous fibrosis and mononuclear infiltration. *Arthritis Rheum.* **38**, 1791–1798.
73. Bocchieri, M. H., Henricksen, P. D., Kasturi, K. N., Muryoi, T., Bona, C. A., and Jimenez, S. A. (1991) Evidence for autoimmunity in the tight skin mouse model of systemic sclerosis. *Arthritis Rheum.* **34**, 599–605.
74. Ong, C., Wong, C., Roberts, C. R., Teh, H. S., and Jirik, F. R. (1998) Anti-IL-4 treatment prevents dermal collagen deposition in the tight skin mouse model of scleroderma. *Eur. J. Immunol.* **28**, 2619–2629.
75. Shulman, H. M., Sullivan, K. M., Weiden, P. L., McDonald, G. B., Striker, G. E., Sale, G. E., et al. (1980) Chronic graft-versus-host syndrome in man. A long-term clinicopathologic study of 20 Seattle patients. *Am. J. Med.* **69**, 204–217.

76. Lawley, T. J., Peck, G. L., Moutsopoulos, H. M., Gratwohl, A. A., and Deisseroth, A. B. (1977) Scleroderma, Sjogren-like syndrome, and chronic graft-versus-host disease. *Ann. Intern. Med.* **87,** 707–709.
77. Jaffee, B. D. and Claman, H. N. (1983) Chronic graft-versus-host disease (GVHD) as a model for scleroderma. I. Description of model systems. *Cell. Immunol.* **77,** 1–12.
78. Declerck, Y., Draper, V., and Parkman, R. (1986) Clonal analysis of murine graft-vs-host disease. II. Leukokines that stimulate fibroblast proliferation and collagen synthesis in graft-vs-host disease. *J. Immunol.* **136,** 3549–3552.
79. Stastny, P., Stembridge, V. A., Vischer, T., and Ziff, M. (1965) Homologous disease in the adult rat, a model for autoimmune disease. II. Findings in the joints, heart, and other tissues. *J. Exp. Med.* **122,** 681–692.
80. Gelpi, C., Martinez, M. A., Vidal, S., Targoff, I. N., and Rodriguez-Sanchez, J. L. (1994) Autoantibodies to a transfer RNA-associated protein in a murine model of chronic graft versus host disease. *J. Immunol.* **152,** 1989–1999.
81. Pals, S. T., Radaszkiewicz, T., Roozendaal, L., and Gleichmann, E. (1985) Chronic progressive polyarthritis and other symptoms of collagen vascular disease induced by graft-vs-host reaction. *J. Immunol.* **134,** 1475–1482.
82. Ytterberg, S. and Schnitzer, T. (1988) Coxsackievirus B1-induced murine polymyositis, in *CRC Handbood of Animal Models for the Rheumatic Diseases* (Greenwald, E. and Diamond, H., eds.), CRC, Boca Raton, pp. 147–156.
83. Cronin, M., Love, L., and Miller, F. (1988) The natural history of encephalomyocarditis virus-induced myositis and myocarditis in mice. *J. Exp. Med.* **168,** 1639–1648.
84. Ytterberg, S., Mahowald, M., and Messner, R. (1987) Coxsackievirus B1-induced polymyositis. Lack of disease in *nu/nu* mice. *J. Clin. Invest.* **80,** 499–506.
85. Klebb, G., Autenrieth, I. B., Haber, H., Gillert, E., Sadlack, B., Smith, K. A., et al. (1996) Interleukin-2 is indispensable for development of immunological tolerance. *Clin. Immunol. Immunopathol.* **81,** 282–286.
86. Shull, M. M., Ormsby, I., Kier, A. B., Pawlowski, S., Diebold, R., Yin, M., et al. (1992) Targeted disruption of the mouse TGF-β1 gene results in multifocal inflammatory disease. *Nature* **359,** 693–699.
87. Dang, H., Geiser, A. G., Letterio, J. J., Nakabayashi, T., Kong, L., Fernandes, G., et al. (1995) SLE-like autoantibodies and Sjögren's syndrome-like lymphoproliferation in TGF-β knockout mice. *J. Immunol.* **155,** 3205–3212.
88. Botto, M., Dell'Agnola, C., Bygrave, A. E., Thompson, E. M., Cook, H. T., Petry, F., et al. (1998) Homozygous C1q deficiency causes glomerulonephritis associated with apoptotic bodies. *Nature Genet.* **19,** 56–59.

III

PATHOGENESIS OF RHEUMATIC DISEASES

20
Systemic Lupus Erythematosus

Stamatis-Nick C. Liossis and George C. Tsokos

Systemic lupus erythematosus (SLE) is a systemic autoimmune disease characterized by chronic inflammatory tissue damage mediated at least in part by immune complexes, autoantibodies, and autoreactive lymphocytes. Although the pathogenesis of SLE is incompletely understood, research efforts have shed light into the complex genetic, environmental, hormonal, and immunoregulatory factors, which are believed to contribute invariably to the development of the disease *(1–3)*.

1. Genetic Factors

One out of every 10 patients with SLE has a first-degree relative with the disease. The relatively high concordance rates for SLE in monozygotic twins (25–57%) compared to the concordance rates in dizygotic twins (2–9%) supports the importance of the host genetic background. It is currently believed that multiple genes confer susceptibility to the expression of the disease in a cumulative manner. Such a concept also encompasses the widely held thought that SLE is a genetically heterogeneous disease (*see also* Chapter 34).

The impact of genetic factors is also underscored by the fact that the incidence and prevalence of the disease differs among races. SLE has a higher incidence and prevalence in African-Americans, Afro-Caribbeans, and East Asians. SLE is not only more common in these populations but also the disease may have a worse overall course and prognosis. Certain clinical (e.g., discoid skin lesions, nephritis) and serological (e.g., anti-Sm autoantibodies) manifestations are more frequent among African-American patients. Ongoing detailed genetic analysis may reveal the molecular basis for such interracial differences.

Previous studies focused on the potential association of SLE with major histocompatibility complex (MHC) alleles or haplotypes. Strong associations have been reported between DR3, DQ2-containing, DR2, and DQ6-containing MHC class II haplotypes. Other genes found in the MHC complex (short arm of human chromosome 6) and comprise the MHC class III have also been associated with SLE. Hereditary deficiencies of early complement components have been associated with lupus. Genes for C2 and C4 map within the MHC, whereas C1q is encoded on chromosome 1. Complement receptor types 1 (CR1) and 2 (CR2) map also on the long arm of chromosome 1, and their expression in SLE red cells and B-lymphocytes,

From: *Current Molecular Medicine: Principles of Molecular Rheumatology*
Edited by: G. C. Tsokos © Humana Press Inc., Totowa, NJ

respectively, has been reported to be decreased. Certain polymorphisms of the promoter of the tumor necrosis factor-α (TNF-α) gene (also encoded within the MHC-III region) in HLA-DR2-positive patients with lupus nephritis are associated with decreased production of TNF-α.

Modern genetic approaches have tackled the study of multigenic human diseases (Chapter 1). Microsatellite markers have been used to screen the whole genome or portions of it in multiplex lupus family members. Previous studies had focused on genetic loci that map on the long arm of chromosome 1. The 1q23 locus is particularly interesting because it harbors at least two genes with potential association with lupus nephritis. Genes FcγRIIA and FcγRIIIA encode the receptors for the Fc fragment of IgG types IIA (CD32) and IIIA (CD16). A well-described polymorphism of the functional domain of FcgRIIA, which consists of a single aminoacid change of an arginine to histidine at position 131, predominates in African-American patients with lupus. This change is associated with defective FcγRIIA function, decreased IgG2 binding, impaired immune-complex handling, and clinically with immune-complex deposition in the kidneys and lupus nephritis in the African-American SLE patients population *(4,5)*.

The first study of lupus families was conducted by Tsao et al. *(6)* who reported a linkage between SLE and the locus 1q41-42. Interestingly, this study was guided to that specific genetic interval because it is syntenic with a known murine lupus-predisposing locus *(2)*. Genes found in the human 1q41-42 locus are not well characterized yet, but it is possible that this genetic marker confers susceptibility to antihistone autoantibody production in humans as it does in lupus-prone mice. The cohorts of multiplex lupus families analyzed in two novel studies are larger. Moser et al. *(7)* studied 94 pedigrees and reported that potential SLE loci (with LOD scores >2) are found at chromosomes 1q23, 1q41, and 11q14-23 in African-Americans. In European-Americans, the potential lupus loci were at 14q11, 4p15, 11q25, 2q32, 19q13, 6q26-27, and 12p12-11. In the combined pedigrees, the potential lupus loci were 1q23, 13q32, 20q13, and 1q31. The stronger linkage was for locus 1q23 in African-Americans. Candidate genes for this interval are those for FcγRIIA, as well as other nearby genes involved in SLE, such as FcγRIIIA, FcγRIIIB, and the ζ chain of the T-cell receptor.

The study by Gaffney et al. *(8)* analyzed 105 sib-pair lupus families almost entirely of European-American origin. This genome-wide microsatellite marker screen revealed that the stronger evidence for linkage was found near the MHC locus at 6p11-q21 and at three additional genetic intervals, at 16q13, 14q21-23, and 20p12. The two latter studies did not use the same microsatellite markers for screening, and it is interesting that there was partial agreement on linkage scores for some, but not all, markers that mapped closely. Moreover, the loci with the strongest linkage reported in one study are not found in the other. The linkage with 1q41-42 was found strong in two of the three studies, but in the first, it is reported that it crosses ethnic barriers, whereas in the other, it predominantly affected the African-American lupus families.

The long arm of human chromosome 1 *(9)* interestingly harbors several of the potential lupus loci found in these genomewide screens and also others that have been implicated in lupus. Such genes are those encoding for FcγRIIA, FcγRIIIA, TCRζ, FasL, interleukin-10 (IL-10), CR1, CR2, and C1q proteins. These molecules have been implicated in SLE either by small-scale genetic or by other-than-genetic studies.

In summary, multiple genetic loci or genes contribute to susceptibility for the development of SLE. The pathogenetic contribution and complex interaction of lupus-susceptibility genes needs to be clarified by additional studies. The precise role and contribution of each of the lupus-related genes should be addressed. The most important of them may represent potential targets for gene therapy in the future.

2. Hormonal Factors

In the prepubertal years, SLE affects boys and girls almost equally. During puberty though, lupus expresses its striking preference for females, an effect that remains steady throughout the reproductive years. There are no data regarding postmenopausal years. It is thus believed that female hormonal factors play at least a permissive role, whereas male hormonal factors play a protective one in the expression of SLE. This has been further supported by studies in murine strains. It has been clearly shown that estrogens have deleterious effects on lupus-prone experimental animals, whereas androgens are protective *(10)*.

There is evidence that the metabolism of endogenous estrogens is abnormal. Patients with SLE and their relatives produce increased amounts of the potent estrogens estrone and estriol because of increased 16α hydroxylation of estradiol and they also have decreased levels of androgens. Although most of our attention is focused on estrogens, other female hormones (e.g., progesterone, prolactin) may play a role. For example, hyperprolactinemia has been correlated with the appearance of such autoantibodies as anti-dsDNA, anti-Sm, and anti-Ro. The role of exogenously provided estrogens was addressed in the Nurses' Health Study, in which it was reported that long-term estrogen replacement therapy was associated with an increased risk for the development of SLE (relative risk = 3.5). Past use of oral contraceptives conferred a slightly increased relative risk of 1.4, but these data refer to a population exposed to the high estrogen content of oral contraceptives. Two newer case-control studies in populations receiving modern (low-dose) oral contraceptives failed to show increased risk for the development of lupus *(11)*.

Generally, estrogens act onto target cells after binding their cytoplasmic estrogen receptors (ER). The estrogen–ER complex acquires transcription factor activity, and following its entrance in the nucleus and its binding on specific estrogen-response elements found in the promoters of specific genes, it modulates the transcription of estrogen-dependent genes. Estrogens exert modulating effects on the immune system by altering the function and activity of T- and B-cells. Whether estrogens augment or inhibit immune cell function is a matter of debate, but in the immune cells of lupus-prone mice, estrogens act clearly as autoimmunity enhancers. It was recently reported that immune cells possess functional ER. Nevertheless, there were no differences between the ER found in lupus immune cells and those found in normal T- and B-lymphocytes and monocytes.

Estrogen receptors are found on the cell-surface membrane as well, and they mediate quite distinct functions compared to those of the classic endoplasmic ER. In murine T-cells, membrane ER, upon binding to estradiol, mediate a rise in the concentration of intracellular calcium ($[Ca^{2+}]_i$), which is a pivotal second messenger. Also, estrogen-response elements are found in the promoters of the protooncogenes c-fos and c-jun.

Estrogens thus affect the transcription of the fos and jun proteins that, when complexed, represent the transcription factor AP-1 *(12)*.

3. Environmental Factors

It is thought that various environmental factors influence a genetically susceptible host triggering the expression of SLE. Factors such as ultraviolet (UV) light, heavy metals, organic solvents, and infections will be discussed here *(10)*.

Exposure to UV light causes photosensitivity (more frequently in the Caucasian lupus population) and is a known disease-exacerbating factor. UV light causes the apoptotic cell death of keratinocytes. This mode of death was shown to be associated with the expression on the cell-surface of the dying keratinocyte of specific autoantigens that were previously "hidden" in the cytoplasm and/or cell nucleus. Autoantigens presented this way in surface membrane blebs of discrete size now become "visible" or accessible for immune recognition and potential targets for immune-mediated attack. The latter may result in local inflammation and the appearance in the circulation of autoantibodies. UV-light irradiation of cultured human keratinocytes induces changes consistent with apoptosis and the autoantigens are clustered in two kinds of bleb of the cell-surface membrane. The smaller blebs contain endoplasmic reticulum, ribosomes, and the (auto)antigen Ro. The larger blebs contain nucleosomal DNA, Ro, and La and the small ribonucleoproteins. This UV-mediated apoptotic cell death may be the molecular basis for the accessibility of hidden intracellular antigens and may explain the flooding of the immune system with autoantigens that activate T- and B-cells *(3)*.

Respirable silica has been previously associated with the appearance of antinuclear antibody and other autoantibodies in the serum and with the development of autoimmune diseases such as scleroderma. Silicosis is an occupationally related disease mostly for men. An analysis of 1130 men from Sweden with silicosis reported significantly more hospitalizations because of SLE and other connective-tissue autoimmune diseases. A prevalence of SLE that was 10 times higher than expected in the general population was reported in another study analyzing 15,000 men with heavy exposure to silica. Inhaled silica particles are phagocytosed by alveolar macrophages and act as a potent stimulus leading to inflammation. It has been hypothesized that increased recruitment and activation of macrophages leads to increased antigen presentation and increased antibody production. Moreover, in vitro silica acts as a polyclonal T-cell activator.

Previous studies reported that the organic solvents found in hair dyes are significantly associated with the development of connective-tissue diseases. However, the Nurses' Health Study did not find an association between hair dye use (even for > 15 yr) and the development of SLE.

Smoking also has been reported to correlate with the development of SLE, as two studies found an increased risk, but in the second (and smaller) one, the increased risk was not significant. Among others, cigaret smoking affects the activity of enzymes involved in estrogen metabolism; thus, it further perplexes the already complex interaction among environmental, hormonal, and genetic factors for the development of SLE.

A common clinical observation has been the development of SLE following an infection; nevertheless, a lupus-causing microorganism has never been identified. It has been hypothesized that an infectious agent(s) can disproportionally trigger an endogenously dysregulated immune system for the development or the exacerbation of SLE (*see* Chapter 2). Among the common pathogens, the herpesvirus Epstein–Barr virus (EBV) has received the most attention. Antibodies against EBV have crossreactivity with the lupus-specific autoantigen Sm. It was recently reported that newly diagnosed young patients with lupus have a significantly higher percentage of seropositivity for EBV infection compared to a control group. Almost all (116 of 117) young patients tested had seroconverted to EBV compared to 70% of their age-, sex-, and race-matched controls. Other herpesviruses tested did not follow this striking pattern. EBV DNA was found in the lymphocytes of all 32 young lupus patients tested, whereas it was present in 23 only of 32 controls. Whether EBV-infected individuals become more susceptible to the development of lupus, or lupus patients are/become more susceptible to EBV infection, or, finally, if a third factor increases susceptibility to both is currently not known *(3,10)*.

4. Drugs And Lupus

Drug-induced lupus has great similarities but also important differences to the idiopathic SLE syndrome. Because it represents a disease entity where the inciting factor is known, exogenous, and fully controllable, it represents a good model for studying aspects of SLE pathogenesis. Drugs that cause the SLE-like syndrome have been reported to induce DNA hypomethylation. Induced autoreactivity of previously non-autoreactive T-cells was first shown with the known DNA hypomethylator 5-azacytidine. Subsequently, it was found that the pharmaceutical agents most commonly associated with the drug-induced lupus, like procainamide and hydralazine, also bind to DNA and inhibit its methylation. The methylation status of a gene is one of the factors that determine the gene transcription rate in general. Thus, it can be assumed that changes in the methylation status of some autoreactivity-related genes contribute to the development of autoimmunity, but this hypothesis has not been substantiated yet.

In idiopathic SLE T-cells, it was reported that DNA is hypomethylated and the activity of the methylation-inducing enzyme, DNA methyltransferase, is decreased. Non-T-cells from patients with SLE did not share this abnormality, which affected only half of the lupus patients tested, and, finally, this abnormality was not disease-specific. Treatment of T-cells with inhibitors of DNA methylation induced the upregulation of the adhesion/costimulatory molecule lymphocyte function-associated antigen-1 (LFA-1). The significance of this event is underscored by studies in animal models in which T-cells overexpressing LFA-1 can mediate the production of anti-dsDNA autoantibodies and the appearance of glomerulonephritis. It is thus possible that drugs inducing DNA hypomethylation can initiate an autoimmune process by upregulating the costimulatory molecule LFA-1. Intracellular adhesion molecule-1 (ICAM-1) is the ligand for LFA-1 and estrogens are known inducers of ICAM-1 upregulation on endothelial cells. It was reported that procainamide induced a more severe disease in female experimental animals compared to procainamide-treated male counterparts, with two to seven times more cells homing to the spleen and higher anti-dsDNA antibody titers.

This example integrates at least two independent lupus-precipitating factors, drugs and estrogens. The exogenous factor (procainamide) caused decreased DNA methylation resulting (among others) in the upregulation of LFA-1 on the surface of T-cells.

This caused disease (or more severe disease) preferably to female animals because their circulating estrogens would make their endothelial cells more susceptible to LFA-1-mediated T-cell binding, resulting in heavier splenic infiltration and higher titers of the pathogenic anti-dsDNA autoantibodies. The extent to which this intriguing example may apply to the human disease is unknown, but LFA-1 was found to be overexpressed on the surface membrane of lupus lymphocytes. Another adhesion molecule, VLA-4, was found to be overexpressed on lupus lymphocytes only in patients suffering from lupus vasculitis. VLA-4-overexpressing lymphocytes displayed enhanced binding to cord vein endothelial cells. It can be assumed that if the expression of VLA-4 partner is upregulated on lupus endothelial cells, this could explain molecularly lupus vasculitis (reviewed in *3*).

5. Anti-DNA Autoantibodies in SLE

Systemic lupus erythematosus is characterized by the production of a large and still growing list of antibodies against an array of non-organ-specific self constituents present principally in the cell nucleus, but also in the cytoplasm, in the cell-surface membrane or even in the circulation. Although in the past it was proposed that the immune response against self was a uniformly harmful event, we now understand that an immune response against self is commonly a part of the normal immune response. This "normal autoimmunity" is a limited and strictly regulated process. Immune cells with autoreactive potential are present in good numbers in the normal subject, and germline genes encoding for antigen receptors of autoreactive T- and B-cells are part of the normal gene repertoire *(13)*.

Therefore, not unexpectedly, antibodies to DNA are produced in the normal host. These are IgM antibodies that bind to single-stranded (denatured) DNA; they have low affinity for DNA and broad crossreactivity with a variety of other self antigens. The production of these natural anti-DNA antibodies is tightly regulated. They do not usually undergo isotype switching and are encoded by germline genes; affinity maturation by the process of somatic mutation does not occur. On the contrary, the anti-DNA antibodies encountered so characteristically in the sera of patients with SLE have quite different features (*see* Chapter 4). They have undergone isotype switching to IgG of the various subclasses, and germline genes do not usually encode them because new aminoacids are introduced into their variable regions to enhance their affinity (somatic mutations and hypermutations). Because DNA is a highly anionic macromolecule, positively charged amino acids are introduced into the autoantibody variable regions, particularly arginine, to enhance DNA binding. Lupus anti-DNA antibodies thus are usually charged, IgG high-affinity and relatively low crossreactivity antibodies that recognize double-stranded (native) DNA (dsDNA) as well; in fact, anti-DNA antibodies that recognize dsDNA exclusively are rather unusual. This is the profile of the anti-dsDNA autoantibodies that are encountered essentially only in patients with SLE. In fact, among the various antinuclear antibody (ANA) specificities encountered in the sera of at least 95% of lupus patients, it is only the anti-dsDNA and the anti-Sm autoantibodies that are virtually specific for SLE.

Anti-dsDNA antibodies are considered pathogenic and they have been shown to cause glomerulonephritis. Even though there are exceptions, pathogenicity of anti-dsDNA antibodies is associated with high complement-fixing capability, high affinity for DNA and other crossreactive antigens, and a highly cationic charge. Circulating DNA–anti-dsDNA immune complexes are trapped in the glomerular basement membrane and the inflammation that follows can cause nephritis. Alternatively, the immune complexes are formed in situ, because the cationic anti-dsDNA antibodies may bind either negatively charged constituents of the glomerular basement membrane itself (laminin, heparan sulfate) or DNA fragments predeposited passively there.

Is DNA the autoantigen? Efforts to induce anti-dsDNA antibodies and glomerulonephritis by immunizations with mammalian, microbial, or viral DNA were not highly successful. Naked DNA is a poor immunogen. On the contrary, when the administered antigen is in the form of chromatin or nucleosomes, then the anti-DNA antibodies produced have an enhanced pathogenic potential. T-Cells from patients with SLE activated by nucleosomes provide help to lupus B-cells to produce anti-dsDNA of the IgG class. In a murine lupus model, the ability to respond to nucleosomes and generate antihistone and anti-DNA antibodies is genetically determined *(10,14)*.

6. Immunoregulatory Factors

A vast literature is devoted to the description of the multiple immune cell abnormalities encountered in SLE. Aberrations of the immune cells are believed to play a major role in lupus pathogenesis. Normally, the immune response takes place under strict regulatory control. Even though the mechanisms involved are incompletely understood, we believe that such control is provided not only by immune cells themselves but also by their products and involve multiple feedback loops *(3)*.

6.1. Helper/Suppressor T-Cell Function Imbalance

The disturbances involved in the production and maintenance of high levels of pathogenic autoantibodies in SLE could result from either increased help provided by specialized helper T-cell subsets, or decreased suppression, or both. Several subsets of T-cells, well characterized phenotypically, have been described to provide excessive help to lupus B-cells for the production of autoantibodies. Besides $CD4^+$ T-cells that provide excessive help, other subsets such as $CD8^+$, $CD3^+CD4^-CD8^-TCR\alpha\beta$ and $CD3^+CD4^-CD8^-TCR\gamma\delta$ T-cells from patients with SLE have been reported to provide help to autologous B-cells to produce anti-DNA autoantibodies. The latter two double-negative subsets are rather unusual in normal subjects, but in SLE, these subpopulations are greatly expanded in the circulation. Because the double-negative T-cell is known as an intermediate cell type during thymic selection, the increased numbers found in the circulation of lupus patients indicates that the processes of intrathymic positive and/or negative selection in SLE is perturbed resulting in tolerance defects *(3)*.

6.2. Th1/Th2-Type Cytokine Imbalance
6.2.1. Decreased Production of Th1-Type Cytokines

The SLE T-cells produce decreased amounts of IL-2 in vitro and this correlates with disease activity. Both $CD4^+$ and $CD8^+$ T-cells contribute to this deficiency. (Table 1) The production of TNF-α from lupus peripheral blood mononuclear cells (PBMC) is deficient. Decreased production of interferon-γ (IFN-γ) also characterizes peripheral blood mononuclear cells from patients with SLE. IL-2, TNF-α, IFN-γ, and IL-12 are

Table 1
Cytokine Abnormalities Encountered in SLE

Cytokine	Increased	Decreased
IL-1		+
TNF-α		+
IFN-γ		+
TGF-β		+
IL-2 (in vitro)		+
IL-2 (in vivo)	+	
IL-6	+	
IL-10	+	
IL-12		+

the Th1-type cytokines. They enhance cytotoxic cell responses and suppress antibody production. More recently, the production of IL-12 was similarly found to be decreased. IL-12 drives the cytokine production profile toward the Th1 type. The production of IL-12 was reportedly not corrected after "resting" the cells for a couple of days; thus, decreased IL-12 production may represent a more central abnormality.

6.2.2. Increased Production of Th2-Type Cytokines

Cytokines of the Th2-type include IL-4, IL-5, IL-6, and IL-10. Their role in general is to promote humoral immunity and suppress cell-mediated immune responses. The production of IL-6, a cytokine that promotes immunoglobulin production by B-cells, in lupus is increased. Also, IL-6 levels in the cerebrospinal fluid of patients with central nervous system lupus is increased, and following successful treatment, IL-6 levels fall. Lupus B-cells secrete large amounts of IL-6 and express increased amounts of IL-6 receptors indicating the presence of an autocrine positive feedback loop. Finally, a disease-accelerating role has been reported following IL-6 infusion in the classic (NZB × NZW) F1 murine lupus model.

Recently, most attention has been drawn on the production and role of IL-10 in lupus. Several studies have convincingly shown that the production of IL-10 is significantly elevated in patients with SLE and that IL-10 overproduction is implicated in the generation of anti-DNA antibodies. Dysregulated IL-10 production characterizes not only lupus patients but also healthy members of lupus multiplex families, as well affecting first-degree and even second-degree relatives of SLE patients. The constitutive production of IL-10 in healthy members of lupus families was 5.9 times higher than the levels of IL-10 found in healthy unrelated control individuals. Moreover, two groups of lupus patients (members and nonmembers of multiplex families) produced 8.5 and 9.1 times, respectively, more IL-10 than normal individuals *(15,16)*.

It was demonstrated that monocytes and an unknown B-cell subset were responsible for IL-10 overproduction in both patients and healthy relatives, whereas IL-10 was absent from B-cells of normal controls. IL-10 is a potent B-cell stimulator and a potent inhibitor of antigen-presenting cell (APC) function. This may explain the defective APC function and B7-1 upregulation previously reported in lupus non-B-cells. The familial pattern of IL-10 dysregulation points toward a potentially intrinsic defect. The human IL-10 gene is located on chromosome 1. In the (NZB × NZW) F1 murine lupus model, one of the disease-predisposing loci is closely linked to the IL-10 gene. Functionally, the importance of IL-10 overproduction was demonstrated by experiments using a monoclonal anti-IL-10 antibody. This anti-IL-10 in vitro diminished the production of anti-dsDNA autoantibodies, to an extent far more significant than that achieved by an anti-IL-6 monoclonal antibody. Furthermore, administration of anti-IL-10 to (NZB × NZW) F1 mice delayed the onset of the lupus-like murine syndrome and restored the production of TNF-α. It is possible that the continuously high levels of IL-10 encountered in lupus are responsible for the decreased production of Th1-type cytokines (IL-10 decreases the production of IL-2, TNF-α, and IFN-γ) and for the perpetuation of the humoral (auto)immune response.

6.3. Antigen Receptor-Mediated Signal Transduction of Lymphocytes in SLE

The immune system has evolved to recognize and respond to antigens that bind to specialized receptors present on the surface of T- and B-lymphocytes (TCR and BCR, respectively). Engagement of TCR or BCR elicits a series of well-regulated interacting intracellular biochemical events that transmit the extracellular signal (encounter of antigen) to the cell nucleus *(17)* *(see* Chapter 5). Because other membrane-receptor-initiated-specific accessory signals are integrated along with the antigen-receptor signal, the outcome of the TCR or BCR pathway can vary considerably. Antigen-receptor crosslinking can result in cell activation, proliferation, secretion of soluble mediators (cytokines or antibodies), phenotypic changes, acquisition of effector functions, anergy, and apoptotic programmed cell death. Because TCR- or BCR-signaling biochemical events principally direct these diverse but equally important outcomes, it was assumed that the diverse cellular aberrations described in lupus patients may reflect the product of signaling biochemical defect(s) that potentially play a central role in SLE pathogenesis.

6.3.1. Aberrant TCR and BCR Signaling in Lupus Lymphocytes

Following the engagement of the antigen receptor either with a specific antigen or with an antireceptor antibody, multiple well-regulated intracellular signaling pathways are triggered in the form of biochemical cascades. A critical event in these cascades is the mobilization of Ca^{2+} from intracellular stores, followed by an influx of Ca^{2+} from the extracellular space. The Ca^{2+} response is shared by many cell types, but the presence of specialized Ca^{2+}-sensitive enzymes and transcription factors found in specific tissues dictates the transcription of cell type-specific genes. Antigen receptor early signaling events (Ca^{2+}, IP3, and protein tyrosine phosphorylation) are increased in lupus T- and B-cells. These abnormalities were present in T-cells despite the fact the TCRζ chain (member of the ζ-family of proteins, part of the hetero-oligomeric TCR/CD3 complex) was missing. Also the cAMP-dependent protein kinase A type I (PKA-I) I is defective in lupus T cells and this may account for the increased Ca^{2+} responses because activation of this enzyme in normal T-cells downregulates Ca^{2+} responses *(3,18,19)*.

6.3.2. Molecular and Functional Consequences of Abnormal Signaling in Lupus Lymphocytes

Clinical disease activity changes reflect immunoregulatory cell changes and for this reason most patients with SLE are treated with immune system-targeting medications. It is thus important to distinguish between immunological parameters characterizing the disease (unrelated to disease activity and/or treatment) and parameters that appear as an outcome of the disease (related to activity and/or treatment). Altogether, the signaling aberrations analyzed earlier (TCR, BCR, CD2-initiated signaling, and TCRζ deficiency) are independent of disease activity, treatment status, and the presence or absence of specific SLE clinical manifestations and may thus represent intrinsic abnormalities of the lupus lymphocyte. These abnormalities are also disease-specific, because they were not found in normal lymphocytes or in lymphocytes from patients with other systemic autoimmune rheumatic diseases. The quite similar lupus T- and B-cell signaling aberrations mentioned earlier could substantiate the hypothesis that a common background underlies some heterogeneous lymphocytic functional defects.

The Ca^{2+} pathway critically influences the NFAT-mediated transcription of genes such as those of CD40-ligand and Fas-ligand (CD40L and FasL). It is thus anticipated that lupus lymphocytes should express more CD40L and FasL on their surface membrane because of their higher Ca^{2+} responses. This is indeed the case, because it has been shown that following activation, lupus T-cells overexpress both FasL and CD40L. CD40L is considered to be a T-cell marker, but lupus B cells display increased CD40L on their surface, which intensely increases following activation. Because both T- and B-cells also express CD40, it is possible that an excessive CD40–CD40L interaction takes place in lupus cell–cell contact *(20)*.

It was shown that cells lacking TCRζ (but expressing an intact CD3ε chain) were not only able to transduce early signaling events, but surprisingly displayed enhanced production of tyrosyl phosphorylated proteins compared to cells that preferentially signaled via the TCRζ chain. Nevertheless, TCRζ− cells displayed decreased IL-2 production. CD3ζ chain deficiency may also account for decreased CD2 signalling and TGF-β production as well as decreased antigen-induced cell death that have been described in lupus cells.

In ζ−/− experimental models, both positive and negative selection of thymocytes is deficient. Decreased negative selection may be responsible for the presence of potent autoreactive T-cells in lupus patients (ζ−/− animals are also autoimmune); decreased positive selection may explain the decreased responses of lupus T-cell to exogenous antigen *(3)*.

6.3.3. CD28/CTLA4: CD80/CD86-Mediated Costimulation in Lupus Immune Cells

In addition to the specific TCR/CD3-mediated signal, at least one costimulatory signal provided by an APC is required for the initiation, maintenance, and/or downregulation of an effective T-cell response. The role of CD40 : CD40L interaction was previously discussed in Chapter 6, and it is currently appreciated as a potential therapeutic target. The importance of this interaction in SLE is underscored by experiments showing that administration of even a single dose of anti-CD40L monoclonal antibody in murine lupus models significantly delayed the appearance of nephritis and substantially improved the survival of such animals without compromising the nonautoimmune response *(20)*.

T-Cell costimulation involves interactions between the CD28 and CTLA4 molecules on the surface of T-cells and their counterreceptors, CD80 (B7-1) and CD86 (B7-2) molecules on APC. CD28 is constitutively detected on the surface of the majority of circulating resting CD4+ T-cells, on half of resting CD8+ T-cells and on some natural-killer (NK) cells; its expression increases following activation. CTLA4 can be detected only on activated T-cells. CD86 is constitutively expressed on resting peripheral monocytes and dendritic cells, but substantial levels of CD80 on these cells are primarily activation induced. CD28- and CTLA4-mediated signals have distinct effects on T-cells, by integrating additional biochemical events in the TCR-signaling pathway. CD28- plus TCR-mediated signals result in secretion of cytokines, upregulation of CTLA4 mRNA, and T-cell proliferation and differentiation. In the absence of CD28-mediated signaling, impaired cytotoxic responses and/or a long-lasting anergic state ensue. In contrast, CTLA4 delivers a downregulatory signal to previously activated T-cells, provided that it functionally couples with the TCRζ chain. It may also mediate deletion in the periphery of autoreactive T-cells that escaped previous deletion in the thymus.

In patients with SLE (active or inactive), the CD28$^+$ peripheral blood T cells of both CD4$^+$ and CD8$^+$ subsets are decreased and the circulating CD28$^-$ T-cell population is expanded. Anti-CD3-induced apoptosis of CD28$^+$ T-cells is significantly accelerated in vitro in SLE, providing a possible explanation for the loss of these cells from the peripheral blood in vivo, whereas apoptosis of CD28$^-$ T-cells is barely detected either in lupus patients or in normal persons. CD28-mediated signaling in lupus T-cells is intact.

Abnormalities in the expression of CD80 and CD86 on the cell surface of peripheral blood B-cells from patients with SLE have also been reported. Levels of CD86 expression on resting and activated lupus B-cells was 7 and 2.5 times greater than the levels of normal B-cells, respectively. CD80 was also significantly overexpressed in activated, but not in resting B-cells from patients with lupus, although at lower than CD86 levels. Therefore, overexpression of costimulatory molecules on circulating B-cells in patients with SLE may play a role in the continuous autoreactive T-cell help to lupus B-cells leading to the production of autoantigens.

On the other hand, non-B APC from patients with SLE but not from normal persons fail to upregulate the in vitro surface expression of CD80 following stimulation with IFN-γ in a disease-independent fashion. Replenishment of functional CD80 molecule in the culture environment significantly increased the responses of SLE T-cells to tetanus toxoid and to an anti-CD3 antibody. Similarly, the decreased responses of lupus T-cells to anti-CD2 are reversed in the presence of adequate CD28-mediated stimulation *(3)*.

Taken together, the above findings suggest that aberrantly regulated and/or expressed costimulatory molecules on T cells and APC at different disease stages in patients with SLE may contribute to pathology. Interrupting the crosstalk of CD28 with CD80- and CD86- may be of clinical value. To test this hypothesis, CD80 and CD86 treated lupus-prone (NZB × NZW) F1 mice with CTLA4–Ig, a soluble recombinant fusion protein that blocks the engagement of CD28. CTLA4–Ig treatment blocked autoantibody production and prolonged the survival of mice, even when it was administered late, during the most advanced stage of clinical illness. In these lupus-prone animals, trials of combined CTLA4–Ig and anti-CD40L mAb treatment gave the most promising of results.

7. Conclusion

Figure 1 is a schematic summary of the pathogenesis of lupus. Notwithstanding its simplicity, it should be noted that multiple genetic, environmental, and hormonal factors instigate a number of cellular and cytokine abnormalities. These abnormalities lead to increased production of autoantibodies, which either directly or after forming complexes with autoantigens and activating complement deposit in tissues and initiate

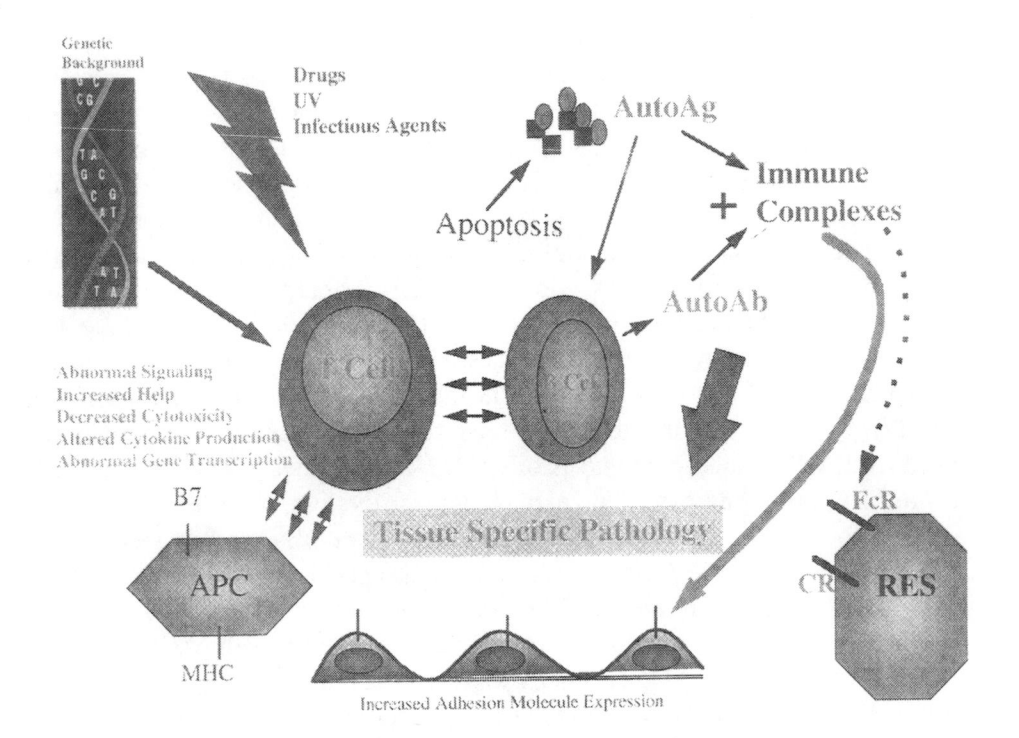

Fig. 1. Schematic summary of the pathogenesis of lupus.

an inflammatory response. Immune complexes are formed in excessive amounts in lupus patients and are cleared a decreased rates because the numbers and or the function of Fc and complement receptors are decreased. In addition, activated T-cells may home inappropriately in tissues and cause pathology (vasculitis).

It is imperative to identify the specific molecular defect(s) encountered in human lupus. This is the only way to design and use any novel and rational treatments, because currently treatment of lupus is largely empiric and more or less unsatisfactory. Novel treatments may include methods to restore immune tolerance (Chapter 32), modulators of cytokine action (as in rheumatoid arthritis, Chapter 31), blocking of cell–cell crosstalk (as with the use of anti-CD40L or CTLA4–Ig, Chapter 6), blocking of calcium-dependent cytoplasmic events (with cyclosporin A, FK506, rapamycin, and other newer compounds, Chapter 29), or lastly, gene therapy (Chapter 34).

References

1. Theofilopoulos, A. N. (1995) The basis of autoimmunity: Part I. Mechanisms of aberrant self-recognition. *Immunol. Today* **16,** 90–98.
2. Theofilopoulos, A. N. (1995) The basis of autoimmunity: Part II. Genetic predisposition. *Immunol. Today* **16,** 150–159.
3. Tsokos, G. C. (1999) Overview of cellular immune function in systemic lupus erythematosus, in *Systemic Lupus Erythematosus*, 2nd ed. (Lahita, R. G., ed.), Churchill Livingstone, New York, pp. 17–54.
4. Salmon, J. E., Millard, S., Schachter, L. A., Arnett, F. C., Ginzler, E. M., Gourley, M. F., et al. (1996) FcgammaRIIA alleles are heritable risk factors for lupus nephritis. *J. Clin. Invest.* **97,** 1348–1354.

5. Wu, J, Edberg, J. C., Redecha, P. B., Bansal, V., Guyre, P. M., Coleman, K., et al. (1997) A novel polymorphism of FcγRIIIa (CD16) alters receptor function and predisposes to autoimmune disease. *J. Clin. Invest.* **100,** 1059–1070.
6. Tsao, B. P., Cantor, R. M., Kalunian, K. C., Chen, C.-J., Singh, R., Wallace, D. J., et al. (1997) Evidence for linkage of a candidate chromosome 1 region to systemic lupus erythematosus (SLE). *J. Clin. Invest.* **99,** 725–731.
7. Moser, L. K., Neas, B. R., Salmon, J. E., Yu, H., Gray-McGuire, C., Asundi, N., et al. (1999) Genome scan of human systemic lupus erythematosus: evidence for linkage on chromosome 1q in African-American pedigrees. *Proc. Natl. Acad. Sci. USA* **95,** 14,869–14,874.
8. Gaffney, P. M., Kearns, G. M., Shark, K. B., Ortmann, W. A., Selby, S. A., Malmgren, M. L., et al. (1999) A genome-wide search for susceptibility genes in human systemic lupus erythematosus sib-pair families. *Proc. Natl. Acad. Sci. USA* **95,** 14,875–14,879.
9. Tsokos, G. C. and Liossis, S. N. C. (1999) Immune cell signaling defects in human lupus: role in activation, anergy and death. *Immunol. Today* **20,** 123–128.
10. Cooper, G. S., Dooley, M. A., Treadwell, E. L., St Clair, E. W., Parks, C. G., and Gilkeson, G. S. (1998) Hormonal, environmental, and infectious risk factors for developing systemic lupus erythematosus. *Arthritis Rheum.* **41,** 1714–1724.
11. Sanchez-Guerrero, J., Liang, M. H., Karlson, E. W., Hunter, D. J., and Golditz, G. A. (1995) Postmenopausal estrogen therapy and the risk for developing systemic lupus erythematosus. *Ann. Intern. Med.* **122,** 430–433.
12. Kammer, G. M. and Tsokos, G. C. (1998) Emerging concepts of the molecular basis for estrogen effects on T lymphocytes in systemic lupus erythematosus. *Clin. Immunol. Immunopathol.* **89,** 192–195.
13. Hahn, B. H. (1998) Antibodies to DNA. *N. Engl. J. Med.* **338,** 1359–1368.
14. Mohan, C., Adams, S., Stanik, V., and Datta, S. K. (1993) Nucleosome: a major immunogen for the pathogenic autoantibody-inducing T cells of lupus. *J. Exp. Med.* **177,** 1367–1381.
15. Llorente, L., Zou, W., Levy, Y., Richaud-Patin, Y., Wijdenes, J., Alcocer-Varela, J., et al. (1995) Role of interleukin 10 in the B lymphocyte hyperactivity and autoantibody production of human systemic lupus erythematosus. *J. Exp. Med.* **181,** 839–844.
16. Llorente, L., Richaud-Patin, Y., Couderc, J., Alarcon-Segovia, D., Ruiz-Soto, R., et al. (1997) Dysregulation of interleukin-10 production in relatives of patients with systemic lupus erythematosus. *Arthritis Rheum.* **40,** 1429–1435.
17. Wange, R. L. and Samelson, L. E. (1996) Complex complexes: signaling at the TCR. *Immunity* **5,** 197–205.
18. Liossis, S. N. C., Kovacs, B., Dennis, G., Kammer, G. M., and Tsokos, G. C. (1996) B cells from patients with systemic lupus erythematosus display abnormal antigen receptor-mediated signal transduction events. *J. Clin. Invest.* **98,** 2549–2557.
19. Liossis, S. N. C., Ding, X. Z., Dennis, G. J., and Tsokos, G. C. (1998) Altered pattern of TCR/CD3-mediated protein-tyrosyl phosphorylation in T cells from patients with systemic lupus erythematosus. Deficient expression of the T-cell receptor zeta chain. *J. Clin. Invest.* **101,** 1448–1457.
20. Datta, S. K. and Kalled, S. L. (1997) CD40-CD40L interaction in autoimmune disease. *Arthritis Rheum.* **40,** 1735–1745.

21

Rheumatoid Arthritis

Richard M. Pope and Harris Perlman

1. Pathology

1.1. Membrane

The normal synovial membrane consists of a synovial lining layer, one to two cell layers deep, that rests on loose areolar connective tissue. The lining layer is comprised of type A macrophage-like synoviocytes and type B fibroblast-like synoviocytes (FLS). There is no discrete basement membrane between the synovial lining and the sublining region. Numerous blood vessels, which are the source of nutrients provided to the normal cartilage and joint space, are present in the sublining region. The junction between the synovial lining and bone and cartilage is a critical region in the pathogenesis of rheumatoid arthritis (RA). Studies have demonstrated the presence of immunocompetent cells overlying and in contact with cartilage and bone in the joints of normal individuals *(1)*. These cells possess markers that indicate the presence of both macrophage-like type A cells and fibroblast-like type B cells, which are not activated in the normal joint.

The synovial membrane of patients with RA demonstrates characteristic changes of chronic inflammation that are not pathognomonic. Synovial lining hyperplasia occurs with an increase in the depth of cells in the lining from 1 to 2 cell layers to as much as 10 or more. The cells in these lesions consist of both type A and type B FLS. There is a marked enrichment of new blood vessels. Whereas 0–3 vessels per high power field may be seen in a normal synovial tissue, there may be more than 15–20 vessels per high-powered field seen in active RA.

A diffuse infiltration with lymphocytes is a characteristic and fairly consistent feature in the tissues of patients with active RA. Within this infiltrate, macrophages and fibroblasts are present. Paravascular infiltrates of lymphocytes may be seen around these blood vessels, the point of ingress into the joint. The paravascular lymphocytic infiltrates are comprised of CD45RO+ ("memory") and CD45RA+ ("naïve") cells *(2)*. Focal aggregates of lymphocytes are present in about 25–30% of biopsies, and granuloma formation, with histologic findings similar to those of rheumatoid nodules, is seen in less than 10% of cases *(3,4)*. Within the lymphoid aggregates or follicles, almost all the T-cells are CD45RO+, and they surround B-lymphocytes that are present in the center of the aggregates. Within the aggregates, there are scattered macrophages. The T-lymphocytes within the aggregates tend to be enriched in CD4+ cells, whereas those from the diffuse infiltrates tend to be enriched in CD8+ T-lymphocytes *(5)*.

From: *Current Molecular Medicine: Principles of Molecular Rheumatology*
Edited by: G. C. Tsokos © Humana Press Inc., Totowa, NJ

Replacement of the loose areolar connective tissue by fibrosis is another common feature of RA. This feature is more common in those biopsies that demonstrate less inflammation. It was once thought that the above-described histologic variations may not fully reflect changes earlier in the disease, as many of the studies employed tissue obtained at the time of arthroplasty. However, more recent studies, which have examined biopsies obtained early in the disease, within the first several months of onset, have observed few differences in the synovial membrane compared to tissue obtained at the time of arthroplasty *(6)*. Additionally, biopsy of asymptomatic, clinically uninvolved joints in patients with established RA has revealed active synovitis *(7)*. Synovial lining hyperplasia, vascular proliferation, and inflammatory cell infiltrates are noted, both early and late in the disease and in asymptomatic joints. Overall, these studies suggest that at the onset of clinical symptoms, RA is already chronic.

Synovial lining hyperplasia, vessel proliferation, and lymphocytic infiltration strongly correlate with clinical activity. In contrast, the degree of fibrosis correlates inversely with the degree of active inflammation observed clinically. A strong correlation was also demonstrated between synovial lining hyperplasia and inflammation in the sublining region, as defined by proliferation of blood vessels and paravascular, focal, and diffuse infiltrates of lymphocytes *(4)*. Of particular relevance to the pathogenesis and prognosis of the disease, the degree of synovial lining hyperplasia and the number of infiltrating macrophages at the time of initial observation correlate with outcome 3 yr later *(8)*. Specifically, the greater the synovial lining hyperplasia and the greater the number of infiltrating macrophages in the synovial lining, the greater the destruction and the worse the outcome, despite the therapy *(8)*.

1.2. Pannus

The pannus is the region of the synovial membrane that invades bone and cartilage, resulting in erosions. At least three types of lesions, two in cartilage and one in bone, have been characterized in RA *(9,10)* (Fig. 1). The first, referred to as the "distinct" cartilage–pannus junction, possesses 40–50% macrophages, as defined by CD68 positivity. As will be described later, these macrophages secrete a variety of pro-inflammatory cytokines and matrix metalloproteinases (MMPs), capable of cartilage destruction. The remaining cells in this pannus are CD68 negative, and many of these cells are likely synovial fibroblasts, which express MMPs. This type of pannus may be very destructive. Electron microscopic analysis of the pannus–cartilage junction in very aggressive lesions has demonstrated the presence of intracellular and membrane-bound collagen, indicating ongoing collagen degradation and phagocytosis *(11)*. Later, the potential relevance of this process to the persistence of the disease will be discussed.

A second type of lesion that may be discerned is the "diffuse" fibroblastic cartilage–pannus junction. This lesion contains predominantly FLS *(10)*, and the margin between cartilage and the pannus has been characterized as diffuse or indistinct. Immunohistology has suggested that preservation of chondrocyte proteoglycans is greater in these lesions, suggesting they are less destructive. It is unknown whether or not there is a transition between these two types of pannus–cartilage junctions in a given patient. In experimental animals, we have observed both types of pannus in the same joint, at the same time.

A third type of lesion is the bone–pannus junction, in which macrophages and osteoclasts appear to be primarily responsible for mediating damage. This region does have

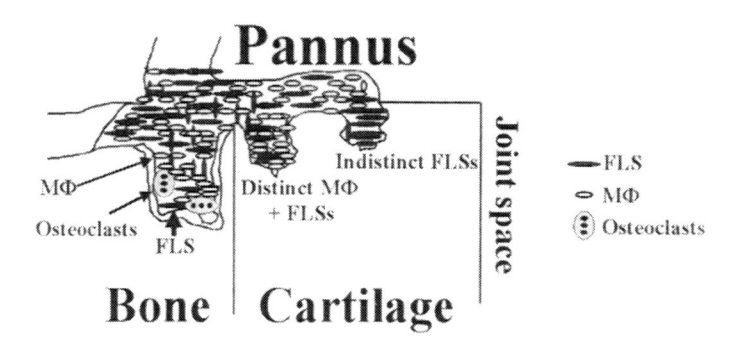

Fig. 1. Three types of pannus have been described in rheumatoid arthritis. Pannus is the region of synovium that invades cartilage and bone. The "distinct" pannus–cartilage junction possesses both macrophages (open ellipses) and fibroblast-like synovial cells (FLS) (solid ellipses) at the leading edge as it erodes into the cartilage. Macrophage derived cytokines such as TNFα and IL-1α and MMPs are abundantly expressed in these lesions. The "indistinct" pannus–cartilage junction possesses primarily fibroblast-like synovial cells. TGF-β and possibly cathepsins have been described in these lesions. The third type of pannus is bone erosion. Macrophages and osteoclasts (ellipses with three dots or nuclei) are highly enriched in this type of pannus. Cathepsins are present in pannus–bone junction.

similarities to the distinct cartilage–pannus junction because it is replete with CD68 positive mononuclear cells, presumably macrophages. Cathepsin L, an enzyme capable of degrading multiple elements of bone and cartilage, including multiple collagens, proteoglycans, and osteonectin, is expressed in macrophages in subchondral bony erosions (12). CD68+ multinucleated osteoclasts, which are tartrate-resistant acid phosphatase and calcitonin receptor positive (9), have been identified in this type of pannus.

2. Initiation

2.1. The Shared Epitope and Antigen Presentation

Susceptibility to RA is strongly associated with MHC class II genes at the HLA-DRβ1 locus (13). Susceptibility is associated with genes that possess the amino acids QRRAA or QKRAA within positions 69 to 74 of the third hypervariable region, called the shared epitope. This motif is present in the DRB1*0401 (Dw4), *0404 (Dw14), *0101(Dw1), and *1001 (Dw10) alleles, but not other DRB1 alleles, including the *0402 (Dw10). Despite the strong associations of these alleles with the presence of RA noted in almost all studies, not all patients with RA possess the shared epitope, and there is variability between ethnic groups. The mechanism by which the shared epitope contributes to the development of RA is also not known. However, the major known function of HLA-DR molecules is the presentation of processed antigen to CD4+ T-lymphocytes. Because the most frequent cell type in RA synovial tissue is T-lymphocytes and they demonstrate markers of activation (HLA-DR, CD69, CD44) and since processed antigen binds at the third hypervariable region, this function of the shared epitope is attractive. However, the antigen(s) that may initiate RA, in the susceptible individual, has remained elusive. Many candidate infectious agents have been examined, including mycoplasma, cytomegalovirus, herpes virus, streptococcus (peptidoglycan), mycobacterium (heat-shock protein), Epstein–Barr virus, parvovirus, and retroviruses, to name some. Despite efforts over more than 20 yr, none of these leads has, to date, proved useful in definitively characterizing an agent responsible for the initiation of RA. The potential role of T cells in the persistence of RA is discussed later in the chapter.

In an attempt to identify disease-associated peptides that might contribute to the pathogenesis of RA, the binding of peptides to the shared epitope was compared with other β1 epitopes. Differences in the peptides bound were noted between the DRB1*0401, disease associated, and the DRB1*0402 which is not associated with RA. These differences mapped to contacts between the peptide and the DR molecule at position 71 within the shared epitope *(14)*. Of interest, one study also identified amino acid 71 as the critical site associated with disease susceptibility *(15)*. These observations are consistent with the potential importance of an antigen presentation function for the shared epitope in the initiation of the disease.

2.2. Molecular Mimicry

It has been hypothesized that an immune response initiated by an organism may lead to crossreactivity because of molecular mimicry, similarities of peptides in the organism, and sequences found in human tissue. Such mechanisms have been elegantly characterized in patients with acute rheumatic fever. It has been postulated that an immune response directed against the HLA-DRβ1 shared epitope, by molecular mimicry, might contribute to the pathogenesis of RA. The QKRAA shared epitope motif is found in the molecules of human pathogens, including the DnaJ protein of *E. coli* and Epstein–Barr virus gp110 *(16)*. It is possible that exposure to these immunogenic antigens possessing the shared epitope, plus other amino acids that are not identical, may lead to the stimulation of T-cells with low affinity for the shared epitope. Repeated stimulation may lead to the development of higher affinity for the shared epitope, and following epitope spreading, chronic autoimmune inflammation may develop *(16)*.

2.3. Altered Antigen Processing

Other mechanisms for the role of the HLA-DRβ1 shared epitope are possible. DnaJ binds to the *E. coli* 70-kDa heat-shock protein (HSP), dnaK, which is homologous to the human 70-kDa HSP, that is upregulated in the RA joint. Binding of DnaJ to the 70-kDa HSP is mediated by the QKRAA motif, within the DnaJ molecule. The *E. coli* HSP70, dnaK, and the human 70-kDa HSP also interact with HLA-DRβ1 alleles containing the shared epitope *(17)*. Because the 70-kDa HSP is a chaperone molecule that targets the movement of protein molecules within the cell, perhaps such an interaction (human 70-kDa HSP with the shared epitope) may interfere with normal antigen processing, allowing for ineffective elimination of an as-yet unidentified initiating agent. This would result in the inability to present an antigen that might protect against RA. Alternatively, during thymic selection, the shared epitope might result in the deletion of T-cells that results in a gap or hole in the immune repertoire, that might result in ineffective elimination of an initiating, infectious agent. If either of these mechanisms was operative, the shared epitope positive individual might not recognize a critical determinant on a disease-promoting organism. However, none of these potential defects has been defined in patients with RA.

Naturally processed peptides have been eluted form shared epitope positive and negative molecules *(18)*. The molecules eluted were autologous in origin and primarily represented HLA class I and II molecules and immunoglobulins, which were not different between the shared epitope positive and negative molecules. An invariant chain, responsible for proper peptide loading within the cell, was found associated with the shared epitope negative, but not positive, molecules. Perhaps the lack of an associated invariant chain may allow inappropriate antigen presentation of exogenous antigen or even autoantigens, that might be relevant to the initiation or persistence of disease. Another possibility has been suggested by work with transgenic animals. Certain nonshared epitope hypervariable region 3 peptides, such as the KDILEDERAAVDTYC epitope from DRB1*0402, might bind to disease associated HLA-DQ molecules (i.e., DQ 4, 5, 7, and 8), limiting or altering immunogenicity and possibly protecting against susceptibility to RA or to more severe disease *(19)*. This mechanism would hypothesize that the shared epitope-containing peptides are not protective.

2.4. Linkage Disequilibrium

Other possible mechanisms for the contribution of HLA-DR to the pathogenesis of RA exist. RA may be viewed as a disease in which the inflammatory response is dysregulated. It is possible that an allele associated with increased or decreased expression or function of a pro- or anti-inflammatory molecule, such as tumor necrosis factor-α (TNF-α) or interleukin-10 (IL-10), might be in linkage disequilibrium with the shared epitope. Associations of polymorphisms of the neighboring TNF locus, with susceptibility to RA, have not produced consistent results. A recent study suggests that a TNF allele may be associated with disease severity when inherited together with the DRβ1 shared epitope *(20)*. Relationships to alleles of other molecules potentially involved in disease pathogenesis have been examined, such as the alleles of the T-cell receptor, IL-10, IL-2, interferon-γ, IL-1β, Bcl-2, and CD40L *(21)*. Studies have looked for enrichment of allele polymorphisms by reverse transcriptase–polymerase chain reaction (RT-PCR) or by microsatellite marker mapping. No strong or definitive associations have been identified to date. Studies employing microsatellite marker mapping in sib pairs with RA are underway to scan the entire genome of patients with RA to determine if there are other areas that might interact with HLA-DR to initiate disease or contribute to disease severity. One recent publication suggests that such areas exist but the nature of the molecule(s) possibly involved have not yet been identified *(22)*.

3. Inflammation

3.1. T-Lymphocytes

3.1.1. Cytokine Expression

T-Lymphocytes are the most frequently observed inflammatory cell in the rheumatoid joint. They are important because of their frequency, the fact that the majority possess not only a memory (CD45RO+) but also an activated phenotype (HLA-DR+, CD44+, CD69+), and because of the MHC class II (which presents antigen to T-cells) association of the disease. These observations all suggest that RA is a T-cell-mediated disease. If this were the case, one might expect to find T-cell mediators of inflammation (e.g., IL-2, interferon-γ, IL-4) and that the disease would respond to therapies that deplete T cells or inhibit T cell activation and function. Most studies have been unable to detect the expression of substantial, constitutive, levels of T-cell mediators of inflammation, such as IL-2, interferon-γ, or IL-4 in rheumatoid synovial tissue or synovial fluid, at the level of either mRNA or protein *(23)*. By *in situ* hybridization, less than 1 in 300 CD3+ lymphocytes produced interferon-γ mRNA and less than 1 in 1000 expressed IL-4 mRNA *(24)*. This suggests that few T-cells are producing cytokines *in vivo*. As will be reviewed later, this does not mean that T-cells are not important if minute levels of T-cell cytokines are adequate, or if physical, cell-to-cell, interaction with other cell types, without the production of T-cell cytokines, is important.

3.1.2. T-Helper Types

T-Cell responses may be divided into Th1 (T helper 1) and Th2. In a Th1, delayed-type hypersensitivity response (e.g., to mycobacterium tuberculosis), cells produce IL-2 and interferon-γ. In the Th2 response (e.g., granulomas induced by schistosoma eggs) cells produce IL-4 and IL-13, which might provide for B-cell help and differentiation, as well as suppression of macrophage activation. In RA, when mRNA is examined, a Th1-type response is observed, although limited by *in situ* hybridization and by RT-PCR *(24)*. Intracellular cytokines are generally not detected constitutively in patient synovial tissue lymphocytes examined by flow cytometry *(25)*. Following stimulation, however, the number of the CD4+ cells synthesizing interferon-γ (Th1) was greater than those expressing IL-4 (Th2). This Th1-type pattern was greater with synovial tissue CD4+ cells, of which most were also CD45R0+, compared to matched peripheral blood CD4+, CD45R0+ cells. Although most studies have found very little in the way of T-cell cytokines constitutively in rheumatoid synovial tissue, even by routine RT-PCR, one group used a very sensitive RT-PCR enzyme-linked immunosorbent assay (ELISA) *(3)*. Tissues were categorized into diffuse lymphocyte infiltration alone, or together with follicular aggregates or granulomas. Only the tissues with follicular aggregates demonstrated a clear-cut Th1-like pattern (high interferon-γ, low IL-4 mRNA). In contrast, both interferon-γ and IL-4 were low when only diffuse infiltrates were seen, and both were high when granulomatous synovitis was present. Because interferon-γ suppresses the Th2-type response, these results are difficult to interpret, but suggest that the usual mechanisms regulating T-cell responses may be altered in RA synovial tissue.

3.1.3. T-Cell Receptor

Studies over many years have attempted to define the specific T-cells responsible for the initiation or the persistence of the disease. One way to determine if there is an antigen-driven T-cell response, is to characterize the T-cell receptor repertoire. Diversity in the T-cell receptor is generated by the combination of α and β chains and further by the joining of one of multiple variable (V) region genes that combine with different diversity (D) and joining (J) regions. As these regions combine, additional diversity occurs by random addition of nucleotides about the diversity region. Peripheral blood, synovial fluid, and synovial tissue have been examined late and early in the course of patients with RA. When the T-cell receptors are sequenced, the T-cells are clearly polyclonal. Nonetheless, evidence for expansion of unique T-cells with identical T-cell receptor sequences have been documented at different areas within the same joint, in different joints, and at different times in the clinical course. Relating these sequences to the pathogenesis of RA is difficult, however, because few similarities in the sequences are observed between patients. Additionally, oligoclonal expansions of CD8 positive T-cells has been observed in normal controls and are not specific to RA.

The mechanisms responsible for the specificity of T-cell responses, even to a defined antigen, may be difficult to define. In RA, in which no disease-inducing antigen has been identified, interpretation of the data is further limited.

3.1.4. Clinical Trials

Many clinical trials directed at depleting or modulating T-cells have been performed in RA. These have included anti-CD4, anti-CD5, toxin-labeled IL-2, anti-CD52 (CAMPATH-1H), and anti-CD7 *(23)*. Generally, in the smaller trials, some benefit was seen. However, in the large controlled trials, such as that with the anti-CD4 monoclonal antibody cM-T412, no benefit was seen at any dose examined *(26)*. Interestingly, when synovial tissue was examined following treatment with CAMPATH-1H, T-cells remained plentiful in the joints, even though the peripheral blood lymphocytes were greatly reduced *(27)*. In one of the cM-T412 studies, a reduction of T-cells was observed in both blood and tissue; however, there was no clinical improvement *(28)*. In these patients, TNF-α and IL-1β were still detected in the synovial tissue following treatment, despite the reduction of CD4+ T-cells. These studies suggest that even if T-cells are important in RA, depletion by the currently available methods is not an effective form of therapy. It is possible that modulation of the T-cell response to favor a Th2 versus a Th1 response, or tolerization to specific responses, might be effective.

3.2. B-Lymphocytes

3.2.1. Affinity Maturation

B-Lymphocytes are detected in lymphoid follicles, which are present in less than half of patients with classical RA. Most, but not all, of these patients are positive for rheumatoid factor, but not all patients with rheumatoid factor have lymphoid follicles in their synovial tissue. Normal germinal centers are populated with proliferating B-cells. With each round of proliferation, mutations in the nucleotide sequence responsible for antigen recognition occur at a rate of about 1 in 1000 base pairs per generation. Normally, the mutations selected result in an increased affinity for the antigen driving the response. The greater the response, the greater the difference from the original germline sequence. These mutations are seen in T-cell-dependent antigen-driven systems, but not in T-independent or non-antigen-driven systems of expansion of B-lymphocytes. Normally within a given follicle, a limited number of specificities are seen and this may become increasingly restricted with further rounds of proliferation. Lymphoid follicles are normally transient in spleen and lymph nodes, but are persistently seen in tonsils, where antigen presentation is recurring *(29)*.

Many of the features of an antigen-driven system as described have been observed in RA synovial tissue *(30)*. B-Cells proliferate in the center of the follicles and are surrounded by CD45R0+, CD45RB^{low} T-cells, which are capable of providing B-cell help *(2)*. Rheumatoid factor production in patients with RA is T-cell dependent. In the mantle zone of the follicle, follicular dendritic cells have been identified. These cells are capable of long-term retention of native antigen and are capable of presentation of antigen to both T- and B-lymphocytes. Normally after exposure to the follicular dendritic cell, the B-cell returns to the central region of the follicle for further rounds of division, mutation, and maturation. In the RA follicle, proliferating nuclear cell antigen is present in the B-cells, indicating that they are not in the resting phase of the cell cycle. Nurse-like cells, capable of protecting B-cells from apoptosis, have also been identified in the rheumatoid joint (Fig. 2) *(31)*.

3.2.2. Rheumatoid Factor

Rheumatoid factors are the characteristic autoantibody detected in 70-80% of patients with RA. Rheumatoid factors sequenced directly from RA synovial tissue or isolated from cells immortalized from the synovial tissue of patients demonstrate hypermutation of the third complementarity-determining regions. Ten or more mutations compared to the germline may be seen in synovial tissue rheumatoid factors *(32)*. These rheumatoid factors demonstrate affinity maturation; that is, they bind more avidly to the Fc portion of the IgG molecule, compared to germline rheumatoid factors (monoclonal rheumatoid factors from patients with lymphoproliferative malignancies). They demonstrate isotype switch; that is, IgG rheumatoid factor production, which is present in the synovial tissue of most patients who are positive for IgM rheumatoid factor, but not those who are rheumatoid factor negative *(29)*. IgG rheumatoid factors also demonstrate affinity maturation. IgG rheumatoid factors are the ultimate autoantibody, forming self-associating IgG rheumatoid factor immune complexes, which likely contribute to the disease. In normal individuals who are immunized or experience an infection, rheumatoid factors are produced, probably to assist in the clearance of immune complexes *(33)*. However, they do not persist and do not undergo affinity maturation. It is possible that in patients with RA, rheumatoid factors are directed against an infecting agent because rheumatoid factors may bind to the Fcγ-binding regions of certain infectious agents, such as herpes virus *(34)*. This suggests that some rheumatoid factors recognize the internal image of the viral Fc receptor that binds to human IgG Fc.

3.2.3. Other Ig Specificities

Rheumatoid factors are only one component of the specificity of immunoglobulins synthesized by the RA synovial tissue. Antibody specificities to a variety of foreign antigens, including bacterial antigens, may be detected in the rheumatoid joint. The local production of these antibodies, versus production at a distant site such as a lymph node, has not been as definitively characterized as it has been for rheumatoid factors. Additionally, important autoantibodies, such as those to type II collagen, are synthesized in the synovial tissue. Immune complexes, of which those possessing rheumatoid factors are plentiful, and autoantibodies, such as those to type II collagen, are capable of depositing in the synovial tissue and cartilage, contributing to the ongoing destruction seen in the rheumatoid joint *(35)*. Evidence for this comes from the direct demonstration of complexes and anti-type II collagen antibodies, deposited together with activated complement components in the cartilage and synovial tissue of patients. High titers of immune complexes and activated complement components are readily detected in the synovial fluids of patients with RA. Together, these observations strongly support an ongoing antigen-driven response in the synovial tissue of patients with RA. The nature of the critical antigen, which may be present on the surface of follicular dendritic cells, has yet to be identified. A further understanding of the antibody specificity may provide important clues for understanding not only the initiation, but, perhaps more importantly, the perpetuation of RA.

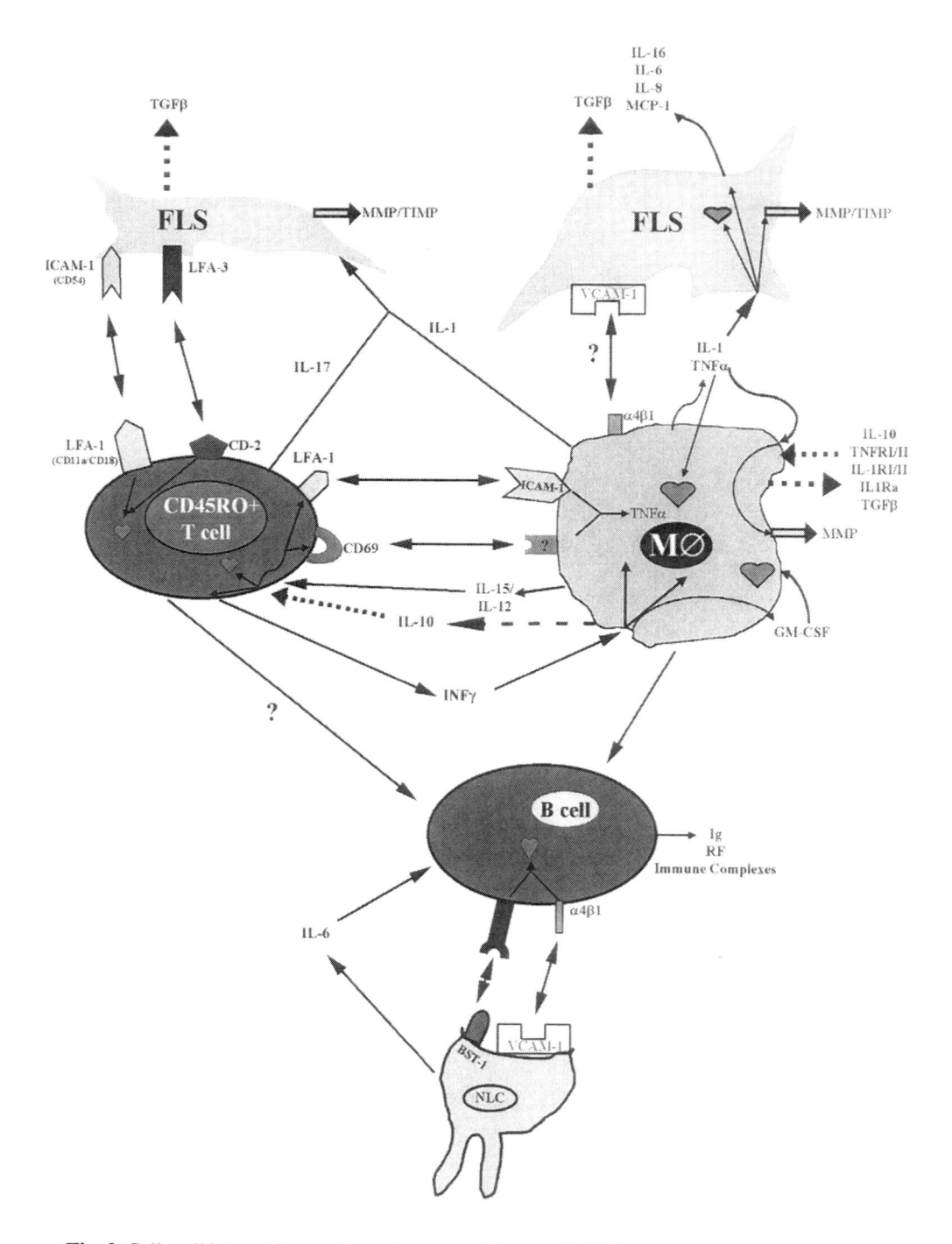

Fig. 2. Cell–cell interactions and cytokines contribute to the inflammatory cascade in rheumatoid arthritis synovial tissue. Five cell types are portrayed: fibroblast-like synoviocytes (FLS), "memory T-lymphocytes (CD45RO+ T-cell), macrophages (Mϕ), B-lymphocytes (B-cell), and nurse-like cells (NLC). The hearts represent the activation of pathways that protect against apoptosis. The one-way arrows indicate the secretion of mediators from one cell that affects the same cell and other cells in an autocrine and paracrine fashion. The solid lines represent activation pathways and the broken lines identify inhibitory pathways. The thick lines identify the expression of destructive proteases, such as the matrix metalloproteinases. The two-way arrows indicate cell–cell interactions.

3.3. Macrophages

3.3.1. Cytokine Expression

Macrophages are present in the synovial lining and the pannus and scattered in the diffuse inflammatory infiltrate in the sublining region. Macrophages are also present scattered within the lymphoid aggregates. In contrast to T-cells, the pro-inflammatory products of macrophages, such as TNF-α, IL-1β, MCP-1, MIP-1α, IL-8, platelet-derived growth factor, IL-15, IL-10, and IL-12 are readily detected in RA synovial tissue macrophages by immunohistochemistry and Western blot analysis of isolated cells *(36–44)*. The presence of these cytokines in the synovial fluid has also been demonstrated functionally, with specificity proven by inhibition with monospecific antibodies. The presence of cytokine mRNA in synovial tissue macrophages has been demonstrated by Northern blot analysis and *in situ* hybridization, indicating that they are the cells producing these cytokines.

Of the cytokines found in the rheumatoid joint, TNF-α is important, because it is capable of inducing cytokines, chemokines and matrix metalloproteinases (MMPs) in an autocrine and paracrine fashion (Fig. 2). In in vitro cultures of synovial tissue, inhibition of TNF-α resulted not only in the reduction of TNF-α in the culture supernatants but also the reduction of IL-1β, IL-6, and IL-8 *(36)*. However, not all investigators have identified the constitutive production of TNF-α in all RA synovial tissue cultures. TNF-α is capable of inducing MMPs not only in an autocrine fashion, but, with IL-1, also in a paracrine fashion by affecting adjacent fibroblasts. MMP-1 (interstitial collagenase), MMP-8 (PMN collagenase), and MMP-9 (92- to 96-kDa gelatinase) contribute to collagen degradation, whereas MMP-3 (stromelysin) contributes to proteoglycan degradation. TNF-α and IL-1 are expressed abundantly in synovial lining macrophages, at the leading edge of the pannus, as the pannus invades bone and cartilage, and in sublining synovial macrophages *(36)*. Cells in the synovial lining and the pannus, both macrophages and fibroblasts, possess TNF-α receptors, indicating that TNF-α may be working in an autocrine and paracrine fashion, locally within the joint. In addition to the MMPs, TNFα and IL-1 also upregulate cytokines and chemokines by synovial fibroblasts, including IL-6, IL-8, MCP-1, and MIP-1α. TNF-α also activates endothelial cells, resulting in the upregulation of adhesion molecules including E-selectin and P-selectin, which contribute to the influx of additional inflammatory cells. IL-1β enhances the production of prostaglandins by fibroblast-like synoviocytes (FLS) by upregulating cycloxygenase 2. IL-1β and TNF-α contribute to joint degradation by enhancing MMP expression by chondrocytes, which enhances collagen and proteoglycan degradation in cartilage. TNF-α and IL-1 are also capable of protecting against the induction of apoptosis in FLS and possibly synovial macrophages (Fig. 2). IL-15, produced by synovial tissue macrophages, is capable of attracting lymphocytes into the joint and of inducing the upregulation of CD69 and LFA-1 on synovial lymphocytes (Fig. 2). As will be discussed later, interaction of these lymphocytes with macrophages is capable of enhancing the expression of TNF-α *(42)*. IL-15 is also capable of protecting lymphocytes from apoptosis.

3.3.2. Chemokines

Chemokines contribute to the inflammation by chemoattraction of inflammatory cells from the peripheral blood into the synovial tissue. There are two families within the chemokine supergene family and each contains two cysteines in the amino terminus of the proteins. Those chemokines that attract primarily monocytes and lymphocytes possess adjoining cysteines (C-C), such as MCP-1 and MIP-1α, whereas those that attract primarily neutrophils possess an additional amino acid between the cysteines (C-X-C), such as IL-8 and epithelial neutrophil-activating protein-78 (ENA-78). All the chemokines mentioned are strongly expressed in RA ST macrophages, either in the lining and/or the sublining regions. They are less strongly expressed by FLS constitutively in vivo, but can be increased in vitro by the addition of TNF-α or IL-1β.

3.3.3. Growth Factors

Granulocyte macrophage colony stimulating factor (GM-CSF), produced locally by FLS and macrophages, also contributes to macrophage differentiation and may contribute to the protection of macrophages from apoptosis (Fig. 2). Because synovial macrophages do not proliferate, they must derive from the peripheral blood monocytes. Immunohistologic studies suggest that macrophages in the synovial lining have become more differentiated, because they express relatively less CD14 (which is decreased during differentiation) and they express MMPs, which occurs to a greater extent in differentiated macrophages. Differentiated macrophages also produce greater quantities of cytokines, compared to monocytes. Platelet-derived growth factor (PDGF) is produced primarily by macrophages and results in the anchorage-independent growth of FLS, a characteristic feature of RA FLS *(43)*. Vascular endothelial growth factor (VEGF) is produced by lining cells and macrophages and is a potent angiogenic factor in the rheumatoid joint. Fibroblast growth factor-1 (FGF-1), is also produced by synovial lining cells, apparently both type A and B, and smooth-muscle cells in RA synovial tissue. FGF-1 also promotes angiogenesis and proliferation, and is a T-cell coactivator *(44)*. FGF-1 receptors are detected on perivascular lymphocytes, suggesting that FGF-1 may contribute to the activation of T-cells as they enter the joint.

3.3.4. Anti-Inflammatory Molecules

Synovial tissue macrophages also produce anti-inflammatory molecules, including IL-10, TGFβ, IL-1R antagonist (IL-1Ra), IL-1 receptors (RI and RII), and TNF receptors (RI or p55 and RII or p75). When synovial fluid is examined, the biological activity of TNF-α and IL-1β is affected by the inhibitors (receptors and IL-1Ra) present. Assays that measure protein (i.e., ELISA) are less likely to be affected, but may be, depending on the specificity of the antibodies used in the assays. When macrophages are activated to produce TNF-α, TNFRI and RII are shed. TNF-α-converting enzyme (TACE), a MMP, is responsible for cleaving both TNF-α and its receptors. In contrast, IL-1Ra is regulated differentially with IL-1β. The interleukin-1-converting enzyme (ICE) is responsible for cleaving pro-IL-1β, resulting in its secretion by monocytic cells. Normally in differentiated macrophages, such as those found in RA synovial tissue, there is a greatly enhanced production of IL1Ra relative to IL-1β. In RA this ratio of IL-1Ra to IL-1β is reduced, suggesting a local dysregulation of macrophages. Soluble IL-1RI and II are also shed following macrophage activation and act as natural inhibitors of IL-1β. Soluble IL-1RII concentration in the peripheral blood correlated inversely with disease activity, suggesting its importance as potential inhibitor of IL-1β *(45)*. In contrast, IL-1Ra correlates positively with disease activity, suggesting that it is less important in damping disease and/or that it is not effective. This positive correlation may be the result of a large excess of IL-1Ra to IL-1β required for effective inhibition. As will be discussed later, IL-1β is not strongly expressed at the pannus–cartilage junction, although IL-1α is *(36)*, perhaps because these macrophages are highly differentiated.

Interleukin-10 is detected abundantly in RA synovial fluid. Although Th2 lymphocytes secrete IL-10, no constitutively expressed IL-10 was detected in RA synovial tissue lymphocytes, although synovial T-cells may exhibit IL-10 mRNA and synthesize IL-10 following stimulation. However, monocytic cells, other than T-cells, were the source for constitutively expressed IL-10 in RA synovial fluid, suggesting that macrophages are the main source for IL-10 in RA. IL-10 is likely an important immunosuppressive molecule because exogenous IL-10 decreased TNF-α, IL-1β, and GM-CSF induced by lipopolysaccharide (LPS) using RA SF mononuclear cells. Additionally, inhibition of IL-10 greatly enhanced the secretion of TNF-α and IL-1β by RA synovial tissue cells *(36,38)*. IL-10 is also chondroprotective, enhancing proteoglycan synthesis. Overall, it would appear there is too little IL-10, and possibly some of the other inhibitory molecules mentioned, locally within the rheumatoid joint, suggesting a potential therapeutic role for IL-10. As will be discussed later, IL-1Ra and TNFRII have already been shown to provide clinical benefit. IL-12 is produced by sublining macrophages and may contribute to the Th1-type response (interferon-γ) seen in the rheumatoid joint *(25)* (Fig. 2). Synovial macrophages also appear to be a major source in vivo for IL-6, which may promote B-cell, T-cell, and monocytic cell differentiation. IL-6 enters the circulation and binds to receptors on hepatocytes, contributing to the typical elevations of the acute-phase reactants (CRP, ESR) seen in patients with active RA. The origin of IL-6 in the joint suggests why changes in acute-phase reactants correspond so closely in a given patient (but not between patients), with changes in disease activity, as measured by number of swollen joints. IL-6 itself may be important in the pathogenesis of RA. Mice in which the IL-6 gene was deleted failed to develop collagen-induced arthritis. However, the lack of the IL-6 gene failed to protect TNF-α transgenic mice from the development of severe destructive arthritis *(46)*.

3.4. Fibroblast-like Synoviocytes

As mentioned earlier, FLS or type B-cells are one of the two major cell types present in the synovial lining in the normal as well as the RA joint. FLS are also present in the sublining region. In the lining, they are in intimate contact with type A macrophage-like cells. FLS are present in the cartilage–pannus junctions and are the major cell type in the diffuse cartilage–pannus junction. In the sublining region, FLS are in intimate contact with other cell types, particularly T-cells in the area of diffuse lymphocytic infiltration. FLS in the lining are distinctive from other fibroblasts in that they possess the enzyme uridine diphosphoglucose dehydrogenase, which is responsible for the production hyaluronic acid, which is secreted into the synovial space.

3.4.1. Cytokines and MMPs

Rheumatoid arthritis FLS are a source of many cytokines, growth factors, and proteinases, which contribute to the inflammation and joint destruction observed in RA. FLS produce IL-6, IL-8, MCP-1, MIP-1α, and IL-16 (a chemoattractant for CD4 positive cells), as well as GM-CSF, and TGF-β *(37,39,40,47–49)*. When RA synovial tissue was examined, IL-6, IL-8, MIP-1α, and MCP-1 were expressed more strongly by synovial macrophages compared to FLS (Fig. 2). The addition of TNF-α or IL-1β to RA FLS in vitro results in the upregulation of these cytokines, suggesting that this is an important mechanism in vivo. MMP-1, MMP-3, and TIMP-1 have been detected in the synovial lining and pannus *(37,50,51)*. Many groups have identified these proteins in cells that appeared morphologically to be FLS. Additionally, in vitro, early passage (passage 1 to 3) FLS still express these proteinases constitutively *(43,52)*. However, after the third passage, the addition of IL-1β and TNF-α is needed for the expression of MMP-1, MMP-3, and TIMP-1. FLS are not the only source of MMPs in RA. CD14 positive macrophages were identified as a source of MMP-1 production, as determined by *in situ* hybridization of RA synovial tissue *(53)*. Furthermore, we have shown that TNF-α regulates the expression of MMP-1 mRNA in monocytic cells in an autocrine fashion *(54)*.

Transforming growth factor-β1 (TGF-β1) and TGF-β2 are present in RA synovial fluid and tissue *(36,43)*. TGF-β receptors are present on synovial tissue lining cells, endothelial cells, and macrophages. TGF-β is important in tissue repair, because it leads to increased collagen synthesis by fibroblasts, perhaps contributing to the increased fibrosis seen in the synovial tissue of patients with RA. TGF-β is capable of suppressing LPS-induced cytokine production when added prior to the stimulus; however, it is not capable of suppressing TNF-α or IL-1β if added after the addition of LPS. Further, addition of exogenous TGF-β did not suppress the spontaneous IL-1β and TNF-α secretion in RA ST, suggesting that it may not be an important immunosuppressive molecule in RA *(36)*. In contrast, TGF-β may contribute to the destruction seen, because injection of TGF-β induced joint inflammation *(36)*. In one study, TGF-β was the only cytokine described at the diffuse fibroblastic cartilage–pannus junction, suggesting that it may contribute to this lesion *(10)*. Alternatively, TGF-β may be responsible for attempted tissue repair, by increasing chondrocyte proteoglycan synthesis.

3.4.2. Transformed Phenotype?

It has been proposed that RA FLS may develop their destructive phenotype, capable of eroding into cartilage, because they are transformed, perhaps by a viral agent *(52)*. The ability of FLS to undergo anchorage-independent growth in vitro and to produce cartilage erosions, without the presence of other cell types when implanted with cartilage in the severe combined immune-deficiency mice, supports this possibility. Human T-cell leukemia virus type I (HTLV-1) is a relevant model for this possibility. HTLV-1 infection can result in a chronic inflammatory arthropathy. A protein called Tax, produced by the HTLV-1 retrovirus, is capable of inducing FLS proliferation and transformation *(55)*, which likely contributes to the arthropathy. However, with RA FLS, the loss of anchorage-independent growth, the transformed phenotype, and the reduction of the spontaneous production of MMPs and IL-6 over time suggest that these cells are responding to the environment of the synovial tissue in RA and are not independently transformed. This phenotype is consistent with prior activation, which persists for several passages, but is eventually lost in vitro. The fact that a number of so-called protooncogenes, such as c-myc, or c-fos, have been detected in FLS is also used as support for FLS transformation. These protooncogenes are transcription factors that are upregulated and/or activated, following an appropriate stimulus. In RA, this activation may be promoted by cytokines such as TNF-α and IL-1 or by cell contact with macrophages or T-lymphocytes (Fig. 2).

4. Inflammatory Cascade

Given the vast array of inflammatory mediators described and their redundancy, identification of which might be most significant in the induction or perpetuation of the disease has been difficult. Therapeutic trials in patients with RA have provided insights into this question.

4.1. Immunoglobulins

Among the first approaches was the removal of immunoglobulins by plasmapheresis. This approach was unsuccessful. However, it is unlikely that this approach was adequate locally within the joint space to reduce antibodies and immune complexes. It is likely that the deposition of immune complexes or autoantibodies such as those to type II collagen is an important amplifying factor, not the driving force, in the pathogenesis of disease. A protein A immunoadsorption column, capable of removing IgG and IgG-containing immune complexes, has recently been approved by the Food and Drug Administration for use in refractory RA.

4.2. T-Lymphocytes

Based on the prominence and activated phenotype of synovial T-cells, a number of approaches to reduce T-cells have been utilized. Among them, depleting antibodies that identify different epitopes on T-lymphocytes, including CD4, CD5, or CD52 (CAMPATH-1H), were effective at the reduction of peripheral T-cells, although patients did not improve significantly (26). Based on animal models, more recent studies with nondepleting anti-CD4 antibodies have been performed. The aim of this approach is to modulate T-cell function, perhaps switching from a Th1 to a Th2 pattern, in hopes of altering the cascade of inflammation, by enhancing the production of inhibitory cytokines such as IL-4. The initial studies were somewhat promising at high doses; however, toxicity prevented continued study at the effective doses. Studies have also been performed with antibodies to the adhesion molecule ICAM-1, in an attempt to reduce trafficking of inflammatory cells into the joint. These studies resulted in modest clinical improvement and a transient increase of lymphocytes in the circulation, suggesting that the T-cells might have been diverted from migration into the joint (56). Although disappointing overall, these studies do not mean that T-cells are not important in the pathogenesis of RA, as will be discussed in Subheading 7.5.–7.7. They mean that this broad-based, nonselective approach was not effective. Preliminary studies are under way to modulate the T-cell repertoire by immunization with peptides representing the T-cell receptors found on activated T-cells in the joints of some patients with RA, in hopes of effecting a long-lasting modulation of the disease (26).

4.3. Macrophage Cytokines

Earlier, we mentioned that in in vitro studies employing RA synovial membranes, inhibition of TNF-α also inhibited IL-1β, IL-6, and IL-8, and inhibition of IL-1 inhibited IL-6 and IL-8 (36), suggesting that both TNF-α and IL-1 may be important. Inhibition of IL-1 has also been used as an approach to treating RA. Recombinant human

IL-1Ra (IL-1 receptor antagonist) binds to IL-1R, preventing IL-1 from binding. At high concentrations, recombinant human IL-1Ra had a modest ameliorative effect on the inflammation, as determined by swelling and pain *(57)*. However, even though the effect of IL-1Ra on inflammation was only modest, it appeared effective at preserving cartilage *(57)*. This is consistent with certain experimental systems in which IL-1Ra was beneficial at preserving chondrocyte and cartilage integrity *(58)*. Further, treatment of monocytic cells with methotrexate, which is clinically effective in the majority of patients with RA, enhances macrophage differentiation and the release of IL-1Ra and sTNFRII and suppresses IL-1β secretion *(59)*.

Treatment with recombinant human IL-1R, type I (IL-1RI), both systemically and intraarticularly did not result in clinical benefit. In fact, a few patients may have become more severely affected with this treatment *(60)*. This is possible because IL-1RI binds more avidly to IL1Ra than to IL-1β, possibly permitting greater bioavailability of IL-1β and increased inflammation. IL-1RII, a nonsignaling decoy molecule that binds avidly to IL-1 but not IL-1Ra, might be more effective at modulation of disease, but it has not been studied.

Currently, the inhibition of TNF-α activity, either by a recombinant chimeric monoclonal antibody or by a bivalent recombinant TNF-α RII (two TNF-α RII molecules attached to a human IgG backbone), has proven clinically effective in a majority of patients with RA *(36)*. A number of very informative studies have been performed with the chimeric monoclonal antibody, which have provided insights into the inflammatory cascade that exists in the rheumatoid joint *(36)*. Within days, a dramatic reduction of circulating C-reactive protein is seen. This is followed by a reduction a joint inflammation over the first couple of weeks. Synovial biopsies done after treatment demonstrate a reduction of inflammatory cells, including T-lymphocytes. A corresponding increase in circulating T-lymphocytes is seen, suggesting that they may no longer be trafficking into the joint tissue. VCAM-1, which is strongly expressed on synovial lining cells and sublining macrophages, is greatly reduced. Additionally, a reduction of E-selectin is seen on the blood vessels in the ST. E-selectin, which contributes to the migration of cells into the ST, is upregulated by TNF-α and is not seen on blood vessels in normal skin. Soluble circulating E-selectin, which may contribute to migration into the joint and to angiogenesis, is also reduced. These observations support the importance of TNF-α in the ongoing inflammation seen in RA. Although very promising, it is too early to be certain how this treatment will affect the long-term course of RA. Further, not all patients respond to strategies to inhibit TNF-α, and only a minority experience dramatic clinical improvement (i.e., a complete remission). This suggests that additional mechanisms contribute to the persistence of disease in most patients and that TNF-α may not be important in all patients. These observations, together with those concerning IL-1Ra, suggest a potential additive or synergistic benefit between the anti-inflammatory effect observed by inhibition of TNF-α and the chondroprotective affect seen with inhibition of IL-1.

5. Transcriptional Regulation

Transcription factors are proteins that generally possess three domains: a DNA-binding domain, a transactivation domain, and another domain, such as a leucine zipper, that provides for specific protein–protein interactions (*see also* Chapter 7). Transcription factors bind to the promoter regions of genes employing their DNA-binding domains, also called the basic domain because of their negative charge. The transactivation domain regulates the expression of the gene in question by interacting with basal transcription factors responsible for the activation of RNA polymerase. Domains such as the leucine zipper domains allow transcription factors to interact with other protein molecules, forming homodimers or heterodimers. Transcription factors exist in cells either constitutively or are synthesized following the appropriate stimulus. Following activation, there is a posttranslational modification, often phosphorylation, that promotes migration to the nucleus and binding to DNA. The DNA sequences in promoter regions to which transcription factors bind are frequently unique, however, different sequences may bind the same transcription factor. For example in the TNF-α promoter, there are three nuclear factor-κB (NF-κB) binding sites, each unique and each able to bind NF-κB with different avidities. The differences in the strength of binding affects how, and under what conditions, each site is able to contribute to the activation of the TNF-α gene. In many situations, an interaction between two or more transcription factors is necessary for the activation of a given gene. For example, the TNF-α promoter is activated in some circumstances by NF-κB alone and in others by the combination of C/EBPβ plus c-Jun *(61)*. RA synovial tissue has been examined for the expression of transcription factors that might be important in the regulation of proinflammatory molecules in macrophages and FLS.

5.1. NF-κB

Nuclear factor-κB (NF-κB) exists, preformed in the cytoplasm of most cell types, as heterodimers composed of p65 or RelA and p50 or NF-κB1. The p50/p65 heterodimers are bound in the cytoplasm to another molecule, called IκB, and this complex is retained in the cytoplasm under resting conditions. Following an appropriate activation signal, which in many cells includes TNF-α or IL-1β, the IκB molecule is phosphorylated and then degraded. This releases the p50/p65 heterodimers to migrate to the nucleus, directed there by means of a nuclear localization signal (a short amino acid sequence), that had been sterically blocked by the IκB. The heterodimers bind to the promoters of many pro-inflammatory genes, including TNF-α, IL-6, IL-8, and others, resulting in activation. The heterodimers also bind to the promoter of IκB, resulting in increased synthesis of IκB, which binds to newly synthesized heterodimer molecules, restoring the balance in the cell. NF-κB p50 and p65 are normally not found in the nucleus, but are only present following activation. NF-κB is essential for viability, because deletion of NF-κB p65 by gene knockout is lethal. Cells from these animals are sensitive to TNF-α-mediated apoptosis, which will be discussed in Subheading 8.

Within the synovial tissue in vivo, nuclear NF-κB was strongly expressed, primarily in lining macrophages and to a lesser degree in some CD14 negative cells, presumably FLS *(62)*. Supporting the importance of ongoing NF-κB activation in macrophages in RA, when IκB was over expressed by infection of RA synovial tissue cells with an adenoviral vector expressing IκB, the constitutive production of TNF-α was greatly reduced *(63)*. Activated NF-κB, as determined by its detection in the nucleus, was also observed in scattered cells in the sublining region and in some blood vessels in the RA joint. These observations are of interest, because they suggest that the activation of NF-κB in the synovial tissue is not normally downregulated following activation, as described above, but is persistent. When NF-κB is activated in vitro, the duration of

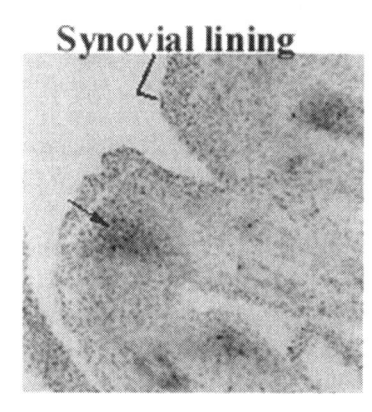

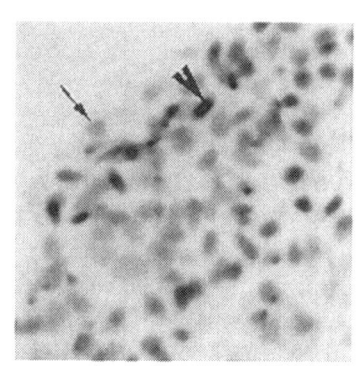

Fig. 3. C/EBPβ is expressed in the nucleus of synovial lining cells in patients with rheumatoid arthritis. In panel A, under low power, the dark stain identifies the presence of C/EBPβ, which can be seen in the synovial lining. Scattered positive cells are seen in the sublining region and in the lymphoid aggregates. In panel B, under high power, the synovial lining can be seen to be seven to nine cells in depth. The arrow identifies the nucleus of a C/EBPβ negative cell, which is stained with Hematoxylin stain. The arrow head identifies a cell positive for C/EBPβ in the nucleus. C/EBPβ (intensely dark staining) is seen in about 40–50% of the nuclei in the synovial lining.

activation is generally limited, in part because new IκB is synthesized following activation of its promoter by NF-κB p50/p65 heterodimers. The mechanism of activation of NF-κB in the rheumatoid joint is unclear. Because NF-κB activation in macrophages can induce TNF-α, but TNF-α itself can induce NF-κB activation, it is possible that in this milieu a self-perpetuating process could be set up if inhibitors that are present are not adequate. IL-4 and IL-10 may function in part by inhibition of NF-κB activation *(64)*.

5.2. C/EBPβ

C/EBPβ (CAAT enhancer-binding protein beta) or NF-IL-6 (nuclear factor IL-6) is also strongly expressed in the nuclei of RA synovial lining macrophages and to a lesser extent in FLS (Fig. 3). C/EBPβ is a bZip protein possessing a basic domain, leucine zipper, and a transactivation domain. Data suggest that under certain conditions, C/EBPβ is capable of regulating a number of pro-inflammatory genes, including TNF-α, IL-1β, IL-6, IL-8, G-CSF, and MMP-1. Mice in which C/EBPβ has been deleted by gene knockout demonstrated defects in phagocytosis and control of certain infections and the expression of G-CSF by macrophages in vitro. These animals also exhibited a defect in the in vivo production of TNF-α. In macrophage cell lines, C/EBPβ cooperates with c-Jun to activate the TNF-α gene in a unique way that does not require the transactivation domain of c-Jun, following stimulation with phorbol myristate acetate (PMA) and LPS *(61)*. Inhibition of C/EBPβ employing a dominant negative version of the molecule that possess the DNA binding and leucine zipper domains, with the transactivation domain deleted, inhibited TNF-α secretion in PMA, and LPS simulated monocyte-differentiated macrophages (unpublished data). Although the precise role of C/EBPβ in RA has not been defined, it is possible that it may be contribute to the

5.3. AP-1

Other transcription factors appear activated in RA synovial tissue. Among the AP-1 (activator protein-1) family members, bZip proteins, c-Jun and c-Fos, have been detected in RA synovial tissue. The nuclear expression of these transcription factors was observed in synovial lining cells that were, generally, CD14 negative, presumably FLS *(62)*. Additional studies have demonstrated that the cells in the synovial lining were actually producing these transcription factors because mRNAs for both c-*jun* and c-*fos* genes were detected in the lining by *in situ* hybridization and by *in situ* reverse transcription *(65)*. Other AP-1 family members jun-B and jun-D have been detected, although less consistently. C-Jun and c-Fos were strongly expressed at the sites of attachment of synovial tissue to bone and cartilage, suggesting their potential importance in the expression of genes responsible for joint destruction *(66)*. Supporting the importance of this observation, mice transgenic for and overexpressing c-*fos*, develop a destructive arthritis, not dependent on T-cells. C-Jun and c-Fos may be important in regulating a number of pro-inflammatory genes in FLS, including ICAM-1 and the MMPs. The difference in the distribution of activated NF-κB, C/EBPβ, and AP-1 transcription factors, detected in the nucleus of various cell types, suggests that different mechanisms of activation may be responsible for the constitutive in vivo expression of pro-inflammatory molecules, expressed in RA synovial fibroblasts and macrophages. Of interest, IL-10 may function by inhibition of NF-κB, AP-1, and C/EBPβ activation *(64)*.

5.4. Mitogen-Activated Protein Kinases

The mitogen-activated protein kinase (MAPK) pathway is a series of kinases that connect the cell surface with the nucleus. It consists of three parallel pathways that interconnect at some levels, capable of resulting in the phosphorylation and activation of c-Jun via the JNK (Jun N-terminal kinase) pathway, of Elk-1/2 and C/EBPβ via the Erk-1/2 (extracellular signal-regulated kinase) pathway, and of ATF-2 (activating transcription factor-2) via the p38 pathway. C-Fos and c-Jun are activated by mitogens, growth factors, and cytokines such as TNF-α and IL-1. The Erk-1/2 pathway is activated by growth factors and by integrin ligation. The oncogene Ras is a proximal kinase in this pathway and may also result in cross-communication with the JNK pathway. Mutations of Ras may result in persistent activation. Ras mutations have been found in the synovial tissue of some patients with RA. Their significance is uncertain because they were also detected in osteoarthritis synovial tissue *(67)*. The cell type(s) expressing the mutated ras was not characterized. The p38 pathway results in the activation of the transcription factor ATF-2, which cooperates with c-Jun. It may be activated by mitogens and cytokines, such as IL-1 and TNF-α.

5.5. c-Myc

Another transcription factor, c-Myc, is broadly expressed in RA synovial tissue, particularly in FLS *(52)*. c-Myc may contribute to regulation of the expression of genes responsible for cell-cycle progression and proliferation, as well as apoptosis. For example, c-Myc is capable of binding heat-shock protein 70 (HSP70) promoter, inducing gene expression under certain conditions *(68)*. HSP70 is upregulated in RA synovial tissue, particularly in the synovial lining. Therefore, c-Myc might contribute to the upregulation of HSP70 in RA. Additionally, heat-shock transcription factor 1 (HSF1), which also contributes to HSP70 expression, is constitutively activated (detected in the nucleus and phosphorylated) in RA synovial tissue *(69)*. In cultured RA FLS, HSF1 was activated by IL-1 and TNF-α. HSP70 is an important chaperonin protein that binds nascent proteins, preventing permanent cell damage and loss of function. In this capacity, HSP70 may contribute to the protection against apoptosis, which will be discussed in Subheading 8. As mentioned earlier, increased HSP70 might also interact with the HLA-DR-β1 shared epitope, potentially interfering with antigen processing.

5.6. STATs

Signal transducer and activator of transcription (STAT) is a family of transcription factors activated by a number of cytokines and growth factors, including IL-6, interferon-γ, and GM-CSF. Following receptor ligation, STATs are activated by janus tyrosine kinases (JAKs). Activated STATs migrate to the nucleus, bind to promoters, and contribute to the regulation of the expression of genes, such as Fc receptors and HLA-DR molecules. RA synovial fluid upregulated the expression of Fcγ RI and RIII, markers of activation on monocytes *(70)*. These synovial fluids also activated STAT-3. Activation of STAT-3 and Fcγ RI was inhibited by an antibody to IL-6. These observations suggest that IL-6, present in high concentration in the RA joint, may contribute to the activation of synovial macrophages, mediated by STAT activation.

5.7. Erg-1

The early growth response 1 gene *(erg-1)*, is a zinc-finger transcription factor that is constitutively upregulated, in RA FLS, compared to osteoarthritis or reactive arthritis *(71)*. It is expressed at low levels in dermal fibroblasts and upregulated transiently by TNF-α. *Erg-1* overexpression persists in RA FLS in vitro over several generations. The upregulation of c-Fos also persists over several generations. Although both c-Fos and Erg-1 upregulation have been associated with proliferation, RA FLS generally proliferate more slowly than dermal fibroblasts, suggesting that Erg-1 may not regulate proliferation in these cells. The genes potentially regulated by Erg-1 have not been clearly defined, although it is coordinately regulated with HSP70, c-Jun, and c-Fos under conditions of stress, such as ischemia *(72)*, which may be relevant to the relatively hypoxic conditions in the rheumatoid joint.

5.8. Transcriptional Regulation in FLS

Recent studies have examined FLS to determine if transcription factors identified in vivo are functionally active in vitro. Functional tests, called electrophoretic mobility gel shift assays (EMSA), are performed by radiolabeling a short piece of double-stranded DNA that represents the DNA-binding site for a transcription factor that is present in any given promoter. Nuclear extracts isolated from the desired cells are mixed with the radiolabeled DNA and electrophoresed on a nondenaturing gel. If the transcription factor has been activated and has migrated to the nucleus, it can bind to the DNA, which will retard the migration of the radiolabeled DNA through the gel (Fig. 4). When this was done with adherent cells from RA synovial tissue, the nuclear

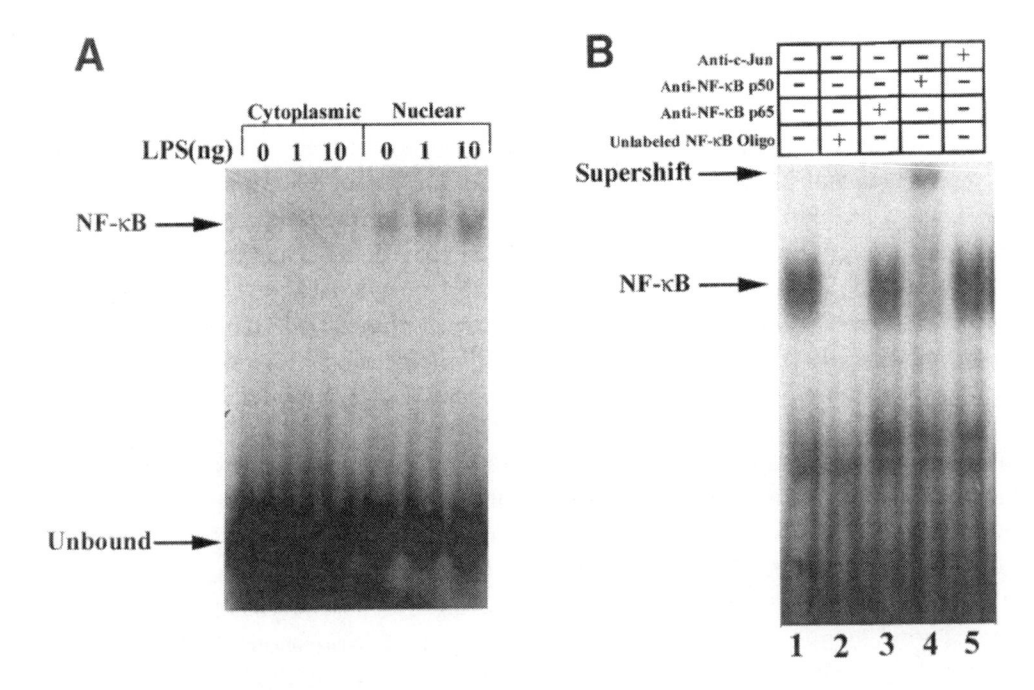

Fig. 4. Activated NF-κB can be detected by its ability to bind to a radiolabeled oligonucleotide. This electrophoretic mobility gel shift assay (EMSA) was performed with a radiolabeled oligonucleotide representing the Ig/HIV NF-κB binding site. In panel A, cells were activated for 1 h with 0, 1, or 10 ng/mL of LPS. The cells were harvested and proteins from the cytoplasm and the nucleus were isolated. If NF-κB is activated, IκB is degraded, freeing NF-κB p65/p50 heterodimers or p50/p50 homodimers to migrate to the nucleus. As can be seen in panel A, no NF-κB complex were available in the cytoplasm to bind to the radiolabeled oligonucleotide, either with or without the addition of LPS. In contrast, when proteins from the nuclear extract were added to the radiolabeled oligonucleotide, they were retained and migrated more slowly in the gel, as indicated by the arrow on the left side of panel A. The free or unbound radiolabeled oligonucleotide migrates more rapidly and is seen at the bottom of the gel. Panel B, generated at a later time-point with nuclear extracts, demonstrates how the composition of the bound complex is identified. The NF-κB binding complex is indicated by the arrow on the left. At the top of the figure are identified the treatments added to the radiolabeled oligonucleotide–nuclear extract complex before adding the complex to the gel. In lane 1, binding by a protein, identified as NF-κB retards the migration of the radiolabeled oligonucleotide in the gel. In lane 2, excess unlabeled NF-κB oligonucleotide inhibits binding of the protein(s) to the radiolabeled oligonucleotide, indicating that it is specific. In lanes 3–5, antibodies to NF-κB p50 or p65 or c-Jun were added, prior to running on the gel. With the anti-p65 and anti-c-Jun, no change is seen in the character of the band, indicating that these proteins were not present. However, the anti-p50 antibody reduced the band, which can now be seen even higher up in the gel, indicating that it was retarded even further or "supershifted." This means that NF-κB p50 homodimers, or p50 bound to a NF-κB protein other than p65, was present in this complex.

extracts bound an oligonucleotide representing the AP-1-binding site of the MMP-1 promoter. Monospecific antibodies identified both c-Jun and c-Fos in these complexes, indicating they were functionally active. This activity was greater than found in osteoarthritis synovial tissue, and it correlated with disease activity as determined by

C-reactive protein *(65)*. The active AP-1 complexes were detected constitutively, with no additional culture or activation of the adherent synovial tissue cells, which included macrophages and FLS. Additionally, if cultured RA FLS are stimulated with IL-1β, the expression of c-Jun and c-Fos protein and activity (ability to bind DNA oligonucleotides) are increased. Under these circumstances, an antisense molecule for *c-fos* inhibited the activation of the MMP-1 promoter, presumably by interfering with the transcription of the mRNA *(73)*. Overexpression of another AP-1 family member, *jun D*, resulted in the reduction of nuclear DNA binding proteins containing c-Jun and c-Fos following activation with TNF-α. Jun D overexpression also resulted in decreased proliferation in response to IL-1β, TNF-α, and PDGF as well as decreased IL-6, IL-8, and MMP-1 secretion in response to TNF-α *(74)*. These observations suggest that proliferation and cytokine and MMP production are regulated in RA FLS by the AP-1 family transcription factors c-Jun and c-Fos, supporting the relevance of the observations made by immunohistochemistry that AP-1 proteins were present in the nucleus in vivo.

More than one mechanism of gene activation may be present simultaneously in a given cell. Even though examination of synovial tissue by immunohistochemistry and the above-described functional studies (EMSA), suggest that c-Jun and c-Fos activation in vivo might be important in the activation of genes in FLS, additional in vitro studies suggest that activation of NF-κB may also be important in this cell type. FLS cloned by limiting dilution such that each clone is likely the progeny of a single cell were selected on the basis of the constitutive production of high or low concentrations of IL-6. A number of transcription factors were examined by EMSA. AP-1 and C/EBPβ complexes capable of binding to radiolabeled oligonucleotides representing the regions of the IL-6 promoter that bind each of these factors was observed constitutively, both in the high and low IL-6-producing clones *(75)*. Only the NF-κB binding complexes, consisting of p50/p65 heterodimers, were expressed more strongly in the FLS clones producing high concentrations of IL-6. This observation suggests that, at least in the clones producing higher concentrations of IL-6, the constitutively activated NF-κB may contribute to the ongoing secretion of IL-6. However, because activated NF-κB was not detected in some of the FLS clones that did secrete IL-6, although at lower concentrations, it is possible that C/EBPβ or AP-1 factors may contribute to the constitutive expression of IL-6 in these cells.

Additional studies have examined the importance of NF-κB activation in the expression of inflammatory mediators by RA FLS in vitro. Although many studies have shown that MMP-1 expression is regulated by an AP-1-binding site in its proximal promoter, a recent study suggests that NF-κB activation may also contribute to the expression of the MMP-1 gene in synovial fibroblasts *(76)*. Additionally, IL-1β and TNF-α induce degradation of IκB and the translocation of NF-κB p65/p50 heterodimers to the nucleus of FLS. The addition of *N*-acetyl-L-cysteine inhibited the activation of NF-κB and the expression of IL-6, IL-8, GM-CSF, and ICAM-1, induced by TNF-α or IL-1β in RA FLS, suggesting that NF-κB activation was important *(77)*. Further, an NF-κB p65 antisense oligonucleotides inhibited the IL-1β-induced expression of the cycloxygenase-2 *(78)*. Cycloxygenase-2 is induced by IL-1β and is responsible for the conversion of arachidonate to prostaglandins (i.e., PGE_2), important mediators of inflammation in RA. We have also observed C/EBPβ expressed in the nucleus of FLS and lining macrophages in RA synovial tissue (Fig. 3). C/EBPβ may regulate a number of proinflammatory genes expressed by fibroblasts, such as IL-6, IL-8, MMP-1, and G-CSF. However, studies have yet to be done to determine the potential of C/EBPβ to contribute to the regulation of these genes in RA FLS.

6. Destruction

The major focus of destruction of bone and cartilage in RA is the pannus. As described earlier, at least three types of lesions can be differentiated, and the mediation of destruction in each appears to be different. The distinct cartilage–pannus junction (Fig. 1) possesses both macrophages and FLS. The macrophages express IL-1α (not IL-1β), TNF-α, IL-6, and GM-CSF. TGF-β and MMP-1 are also expressed in these lesions. A likely scenario in the diffuse lesion is that macrophages are induced to express proinflammatory cytokines, such as TNF-α and IL-1α, inducing MMP-1 and MMP-3, in both FLS and macrophages. In the less aggressive diffuse fibroblastic cartilage–pannus junction, macrophages and their inflammatory mediators are not readily detected *(10,36)*. Only TGF-β is seen. It is not clear which MMPs are present in these lesions. Because TGF-β possesses both inflammatory and reparative properties, it is unclear if this represents a healing or an actively destructive phase. Nonetheless, it is clear from immunohistochemistry, and from studies performed in vitro that macrophages plus FLS produce greater destruction together compared to either cell type alone *(10,36,64,79)*.

Cathepsins K and L have been detected in the bone and cartilage pannus of patients with RA *(12,80)*. Cathepsins are cysteine proteinases capable of cleaving collagen, elastin, proteoglycans, and fibronectin. Although present in the pannus–cartilage junction, the contribution to a discrete versus a diffuse pannus, or both, has not been characterized. However, in the severe combined immune deficiency (SCID) model in which RA synovial tissue and cartilage are coimplanted, cathepsin L and B were strongly expressed by fibroblasts eroding into the cartilage *(81)*. Macrophages were rare in these implants, similar to the diffuse cartilage–pannus, suggesting that cathepsins might contribute to the destruction seen in the diffuse lesion. In addition to the ability of the synovial tissue to induce destruction directly by proteinases, the inflammatory mediators present in the cartilage–pannus lesion may affect cartilage at a distance. TNF-α and IL-1 can induce proteoglycan degradation in the cartilage and induce the chondrocyte to synthesize MMPs that are capable of enhancing cartilage destruction. In contrast, TGF-β and IL-10 may have a protective effect by enhancing proteoglycan and collagen synthesis.

Subchondral bony erosions are characteristic of RA. It seems that less attention has been paid to the pannus–bone lesions seen in RA, perhaps because of the difficulty of working with bone. Nonetheless, this lesion is critical and its presence is the harbinger of a poor prognosis. The pannus–bone junction is replete with mononuclear cells that are CD68 positive, likely of macrophage origin. Cathepsin L is strongly expressed by mononuclear cells and cathepsin K by osteoclasts in these lesions *(12)*. This proteinase is capable of degrading bone, including type I collagen and osteocalcin. We are not aware of published studies documenting the presence of the pro-inflammatory cytokines in these lesions. The presence of multinucleated giant cells has been documented in the pannus–bone lesions of patients with RA. These cells express tartrate-resistant acid phosphatase and calcitonin receptors, indicating that they are true osteoclasts *(9)*. It is likely that IL-1, IL-11, and IL-6, known to be present in the adjacent cartilage–pannus lesions, might contribute to the differentiation of osteoclasts from macrophages. It appears that the expression of the calcitonin receptor, essential for identification as an osteoclast, only occurs after contact with bone. Macrophages may prepare or roughen the bone surface that allows for the development of osteoclasts *(79)*. Osteoclasts uniquely contribute to the destruction of bone by their ability to remove the mineral content allowing the proteinases, such as cathepsins L and K, to degrade the matrix more readily.

7. Persistence

Once initiated, why does RA persist? Normally, an inflammatory response results in the removal of the offending agent and resolution of the inflammation. It is possible that in certain individuals, once initiated, the local milieu of the RA joint may contribute to the persistence of the disease. In the normal joint, types A and B lining cells are present adjacent to the cartilage bone junction, and no inflammatory response develops. Earlier in this chapter, the ability of soluble cytokines, such as TNF-α and IL-1β, to affect other cells locally, to contribute to an inflammatory cascade, was described. What mechanisms might contribute to the persistence of the expression of these inflammatory mediators? Interactions between cells in the synovial tissue might lead to persistence. For example, cognate interactions between cells, particularly if one or both of the cell types has already been partially activated, might contribute to the persistence of RA. It is possible that cell–cell interaction during migration into the joint may also contribute to this process. Another interaction that may contribute to the persistence of disease activity and destruction is the interaction of the cells of the lining with bone and cartilage, by adhesion molecules (such as VCAM-1) or by integrins, which are upregulated in RA synovial tissue.

The example of chronic Lyme arthritis should be kept in mind when considering this paradigm. Chronic Lyme arthritis may develop in the predisposed individual who possesses the HLA-DRβ1 shared epitope associated with RA. However, following appropriate treatment with antibiotics, the organism can no longer be detected in the joint, and the synovitis generally resolves. Histologically, Lyme arthritis and RA cannot be distinguished. Why does the chronic inflammation of Lyme arthritis, even in a shared-epitope-positive individual, resolve, whereas RA does not? One explanation may be that there is an ongoing infection that has not been characterized. If identified and treated, perhaps RA would not persist. It is possible that other factors, perhaps genetically inherited, might contribute to the dysregulation resulting in chronic inflammation.

7.1. Interaction with Endothelial Cells

Cell–cell interactions may contribute to the perpetuation of RA. Lymphocytes, neutrophils, and monocytes migrate into the synovial tissue because of the interactions with adhesion molecules on synovial endothelial cells *(82)*. E-selectin, P-selectin, VCAM-1, ICAM-1 and the CS-1 region of fibronectin are expressed on synovial endothelial cells, in part because of the action of TNF-α, secreted locally. As inflammatory cells traverse the vessels, they interact with adhesion molecules on the vessels, resulting in rolling (weak attachment due to selectins), firm attachment, and then diapedesis or migration through the vessel. LFA-1 (a β2 integrin) is present on peripheral blood lymphocytes, and while rolling, the molecule is induced to a high activity state, allowing for stronger interaction with ICAM-1 *(83)*. Other molecules involved in the adhesion of lymphocytes to synovial tissue endothelial cells, as determined by the inhibition of binding by monospecific antibodies, include VLA-4 (α4β1)/VCAM-1 (CD106) and VLA-4/CS-1 fibronectin interactions. The interaction of P-selectin on endothelial cells with its counterreceptor on monocytes is important for the binding of monocytes to RA synovial tissue endothelial cells, whereas E- and L-selectin are less important *(84)*. As cells adhere to the endothelium and migrate into the joint, they may become activated. Although this has not been demonstrated specifically in the synovial tissue, the interaction of monocytes with P-selectin resulted in the activation of NF-κB and, in the presence of platelet-activating factor, the expression of TNF-α and MCP-1 *(85)*. This may be very relevant in RA, because just the binding of the monocytes to P-selectin, upregulated on the endothelial cell, may be enough to sensitize the monocytes to respond further in the pro-inflammatory environment of the rheumatoid joint.

7.2. Adhesion Molecule and Integrin Ligation

The integrin α6β1 plus its ligand laminin are upregulated in RA synovial lining. Also, α5β1 and αvβ5, vitronectin-fibronectin receptors, are expressed on most synovial lining cells and FLS *(82,86)*. VCAM-1 and ICAM-1 are strongly expressed on RA synovial lining cells. Adhesion molecules and integrins not only regulate the interaction between cells, providing structure, but they also regulate the migration of cells through the tissue, as well as their retention or egress. Once in the synovial tissue, interaction of inflammatory cells with matrix molecules such as fibronectin, vitronectin, or collagen may contribute to their retention and activation. For example, synovial fluid lymphocytes may interact, via the integrins VLA-4 (α4β1) and VLA-5 (α5β1), with fibronectin, which is secreted by synovial fibroblasts. It is possible that this interaction could contribute to the retention of the lymphocytes in the synovial tissue. Ligation of integrins by interaction with extracellular matrix proteins such as fibronectin, vitronectin, collagen, or laminin is capable of providing activation signals to cells that are important in survival, proliferation, and expression of proteinases such as MMP-1 *(86)*. Integrin ligation is capable of activating MAP kinase pathways, resulting in the activation of transcription factors such as Elk-1/2, C/EBPβ, and c-Jun. Activation of these transcription factors may contribute to the regulation of the expression of the pro- or anti-inflammatory molecules found in RA synovial tissue.

7.3. FLS and Synovial Lining

Interaction of RA FLS with fibronectin, which is mediated primarily by αvβ5 and α5β1 integrin receptors, results in increased proliferation of FLS in response to PDGF and decreased MMP-1 secretion *(86)*. However, if the cytoskeletal attachments that occur in RA FLS after integrin ligation by fibronectin are disrupted, as might occur because of the change in cell shape in the synovial lining, integrin ligation acts synergistically with TNF-α to increase MMP-1 expression *(86)*. This might contribute to the enhanced MMP-1 expression seen in the RA synovial lining and pannus. Interaction between FLS, mediated by VCAM-1, and cartilage and bone in the pannus may contribute to the destruction observed in the pannus. When RA FLS alone plus cartilage were engrafted into mice that were severe combined immune deficient (SCID), the

FLS eroded into the cartilage, which may represent a model of the diffuse cartilage–pannus. At the leading edge of the erosion by the FLS, VCAM-1 was strongly expressed together with cathepsins L and B, supporting the importance of VCAM-1 in this experimental model of cartilage erosion *(81)*. Perhaps contact with cartilage in this model results in persistent activation, perhaps mediated through VCAM-1, although such a mechanism has yet to be defined. Interaction of FLS with cartilage may also involve CD44 *(87)*. Ligation of CD44, perhaps by hyaluronic acid, might also contribute to FLS activation.

7.4. Monocytes and Macrophages

Monocytes and macrophages express a number of integrins including β1 (α2β1, α4β1, α5β1), β2 (LFA-1, CD11a/CD18, and Mac-1, CD11b, CD18), and αv (αvβ3, αvβ5). The interaction of macrophages with fibronectin present in the extracellular matrix via the α5β1-integrin receptor (upregulated during macrophage differentiation) has been shown to result in the secretion of IL-1β *(88,89)*. Ligation of collagen to the α2β1-integrin receptor also contributes to the expression of IL-1β by monocytes *(88)*. Ligation of α5β1 by fibronectin may also increase the expression of MMP-9 in macrophages *(90)*. Cells phagocytosing intact cartilage collagen fragments can be seen in a very aggressive cartilage–pannus lesions *(11)*. It is possible that the uptake of soluble collagen or the phagocytosis of cartilage and bone fragments in more aggressive lesions may lead to the expression of cytokines such as IL-1 and TNF-α, and MMPs, thereby leading to a self-perpetuating process. An additional mechanism of increasing cytokine gene expression in synovial tissue macrophages, unrelated to integrins, is the phagocytosis of human HSP60 by human macrophages. Human HSP60 is capable of inducing the secretion of TNF-α, in the absence of antigen-specific sensitization *(91)*. Additionally, HSP60 also induced IL-15 and IL-12 expression, which promotes Th1-type responses, as seen in the rheumatoid joint. HSP60 is upregulated in RA synovial tissue.

7.5. T-Lymphocyte–FLS Interaction

Lymphocytes interact with FLS, particularly in the sublining region. This interaction may be mediated by VCAM-1, ICAM-1, and LFA-3 on the FLS, and by VLA-4, LFA-1, and CD2 (respectively) on the lymphocytes (Fig. 2). A recent study used lymphocytes from patients that were activated in vitro and then fixed *(92)*. When these activated lymphocytes were added to FLS, PGE$_2$, TIMP-1, and MMP-1 were secreted. MMP-1 was expressed in quantities greater than TIMP-1, which would favor MMP-1 activity. Also, MMP-1 was expressed over a long period of time, whereas the expression of TIMP-1 was brief. These observations provide insights into a potential mechanism that may help explain why, in RA, although both MMP-1 and TIMP-1 are expressed by the same cells, the ratio of MMP-1 to TIMP-1 in the synovial fluid and circulation is greater than seen in normal controls or in osteoarthritis. Additionally, the quantity of MMP-1 secreted by FLS in response to activated T-cells was greater than that associated with an optimal concentration of IL-1β, suggesting the potential importance of these cellular interactions in the rheumatoid joint. The degree to which synovial lymphocytes, without additional activation, might support this process is unclear.

7.6. Monocyte–T-Lymphocyte Interactions

Monocytes and T-cells interact in the areas of diffuse infiltration as well as in the lymphoid aggregates. Although previously activated lymphocytes may migrate more readily, our earlier studies showed that naïve (CD45RA+) and memory (CD45RO+) T-cells both enter the joint and may be seen comparably in and adjacent to the blood vessels. FGF-1 receptors are present on perivascular lymphocytes, suggesting that migration locally might contribute to the expression of these receptors. FGF-1 is a coactivator of T-cells, suggesting that FGF-1 might also contribute to the activated phenotype seen in RA synovial tissue *(44)*. As with monocytes, it is possible that interactions with endothelial cells during binding and diapedesis may contribute to the initial activation of these lymphocytes. By the time the T-cells migrate away from the area of the blood vessel, they essentially all have acquired the CD45R0+ or "memory" phenotype. T-Cells acquire additional activation markers, including CD44, HLA-DR, and CD69. Although this activated phenotype can occur during antigen-specific activation, inflammatory cytokines produced within the rheumatoid joint, such as FGF-1, TNF-α, and IL-15, may contribute to the activated phenotype, even in the absence of a specific antigenic stimulus. Lymphocytes activated in vitro by mitogens induced IL-1β, MMP-1, and 92-kDa gelatinase (MMP-9) in monocytes, via direct contact, suggesting a possible mechanism in RA *(64,93,94)*. Additionally, the cognate interaction between T-cells, incubated with IL-15, which is secreted by RA synovial tissue macrophages and monocytes, resulted in increased TNF-α secretion *(42)* (Fig. 2). In these studies, the interaction between normal peripheral blood T-cells and monocytes, without the addition of IL-15, did not induce TNF-α, indicating that the cognate interaction of normal T-cells and monocytes alone was not sufficient to induce TNF-α secretion. However, synovial fluid lymphocytes taken directly out of the joints of patients were capable of stimulating TNF-α secretion by monocytes, suggesting that these cells had already been adequately activated. If the synovial fluid lymphocytes were cultured in vitro prior to addition to the monocytes, the ability to induce TNF-α was lost but could be restored or maintained by IL-15, suggesting that the synovial lymphocytes had been activated in vivo by IL-15. The T-cell–macrophage interactions were mediated by LFA-1 and CD69 on the lymphocyte and by ICAM-1 and a counterreceptor for CD69 on the macrophage (Fig. 2). In summary, as lymphocytes enter the synovial tissue, macrophage-derived FGF-1, TNF-α, and IL-15 might contribute to an activated, "memory" phenotype, without antigen-specific activation. These cells may then come in contact with recently recruited monocytes, which have been sensitized by interaction with P-selectin on endothelial cells. Monocyte–lymphocyte cell–cell interactions might then lead to the continued production of pro-inflammatory cytokines, such as TNF-α, in the sublining region, which is observed by immunohistochemistry.

7.7. Antigen-Specific T-Cells

Another possible source for the persistence of RA is the generation of antigen-specific T-cells that might drive the inflammatory process. It is possible that following the initial joint destruction, a self-perpetuating process might develop if antigen-specific T-cells were generated by persistent exposure to locally expressed antigens, exposed by the inflammatory process. We examined this possibility by characterizing the T-cell response to HSP60. We observed a strong response to mycobacterial HSP60 with synovial fluid, compared to peripheral blood, T-lymphocytes of patients with RA. In contrast, the response to tetanus toxoid was much greater with peripheral blood lymphocytes. However, this difference was not the result of crossreactivity with human HSP60, because the synovial fluid lymphocytes responded much less to it than to the mycobacterial HSP60 *(95)*. Subsequent studies have demonstrated that T-cell clones that respond to the mycobacterial antigen do not respond to epitopes that are conserved in the human protein. T-Cell and B-cell responses to other autoantigens have been detected in the rheumatoid joint. Of these, MHC class II-restricted T-cell responses to human type II collagen have been clearly documented, to a greater extent in patients compared to normal controls. However, specificity to type II collagen is seen with the synovial fluid lymphocytes of only a limited number of patients *(96)*. T-Cell responses to additional joint constituents, including a synovial fluid protein p205, solubilized antigen from synovial cells, and solubilized antigens from chondrocytes, have been described *(97–100)*. These observations suggest that after joint destruction is initiated, antigen-specific T-cells may develop and contribute to the persistence of the disease.

Although current therapies directed against cytokines (TNF-α and IL-1) are effective temporarily, no treatment has been capable of inducing a disease remission. Perhaps if the initial destruction of cartilage and bone can be prevented, the disease would not persist. Of interest in this regard, the early treatment of RA, which may be more effective than therapy given once destruction has occurred, may provide an insight. In a recent study, treating patients with RA with minocycline early, which may work as a MMP inhibitor, resulted in greater than 20% complete remission at 1 yr *(101)*. Perhaps, this early, and admittedly short term, remission prior to joint destruction might prevent the chronicity of this disease, perhaps by preventing the local development of T-cells specific to the joint constituents.

A recent study has addressed, in a novel way, the potential importance of T-cells driving the inflammatory cascade in the rheumatoid joint, without addressing whether it is caused by cognate cell–cell interactions or antigen-specific T-cells. In this study, RA synovial tissue was placed into SCID mice, and the persistence of the synovitis was determined in relation to the presence or absence of T-cells *(102)*. Following implantation of RA synovial tissue, the mice were treated with a control or an anti-CD2 antibody to deplete T-cells. The tissue was examined over time for the presence of TNF-α, IL-1β, interferon-γ, IL-15, MMP-1, and MMP-3. Treatment with anti-CD2 decreased the number of T-cells and interferon-γ, which was measured by a sensitive RT-PCR ELISA. The cytokines of macrophage origin, IL-1β, TNF-α, and IL-15, as well as MMP-1 and MMP-3 were greatly reduced following anti-CD2 treatment. Whether or not the MMP-1 and MMP-3 was derived from macrophages or FLS was not determined. CD4+ synovial tissue T-cells or interferon-γ could restore or maintain the expression of the macrophage-derived cytokines and MMPs. These observations support the potential importance of T-cells in maintaining the inflammatory cascade observed in RA. The question raised by these observations is how could the inflammatory response be so dependent on T-cells, and yet most groups have detected little or no interferon-γ protein or mRNA in RA synovial tissue? It is possible that only a very few cells are necessary to drive the response. It is also possible that the expression of interferon-γ is brief and therefore difficult to detect. Also, how can these observations be reconciled with the lack of response in patients to anti-CD4 treatment? It is possible that the depletion necessary to achieve a clinically significant reduction of inflammation was not achieved in the clinical trials mentioned earlier. Also of interest, patients with RA did not flare when treated with interferon-γ, which might have been expected if the synovitis was interferon-γ dependent. Further studies that effectively deplete or modulate the relevant T-cell subsets in the rheumatoid joint will be required to settle this issue.

7.8. Macrophage–FLS Interactions

The interaction between macrophages and FLS in the synovial lining is a characteristic feature in RA, as well as the normal joint. Monocytes interact with FLS to induce ICAM-1 and VCAM-1 on the FLS. This effect was inhibited by antibody to TNF-α, suggesting that this cytokine was released by the monocytes following the cognate interactions. Coculture of monocytic cell lines with FLS has been shown to enhance cartilage degradation. TNF-α, IL-1β, and IL-6 contributed to the effects observed and cell–cell interaction of FLS and monocytic cells was not essential (87). FLS contact with cartilage was necessary for cartilage damage, however. CD44, the hyaluronate receptor, was necessary for the attachment of the FLS to the cartilage. Recently, ligation of CD44 on RA FLS resulted in the upregulation of VCAM-1 at the transcriptional level, which enhanced the ability of FLS to interact with T-cells and macrophages via the VLA-4 integrin (α4β1) (103), setting up a potential cascade of cellular interactions (Figure 2). These observations suggest that macrophage–FLS interactions enhance cartilage destruction and can enhance the ability of FLS to interact with T-cells. As mentioned earlier, the T-cell–FLS interactions may enhance MMP expression and activity.

8. Apoptosis and Persistence of RA

8.1. Synovial Tissue

The regulation of apoptosis in the RA joint may contribute to the perpetuation of the disease. Although the reported studies on RA apoptosis are conflicting (104–107), it appears that apoptosis is not increased in RA synovial tissue (105–107). Studies using end labeling to measure DNA fragmentation demonstrated macrophage-positivity (104) and sublining fibroblast-positivity, originally interpreted as apoptosis (104,106). However, electron microscopic (EM) examination, a more definitive measure of apoptosis, revealed few cells that displayed morphological evidence of cell death (105,106), suggesting that the amount of apoptosis might have been overestimated in the original studies. Together, these observations suggest that the positive studies noted earlier, may represent DNA fragmentation resulting from the local environment by mediators such as cytokines, MMPs, and reactive oxygen species. No study has described apoptotic bodies in macrophages or in synovial fluid. These data suggest that insufficient apoptosis may contribute to the persistence of RA, though the mechanism is unclear.

8.2. FLS

The tumor-suppressor gene product, p53, is upregulated in intimal lining cells (108). The fact that p53 is upregulated suggests that it may have been induced by DNA damage, as mentioned in the preceding paragraph. Somatic mutations in p53 have also been reported in RA-FLSs (109), suggesting that a subset of FLSs possess an inactivated form of p53. Inactivation of wild-type p53 in FLSs might render them more resistant to apoptotic stimuli, because one role of wild-type p53 is to promote apoptosis (110).

These data suggest that inhibition or inactivation of p53 activity might allow FLSs to become more resistant to apoptotic stimuli.

Ligation of the death receptors, Fas or TNFRI, by Fas ligand, or by TNF-α, may induce apoptosis in certain cell types. However, apoptosis following death receptor ligation may be blocked by the upregulation of antiapoptotic molecules (e.g., Bcl-2 or Bcl-xL) or a reduction of those that are proapoptotic (e.g., caspases). The ability to induce apoptosis in RA FLS by ligation of the death receptors has been examined. RAFLSs express Fas receptor on the cell surface *(106)*. Furthermore, ligation of Fas with an antibody induced apoptosis in RA FLS *(18,74,111)*. In addition, analysis of the effects of cytokines on Fas-induced cell death demonstrated that both TNF-α and IL-1β, which promote FLS proliferation, also inhibited RA FLS apoptosis (Fig. 2). This protection was associated with Bcl-2 upregulation and downregulation of caspases 2 and 3 *(112)*. Furthermore, TGF-β also inhibited Fas-induced apoptosis in RA FLSs, and this protection correlated with Bcl-2 upregulation *(113)*. These data demonstrate that Fas is expressed on RA FLSs, and addition of pro- or anti-inflammatory cytokines inhibits Fas-induced apoptosis.

8.3. Macrophages

Synovial tissue macrophages also appear resistant to apoptosis. Although activation of NF-κB, potentially by TNF-α, protects monocytes from apoptosis (Fig. 2), the role of NF-κB in the protection of differentiated macrophages against TNF-α-mediated apoptosis is less clear. Interferon-γ may contribute to the expression of GM-CSF production by macrophages, which may protect synovial macrophages from cell death *(102)* (Fig. 2). Also, TNF-α and IL-1β increase the expression of GM-CSF by RA FLS *(43)*.

8.4. T-Lymphocytes

Activated T-cells undergo apoptosis resulting from growth factor withdrawal or activation of the death receptor pathway (i.e., Fas). Synovial fluid T-cells from patients with RA, when placed in culture in vitro, undergo spontaneous apoptosis, which can be reversed by culturing with IL-2Rγ cytokines, including IL-2 and IL-15, or by coculturing with synovial fibroblasts (Fig. 2). In RA, synovial tissue T-cell apoptosis is not seen, despite the phenotype CD45RO^{bright}, CD45RB^{dull}, which identifies a highly differentiated T-cell, which is susceptible to apoptosis *(114)*. Because IL-15 and FLS are present in RA synovial tissue, either might lead to protection. IL-10 derived from macrophages may also protect T-cells from apoptosis (Fig. 2). However, the expression of Bcl-2 is reduced in synovial compared to peripheral blood T-lymphocytes. In contrast, another Bcl-2 family member, Bcl-x$_L$, is upregulated in freshly isolated RA synovial fluid lymphocytes compared to those from the peripheral blood. A relative increase of Bcl-x$_L$ compared to Bcl-2 occurs following T-cell interaction with FLS, not incubation of T-cells with IL-15. These observations suggest that T-cell interaction with FLS may be important in the protection against apoptosis of T-cells in the RA joint.

8.5. Enhanced Apoptosis May Be Beneficial

A potential role for induction of apoptosis as a therapeutic approach in autoimmune diseases, particularly RA, has been proposed by many authors *(111,115)*, and recent observations support this hypothesis. NF-κB inhibition by an IκBα-expressing adenovirus enhanced apoptosis in the streptococcal cell-wall arthritis model, whereas inhibition by NF-κB decoy oligonucleotides ameliorated the arthritis in this model *(116)*. Additionally, increased apoptosis was associated with reduced inflammation and clinical improvement following Fas ligation in HTLV-1 tax transgenic mice and in collagen-induced arthritis *(117,118)*. Furthermore, Fas ligation resulted in apoptosis and reduced inflammation in RA explants in SCID mice *(119)*, supporting the potential therapeutic value of increased apoptosis. In addition to inhibiting cytokine expression, which may be mediated by adenosine release locally, methotrexate may also promote apoptosis. Methotrexate induced apoptosis of activated lymphocytes, by a mechanism other than ligation of the Fas receptor *(120)*. These observations suggest that increasing apoptosis locally may be an effective approach for the treatment of RA. Increasing the expression of Fas ligand, inhibition of NF-κB activation, or downregulation of antiapoptotic molecules such as Bcl-2 are potential approaches that might be effective locally in the rheumatoid joint.

9. Summary

Rheumatoid arthritis occurs in a genetically susceptible individual, generally in an insidious manner, usually without other symptoms, which would help identify an inciting cause. At the time of presentation to the physician, the inflammation in the joint is chronic with a polyclonal T-cell response and the expression of multiple pro-inflammatory cytokines and destructive MMPs by macrophages and FLS. There is reason to believe that early, effective treatment may reduce the frequency of persistent disease, possibly by preventing the development of antigen-specific T-cells directed at breakdown components of the joint, such as type II collagen or chondrocyte-specific antigens. Our current knowledge would suggest that macrophages are important in the persistence of RA. It is clear that the specific inhibition of TNF-α and, to a lesser degree, IL-1 results in reduced inflammation and symptoms. IL-1 inhibition may provide chondroprotection, although the effects of TNF inhibition on joint integrity remain to be determined. The very interesting question is: Why are macrophages expressing TNF-α and IL-1? It is possible that T-cells, either by cell–cell contact and/or the secretion of interferon-γ, might contribute, following the possible priming of monocytes, by interaction with P-selectin on endothelial cells as they enter the joint. Additionally, interaction with FLS, mediated by α4β1/VCAM-1, might also contribute to the persistence macrophage activation. The interaction of macrophages with structural matrix molecules, in synovium and cartilage or bone, such as fibronectin and collagen, mediated by integrin receptors such as α5β1 might also contribute to the upregulation of cytokines and MMPs. The expression of chemokines and MMPs by FLS appears to result in large part because of actions of TNF-α and IL-1. Cell–cell interactions of FLS with macrophages and with T-cells may also contribute to their activation. This is an exciting time in the study of RA. Because of the tools of molecular and cellular biology, specific abnormalities in the rheumatoid joint, once identified, can be modified in a specific fashion, such as the specific inhibition of TNF, which is now clinically available. It is likely that additional specific and effective treatments will be forthcoming, based on molecular mechanisms, which will be identified by current, ongoing research.

References

1. Allard, S. A., Bayliss, M. T., and Maini, R. W. (1990) Synovium–cartilage junction of the normal knee: implications for joint destruction and repair. *Arthritis Rheum.* **33**, 1170–1179.
2. Koch, A. E., Robinson, P. G., Radosevich, J. A., and Pope, R. M. (1990) Distribution of CD45RA and CD45RO T-lymphocyte subsets in rheumatoid arthritis synovial tissue. *J. Clin. Immunol.* **10**, 192–199.
3. Klimiuk, P. A., Goronzy, J. J., Bjornsson, J., Beckenbaugh, R. D., and Weyand, C. M. (1997) Tissue cytokine patterns distinguish variants of rheumatoid synovitis. *Am. J. Pathol.* **151**, 1311–1319.
4. Rooney, M., Condell, D., Quinlan, W., Daly, L., Whelan, A., Feighery, C., et al. (1988) Analysis of the histologic variation of synovitis in rheumatoid arthritis. *Arthritis Rheum.* **31**, 956–963.
5. Kurosaka, T. and Ziff, M. (1983) Immunoelectron microscopic study of the distribution of T cell subsets in rheumatoid synovium. *J. Exp. Med.* **158**, 1191–1210.
6. Yousseff, P. P., Kruan, M., Breedveld, F., Bresnihan, B., Cassidy, N., Cunnane, G., et al. (1998) Quantitative microscopic analysis of inflammation in rheumatoid arthritis synovial membrane samples selected at arthroscopy compared with samples obtained blindly by needle biopsy. *Arthritis Rheum.* **41**, 663–669.
7. Zvaifler, N. J., Boyle, D., and Firestein, G. S. (1994) Early synovitis—synoviocytes and mononuclear cells. *Semin. Arthritis Rheum.* **23**, 11–16.
8. Mulherin, D., Fitzgerald, O., and Bresnihan, B. (1996) Synovial tissue macrophage populations and articular damage in rheumatoid arthritis. *Arthritis Rheum.* **39**, 115–124.
9. Gravallese, E. M., Harada, Y., Wang, J.-T., Gorn, A. H., Thornhill, T. S., and Goldring, S. R. (1998) Identification of cell types responsible for bone resorption in rheumatoid arthritis and juvenile rheumatoid arthritis. *Am. J. Pathol.* **152**, 943–951.
10. Chu, C. Q., Field, M., Allard, S., Abney, E., Feldmann, M., and Maini, R. N. (1992) Detection of cytokines at the cartilage/pannus junction in patients with rheumatoid arthritis: implications for the role of cytokines in cartilage destruction and repair. *Br. J. Rheumatol.* **31**, 653–661.
11. Harris, E. D., Jr., Glauert, A. M., and Murley, A. H. G. (1977) Intracellular collagen fibers at the pannus-cartilage junction in rheumatoid arthritis. *Arthritis Rheum.* **20**, 657–665.
12. Iwata, Y., Mort, J. S., Tateishi, H., and Lee, E. R. (1997) Macrophage cathepsin L, a factor in the erosion of subchondral bone in rheumatoid arthritis. *Arthritis Rheum.* **40**, 499–509.
13. Weyand, C. M., McCarthy, T. G., and Goronzy, J. J. (1995) Correlation between disease phenotype and genetic heterogeneity in rheumatoid arthritis. *J. Clin. Invest.* **95**, 2120–2126.
14. Hammer, J., Gallazzi, F., Bono, E., Karr, R. W., Guenot, J., Valsasnini, P., et al. (1995) Peptide binding specificity of HLA-DR4 molecules: correlation with rheumatoid arthritis association. *J. Exp. Med.* **181**, 1847–1855.
15. Perdriger, A., Guggenbuhl, P., Chales, G., Le Dantec, P., Yaouanq, J., Genetet, B., et al. (1996) The role of HLA-DR-DR and HLA-DR-DP interactions in genetic susceptibility to rheumatoid arthritis. *Hum. Immunol.* **46**, 42–48.
16. Albani, S. and Carson, D. A. (1996) A multistep molecular mimicry hypothesis for the pathogenesis of rheumatoid arthritis. *Immunol. Today* **17**, 466–470.
17. Auger, I., Escola, J. M., Gorvel, J. P., and Roudier, J. (1996) HLA-DR4 and HLA-DR10 motifs that carry susceptibility to rheumatoid arthritis bind 70-kD heat shock proteins. *Nature Med.* **2**, 306–310.
18. Kirschmann, D. A., Duffin, K. L., Smith, C. E., Welply, J. K., Howard, S. C., Schwartz, B. D., et al. (1995) Naturally processed peptides from rheumatoid arthritis associated and non-associated HLA-DR alleles. *J. Immunol.* **155**, 5655–5662.

19. Zanelli, E., Krco, C. J., and David, C. S. (1997) Critical residues on HLA-DRB1*0402 HV3 peptide for HLA-DQ8-restricted immunogenicity. *J. Immunol.* **158,** 3545–3551.
20. Mu, H., Chen, J. J., Jiang, Y., King, M.-C., Thomson, G., and Criswell, L. A. (1999) Tumor necrosis factor α microsatellite polymorphism is associated with rheumatoid arthritis severity through an interaction with the HLA-DRB1 shared epitope. *Arthritis Rheum.* **42,** 438–442.
21. John, S., Myerscough, A., Marlow, A., Hajeer, A., Silman, A., Ollier, W., et al. (1998) Linkage of cytokine genes to rheumatoid arthritis. Evidence of genetic heterogeneity. *Ann. Rheum. Dis.* **57,** 361–365.
22. Cornelis, F., Faure, S., Martinez, M., Prud'homme, J.-F., Fritz, P., Dib, C., Alves, H., et al. (1998) New susceptibility locus for rheumatoid arthritis suggested by a genome-wide linkage study. *Proc. Natl. Acad. Sci. USA* **95,** 10,746–10,750.
23. Fox, D. A. (1997) The role of T cells in the immunopathogenesis of rheumatoid arthritis: new perspectives. *Arthritis Rheum.* **40,** 598–609.
24. Simon, A. K., Seipelt, E., and Sieper, J. (1994) Divergent T-cell cytokine patterns in inflammatory arthritis. *Proc. Natl. Acad. Sci. USA* **91,** 8562–8566.
25. Morita, Y., Yamamura, M., Kawashima, M., Harada, S., Tsuji, K., Shibuya, K., et al. (1998) Flow cytometric single-cell analysis of cytokine production by CD4+ T cells in synovial tissue and peripheral blood from patients with rheumatoid arthritis. *Arthritis Rheum.* **41,** 1669–1676.
26. Moreland, L. W., Heck, L. W., Jr., and Koopman, W. J. (1997) Biologic agents for treating rheumatoid arthritis: concepts and progress. *Arthritis Rheum.* **40,** 397–409.
27. Ruderman, E. M., Weinblatt, M. E., Thurmond, L. M., Pinkus, G. S., and Gravallese, E. M. (1995) Synovial tissue response to treatment with Campath-1H. *Arthritis Rheum.* **38,** 254–258.
28. Tak, P. P., van der Lubbe, P. A., Cauli, A., Daha, M. R., Smeets, T. J. M., Kluin, P. M., et al. (1995) Reduction of synovial inflammation after anti-CD4 monoclonal antibody treatment in early rheumatoid arthritis. *Arthritis Rheum.* **38,** 1457–1465.
29. Pope, R. M. and McDuffy, S. J. (1979) IgG rheumatoid factor. *Arthritis Rheum.* **22,** 988–998.
30. Randen, I., Mellbye, O. J., Forre, O., and Natvig, J. B. (1995) The identification of germinal centres and follicular dendritic cell networks in rheumatoid synovial tissue. *Scand. J. Immunol.* **41,** 481–486.
31. Shimaoka, Y., Attrep, J. F., Hirano, T., Ishihara, K., Suzuki, R., Toyosaki, T., et al. (1998) Nurse-like cells from bone marrow and synovium of patients with rheumatoid arthritis promote survival and enhance function of human B cells. *J. Clin. Invest.* **102,** 606–618.
32. Mageed, R. A., Borretzen, M., Moyes, S. P., Thompson, K. M., and Natvig, J. B. (1997) Rheumatoid factor autoantibodies in health and disease. *Ann. NY Acad. Sci.* **815,** 296–311.
33. Posnett, D. N. and Edinger, J. (1997) When do microbes stimulate rheumatoid factor? *J. Exp. Med.* **185,** 1721–1723.
34. Tsuchiya, N., Malone, C., Hutt-Fletcher, L. M., and Williams, R. C., Jr. (1991) Rheumatoid factors react with Fab fragments of monoclonal antibodies to herpes simplex virus types 1 and 2 Fcγ-binding proteins. *Arthritis Rheum.* **34,** 846–855.
35. Klareskog, L. and Olsson, T. (1990) Autoimmunity to collagen II and myelin basic protein: comparative studies in humans and rodents. *Immunol. Rev.* **118,** 285–310.
36. Feldmann, M., Brennan, F. M., and Maini, R. N. (1996) Role of cytokines in rheumatoid arthritis. *Annu. Rev. Immunol.* **14,** 397–440.
37. Firestein, G. S., Alvaro-Garcia, J. M., and Maki, R. (1990) Quantitative analysis of cytokine gene expression in rheumatoid arthritis. *J. Immunol.* **144,** 3347–3353.
38. Katsikis, P. D., Chu, C. Q., Brennan, F. M., Maini, R. N., and Feldmann, M. (1994) Immunoregulatory role of interleukin 10 in rheumatoid arthritis. *J. Exp. Med.* **179,** 1517–1527.

39. Koch, A. E., Kunkel, S. L., Burrows, J. C., Evanoff, H. L., Haines, G. K., Pope, R. M., et al. (1991) Synovial tissue macrophage as a source of the chemotactic cytokine IL-8. *J. Immunol.* **147,** 2187–2195.
40. Koch, A. E., Kunkel, S. L., Harlow, L. A., Mazarakis, D. D., Haines, G. K., Burdick, M. D., et al. (1994) Epithelial neutrophil activating peptide-78: a novel chemotactic cytokine for neutraphils in arthritis. *J. Clin. Invest.* **94,** 1012–1018.
41. Morita, Y., Yamamura, M., Nishida, K., Harada, S., Okamoto, H., Inoue, H., et al. (1998) Expression of interleukin-12 in synovial tissue from patients with rheumatoid arthritis. *Arthritis Rheum.* **41,** 306–314.
42. McInnes, I. B., Leung, B. P., Sturrock, R. D., Field, M., and Liew, F. Y. (1997) Interleukin-15 mediates T cell-dependent regulation of tumor necrosis factor-α production in rheumatoid arthritis. *Nature Med.* **3,** 189–195.
43. Koch, A. E., Kunkel, S. L., and Strieter, R. M. (1995) Cytokines in rheumatoid arthritis. *J. Invest. Med.* **43,** 28–38.
44. Byrd, V., Zhao, X.-M., McKeehan, W. L., Miller, G. G., and Thomas, J. W. (1996) Expression and functional expansion of fibroblast growth factor receptor T cells in rheumatoid synovium and peripheral blood of patients with rheumatoid arthritis. *Arthritis Rheum.* **39,** 914–922.
45. Jouvenne, P., Vannier, E., Dinarello, C. A., and Miossec, P. (1998) Elevated levels of soluble interleukin-1 receptor type II and interleukin-1 receptor antagonist in patients with chronic arthritis. *Arthritis Rheum.* **41,** 1083–1089.
46. Alonzi, T., Fattori, E., Lazzaro, D., Costa, P., Probert, L., Kollias, G., et al. (1998) Interleukin 6 is required for the development of collagen-induced arthritis. *J. Exp. Med.* **187,** 461–468.
47. Franz, J. K., Kolb, S. A., Hummel, K. M., Lahrtz, F., Neidhart, M., Aicher, W. K., et al. (1998) Interleukin-16, produced by synovial fibroblasts, mediates chemoattraction for CD4+ T lymphocytes in rheumatoid arthritis. *Eur. J. Immunol.* **28,** 2661–2671.
48. Koch, A. E., Kunkel, S. L., Harlow, L. A., Johnson, B., Evanoff, H. L., Haines, G. K., et al. (1992) Enhanced production of monocyte chemoattractant protein-1 in rheumatoid arthritis. *J. Clin. Invest.* **90,** 772–779.
49. Koch, A. E., Kunkel, S. L., Harlow, L. A., Mazarakis, D. D., Haines, G. K., Burdick, M. D., et al. (1994) Macrophage inflammatory protein-1α: a novel chemotactic cytokine for marcrophages in rheumatoid arthritis. *J. Clin. Invest.* **93,** 921.
50. Okada, Y., Takeuchi, N., Tomita, K., Nakanishi, I., and Nagase, H. (1989) Immunolocalisation of matrix metalloproteinase 3 (stromelysin) in rheumatoid synovioblasts (B cells): correlation with rheumatoid arthritis. *Ann. Rheum. Dis.* **48,** 645–653.
51. Woolley, D. E., Crossley, M. J., and Evanson, J. M. (1977) Collagenase at sites of cartilage erosion in the rheumatoid joint. *Arthritis Rheum.* **20,** 1231–1239.
52. Firestein, G. S. (1996) Invasive fibroblast-like synoviocytes in rheumatoid arthritis. *Arthritis Rheum.* **39,** 1781–1790.
53. McCachren, S. S., Haynes, B. F., and Niedel, J. E. (1990) Localization of collagenase mRNA in rheumatoid arthritis synovium by in situ hybridization histochemistry. *J. Clin. Immunol.* **10,** 19–27.
54. Callaghan, M. M., Lovis, R. M., Rammohan, C., Lu, Y., and Pope, R. (1996) Autocrine regulation of collagenase gene expression by TNFα in U937 cells. *J. Leukocyte Biol.* **59,** 125.
55. Aono, H., Fujisawa, K., Hasunuma, T., Marriott, S. J., and Nishioka, K. (1998) Extracellular human T cell leukemia virus type I tax protein stimulates the proliferation of human synovial cells. *Arthritis Rheum.* **41,** 1995–2003.
56. Davis, L. S., Kavanaugh, A. F., Nichols, L. A., and Lipsky, P. E. (1995) Induction of persistent T cell hyporesponsiveness in vivo by monoclonal antibody to ICAM-1 in patients with rheumatoid arthritis. *J. Immunol.* **154,** 3525–3537.

57. Bresnihan, B., Alvaro-Gracia, J. M., Cobby, M., Doherty, M., Domljan, Z., Emery, P., et al. (1998) Treatment of rheumatoid arthritis with recombinant human interleukin-1 receptor antagonist. *Arthritis Rheum.* **41,** 2196–2204.
58. Muller-Ladner, U., Roberts, C. R., Franklin, B. N., Gay, R. E., Robbins, P. D., Evans, C. H., et al. (1997) Human IL-1Ra gene transfer into human synovial fibroblasts is chondroprotective. *J. Immunol.* **158,** 3492–3498.
59. Seitz, M., Zwicker, M., and Loetscher, P. (1998) Effects of methotrexate on differentiation of monocytes and production of cytokine inhibitors by monocytes. *Arthritis Rheum.* **41,** 2032–2038.
60. Drevlow, B. E., Lovis, R., Haag, M. A., Sinacore, J. M., Jacobs, C., Blosche, C., et al. (1996) Recombinant human interleukin-1 receptor type I in the treatment of patients with active rheumatoid arthritis. *Arthritis Rheum.* **39,** 257–265.
61. Zagariya, A., Mungre, S., Lovis, R., Birrer, M., Ness, S., Thimmapaya, B., et al. (1998) Tumor necrosis alpha gene regulation: enhancement of C/EBPβ-induced activation by c-Jun. *Mol. Cell. Biol.* **18,** 2815–2824.
62. Handel, M. L., McMorrow, L. B., and Gravallese, E. M. (1995) Nuclear factor-κB in rheumatoid synovium. *Arthritis Rheum.* **38,** 1762–1770.
63. Foxwell, B., Browne, K., Bondeson, J., Clarke, C., DeMartin, R., Brennan, F., et al. (1998) Efficient adenoviral infection with IκBα reveals that macrophage tumor necrosis factor α production in rheumatoid arthritis is NF-κB dependent. *Proc. Natl. Acad. Sci. USA* **95,** 8211–8215.
64. Burmester, G. R., Stuhlmuller, B., Keyszer, G., and Kinne, R. W. (1997) Mononuclear phagocytes and rheumatoid synovitis. *Arthritis Rheum.* **40,** 5–18.
65. Asahara, H., Fujisawa, K., Kobata, T., Hasunuma, T., Maeda, T., Asanuma, M., et al. (1997) Direct evidence of high DNA binding activity of transcription factor AP-1 in rheumatoid arthritis synovium. *Arthritis Rheum.* **40,** 912–918.
66. Schroen, D. J. and Brinckerhoff, C. E. (1996) Inhibition of rabbit collagenase (matrix metalloproteinase-1; MMP-1) transcription by retinoid receptors: evidence for binding of RARs/RXRs to the -77 AP-1 site through interactions with c-Jun. *J. Cell. Physiol.* **169,** 320–332.
67. Roivainen, A., Jalava, J., Pirila, L., Yli-Jama, T., Tiusanen, H., and Toivanen, P. (1997) H-ras oncogene point mutations in arthritis synovium. *Arthritis Rheum.* **40,** 1636–1643.
68. Lin, H., Head, M., Blank, M., Han, L., Jin, M., and Goodman, R. (1998) Myc-mediated transactivation of HSP70 expression following exposure to magnetic fields. *J. Cell. Biol.* **69,** 181–188.
69. Schett, G., Redlich, K., Xu, Q., Bizan, P., Groger, M., Tohidast-Akrad, M., et al. (1998) Enhanced expression of heat shock protein 70 (hsp70) and heat shock factor 1 (HSF1) activation in rheumatoid arthritis synovial tissue. Differential regulation of hsp70 expression and hsf1 activation in synovial fibroblasts by proinflammatory cytokines, shear stress, and antiinflammatory drugs. *J. Clin. Invest.* **102,** 302–311.
70. Sengupta, T. K., Chen, A., Zhong, Z., Darnell, J. E. J., and Ivashkiv, L. B. (1995) Activation of monocyte effector genes and STAT family transcription factors by inflammatory synovial fluid is independent of interferon gamma. *J. Exp. Med.* **181,** 1015–1025.
71. Aicher, W. K., Heer, A. H., Trabandt, A., Bridges, S. L., Jr., Schroeder, H. W., Jr., Gay, R. E., et al. (1994) Overexpression of zinc-finger transcription factor Z-225/Egr-1 in synoviocytes from rheumatoid arthritis patients. *J. Immunol.* **152,** 5940.
72. Plumier, J. C., Robertson, H. A., and Currie, R. W. (1996) Differential accumulation of mRNA for immediate early genes and heat shock genes in heart after ischaemic injury. *J. Mol. Cell. Cardiol.* **28,** 1251–1260.

73. Lafyatis, R., Kim, S.-J., Angel, P., Roberts, A. B., Sporn, M. B., Karin, M., et al. (1990) Interleukin-1 stimulates and all-trans-retinoic acid inhibits collagenase gene expression through its 5' activator protein-1-binding site. *Mol. Endocrinol.* **4,** 973–980.
74. Wakisaka, S., Suzuki, N., Saito, N., Ochi, T., and Sakane, T. (1998) Possible correction of abnormal rheumatoid arthritis synovial cell function by jun D transfection in vitro. *Arthritis Rheum.* **41,** 470–481.
75. Miyazawa, K., Mori, A., Yamamoto, K., and Okudaira, H. (1998) Constitutive transcription of the human interleukin-6 gene by rheumatoid synoviocytes. *Am. J. Pathol.* **152,** 793–803.
76. Vincenti, M. P., Coon, C. I., and Brinckerhoff, C. E. (1998) Nuclear factor κB/p50 activates an element in the distal matrix metalloproteinase 1 promoter in interleukin-1β-stimulated synovial fibroblasts. *Arthritis Rheum.* **41,** 1987–1994.
77. Sakurada, S., Kato, T., and Okamoto, T. (1996) Induction of cytokines and ICAM-1 by proinflammatory cytokines in primary rheumatoid synovial fibroblasts and inhibition by N-acetyl-L-cysteine and aspirin. *Int. Immunol.* **8,** 1483–1493.
78. Crofford, L. J., Tan, B., McCarthy, C. J., and Hla, T. (1997) Involvement of nuclear factor κB in the regulation of cyclooxygenase-2 expression by interleukin-1 in rheumatoid synoviocytes. *Arthritis Rheum.* **40,** 226–236.
79. Janusz, M. J. and Hare, M. (1993) Cartilage degradation by cocultures of transformed macrophage and fibroblast cell lines. *J. Immunol.* **150,** 1922–1931.
80. Hummel, K. M., Petrow, P. K., Franz, J. K., Muller-Ladner, U., Aicher, W. K., Gay, R. E., et al. (1998) Cysteine proteinase cathepsin K mRNA is expressed in synovium of patients with rheumatoid arthritis and is detected at sites of synovial bone destruction. *J. Rheumatol.* **25,** 1887–1894.
81. Muller-Ladner, U., Kriegsmann, J., Franklin, B. N., Matsumoto, S., Geiler, T., Gay, R. E., et al. (1996) Synovial fibroblasts of patients with rheumatoid arthritis attach to and invade normal human cartilage when engrafted into SCID mice. *Am. J. Pathol.* **149,** 1607–1615.
82. Szekanecz, Z., Szegedi, G., and Koch, A. E. (1996) Cellular adhesion molecules in rheumatoid arthritis: regulation by cytokines and possible clinical importance. *J. Invest. Med.* **44,** 124–135.
83. Diaz-Gonzalez, F. and Sanchez-Madrid, F. (1998) Inhibition of leukocyte adhesion: an alternate mechanism of action for anti-inflammatory drugs. *Immunol. Today* **19,** 169–172.
84. Grober, J. S., Bowen, B. L., Ebling, H., Athey, B., Thompson, C. B., Fox, D. A., et al. (1993) Monocyte-endothelial adhesion in chronic rheumatoid arthritis: in situ detection of selectin and integrin-dependent interactions. *J. Clin. Invest.* **91,** 2609–2619.
85. Weyrich, A. S., McIntyre, T. M., McEver, R. P., Prescott, S. M., and Zimmerman, G. A. (1995) Monocyte tethering by P-selectin regulates monocyte chemotactic protein-1 and tumor necrosis factor-α secretion. *J. Clin. Invest.* **95,** 2297–2303.
86. Sarkissian, M. and Lafyatis, R. (1999) Integrin engagement regulates proliferation and collagenase expression of rheumatoid synovial fibroblasts. *J. Immunol.* **162,** 1772–1779.
87. Scott, B. B., Weisbrot, L. M., Greenwood, J. D., Bogoch, E. R., Paige, C. J., et al. (1997) Rheumatoid arthritis synovial fibroblast and U937 macrophage/monocyte cell line interaction in cartilage degradation. *Arthritis Rheum.* **40,** 490–498.
88. Pacifici, R., Roman, J., Kimble, R., Civitelli, R., Brownfield, C. M., and Bizzarri, C. (1994) Ligand binding to monocyte $\alpha_5\beta_1$ integrin activates the $\alpha_2\beta_1$ receptor via the α_5 subunit cytoplasmic domain and protein kinase C. *J. Immunol.* **153,** 2222.
89. Yurochko, A. D., Liu, D. Y., Eierman, D., and Haskill, S. (1992) Integrins as a primary signal transduction molecule regulating monocyte immediate-early gene induction. *Proc. Natl. Acad. Sci. USA* **89,** 9034–9038.

90. Xie, B., Laouar, A., and Huberman, E. (1998) Autocrine regulation of macrophage differentiation and 92-kDa gelatinase production by tumor necrosis factor-α via $\alpha_5\beta_1$ integrin in HL-60 cells. *J. Biol. Chem.* **273**, 11,583–11,588.
91. Chen, W., Syldath, U., Bellmann, K., Burkart, V., and Kolb, H. (1999) Human 60-kDa heat-shock protein: a danger signal to the innate immune system. *J. Immunol.* **162**, 3212–3219.
92. Burger, D., Rezzonico, R., Li, J.-M., Modoux, C., Pierce, R. A., Welgus, H. G., et al. (1998) Imbalance between interstitial collagenase and tissue inhibitor of metalloproteinases 1 in synoviocytes and fibroblasts upon direct contact with stimulated T lymphocytes. *Arthritis Rheum.* **41**, 1748–1759.
93. Lacraz, S., Isler, P., Vey, E., Welgus, H. G., and Dayer, J.-M. (1994) Direct contact between T lymphocytes and monocytes is a major pathway for induction of metalloproteinase expression. *J. Biol. Chem.* **269**, 22,027–22,033.
94. Miltenburg, A. M. M., Lacraz, S., Welgus, H. G., and Dayer, J.-M. (1995) Immobilized anti-CD3 antibody activates T cell clones to induce the production of interstitial collagenase, but not tissue inhibitor of metalloproteinases, in monocytic THP-1 cells and dermal fibroblasts. *J. Immunol.* **154**, 2655–2667.
95. Pope, R. M., Lovis, R. M., and Gupta, R. S. (1992) Activation of synovial fluid T lymphocytes by 60-kd heat-shock proteins in patients with inflammatory synovitis. *Arthritis Rheum.* **35**, 43–48.
96. Desai, S. V., Dixit, S., and Pope, R. M. (1989) Limited proliferative response to type II collagen in rheumatoid arthritis. *J. Rheumatol.* **16**, 1310–1314.
97. Alsalameh, S., Mollenhauer, J., Hain, N., Stock, K.-P., Kalden, J. R., and Burmester, G. R. (1990) Cellular immune response toward human articular chondrocytes. *Arthritis Rheum.* **33**, 1477–1486.
98. Guerassimov, A., Zhang, Y., Banerjee, S., Cartman, A., Leroux, J.-Y., Rosenberg, L. C., et al. (1998) Cellular immunity to the G1 domain of cartilage proteoglycan aggrecan is enhanced in patients with rheumatoid arthritis but only after removal of keratan sulfate. *Arthritis Rheum.* **41**, 1019–1025.
99. Hain, N. A. K., Stuhlmuller, B., Hahn, G. R., Kalden, J. R., Deutzmann, R., and Burmester, G. R. (1996) Biochemical characterization and microsequencing of a 205-kDa synovial protein stimulatory for T cells and reactive with rheumatoid factor containing sera. *J. Immunol.* **157**, 1773–1780.
100. Toyosaki, T., Tsuruta, Y., Yoshioka, T., Takemoto, H., Suzuki, R., Tomita, T., et al. (1998) Recognition of rheumatoid arthritis synovial antigen by CD4+, CD8– T cell clones established from rheumatoid arthritis joints. *Arthritis Rheum.* **41**, 92–100.
101. O'Dell, J. R., Haire, C. E., Palmer, W., Drymalski, W., Wees, S., Blakely, K., et al. (1997) Treatment of early rheumatoid arthritis with minocycline or placebo. *Arthritis Rheum.* **40**, 842–848.
102. Klimiuk, P. A., Yang, H., Goronzy, J. J., and Weyand, C. M. (1999) Production of cytokines and metalloproteinases in rheumatoid synovitis is T cell dependent. *Clin. Immunol.* **90**, 65–78.
103. Fujii, K., Tanaka, Y., Hubscher, S., Saito, K., Ota, T., and Eto, S. (1999) Cross-linking of CD44 on rheumatoid synovial cells up-regulates VCAM-1. *J. Immunol.* **162**, 2391–2398.
104. Firestein, G. S. (1995) Apoptosis in rheumatoid arthritis synovium. *J. Clin. Invest.* **96**, 1631–1638.
105. Matsumoto, S., Muller-Ladner, U., Gay, R. E., Nishioka, K., and Gay, S. (1996) Ultrastructural demonstration of apoptosis, Fas and Bcl-2 expression of rheumatoid synovial fibroblasts. *J. Rheum.* **23**, 1345–1352.
106. Nakajima, T., Aono, H., Hasunuma, T., Yamamoto, K., Shirai, T., Hirohata, K., et al. (1995) Apoptosis and functional Fas antigen in rheumatoid arthritis synoviocytes. *Arthritis Rheum.* **38**, 485–91.

107. Sugiyama, M., Tsukazaki, T., Yonekura, A., Matsuzaki, S., Yamashita, S., and Iwasaki, K. (1995) Localization of apoptosis and expression of apoptosis related proteins in the synovium of patients with rheumatoid arthritis. *Ann. Rheum. Dis.* **55,** 442–449.
108. Firestein, G. S., Nguyen, K., Aupperle, K. R., Yeo, M., Boyle, D. L., and Zvaifler, N. J. (1996) Apoptosis in rheumatoid arthritis: p53 overexpression in rheumatoid arthritis synovium. *Am. J. Pathol.* **149,** 2143–2151.
109. Firestein, G. S., Echeverri, F., Yeo, M., Zvaifler, N. J., and Green, D. R. (1997) Somatic mutations in the p53 tumor suppressor gene in rheumatoid arthritis synovium. *Proc. Natl. Acad. Sci. USA* **94,** 10,895–10,900.
110. Aupperle, K. R., Boyle, D. L., Hendrix, M., Softor, E. A., Zvaifler, N. J., Barbosa, M., et al. (1998) Regulation of synoviocyte proliferation, apoptosis and invasion by the p53 tumor suppressor gene. *Am. J. Pathol.* **152,** 1091–1098.
111. Nishioka, K., Hasunuma, T., Kato, T., Sumida, T., and Kobata, T. (1998) Apoptosis in rheumatoid arthritis: a novel pathway in the regulation of synovial tissue. *Arthritis Rheum.* **41,** 1–9.
112. Wakisaka, S., Suzuki, N., Takeba, Y., Shimoyama, Y., Nagafuchi, H., Takeno, M., et al. (1998) Modulation by proinflammatory cytokines of Fas/Fas ligand-mediated apoptotic cell death of synovial cells in patients with rheumatoid arthritis. *Clin. Exp. Immunol.* **114,** 119–128.
113. Kawakawi, A., Eguchi, K., Matsuoka, N., Tsuboi, M., Kawabe, Y., Aoyagi, T., et al. (1996) Inhibition of Fas antigen-mediated apoptosis of rheumatoid synovial cells in vitro by transforming growth factor β1. *Arthritis Rheum.* **39,** 1267–1276.
114. Salmon, M., Scheel-Toellner, D., Huissoon, A. P., Pilling, D., Shamsadeen, N., Hyde, H., et al. (1997) Inhibition of T cell apoptosis in the rheumatoid synovium. *J. Clin. Invest.* **99,** 439–446.
115. Mountz, J. D., Wu, J., Cheng, J., and Zhou, T. (1994) Autoimmune disease: a problem of defective apoptosis. *Arthritis Rheum.* **37,** 1415–1420.
116. Miagkov, A. V., Kovalenko, D. V., Brwon, C., Didsbury, J. R., Cogswell, J. P., Stimpson, S. A., et al. (1998) NF-κB activation provides the potential link between inflammation and hyperplasia in the arthritic joint. *Proc. Natl. Acad. Sci. USA* **95,** 13,859–13,864.
117. Fujisawa, K., Asahara, H., Okamoto, K., Aono, H., Hasunuma, T., Kobata, T., et al. (1996) Therapeutic effect of the anti-Fas antibody on arthritis in HTLV-1 tax transgenic mice. *J. Clin. Invest.* **98,** 271–278.
118. Zhang, H., Yang, Y., Horton, J. L., Samoilova, E. B., Judge, T. A., Turka, L. A., et al. (1997) Amelioration of collagen-induced arthritis by CD-95 (Apo-1/Fas)-ligand gene transfer. *J. Clin. Invest.* **100,** 1951–1957.
119. Okamoto, K., Asahara, H., Kobayahi, T., Matsuno, H., Hasuno, T., Kobata, T., et al. (1998) Induction of apoptosis in the rheumatoid synovium by Fas ligand gene transfer. *Gene Ther.* **5,** 331–338.
120. Genestier, L., Paillot, R., Fournel, S., Ferraro, C., Miossec, P., and Revillard, J.-P. (1998) Immunosuppressive properties of methotrexate: apoptosis and clonal deletion of activated peripheral T cells. *J. Clin. Invest.* **102,** 322–328.

22

Inflammatory Myopathies

Norbert Goebels and Reinhard Hohlfeld

1. Introduction

The (idiopathic) inflammatory myopathies are a heterogenous group of diseases, including dermatomyositis (DM), different forms of polymyositis (PM), and inclusion-body myositis (IBM) (reviewed in refs. *1–4*). Clinically, DM is distinguished from PM and IBM by characteristic skin manifestations. A microscopic feature highly characteristic of DM is perifascicular atrophy, which is due to degeneration of muscle fibers at the periphery of muscle fascicles secondary to microvascular damage. Quantitative morphological analyses suggest that depletion of capillaries is one of the earliest changes in DM. Immunofluorescence studies revealed the deposition of complement in or around microvascular endothelium in a significant proportion of capillaries *(5)*. These observations support the concept that an antibody- or immune-complex-mediated response against a vascular–endothelial component is a primary pathogenetic mechanism in DM.

In contrast, in PM and IBM there is a conspicuous endomysial inflammatory exudate containing mainly CD8$^+$ T-cells and macrophages that surround and focally invade non-necrotic muscle fibers. Immunoelectron microscopy demonstrated that CD8$^+$ T-cells and macrophages traverse the basal lamina, focally compress the fiber, and, ultimately, replace entire segments of muscle fiber *(6)*. All of the invaded fibers and some noninvaded fibers express increased amounts of HLA class I, but not class II molecules (reviewed in refs. *1* and *2*). By contrast, normal muscle fibers do not express detectable amounts of human leukocyte antigen (HLA) class I or class II antigens. Taken together, these observations are consistent with an HLA class-I-restricted cytotoxic T-lymphocyte (CTL)-mediated response against antigen(s) expressed on muscle fibers in PM and IBM. Consistent with this hypothesis, CD8$^+$ T-cells expanded from the muscles of patients with different inflammatory myopathies may show low but significant cytotoxicity against autologous cultured myotubes *(7)*.

2. Histological Features

In PM the endomysial inflammatory infiltrate is typically dominated by CD8$^+$ T-lymphocytes, which surround, invade, and eventually destroy muscle fibers (Fig. 1). In a rare subtype of PM, the infiltrate consists of $\gamma\delta$ T-lymphocytes *(8)*. In contrast to noninflamed muscle, the invaded muscle fibers express HLA class I molecules. This is

From: *Current Molecular Medicine: Principles of Molecular Rheumatology*
Edited by: G. C. Tsokos © Humana Press Inc., Totowa, NJ

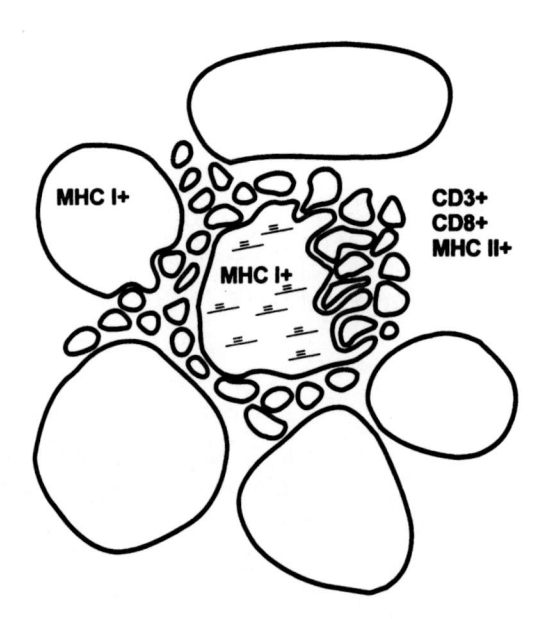

Fig. 1. Schematic representation of the typical histological changes observed in polymyositis. T-Cells surround and invade a muscle fiber. The majority of the autoinvasive T-cells are CD3+CD8+. All invaded muscle fibers and some that are noninvaded show surface reactivity for MHC class I. (Modified from ref. *1*.)

a prerequisite for the immunological interaction with CD8+ T-cells. The different stages of CTL-mediated myocytotoxicity were analyzed by immunoelectron microscopy *(6)*. Initially, CD8+ cells and macrophages abut on and send spikelike processes into nonnecrotic muscle fibers. Subsequently, an increasing number of CD8+ cells and macrophages traverse the basal lamina and focally replace the fiber.

Dermatomyositis is characterized by perivascular and perifascicular infiltrates consisting predominantly of B-lymphocytes, macrophages, and CD4+ T-lymphocytes. Immunohistochemistry shows immune complexes and C5b9 complement (membrane-attack complex) on small blood vessels, suggesting a humoral immune effector mechanism *(5)*. The immune processes affecting the muscle microvasculature lead to a reactive proliferation of endothelial cells and a reduction of muscle capillaries. Electronmicroscopy demonstrates tubulovesicular inclusions in endothelial cells. Capillary changes are thought to be the cause of the characteristic perifascicular muscle fiber atrophy in DM (Fig. 2). Perifascicular atrophy is diagnostic for DM, even in the absence of an inflammatory infiltrate. As in PM, the molecular target of the autoimmune reaction in DM has not yet been defined.

In IBM, eosinophilic inclusions are found in the cytoplasm and nuclei. Irregular "rimmed vacuoles" are present in 2–70% of the muscle fibers *(9)*. In sporadic IBM, endomysial infiltrates dominated by CD8+ T-lymphocytes resemble those seen in PM. In familial IBM, inflammatory changes are absent ("familial inclusion body myopathy"). The inclusions represent an accumulation of proteins, some of which contain proteins also found in Alzheimer's disease (10–12). Electronmicroscopically, the inclusions appear as 15- to 21-nm helical filaments and 6- to 10-nm amyloidlike fibrils.

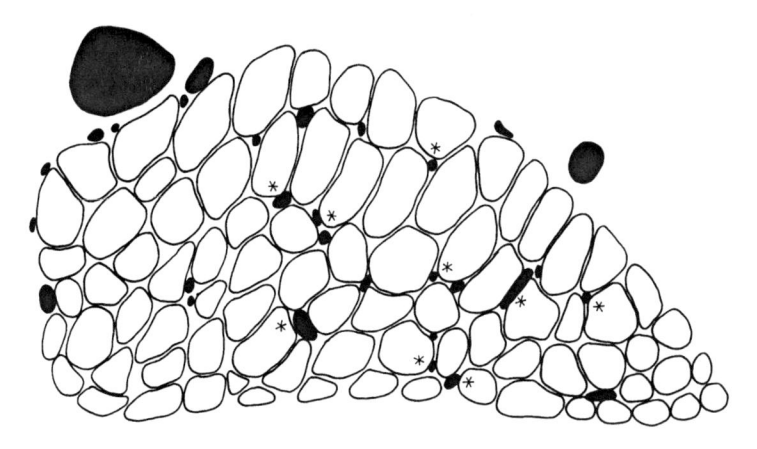

Fig. 2. Typical histological changes of dermatomyositis. Muscle fibers are shown in white, blood vessels in black. Note atrophic fibers at the edge of the fascicle (perifascicular atrophy). Clusters of capillaries and venules stain positively for complement membrane attack complex (MAC). The capillary density is significantly reduced. (From ref. *1*.)

3. Expression of Cytokines and Adhesion Molecules in Muscle Lesions

Using reverse transcriptase–polymerase chain reaction (RT-PCR), Lundberg et al. *(13)* found moderate to strong expression of IL-4 in PM, whereas IL-4 expression was low or absent in IBM and DM. Granulocyte–macrophage colony-stimulating factor (GM-CSF) and transforming growth factor-β (TGF-β) were expressed in most inflammatory myopathy cases but not in noninflammatory controls. Confalonieri et al. *(14)* reported that TGF-β1 is expressed significantly more strongly in DM than in PM and controls. By immunohistochemistry, TGF-β1 was localized mainly in connective tissue, indicating a possible relationship with connective-tissue proliferation. Using immunohistochemical techniques, Lundberg et al. *(15)* found prominent expression of interleukin-1α (IL-1α), (IL-1β), and TGF-β isoforms in PM, IBM, and DM, but not in normal control muscle. IL-1α was expressed in endothelial cells and inflammatory cells, whereas IL-1β was expressed only in inflammatory cells, not in blood vessel walls. TGF-β1 and TGF-β3 were expressed mainly in inflammatory cells and muscle fiber membranes. TGF-β2 was found in endothelial cells and inflammatory cells. Tews and Goebel *(16)* detected IL-1α, IL-β, IL-2, IL-4, tumor necrosis factor-α (TNF-α), TNF-β, and interferon-γ in a proportion of inflammatory cells, and IL-1α, IL-β, IL-2, and TNF-α also in muscle fibers. Tateyama et al. *(17)* identified TNF-α in inflammatory cells in several PM cases.

Cell adhesion molecules, many of which are inducible by cytokines, participate in target–effector cell interactions in cell-mediated cytotoxicity and in leukodiapedesis in inflammatory diseases. De Bleecker and Engel *(18)* demonstrated that intercellular adhesion molecule-1 (ICAM-1) is strongly induced on the surfaces of non-necrotic muscle fibers where they are invaded by autoaggressive cells, suggesting that it serves as an important ligand for these cells. In DM, ICAM-1 was strongly expressed on endothelial cells of perimysial arterioles and venules and on some perifascicular capillaries. In the other myopathies, vascular ICAM-1 expression was restricted to endothelia of capillaries surrounded by inflammatory cells, suggesting that this ligand is differentially activated in DM *(18)*. Additional studies of adhesion molecule expression in inflammatory myopathies have been reported *(19–21)*.

It is likely that myoblasts (and perhaps also mature muscle fibers) can be a source of various cytokines, both in vitro and in vivo. The complete spectrum of cytokines that can be produced by human myoblasts has not yet been established. One example of a cytokine that can be induced in myoblasts is interleukin-6 *(22)*.

Despite some discrepancies between the different studies, which are probably explained by methodological problems, it is safe to conclude that in the inflammatory myopathies, many inflammatory cells, muscle fibers, and endothelial cells express a complex array of different cytokines. The local production of cytokines is likely to induce several cell interaction and adhesion molecules on these tissue elements.

4. Phenotype and Activation State of Inflammatory T-Cells

In IBM and PM, approximately one-third of all autoinvasive cells and about one-half of the CD8+ autoinvasive T cells are HLA-DR+, suggesting that they have been activated *(23)*. The vast majority of the inflammatory CD4+ and CD8+ T-cells display the phenotype of memory T-cells; that is, they express the RO isoform of the leukocyte common antigen CD45 *(24)*. The intensity of the CD45RO signal was similar in all CD8+ T-cells, regardless of their position relative to the invaded muscle fiber surface. A similar expression pattern was noted for the leukocyte function-associated antigen (LFA)-1 *(18,25)*. LFA-1 (CD11a/CD18) is a $\beta 2$ integrin that has a key role in mediating leukocyte adhesion to endothelium and T-cell adhesion to target cells. ICAM-1, a ligand of LFA-1, was upregulated, especially on T-cells in the vicinity of invaded muscle fibers, suggesting that the expression of CD45RO and ICAM-1 is differentially regulated *(18)*. Indeed, LFA-1 is mainly constitutively expressed, whereas ICAM-1 is widely inducible on B- and T-cells. Taken together, these results establish that the autoaggressive (autoinvasive) T-cells in the inflammatory lesions of PM and IBM muscle represent activated CD8+ memory T-cells.

5. T-Cell Receptor Repertoire of Autoaggressive T-Cells

The characteristic lesion of PM and IBM has several features that make it an ideal paradigm to study CD8+ T-cell-mediated immunopathology. The muscle fiber target cells can be readily distinguished from the effector T-cells. Further, different populations of inflammatory T-cells can be discerned: one population, which deeply invades muscle fibers (the autoaggressive or autoinvasive T-cells), and another, which remains in interstitial areas and therefore seems to represent regulatory or bystander cells (the interstitial T-cells).

Bender et al. *(26)* combined two independent PCR techniques with immunohistochemistry to characterize the T-cell receptor (TCR) repertoire of inflammatory cells in the muscle of a patient with typical PM. PCR revealed a preferential usage of TCR Vα33.1, Vβ13.1, and Vβ5.1. Six of six TCR Vα33.1+ cDNA clones and five of seven Vβ13.1+ clones had identical nucleotide sequences. In contrast, the Vβ5.1+ TCR were more heterogeneous. No TCR sequences could be amplified from noninflammatory control muscle. Furthermore, none of the TCR sequences found in PM muscle could be detected in blood from the same patient or from a normal control subject. Immunohistochemistry using monoclonal antibodies (mAb) specific for Vβ5.1 or Vβ13.1 confirmed that Vβ5.1 and Vβ13.1 were overrepresented in the muscle lesions. Thirty-two percent of *all* CD8+ T-cells were Vβ13.1+, and 16% were Vβ5.1+. However, approximately 60% of the CD8+ T-cells that *invaded* muscle fibers were Vβ13.1+, whereas less than 10% were Vβ5.1+. These findings are consistent with the results of previous studies, which, however, did not combine sequence with histological analysis of TCR Vβ expression *(27–29)*. Differences in TCR usage in the different studies presumably reflect differences between individual patients (e.g., different HLA types).

A possible clue to the nature of the suspected autoantigen(s) was provided by the discovery of a rare variant of PM. In this variant, CD3+CD4−CD8−TCRγδ+ T-cells surrounded and invaded non-necrotic muscle fibers in the same way as CD3+CD8+TCRαβ+ T-cells in the more common forms of PM *(8)*. The autoaggressive myocytotoxic γδ T-cells were essentially monoclonal and expressed an unusual Vγ3Jγ1Cγ1–Vδ2Jδ3Cδ disulfide-linked TCR *(30)*. In γδ T-cell-mediated PM, all muscle fibers expressed MHC class I antigen and showed intense reactivity with a monoclonal antibody specific for the 65-kDa heat-shock protein (hsp) *(31)*. One possible implication of the striking colocalization of γδ T-cells with the 65-kDa hsp is that the autoinvasive γδ T-cells recognize hsp determinants on muscle fibers. Therefore, hsp may be considered as a candidate autoantigen in some inflammatory myopathies.

A number of studies have addressed the T-cell repertoire expressed in IBM muscle, using immunohistochemistry *(29)* or PCR *(32,33)*. Lindberg et al. *(29)* compared the expression of TCR V genes in IBM, PM, and DM, using 10 different TCR Vβ-specific monoclonal antibodies. The most abundant TCR Vβ elements detected with these mAbs were Vβ3 and Vβ19. TCR sequences were not reported *(29)*. Using PCR with TCR V-family-specific primers, O'Hanlon et al. *(32)* analyzed the TCR repertoire in muscle biopsy specimens from 13 IBM patients. On average, six to seven TCR Vβ families were detected per specimen. Vβ3 and Vβ6 were detected more frequently than the other Vβ families. Sequence analysis of the expressed Vβ3 and Vβ6 receptors was performed on three patients. In one patient, both the Vβ3 and Vβ6 sequences were heterogeneous. This raised the possibility of a superantigen effect *(32)*. However, in the two other patients, 5 of the 10 sequenced Vβ3 cDNA clones were identical *(32)*. This would be more consistent with clonally dominant T-cells recognizing a defined antigen. An additional argument against a superantigen effect is that superantigens typically activate CD4+ T-cells by bridging the TCR to HLA class II molecules expressed on other cells *(34,35)*. However, muscle fibers do not normally express detectable levels of HLA class II even in an inflammatory environment *(36,37)* and the autoinvasive T cells in muscle are CD8+ rather than CD4+ *(1)*. Using RT-PCR, Fyhr et al. *(33)* found a limited repertoire of TCRs expressed in muscle of six analyzed patients. TCR Vβ3, 5.2, 8, 12, 14, and 22 were each expressed in at least three cases. No TCR sequences were reported and PCR was not combined with immunohistochemistry. Finally, using a combination of PCR and immunohistochemistry, we found a high degree of clonal restriction of TCR Vβ families expressed by *autoinvasive* CD8+ T-cell clones in IBM *(38)*. In conclusion, the presently available data indicate that the TCR repertoire expressed in muscle is similar in IBM and PM: The autoaggressive T-cells are oligoclonal, suggesting that they recognize a limited number of HLA class-I-associated antigenic peptides.

Apart from inflammatory changes, microscopic findings in IBM include rimmed vacuoles, congophilic amyloid deposits typically near or within the vacuoles and occasionally in nuclei, necrotic and regenerating fibers, small groups of atrophic fibers, and mitochondrial abnormalities *(10,12,39,40)*. The relative significance of these alterations and their possible relation to the inflammatory changes are presently debated *(10)*. That non-necrotic muscle fibers invaded by T-cells are several-fold more frequent than fibers displaying other pathologic alterations *(41)* suggests that, despite refractoriness to immunotherapy, immune mechanisms play an important role in the pathogenesis of IBM.

This notion is further supported by the strong association of IBM with the major histocompatibility complex (MHC) antigens HLA-DR3, DR52, and B8 *(42)* and the known association with other autoimmune diseases (for reviews of IBM, *see* refs. *3,10,12,39,40* and *43*).

6. Cytotoxic Effector Mechanisms

The precise mechanism by which the invading CD8+ T-cells kill muscle fibers in PM and IBM are still unknown. There is evidence that a perforin- and secretion-dependent mechanism contributes to the muscle fiber injury. Perforin has been localized in inflammatory T-cells by immunohistochemistry *(44,45)* and by *in situ* hybridization *(46)*. In PM but not DM, the autoinvasive T cells orient their perforin-containing cytotoxic granules toward the target muscle fiber *(45)*, providing suggestive evidence that secretion of this cytotoxic effector molecule contributes to muscle fiber injury.

Perforin is not the only potentially cytotoxic molecule expressed in inflammatory myopathies. For example, muscle fibers in myositis display distinct upregulation both of inducible and neuronal nitric oxide synthase (NOS). It may be speculated that the enhanced expression of NOS with production of nitric oxide contributes to oxidative stress, mediating muscle fiber damage.

In the early stages of muscle fiber invasion in PM and IBM, the surface membrane of muscle fibers appears to remain intact at the light microscopic *(23)* and electron-microscopic *(6)* level. Porelike structures could not be detected in the sarcolemma of muscle fibers attacked by T-cells in PM *(6)*. One possible explanation is that perforin pores/channels on nucleated cells in vivo are smaller in size than the pores generated in vitro on erythrocytes and other target cells by the addition of purified perforin. Perforin pores containing less than 10–20 monomers would escape detection by electron microscopy *(47)*. Another explanation for the lack of morphologically visible muscle cell damage is that the surface membrane of the muscle fiber is rapidly repaired at least during the early stages of muscle fiber invasion. Repair could occur, for example, by shedding or endocytosis of pore-damaged membrane (reviewed in ref. *48*).

As pointed out by Arahata and Engel *(6)*, it is interesting to note that the volume of a 25-mm-long and 50-µm-wide muscle fiber is nearly 28,000-fold larger than, for example, that of a spherical 15-µm tumor cell. Perforin pores would allow the influx of calcium. Consistent with this assumption is the observation that invaded muscle fibers show signs of focal myofibrillar degeneration near invading cells *(6)*. These changes could be a consequence of membrane insertion of perforin and focal protease activation *(6)*. Another indirect sign of muscle fiber damage is the intense focal regenerative activity noted in areas immediately adjacent to autoinvasive T-cells *(6)*.

In addition to perforin-dependent killing, cytotoxic T-cells can kill by a nonsecretory, ligand-mediated mechanism. This second killing mechanism requires the interaction between Fas (expressed on the target cell) and Fas ligand (expressed on the T-cell). Fas-mediated cytotoxicity is thought to induce programmed cell death (apoptosis) rather than necrosis, although it is not always possible to relate the different modes and mechanisms of cell death to specific morphological features and triggering events. The special properties of muscle fibers as giant syncytial cells with hundreds of nuclei further complicate the classification of any morphological changes as "necrosis" or "apoptosis."

In several studies, different groups of investigators found no evidence that apoptosis is a mechanism of muscle fiber injury in human inflammatory myopathies *(49,50)* or dystrophies *(51)*. On the other hand, in PM, DM, and IBM, many muscle fibers express Fas *(49)*. What could explain the discrepancy between the expression of the Fas "death receptor" on muscle fibers and the absence of signs of apoptosis? One possibility is that muscle fibers are intrinsically resistant to Fas-mediated classical apoptosis, at least in vivo. Resistance could be related to the peculiar properties of syncytial muscle fibers discussed earlier, or to the expression of specific inhibitory factors such as Bcl-2, or both. Indeed, the majority of Fas$^+$ fibers coexpress Bcl-2 *(49)*. Bcl-2 and another antiapoptotic protein, Bcl-x, have also been localized in atrophic muscle fibers in late-onset spinal muscular atrophy *(52)*. Bcl-2 protects against Fas-based but not perforin-based T-cell-mediated cytolysis *(53)*. The exact mechanisms of Bcl-2-mediated protection need yet to be defined, but it has been proposed that Bcl-2 binds and inactivates various apoptosis-inducing factors, including Bax *(54)*.

Fas expression was observed not only in muscle fibers but also in inflammatory cells in PM, IBM, DM, and Duchenne muscular dystrophy *(49)*. Immunologically naive peripheral T-cells are known to express little or no Fas on their surface, whereas previously activated memory T-cells express relatively high amounts of cell-surface Fas (reviewed in ref. 55). Interestingly, Fas expression in lymphocytes can have different functional consequences. In freshly isolated T-cells, ligation of Fas with anti-Fas mAb leads to enhanced proliferation, increased expression of activation markers and production of cytokines such as interleukin-2, interferon-γ, and TNF-α *(55)*. By contrast, chronically activated T-cells are susceptible to Fas-mediated apoptosis *(55,56)*. It is therefore thought that Fas is an important factor in the homeostatic regulation of immune responses: Fas-mediated costimulation seems to contribute to clonal expansion and effector function of T-cells during the early stage of an immune response. Later, Fas-mediated apoptosis helps to eliminate chronically activated T-cells *(55)*. It appears that although a proportion of inflammatory cells do express Fas, like muscle fibers they are protected from apoptosis by Bcl-2 or other antiapoptotic molecules.

The observation that the autoinvasive T-cells express and orient perforin toward target muscle fibers is consistent with a secretion- and perforin-dependent cytotoxic mechanism. On the other hand, although many muscle fibers express Fas, the nuclear changes typical for apoptosis are essentially absent in the inflammatory myopathies. Resistance to Fas-mediated injury could be related to the expression of specific protective factors. Indeed, in PM and IBM, the majority of Fas-positive muscle fibers coexpress Bcl-2, a protein known to protect from apoptosis.

7. Immunological Properties of Cultured Muscle Cells

Tissue culture systems are a powerful tool for the study of the functional aspects of cell-mediated myocytotoxicity. Human myogenic stem cells (myoblasts) can be isolated and purified from muscle biopsy specimens and expanded in culture *(57)*. In contrast to fibroblasts, myoblasts express the cytoskeletal protein desmin and the neural cell adhesion molecule N-CAM (CD56/Leu 19/NKH-1) *(1)*. Myoblasts constitutively express HLA class I antigens and a low level of lymphocyte function-associated (LFA) molecule 3 (LFA-3, CD58). TNF-α, a cytokine secreted by macrophages, T-cells and natural killer (NK) cells induces myoblasts to express the intercellular adhesion molecule-1 (ICAM-1, CD54) *(57)*. γ-Interferon-γ (IFN-γ), a cytokine secreted by T-cells and NK cells, induces myoblasts to express HLA-DR and ICAM-1 *(57–59)*. HLA-DP and HLA-DQ are also inducible by IFN-γ, but the kinetics of induction and the levels of expression vary with the different HLA class II molecules *(57)*. Both TNF-α and IFN-γ are expressed in inflammatory myopathies together with other pro-inflammatory cytokines. Further, various cell adhesion molecules have been detected in muscle, suggesting that the in vitro models adequately reflect the situation in vivo.

8. Interaction Of Myoblasts and CD8+ Cytotoxic T-Cells

Cultured myotubes and myoblasts express HLA class I molecules. This qualifies them as potential targets of CD8$^+$ CTL. Lysis of myotubes by CTL was shown in different experimental situations. On the one hand, myotubes were lysed by allogeneic CD8$^+$ CTL lines raised against the allogeneic HLA antigens expressed by the myotubes *(60)*. Autologous control myotubes were not lysed. Lysis involved the recognition of allogeneic HLA class I antigens because it was completely blocked by a monoclonal antibody against a monomorphic determinant of HLA class I *(60)*. Furthermore, myotubes were lysed by autologous polyclonal CD8$^+$ T-cell lines directly expanded from muscle of patients with different inflammatory myopathies *(7)*. The results obtained in this model system clearly establish that cultured myotubes are fully susceptible to HLA class I restricted lysis by CD8$^+$ CTL. The autoreactive myocytotoxicity is consistent with the hypothesis that some of the CTL isolated from muscle recognize the same antigen on myotubes in vitro that they recognize on muscle fibers in vivo.

9. Interaction of Myoblasts and CD4+ T-Cells: Myoblasts as Antigen-presenting Cells

Antigen presentation to CD4$^+$ T-cells depends on the constitutive or induced expression of HLA class II on the presenting cell. Because myoblasts can be induced to express HLA class II by IFN-γ, we tested the ability of highly purified human myoblasts to present various protein antigens to autologous CD4$^+$ T-cell lines specific for tuberculin, tetanus toxoid, or myelin basic protein *(57)*. Noninduced myoblasts or myoblasts treated with TNF-α alone could not present any of these antigens to T-cells. However, interferon-γ-treated myoblasts induced antigen-specific T-cell proliferation and were killed by the T-cells only in the presence of the relevant antigen *(57)*. Antigen-specific lysis was reduced to background level by adding the anti-HLA-DR monoclonal antibody L-243. These results suggest that HLA class II-positive human myoblasts can act as facultative local antigen-presenting cells in muscle by providing the signals necessary to trigger both antigen-specific lysis and T-cell proliferation. It is difficult to demonstrate HLA-DR by immunohistochemistry on the surface of human muscle fibers in inflammatory lesions, but this does not necessarily imply that HLA-DR is absent *(61)*.

10. Summary

The inflammatory myopathies are a heterogenous group of disorders, including dermatomyositis (DM), polymyositis (PM), and inclusion body myositis (IBM). In DM, muscle fiber injury is secondary to an antibody- or immune-complex-mediated immune response against a vascular–endothelial component. In PM and IBM, initially nonnecrotic muscle fibers are invaded and eventually destroyed by $CD8^+$ T-cells and macrophages. The results of the studies reviewed here are consistent with the following sequence of pathogenetic events in PM and IBM. First, some muscle fibers, which do not constitutively express detectable levels of MHC class I, are induced to express MHC class I- and class II-associated (auto)antigen(s). Next, the MHC class I-positive muscle fibers are surrounded by $CD8^+$ T-cells, some of which traverse the basal lamina of the muscle fiber and contact the muscle fiber surface. After recognition of "their" antigen, the $CD8^+$ T-cells become activated and secrete perforin and perhaps other cytotoxic effector molecules. T-cell receptor (TCR) analyses revealed that the autoaggressive T-cells are oligoclonal. In inflammatory lesions, muscle fibers express a number of cytoplasmic and surface molecules that are not detectable in normal muscle fibers. These molecules, which include HLA class I antigens, heat-shock proteins, adhesion molecules, and Fas, are probably induced by locally secreted cytokines. Although many of the muscle fibers invaded by $CD8^+$ T-cells express the Fas "death receptor," signs of apoptosis are absent. However, the autoaggressive $CD8^+$ T-cells possess perforin-containing granules, which they orient toward the contact zone with the target muscle fiber. This is consistent with a perforin- and secretion-dependent mechanism of muscle fiber injury in PM.

Acknowledgments

The authors' studies were supported by the Deutsche Forschungsgemeinschaft (SFB 217, C13), Wilhelm-Sander Stiftung (94.068.1), and Max Planck Society. The Institute for Clinical Neuroimmunology is supported by the Hermann and Lilly Schilling Foundation.

References

1. Hohlfeld, R. and Engel, A. G. (1994) The immunobiology of muscle. *Immunol. Today* **15**, 269–274.
2. Engel, A. G., Hohlfeld, R., and Banker, B. Q. (1994) The polymyositis and dermatomyositis syndromes, in *Myology* (Engel, A. G. and Franzini-Armstrong, C., eds.), McGraw-Hill, New York, pp. 1335–1383.
3. Dalakas, M. C. and Sivakumar, K. (1996) The immunopathologic and inflammatory differences between dermatomyositis, polymyositis and sporadic inclusion body myositis. *Curr. Opin. Neurol.* **9**, 235–239.
4. Mantegazza, R., Bernasconi, P., Confalioneri, P., and Cornelio, D. (1997) Inflammatory myopathies and systematic disorders: a review of immunopathogenic mechanisms and clinical features. *J. Neurol.* **244**, 277–287.

5. Mendell, J. R., Garcha, T. S., and Kissel, J. T. (1996) The immunopathogenic role of complement in human muscle disease. *Curr. Opin. Neurol.* **9,** 226–234.
6. Arahata, K. and Engel, A. G. (1986) Monoclonal antibody analysis of mononuclear cells in myopathies III. Immunoelectron microscopy aspects of cell-mediated muscle fiber injury. *Ann. Neurol.* **19,** 112–125.
7. Hohlfeld, R. and Engel, A. G. (1991) Coculture with autologous myotubes of cytotoxic T cells isolated from muscle in inflammatory myopathies. *Ann. Neurol.* **29,** 498–507.
8. Hohlfeld, R., Engel, A. G., Ii, K., and Harper, M. C. (1991) Polymyositis mediated by T lymphocytes that express the γ/δ receptor. *N. Engl. J. Med.* **324,** 877–881.
9. Dalakas, M. C. (1995) Immunopathogenesis of inflammatory myopathies. *Ann. Neurol.* **37,** S74–S86.
10. Griggs, R. C., Askanas, V., DiMauro, S., Engel, A. G., Karpati, G., Mendell, J. R., et al. (1995) Inclusion body myositis and myopathies. *Ann. Neurol.* **38,** 707–713.
11. Askanas, V. (1997) New developments in heredity inclusion body myopathies. *Ann. Neurol.* **41,** 421–422.
12. Askanas, V., Engel, W. K., and Mirabella, M. (1994) Idiopathic inflammatory myopathies. Inclusion-body myositis, polymyositis, and dermatomyositis. *Curr. Opin. Neurol.* **7,** 48–456.
13. Lundberg, I., Brengman, J. M., and Engel, A. G. (1995) Analysis of cytokine expression in muscle in inflammatory myopathies. Duchenne dystrophy and non-weak controls. *J. Neuroimmunol.* **63,** 9–16.
14. Confalonieri, P., Bernasconi, P., Cornelio, F., and Mantegazza, R. (1997) Transforming growth factor-β1 in polymyositis and dermatomyositis correlates with fibrosis but not with cell infiltrate. *J. Neuropathol. Exp. Neurol.* **56,** 479–484.
15. Lundberg, I., Ulfgren, A.-K., Nyberg, P., Andersson, U., and Klareskog, L. (1997) Cytokine production in muscle tissue of patients with idiopathic inflammatory myopathies. *Arthritis Rheum.* **40,** 865–874.
16. Tews, D. S. and Goebel, H. H. (1996) Cytokine expression profile in idiopathic inflammatory myopathies. *J. Neuropathol. Exp. Neurol.* **55,** 342–347.
17. Tateyama, M., Nagano, I., Yoshioka, M., Chida, K., Nakamura, S., and Itoyama, Y. (1997) Expression of tumor necrosis factor-a in muscles of polymyositis. *J. Neurol. Sci.* **146,** 45–51.
18. De Bleecker, J. L. and Engel, A. G. (1994) Expression of cell adhesion molecules in inflammatory myopathies and Duchenne dystrophy. *J. Neuropathol. Exp. Neurol.* **53,** 369–376.
19. Bartoccioni, E., Gallucci, S., Scuderi, F., Ricci, E., Servidei, S., Broccolini, A., et al. (1994) MHC class I, MHC class II and intercellular adhesion molecule-1 expression in inflammatory myopathies. *Clin. Exp. Immunol.* **95,** 166–172.
20. Tews, D. S. and Goebel, H. H. (1995) Expression of cell adhesion molecules in inflammatory myopathies. *J. Neuroimmunol.* **59,** 185–194.
21. Cid, M.-C., Grau, J.-M., Casademont, J., Tobías, E., Picazo, A., Coll-Vinent, B., et al. (1996) Leucocyte/endothelial cells adhesion receptors in muscle biopsies from patients with idiopathic inflammatory myopathies. *Clin. Exp. Immunol.* **104,** 476–473.
22. Gallucci, S., Provenzano, C., Mazzarelli, P., Scuderi, F., and Bartoccioni, E. (1998) Myoblasts produce IL-6 in response to inflammatory stimuli. *Int. Immunol.* **10,** 267–273.
23. Engel, A. G. and Arahata, K. (1984) Monoclonal antibody analysis of mononuclear cells in myopathies. II Phenotypes of autoinvasive cells in polymyositis and inclusion body myositis. *Ann. Neurol.* **16,** 209–216.
24. De Bleecker, J. L. and Engel, A. G. (1995) Immunocytochemical study of CD45 T cell isoforms in inflammatory myopathies. *Am. J. Pathol.* **146,** 1178–1187.
25. Iannone, F., Cauli, A., Yanni, G., Kingsley, G., Isenberg, D. A., Corrigall, V. M., et al. (1996) T lymphocyte immunophenotyping in polymyositis and dermatomyositis. *Br. J. Rheumatol.* **35,** 839–845.

26. Bender, A., Ernst, N., Iglesias, A., Dornmair, K., Wekerle, H., and Hohlfeld, R. (1995) T cell receptor repertoire in polymyositis: clonal expansion of autoaggressive CD8 T cells. *J. Exp. Med.* **181,** 1863–1868.
27. Mantegazza, R., Andreetta, F., Bernasconi, P., Baggi, F., Oksenberg, J. R., Simoncini, O., et al. (1993) Analysis of T cell receptor repertoire of muscle-infiltrating T lymphocytes in polymyositis. *J. Clin. Invest.* **91,** 2880–2886.
28. O'Hanlon, T. P., Dalakas, M. C., Plotz, P. H., and Miller, F. W. (1994) Predominant TCR-αβ variable and joining gene expression by muscle-infiltrating lymphocytes in the idiopathic inflammatory myopathies. *J. Immunol.* **152,** 2569–2576.
29. Lindberg, C., Oldfors, A., and Tarkowski, A. (1994) Restricted use of T cell receptor V genes in endomysial infiltrates of patients with inflammatory myopathies. *Eur. J. Immunol.* **24,** 2659–2663.
30. Pluschke, G., Rüegg, D., Hohlfeld, R., and Engel, A. G. (1992) Autoaggressive myocytotoxic T lymphocytes expressing an unusual γ/δ T cell receptor. *J. Exp. Med.* **176,** 1785–1789.
31. Hohlfeld, R. and Engel, A. G. (1992) Expression of 65-kd heat shock proteins in the inflammatory myopathies. *Ann. Neurol.* **32,** 821–823.
32. O'Hanlon, T. P., Dalakas, M. C., Plotz, P. H., and Miller, F. W. (1994) The αβ T-cell receptor repertoire in inclusion body myositis: diverse patterns of gene expression by muscle-infiltrating lymphocytes. *J. Autoimmun.* **7,** 321–333.
33. Fyhr, I.-M., Moslemi, A.-R., Tarkowski, A., Lindberg, C., and Oldfors, A. (1996) Limited T cell receptor V gene usage in inclusion body myositis. *Scand. J. Immunol.* **43,** 109–114.
34. Fleischer, B. (1995) Superantigens. *Acta Pathol. Microbiol. Immunol. Scand. (C)* **102,** 3–12.
35. Kotzin, B. L., Leung, D. Y. M., Kappler, J., and Marrack, P. (1995) Superantigens and their potential role in human disease. *Adv. Immunol.* **54,** 99–166.
36. Karpati, G., Pouliot, Y., and Carpenter, S. (1988) Expression of immunoreactive major histocompatibility complex products in human skeletal muscles. *Ann. Neurol.* **23,** 64–72.
37. Emslie-Smith, A. M., Arahata, K., and Engel, A. G. (1989) Major histocompatibility complex class I antigen expression, immunolocalization of interferon subtypes, and T cell-mediated cytotoxicity in myopathies. *Hum. Pathol.* **20,** 224–231.
38. Bender, A., Behrens, L., Engel, A. G., and Hohlfeld, R. (1998) T-cell heterogeneity in muscle lesions of inclusion body myositis. *J. Neuroimmunol.* **84,** 86–91.
39. Mikol, J. and Engel, A. G. (1994) Inclusion body myositis, in *Myology. Basic and Clinical.* (Engel, A. G. and Franzini-Armstrong, C., eds.), McGraw-Hill, New York, pp. 1384–1398.
40. Carpenter, S. (1996) Inclusion body myositis. *J. Neuropathol. Exp. Neurol.* **55,** 1105–1114.
41. Pruitt, J. N., Showalter, C. J., and Engel, A. G. (1996) Sporadic inclusion body myositis: counts of different types of abnormal fibers. *Ann. Neurol.* **39,** 139–143.
42. Garlepp, M. J., Laing, B., Zilko, P. J., Ollier, W., and Mastaglia, F. L. (1994) HLA associations with inclusion body myositis. *Clin. Exp. Immunol.* **98,** 40–45.
43. Garlepp, M. J. and Mastaglia, F. L. (1996) Inclusion body myositis. *J. Neurol. Neurosurg. Psychiatr.* **60,** 251–255.
44. Orimo, S., Koga, R., Nakamura, K., Arai, M., Tamaki, M., Sugita, H., et al. (1994) Immunohistochemical analysis of perforin and granzyme A in inflammatory myopathies. *Neuromusc. Disord.* **4,** 219–226.
45. Goebels, N., Michaelis, D., Engelhardt, M., Huber, S., Bender, A., Pongratz, D., et al. (1996) Differential expression of perforin in muscle-infiltrating T cells in polymyositis and dermatomyositis. *J. Clin. Invest.* **97,** 2905–2910.
46. Cherin, P., Herson, S., Crevon, M. C., Hauw, J.-J., Cervera, P., Galanaud, P., et al. (1996) Mechanisms of lysis by activated cytotoxic cells expressing perforin and granzyme-b genes and the protein TIA-I in muscle biopsies of myositis. *J. Rheumatol.* **23,** 1135–1142.
47. Liu, C.-C., Walsh, C. M., and Young, J. D. E. (1995) Perforin: Structure and Function. *Immunol. Today* **16,** 194–201.

48. Henkart, P. A. (1994) Two pathways and multiple effector molecules. *Immunity* **1,** 343–346.
49. Behrens, L., Bender, A., Johnson, M. A., and Hohlfeld, R. (1997) Cytotoxic mechanisms in inflammatory myopathies. Co-expression of Fas and protective Bcl-2 in muscle fibers and inflammatory cells. *Brain* **120,** 929–938.
50. Schneider, C., Gold, R., Dalakas, M. C., Schmied, M., Lassmann, H., Toyka, K. V., et al. (1996) MHC class I mediated cytotoxicity does not induce apoptosis in muscle fibers nor in inflammatory CT cells: studies in patients with inclusion body myositis. *J. Neuropathol. Exp. Neurol.* **55,** 1205–1209.
51. Inukai, A., Kobayashi, Y., Ito, K., Doyu, M., Takano, A., Honda, H., et al. (1997) Expression of Fas antigen is not associated with apoptosis in human myopathies. *Muscle Nerve* **20,** 702–709.
52. Tews, D. S. and Goebel, H. H. (1997) Apoptosis-related proteins in skeletal muscle fibers of spinal muscular atrophy. *J. Neuropathol. Exp. Neurol.* **56,** 150–156.
53. Lee, R. K., Spielman, J., and Podack, E. R. (1996) *bcl*-2 protects against Fas-based but not perforin-based T cell-mediated cytolysis. *Int. Immunol.* **8,** 991–1000.
54. Farrow, S. N. and Brown, R. (1996) New members of the Bcl-2 Family and their protein partners. *Curr. Opin. Genet. Dev.* **6,** 45–49.
55. Lynch, D. H., Ramsdell, F., and Alderson, M. R. (1995) Fas and FasL in the homeostatic regulation of immune responses. *Immunol. Today* **16,** 569–574.
56. Brunner, T., Mogil, R. J., LaFace, D., Yoo, N. J., Mahboubi, A., Echeverri, F., et al. (1995) Cell-autonomous Fas (CD95)/Fas-ligand interaction mediates activation-induced apoptosis in T-cell hybridomas. *Nature* **373,** 441–444.
57. Goebels, N., Michaelis, D., Wekerle, H., and Hohlfeld, R. (1992) Human myoblasts as antigen presenting cells. *J. Immunol.* **149,** 661–667.
58. Hohlfeld, R. and Engel, A. G. (1990) Induction of HLA-DR expression on human myoblasts with interferon-gamma. *Am. J. Pathol.* **136,** 503–508.
59. Mantegazza, R., Hughes, S. M., Mitchell, D., Travis, M., Blau, H. M., and Steinman, L. (1991) Modulation of MHC class II antigen expression in human myoblasts after treatment with IFN-γ. *Neurology* **41,** 1128–1132.
60. Hohlfeld, R. and Engel, A. G. (1990) Lysis of myotubes by alloreactive cytotoxic T cells and natural killer cells. Relevance to myoblast transplantation. *J. Clin. Invest.* **86,** 370–374.
61. Lindberg, C., Oldfors, A., and Tarkowski, A. (1995) Local T-cell proliferation and differentiation in inflammatory myopathies. *Scand. J. Immunol.* **41,** 421–426.

23
Systemic Sclerosis

Timothy M. Wright

1. Introduction

Systemic sclerosis (SSc) or scleroderma is an autoimmune connective tissue disease of as-yet unknown etiology. Clinically, SSc is one of a group of illnesses that represent a spectrum of inflammatory and fibrotic diseases with related features. These other disorders include eosinophilia myalgia syndrome, toxic oil syndrome, eosinophilic fasciitis, morphea, and linear scleroderma (reviewed in ref. *1*). SSc is now generally divided into two major clinical subsets: limited SSc and diffuse SSc, based on the extent of skin involvement. Diffuse SSc involves the skin proximal to the elbow or knee and frequently involves the trunk, whereas limited SSc involves skin of the hands, forearms, legs below the knees, and face. The course and prognosis are quite variable from patient to patient and are related to disease subset, with diffuse disease having a worse prognosis. The overall mortality of SSc is reported to be 50% at 10 yr *(2)*.

The two major SSc clinical subsets differ significantly in clinical and laboratory features. For example, in limited SSc, Raynaud's phenomenon usually antedates the onset of skin thickening by many years, often decades, whereas in diffuse SSc, the onset of Raynaud's is usually within 1 yr of cutaneous changes and may occur after the onset of digital swelling or fibrosis. Pulmonary hypertension is a common late manifestation of limited SSc, whereas pulmonary interstitial fibrosis, scleroderma renal crisis, myocardial involvement, and tendon friction rubs occur more frequently in diffuse SSc patients *(3)*. The constellation of cutaneous calcinosis, Raynaud's phenomenon, esophageal dysmotility, sclerodactyly, and telangiectases, once felt to define a more "benign" subset of SSc patients with limited cutaneous involvement (CREST), has proven less valuable in distinguishing SSc clinical subsets because of the similar frequency of these clinical findings over the course of the disease in patients with diffuse SSc *(3)*. It is also important to note that a small group of patients develop internal organ involvement indistinguishable from SSc without clinical evidence of skin fibrosis (referred to as systemic sclerosis sine scleroderma).

The presence of specific serum autoantibodies is also highly correlated with SSc clinical subsets *(3)*. Diffuse SSc is frequently accompanied by serum antibodies directed against DNA topoisomerase I (also known as Scl-70), RNA polymerases I and III, or U3 RNP/fibrillarin, whereas limited SSc patients most often have anticentromere antibodies. An interesting feature of the autoantibodies in SSc patients is that in contrast to other autoim-

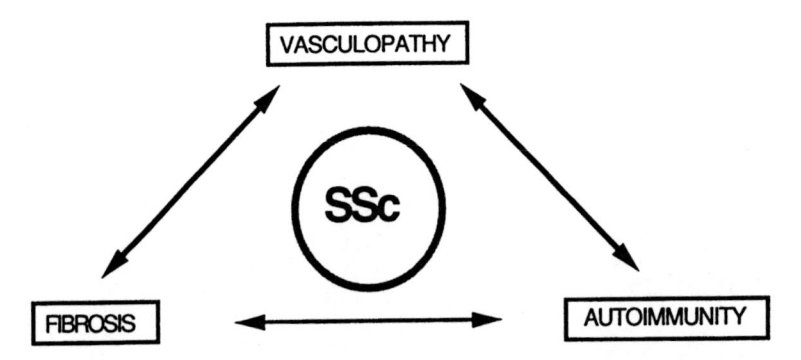

Fig. 1. Major components in SSc pathogenesis.

mune diseases such as systemic lupus erythematosus (SLE), Sjögren's syndrome, and rheumatoid arthritis in which more than one autoantibody specificity is frequently encountered in the same patient, the autoantibodies in SSc are nearly always mutually exclusive.

2. Overview Of SSc Pathogenesis

It is in the context of this background that one must consider the pathogenesis of SSc. Whether SSc represents a single disease entity that is modified by host genetic factors or is a cluster of diseases with similar clinical features, yet having distinct etiologies and discrete clinical and laboratory features, remains to be defined. For the purpose of this chapter, the former hypothesis will be assumed to be correct. However, where clearly apparent, the differences between the pathogenetic processes of limited and diffuse SSc subsets will be described. As is the case with most of the "autoimmune" diseases, the precise pathogenesis of SSc remains obscure. Clues to the pathogenesis of SSc arise from the unique characteristics of this multisystem disease. The hallmarks of SSc are vasculopathy, a systemic inflammatory process accompanied by autoimmune T- and B-cell responses directed against specific nuclear antigens, and widespread tissue fibrosis involving skin and internal organs. Because these three processes appear simultaneously in most SSc patients, it has been difficult to determine a causal pathogenetic relationship, if any, between these disease manifestations.

The pathogenesis of SSc can be divided, therefore, into three main components: vascular, autoimmune, and fibrotic, as depicted in Fig. 1. The bidirectional arrows between components denote the potential interrelatedness in the pathogenesis of SSc. Vascular changes, in particular endothelial cell activation, can result in increased leukocyte trafficking and activation in the skin and internal organs. Vasospasm, as occurs in Raynaud's phenomenon, can lead to ischemia–reperfusion injury and may result in an exaggerated wound-healing response by fibroblasts leading to tissue fibrosis. Activated lymphocytes elaborate a variety of soluble mediators (cytokines) and upregulate surface ligands that can promote fibroblast matrix production and alter the properties of vascular endothelium and smooth muscle. Fibroblasts from SSc lesional skin produce excess matrix and, likewise, upregulate cytokine production and surface protein expression that can stimulate lymphocytes and vascular endothelium.

In the following sections of this chapter, these three components will be presented in detail, with an emphasis on how the molecular aspects of each component relate to clinical manifestations and overall disease pathogenesis.

3. Vasculopathy In SSc

One of the earliest histopathologic changes in SSc skin is the swelling of endothelial cells and perivascular mononuclear cell accumulation *(4,5)*. This is frequently associated with vasospasm and vascular hyperreactivity manifested by Raynaud's phenomenon. In many tissues, an obliterative vasculopathy ensues with myointimal cell proliferation and vascular fibrosis. The clinical manifestations of these vascular changes include Raynaud's phenomenon, dermal edema, pulmonary hypertension, renal insufficiency (scleroderma renal crisis), and digital ischemic ulcers. Other vascular changes seen commonly in SSc, such as telangiectases and nailfold capillary abnormalities may be related to altered angiogenesis resulting from the obliterative vasculopathy.

There is considerable evidence favoring a role for both endothelial cell injury and vascular hyperactivity in the pathogenesis of SSc *(6,7)*. The basis for these processes in SSc, however, is not fully understood. Endothelial injury may result from circulating soluble mediators (cytokines such as tumor necrosis factor [TNF] or cytotoxic enzymes such as Granzyme A) that result from an immune response to altered (e.g., by a toxin) or possibly infected (e.g., viral) endothelium. Alternatively, the endothelium may not be the primary target of the immune response; rather, elevated serum levels of toxic mediators may secondarily affect the endothelium, resulting in damage and/or activation. The downstream effects of vascular hyperactivity, or vasospasm, include tissue ischemia, endothelial damage, thrombosis, fibrosis, and neovascularization. There may be an intrinsic abnormality in the response of vascular smooth muscle to vasoconstrictor stimuli in SSc, as suggested by a 100-fold increased sensitivity to α-2 adrenoreceptor stimulation of dermal arterioles from uninvolved SSc skin compared to vessels from normal controls *(7)*. Following vasospasm, reperfusion leads to the generation of reactive oxygen species that can further damage tissues and may result in fibrosis. In this regard, Stein et al. demonstrated increased levels of urinary F_2-isoprostane metabolites (derived from the nonenzymatic, oxygen-free radical-catalyzed peroxidation of arachidonic acid) in samples from SSc patients *(8)*.

Increased serum levels of endothelial-derived factors, markers of endothelial injury and activation, have been reported in SSc patients. One of these, endothelin-1, was found to be present in higher levels in sera from patients with diffuse SSc compared to limited SSc patients and healthy controls *(9)*. Endothelin-1 has multiple effects including vasoconstriction, vascular smooth-muscle cell and fibroblast proliferation, and stimulation of collagen production by fibroblasts *(10)*. Another important endothelium-derived mediator is nitric oxide (NO), also known as endothelium-derived relaxing factor (EDRF). Nitric oxide is an essential modulator of vascular smooth-muscle tone and its production by endothelial cells is regulated by a complex interplay of mechanical forces, neuropeptide mediators, and other endothelial activators derived from platelets and the coagulation cascade *(7,10)*. Increased levels of NO have been reported in SSc patients, although whether this is the result of chronic endothelial injury or inflammation remains to be elucidated *(11)*.

The endothelial surface is also modified in SSc to promote inflammation and coagulation. The endothelium plays an important role in leukocyte trafficking via the upregulation of adhesion molecules such as endothelial leukocyte adhesion molecule-1

Table 1
Major Autoantibody Specificities in SSc

Limited SSc	Diffuse SSc	SSc overlap
Centromere proteins	DNA topoisomerase I	PM-Scl
Th RNP/RNase MRP	RNA polymerase I, III complexes	U1 RNP
	U3 RNP/fibrillarin	U3 RNP/fibrillarin

(ELAM-1, E-selectin, CD62E) and intercellular adhesion molecule-1 (ICAM-1, CD54). Increased levels of circulating soluble forms of ICAM-1 and ELAM-1, reflective of endothelial activation, have been observed in SSc (10). It is likely that the increased expression of adhesion molecules is responsible for the perivascular accumulation of lymphocytes and monocytes seen in early SSc lesions (4,5). The procoagulant property of activated endothelium in SSc is demonstrated by increased circulating levels of von Willebrand factor, an endothelium-derived pro-coagulant, and by evidence of in vivo platelet activation, including increased β thromboglobulin and platelet factor 4 (10,12).

It is important to consider that although it is tempting to speculate that the primary event in the pathogenesis of SSc is endothelial injury with associated vascular hyperactivity, there is not always a direct correlation between the location of vascular changes and tissue fibrosis, nor does vascular hyperactivity as evidenced by Raynaud's phenomenon bear a direct relationship to tissue damage. In fact, primary Raynaud's disease is a relatively common illness and only a small proportion of these patients progress to SSc (7). Furthermore, secondary Raynaud's occurs in a variety of autoimmune diseases and in these settings it is not associated with tissue fibrosis. It is possible that the vascular injury in SSc is qualitatively different than these other illnesses, thereby resulting in unique downstream inflammatory and postinflammatory (i.e., fibrotic) events, and that variability of the extent of vascular abnormalities within the tissues of an SSc patient may be responsible for the imperfect correlation with tissue damage.

4. Autoimmunity In SSc

One of the features that relates SSc to the other autoimmune connective-tissue diseases is the presence of serum antibodies directed against self proteins. Although a direct role for these autoantibodies in the pathogenesis of SSc is unclear, there is growing evidence that the generation of these autoantibodies is dependent on self-reactive T-lymphocytes (13). The stimulation of autoreactive T-cells by as-yet unknown mechanisms may be responsible for the production of soluble and cell-surface mediators that result in fibroblast and endothelial cell activation. The autoantibodies, therefore, serve as markers of this ongoing autoimmune stimulation.

Approximately 95% of SSc patients have defined serum autoantibodies. The specificity of these antibodies has important correlations with disease subset and organ system involvement (3). For example, as shown in Table 1, the diffuse disease subset of SSc is associated with anti-DNA topoisomerase I, anti-RNA polymerase, and anti-U3 RNP/fibrillarin autoantibodies, whereas the limited SSc subset is associated with the presence of serum antibodies specific for centromere proteins and the nucleolar ribonuclear protein complex Th RNP, which is identical to the mitochondrial RNA processing enzyme designated RNase MRP *(14)*. When SSc patients have prominent clinical features characteristic of other connective tissue diseases (overlap) such as myositis or systemic lupus erythematosus, this is associated with anti-PM-Scl (myositis), U3 RNP (myositis), or U1 RNP (systemic lupus erythematosus) antibodies *(3)*. With rare exception, the presence of serum autoantibodies in SSc is mutually exclusive. Clearly, the specificity of these autoantibodies for SSc and their correlation with distinct clinical subsets and internal organ involvement indicates that the process responsible for their production is likely to be important in disease pathogenesis.

An interesting feature of the proteins targeted by the autoantibodies in SSc is their presence within the nucleolus of the cell *(14)*. Recently, Rosen and colleagues proposed an hypothesis to explain the localization of SSc autoantigens in the nucleolus *(15)*. According to their hypothesis, cleavage of SSc-associated autoantigens may occur in vivo as a result of metal-catalyzed oxidation reactions resulting in the generation of peptides containing cryptic epitopes not normally exposed to the immune system and for which there is no self tolerance. The cleavage process, therefore, could be downstream of ischemia–reperfusion, which is a common feature of SSc. Ischemia–reperfusion, as occurs with the reversible vasospasm of Raynaud's phenomenon, would generate reactive oxygen species necessary for the reaction. It has been proposed that this chemical reaction would target primarily nucleolar proteins (i.e., SSc autoantigens), because the nucleolus is the subcellular site of metal deposition (e.g., iron or copper) involved in catalyzing the cleavage *(15)*. Their studies demonstrated metal and reactive-oxygen-species-dependent cleavage of DNA topoisomerase I, the large subunit of RNA polymerase II, NOR-90, and the 70-kDa subunit of U1 RNP. Interestingly, U3 RNP/fibrillarin was resistant to cleavage by this reaction; however, it did undergo formation of intermolecular and intramolecular disulfide bonds that could result in altered antigenic properties *(15)*.

Another potential mechanism for the break in tolerance to self proteins is the presence of immune cell microchimerism resulting in an illness resembling graft-versus-host disease (GVHD) *(16)*. Experimental data support the hypothesis that microchimerism resulting from the persistence of fetal cells circulating in the blood of women years after childbirth is more frequent among women who develop SSc *(17)*. Artlett et al. using a Y-chromosome-specific polymerase chain reaction (PCR) assay also demonstrated the presence of male cells in skin biopsies of female SSc patients, whereas skin samples from healthy controls were uniformly negative *(17)*. Although the clinical and laboratory features of GVHD and SSc differ in many respects, there are enough similarities to warrant further exploration of this intriguing hypothesis.

The mechanism leading to the loss of self tolerance in SSc is not defined. However, there is now a considerable body of data indicating that autoreactive T-cells are present in the blood and lungs of SSc patients and that they appear activated in comparison to their counterparts in healthy controls *(18,19)*. Kuwana et al. characterized the autoreactive T-cells specific for DNA topoisomerase I from SSc patients and healthy controls and found them to have a limited T-cell-receptor repertoire *(20)*. These autoreactive CD4+ T-cells were capable of stimulating B-cells from SSc patients to generate anti-DNA topoisomerase antibodies in an antigen-dependent manner *(13)*. Analysis of cytokine production by DNA topoisomerase-I-specific T-cell clones from SSc patients and controls indicated that SSc patients were more likely to have T-cells

Table 2
Cytokines Implicated in the Fibrosis of SSc

Cytokine	Potential cellular source(s) in SSc
CTGF	Fibroblasts
IL-1	Endothelium, fibroblasts, macrophages
IL-4	Mast cells, T-cells
IL-6	Endothelial cells, fibroblasts, T-cells, mast cells, macrophages
PDGF	Endothelial cells, fibroblasts, macrophages, platelets
TGF-β	Endothelial cells, fibroblasts, macrophages, platelets, T-cells

with defined phenotypes (Th2 > Th1) rather than a naive (Th0) phenotype seen predominantly in healthy controls (21).

Yurovsky et al. found increased numbers of activated CD8+ T-cells in bronchoalveolar lavage BAL samples from SSc patients and detected skewing of their T-cell-receptor repertoire suggestive of an antigen-driven oligoclonal expansion (19). As will be discussed further in the section on tissue fibrosis, Th2-cell-derived cytokines, in particular transforming growth factor-β (TGF-β), interleukin-4 (IL-4), and IL-6, can stimulate fibroblasts to increase matrix production, thereby providing a potential link between the autoimmune and fibrotic processes observed in SSc.

5. Mechanisms of Tissue Fibrosis

The pathologic feature that distinguishes SSc from the other autoimmune rheumatic diseases is the development of extensive tissue fibrosis. Studies on the histopathologic changes in SSc skin and in vitro analysis of fibroblasts from SSc patients have demonstrated increases in numerous matrix components including types I, III, V, VI, and VII collagens, fibronectin, tenascin, osteonectin/SPARC, fibrillin, and glycosaminoglycan (22). The regulation of matrix protein gene expression is presented in Chapter 11; therefore, the focus of this section will be on the cellular and molecular mechanisms leading to fibroblast activation and increased matrix production.

The fibrosis that occurs in SSc can involve many tissues, including the dermis, myocardium, skeletal muscle, lungs, tendon sheaths, and gastrointestinal tract. There is now a general consensus that the fibrotic response follows an insidious low-grade inflammation in these tissues comprised primarily of a mononuclear cell inflammatory infiltrate. Studies of skin lesions in SSc have demonstrated the presence of CD4+ T-cells (5) and increased numbers of degranulated mast cells (23). Both T-cells and mast cells are known to produce a variety of soluble mediators capable of stimulating fibroblast proliferation and increased matrix protein production. Most notable among these factors are the cytokines IL-4, IL-6, and TGF-β, which are secreted by activated T-cells and mast cells, and the mast cell products histamine and tryptase (24,25).

In addition to activated T-cells and mast cells, many other cells, including endothelial cells, macrophages, dendritic cells, and fibroblasts themselves, may contribute to the cytokine milieu that results in the fibrotic response observed in SSc. A list of the cytokines that have been shown to be increased in SSc skin tissue or in cultures of SSc skin fibroblasts is shown in Table 2. Of note is the fact that many of the cytokines listed are produced by fibroblasts and can promote fibroblast proliferation and/or increased matrix synthesis, thereby acting as autocrine or paracrine factors. The presence of autocrine/paracrine pathways may explain the persistent "fibrogenic" phenotype of SSc lesional fibroblasts in vitro characterized by increased proliferation and matrix protein synthesis over several passages in culture *(26,27)*.

Two autocrine/paracrine pathways have been described in SSc fibroblasts that may contribute to tissue fibrosis. The first pathway involves TGF-β, which may be produced by infiltrating T-cells and activated macrophages in SSc lesional skin. TGF-β can stimulate its own production in fibroblasts and also stimulates connective tissue growth factor (CTGF) and platelet-derived growth factor (PDGF) synthesis. Increased expression of TGF-β in SSc skin has been demonstrated using immunohistochemical and *in situ* hybridization techniques *(22)*. Recent evidence suggests that many of the downstream effects of TGF-β on fibroblast proliferation and collagen synthesis may be mediated by PDGF and CTGF *(28,29)*. The second autocrine/paracrine pathway includes IL-1, IL-6, and PDGF *(30)*. The expression of IL-1α in SSc fibroblasts, which is not normally expressed in quiescent dermal fibroblasts, was correlated with increased expression of the downstream cytokines IL-6 and PDGF. The relationship between these cytokines was investigated using antisense IL-1α oligonucleotides to treat cultured SSc lesional fibroblasts. The antisense oligonucleotides transiently reduced IL-1α expression as well as that of IL-6 and PDGF. Increased IL-1α expression in vivo was demonstrated by immunohistochemistry in SSc lesional skin *(30)*. Recent studies which involve stable transfection of SSc lesional fibroblasts with an expression construct encoding antisense IL-1α mRNA to chronically suppress IL-1α protein expression indicate that this cascade is directly related to proliferation and collagen production in SSc fibroblasts in vitro (Wright and Kawaguchi, unpublished).

6. Conclusion

The pathogenesis of SSc is highly complex and involves the interaction of three primary disease processes: vasculopathy, autoimmunity, and tissue fibrosis. The crosstalk between these processes is the result of a network of cellular interactions mediated by soluble (e.g., cytokines) and cell surface (e.g., adhesion molecules) factors. The initiating event leading to the disease phenotype we refer to as SSc remains elusive; however, clues abound in our current knowledge of the three main pathogenetic mechanisms. The expanding information about the pathogenesis of SSc offers new possibilities for therapeutic intervention in the near future.

References

1. Varga, J. and Kahari, V. (1997) Eosinophilia–myalgia syndrome, eosinophilic fasciitis, and related fibrosing disorders. *Curr. Opin. Rheum.* **9,** 562–570.
2. Silman, A. J. (1991) Epidemiology of scleroderma. *Ann. Rheum. Dis.* **50,** 846–853.
3. Medsger, T. A., Jr. and Steen, V. D. (1996) Classification, prognosis, in *Systemic Sclerosis* (Clements, P. J. and Furst, D. E., eds.), Williams & Wilkins, Baltimore, MD, pp. 51–64.
4. Fleischmajer, R., Perlish, J. S., and Reeves, J. R. T. (1976) Cellular infiltrates in scleroderma skin. *Arthritis Rheum.* **20,** 975–984.
5. Roumm, A. D., Whiteside, T. L., Medsger, T. A., Jr., and Rodnan, G. P. (1984) Lymphocytes in the skin of patients with systemic sclerosis: quantification, subtyping, and clinical correlations. *Arthritis Rheum.* **27,** 645–653.

6. Kahaleh, M. B. and Fan P. (1997) Mechanism of serum-mediated endothelial injury in scleroderma: identification of a granular enzyme in scleroderma skin and sera. *Clin. Immunol. Immunopathol.* **83,** 32–40.
7. Wigley, F. M. (1996) Raynaud's phenomenon and other features of scleroderma, including pulmonary hypertension. *Curr. Opin. Rheum.* **8,** 561–568.
8. Stein, C. M., Tanner, S. B., Awad, J. A., Roberts, L. J., and Morrow, J. (1996) Evidence of free radical-mediated injury (Isoprostane overproduction) in scleroderma. *Arthritis Rheum.* **39,** 1146–1150.
9. Yamane, K., Miyauchi, T., Suzuki, N., Yuhara, T., Akama, T., Suzuki, H., et al. (1992) Significance of plasma endothelin-1 levels in patients with systemic sclerosis. *J. Rheum.* **19,** 1566–1571.
10. Kahaleh, M. B. (1995) The vascular endothelium in scleroderma. *Int. Rev. Immunol.* **12,** 227–245.
11. Yamamoto, T., Katayama, I., and Nishioka, K. (1998) Nitric oxide production and inducible nitric oxide synthase expression in systemic sclerosis. *J. Rheum.* **25,** 314–317.
12. Kahaleh, B. and Matucci-Cerinic, M. (1995) Raynaud's phenomenon and scleroderma: dysregulated neuroendothelial control of vascular tone. *Arthritis Rheum.* **38,** 1–4.
13. Kuwana, M., Medsger, T. A., Jr., and Wright, T. M. (1995) T–B cell collaboration is essential for the autoantibody response to DNA topoisomerase I in systemic sclerosis. *J. Immunol.* **155,** 2703–2714.
14. Lee, B. and Craft, J. E. (1995) Molecular structure and function of autoantigens in systemic sclerosis. *Int. Rev. Immunol.* **12,** 129–144.
15. Rosen, A., Casciola-Rosen, L., and Wigley, F. (1997) Role of metal-catalyzed oxidation reactions in the early pathogenesis of scleroderma. *Curr. Opin. Rheum.* **9,** 538–543.
16. Nelson, J. L. (1998) Microchimerism and the pathogenesis of systemic sclerosis. *Curr. Opin. Rheum.* **10,** 564–571.
17. Artlett, C. M., Smith, J. B., and Jimenez, S. A. (1998) Identification of fetal DNA and cells in skin lesions from women with systemic sclerosis. *N. Engl. J. Med.* **338,** 1186–1191.
18. Kuwana, M., Medsger, T. A., Jr., and Wright, T. M. (1995) T cell proliferative response induced by DNA topoisomerase I in patients with systemic sclerosis and healthy donors. *J. Clin. Invest.* **96,** 586–596.
19. Yurovsky, V. V., Wigley, F. M., Wise, R. A., and White, B. (1996) Skewing of the CD8+ T-cell repertoire in the lungs of patients with systemic sclerosis. *Hum. Immunol.* **48,** 84–97.
20. Kuwana, M., Medsger, T. A., Jr., and Wright, T. M. (1997) Highly restricted TCR α/β usage by autoreactive human T cell clones specific for DNA topoisomerase I: recognition of an immunodominant epitope. *J. Immunol.* **158,** 485–491.
21. Kuwana, M., Medsger, T. A. Jr., and Wright, T. M. (2000) Analysis of soluble and cell surface factors regulating anti-DNA topoisomerase I autoantibody production demonstrates synergy between Th1 and Th2 autoreactive T cells. *J. Immunol., in Press.*
22. Varga, J. and Bashey, R. I. (1995) Regulation of connective tissue synthesis in systemic sclerosis. *Int. Rev. Immunol.* **12,** 187–199.
23. Hawkins, R. A., Claman, H. N., Clark, R. A., and Steigerwald, J. C. (1985) Increased dermal mast cell populations in progressive systemic sclerosis: a link in chronic fibrosis? *Ann. Intern. Med.* **102,** 182–186.
24. Postlethwaite, A. E. (1995) Role of T cells and cytokines in effecting fibrosis. *Int. Rev. Immunol.* **12,** 247–258.
25. Gruber, B. L. (1995) Mast cells: accessory cells which potentiate fibrosis. *Int. Rev. Immunol.* **12,** 259–279.

26. LeRoy, E. C. (1974) Increased collagen synthesis by scleroderma skin fibroblasts in vitro: a possible defect in the regulation or activation of the scleroderma fibroblast. *J. Clin. Invest.* **54,** 880–889.
27. Buckingham, R. B., Prince, R. K., Rodnan, G. P., and Taylor, F. (1978) Increased collagen accumulation in dermal fibroblast cultures from patients with progressive systemic sclerosis (scleroderma). *J. Lab. Clin. Med.* **92,** 5–21.
28. Silver, R. M. (1995) Interstitial lung disease of systemic sclerosis. *Int. Rev. Immunol.* **12,** 281–291.
29. Igarashi, A., Nashiro, K., Kikuchi, K., Sato, S., Ihn, H., Fujimoto, M., et al. (1996) Connective tissue growth factor gene expression in tissue sections from localized scleroderma, keloid, and other fibrotic skin disorders. *J. Invest. Dermatol.* **106,** 729–733.
30. Kawaguchi, Y., Hara, M., and Wright, T. M. (1999) Endogenous IL-1α from systemic sclerosis fibroblasts induces IL-6 and PDGF-A. *J. Clin. Invest.* **103,** 1253–1260.

24
Vasculitis

Jörg J. Goronzy and Cornelia M. Weyand

1. Introduction

Vasculitides are a heterogeneous group of diseases characterized by inflammatory cell infiltrates and structural injury of blood vessel walls. The clinical significance of vasculitic syndromes directly relates to their potential to threaten the integrity of blood supply to tissues. In essence, blood vessel wall inflammation and destruction can cause aneurysm formation, rupture, and hemorrhage or can lead to stenosis and occlusion with subsequent infarction of dependent organs. The risk of life-threatening complications and the systemic nature of inflammatory blood vessel diseases emphasize the need for prompt diagnosis and treatment in patients suspected of suffering from vasculitis.

To standardize the diagnostic and therapeutic approach to patients with inflammatory vasculopathies, a series of major vasculitis categories has been defined (Table 1) *(1)*. This categorization makes use of a unique feature of these entities, namely their tendency to target specific vascular beds, usually defined by the size of the affected arteries and veins (Fig. 1). Small blood vessels, such as capillaries, venules, and arterioles, are the primary sites of inflammation in cutaneous leukocytoclastic angiitis, essential cryoglobulinemic vasculitis, and Henoch–Schönlein purpura. Most commonly, these small-vessel vasculitides cause manifestations in the skin, but also affect major organs, particularly the kidneys, when they display a more generalized pattern of involvement. Small to medium-sized blood vessels, including muscular arteries, are attacked in Wegener's granulomatosis, Churg–Strauss syndrome, and microscopic polyangiitis. Consequently, these are often associated with major organ disease. Necrosis of the walls of medium-sized vessels also occurs in polyarteritis nodosa (PAN) and Kawasaki disease. Inflammation of the aorta and its major branches is a characteristic feature of two vasculitic entities, giant-cell arteritis (GCA) and Takayasu's arteritis (TA). Categorizing the systemic vasculitides according to the size of the affected blood vessel has proven clinically useful. Pathophysiological criteria were not included in the definitions of the vasculitic entities. However, it can be assumed that this categorization of the vasculitic syndromes is also mechanistically relevant and that each follows its own pathogenic rules with uniqueness in etiology and pathomechanisms.

The last decade has seen remarkable progress in approaching these clinically fascinating diseases. New concepts have been developed that have permitted a novel pathogenic view of inflammatory vasculopathies *(2,3)*. The two major partners in vasculitis,

From: *Current Molecular Medicine: Principles of Molecular Rheumatology*
Edited by: G. C. Tsokos © Humana Press Inc., Totowa, NJ

Table 1
Histological Features of Major Vasculitides

Vasculitis	Histopathology of vascular inflammation	Extravascular pathology
Cutaneous leukocytoclastic angiitis	Fibrinoid necrosis of arterioles, capillaries, and venules with leukocytoclasis and RBC extravasation	–
Cryoglobulinemic vasculitis	Immunocomplex deposition and leukocytoclastic vasculitis in small vessels	Diffuse proliferative glomerulonephritis
Henoch-Schönlein purpura	Fibrinoid necrosis of small vessels with leukocytoclasis, in particular, of skin and gastrointestinal vessels	Glomerulonephritis, arthritis
Microscopic polyangiitis	Necrotizing vasculitis of small vessels with few immunocomplexes and with preferential involvement of lungs and kidneys	Necrotizing glomerulonephritis
Wegener's granulomatosis	Necrotizing vasculitis of medium-sized arteries, small vessels, and veins	Granulomatosus inflammation of the respiratory tract, necrotizing glomerulonephritis
Churg-Strauss vasculitis	Necrotizing vasculitis of medium-sized arteries and small vessels	Eosinophil-rich granulomatous inflammation of the respiratory tract, asthma
Polyarteritis nodosa	Fibrinoid necrosis and mixed cellular infiltrate of medium-sized vessels with elastic membrane destruction and aneurysm formation	Glomerulonephritis
Kawasaki disease	Non-necrotizing polyarteritis of medium-sized muscular arteries	Mucocutaneous lymph node syndrome
Giant cell arteritis	Granulomatous arteritis with lymphocyte/macrophage infiltrate of large- and medium-sized arteries with preference for extracranial branches of the carotid artery	–
Takayasu's arteritis	Granulomatous inflammation (lymphocytes/macrophages) of aorta and its major branches	–

the blood vessel wall and the infiltrating inflammatory cells, are connected by complex molecular pathways that define the biological principle of leukocyte adhesion, migration, and extravasation. To fulfill their tasks in tissue surveillance, leukocytes must be

Vasculitic syndrome	Vascular involvement
	aorta / large to mid-size arteries / small arteries / arterioles / capillaries / venules / veins
Cutaneous leukocytoclastic vasculitis	arterioles–venules
Henoch-Schönlein purpura	small arteries–venules
Cryoglobulinemic vasculitis	small arteries–venules
Microscopic polyangiitis	small arteries–venules
Wegener's granulomatosis	large to mid-size arteries–veins
Churg-Strauss vasculitis	large to mid-size arteries–veins
Polyarteritis nodosa	large to mid-size arteries–small arteries
Kawasaki disease	large to mid-size arteries–small arteries
Giant cell arteritis	aorta–large to mid-size arteries
Takayasu's arteritis	aorta–large to mid-size arteries

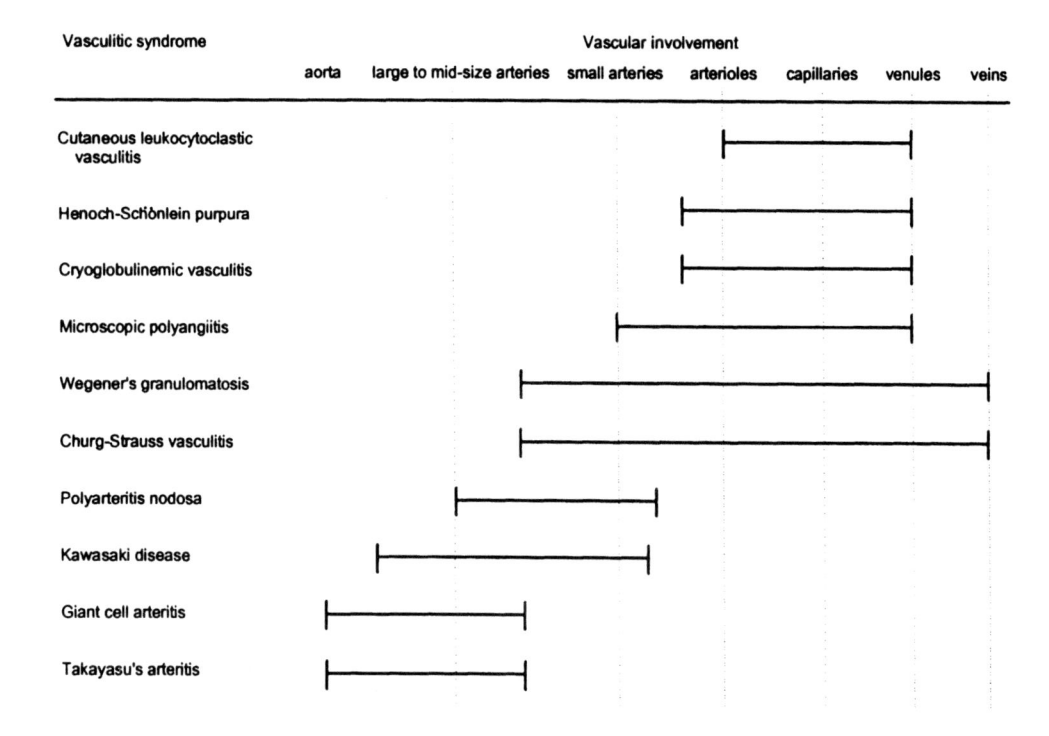

Fig. 1. Vasculitic syndromes and their preferential vascular involvement.

able to adhere to and migrate through the blood vessel endothelial layer. Under physiological conditions, leukocytes leave the vessel wall and the perivascular region and migrate into the avascular areas of the dependent tissue. This process is obviously critical in vasculitis, and abnormal regulation of adhesion molecule expression has been proposed to play a pathophysiological role in small vessel disease. Another area of progress relates to the definition and improved functional characterization of autoantibodies, such as antineutrophil cytoplasmic antibodies (ANCA), that possibly have direct involvement in mediating inflammation inside and outside the vessel wall. Finally, attention has been drawn to the particular type of vessel destruction associated with large artery disease. In the large vessel arteritides, tissue damage not only emerges from the structural disruption of wall components but, more importantly, from the response of the artery to the inflammatory injury. Specifically, an abrupt hyperproliferative response of the arterial media and intima leads to the formation of hyperplastic intima and subsequent luminal occlusion. Arteritis-induced intimal hyperplasia possibly shares a pathogenic mechanism with atheromatous disease, so far defined as a noninflammatory vascular disease, raising the interesting possibility that the response pattern of the attacked blood vessel is a critical determinant in the clinical manifestations of vasculitis.

2. Leukocyte-Endothelial Interaction, Leukocyte Extravasation, and Vasculitis

Leukocytes are a mobile tissue and have the remarkable ability to leave the circulation, to enter peripheral lymphoid organs, and penetrate into inflamed tissue. The processes of adherence and extravasation are governed by a multitude of molecules that act in a coordinated fashion (4,5). An appealing disease model proposes that homing mechanisms regulating the physiologic extravasation of leukocytes are aberrantly regulated in small-vessel vasculitis, leading to the accumulation of inflammatory cells in the blood vessel wall. Most of the molecules involved in leukocyte adhesion and migration can be assigned to one of five superfamilies: selectins, sialomucins (ligands for selectins), integrins, immunoglobulin-like molecules (bind to integrins), and proteoglycans. The current paradigm holds that adhesion of leukocytes to endothelial cells is a multistep cascade. The majority of leukocytes flow freely in the bloodstream at a high velocity. Some cells in the marginal stream make transient contact with the vascular lining and start tethering and rolling. This initial binding is mediated by selectins and sialomucins expressed on leukocytes and endothelial cells, respectively. Selectins are constitutively expressed proteins that are N-glycosylated and carry a lectin domain. The lectin domain interacts with glycoproteins that contain abundant oligosaccharide augmentation. Sialomucins, which are selectin ligands, have multivalent binding sites presented on a rigid rod that extends above the cell surface into the bloodstream to facilitate binding of circulating cells. The lectin–oligosaccharide interactions are characterized by rapid association and dissociation kinetics and are, therefore, ideally suited to establish transient contact and to slow circulating cells.

Initially, leukocyte binding is transient and fully reversible. To firmly adhere to endothelial cells, leukocytes must be activated. Activation signals generally come from chemoattractants that are locally produced and can be trapped on endothelial cells. Chemokines are a group of chemoattractive cytokines that have been subgrouped on the basis of spacing of conserved cysteine residues. C-C chemokines (containing two adjacent cysteines) act on mononuclear cells, whereas C-X-C chemokines mainly target neutrophils. Many chemoattractants bind to proteoglycans that serve as reservoirs and increase the half-lives and local concentrations of these mediators at the site of leukocyte extravasation. As a general rule, neutrophils, monocytes, and T-cell subsets differ in the panel of chemokine receptors they express. Notably, lymphocytes lack cell-surface receptors for some classical chemoattractants such as complement component C5a and platelet-activating factor (PAF), both of which have pivotal roles in neutrophil extravasation.

Rolling leukocytes, if activated, come to a stable arrest and stick to the endothelial cells sufficiently to withstand the shear forces of the bloodstream. This firm adhesion is mediated by the interaction of integrins and immunoglobulin-like molecules (ICAMs, VCAMs). Additional receptor–ligand pairs have a role in this adhesion step—in particular, CD44 binding to proteoglycans. Finally, the cells have to penetrate the interendothelial junction and the basement membrane. Proteolytic enzymes are likely to be involved in this process; however, the exact mechanism and its regulation are poorly understood.

The model of a multistep adhesion cascade has been primarily developed using neutrophils, but has principally been applicable to lymphocyte homing to primary lymphoid organs. It is likely that similar mechanisms apply to leukocyte extravasation in small-vessel vasculitis; however, some important differences cannot be ignored. First, physiological lymphocyte homing mainly occurs in small venules, whereas vasculitides such as leukocytoclastic vasculitis, Henoch–Schönlein purpura, and cryoglobulinemic vasculitis target arterioles, capillaries, and venules. Microscopic polyangiitis and Wegener's granulomatosis affect small arteries in addition to the microvasculature. Obviously, the blood flow in these vascular beds is greater and the shear forces are less amenable to adhesion. Hemodynamic changes such as vasodilatation, decrease in blood flow, turbulences in the marginal bloodstream, or increased viscosity have to occur to allow for stable endothelial cell–leukocyte interactions. Second, postcapillary venules have an endothelium specialized to facilitate leukocyte extravasation. Endothelial cells in these venules have a plump, cuboidal shape, and the vessels are referred to as high-endothelial venules. Normal endothelial cells, after activation, can mimic some of the features of high endothelial cells; however, it is likely that they differ in the genetic regulation and expression of the molecules relevant to blood vessel wall transmigration.

The functional activity of adhesion molecules is regulated at multiple levels. Obviously, expression of a given molecule is a prerequisite of its function. Most adhesion molecules are absent on endothelial cells under physiological conditions, but can be readily upregulated in response to inflammatory cytokines. Cytokines such as interleukin-1 (IL-1) and tumor necrosis factor-α (TNF-α) are rather promiscuous and induce the expression of a variety of adhesion molecules including the immunoglobulin-like ICAM and VCAM molecules as well as E-selectin. Other cytokines, such as interferon-γ (IFN-γ), are more selective, and different combinations of cytokines can yield specific patterns of adhesion molecule expression. Stimuli other than cytokines that can also induce the expression of adhesion molecules on endothelial cells include oxygen radicals, complement factor C5a, and mechanostimulation. Many of these stimuli have been shown to be functional in vasculitic syndromes: (1) cytokine production, in particular production of IL-1 and TNF-α by monocytes and macrophages, is a common event in inflammatory responses; (2) complement can be activated after immunocomplex deposition, resulting in the generation of C5a; (3) changes in turbulence and vessel caliber may cause mechanostimulation of endothelial cells; and (4) antiendothelial antibodies may directly stimulate endothelial cells. Thus, mechanisms are in place in vasculitic syndromes to explain upregulation of the adhesion cascade and leukocyte extravasation. Not surprisingly, expression of ICAM, VCAM, and E-selectin has been shown on endothelial cells in vasculitic tissue.

Expression of a relevant adhesion molecule is generally not sufficient to effectively trap leukocytes. Modifications are necessary to increase the affinity and avidity of the leukocyte–endothelial cell interaction. Posttranslational modification of adhesion molecules is central to their functional activity. The most evident example is the glycosylation of selectins that is a prerequisite for their function. The regulation of glycosylation is not well defined, but tissue-specific expression of enzymes, such as sialyltransferases, fucosyltransferases, and sulfotransferases, is likely to have a major impact on the function of selectins. Integrins require a conformational change to be functionally active. Local clustering of adhesion molecules on endothelial cells, either by oligomerization of single molecules or by generating microdomains with high cell-surface density of adhesion molecules, can significantly increase the avidity of the interaction with leukocytes. All of these mechanisms are likely to be important in promoting the extravasation of leukocytes in small-vessel vasculitis, although their exact contribution has not been defined for any of the vasculitic syndromes. In particular, it is unknown whether an aberration in one of these pathways is primarily causative in

Vasculitic syndrome	Pathological immunocomplex formation		Defect in immunocomplex clearance
	Antigen	Antibody	
Serum sickness	Exogenous	Polyclonal	−
Cutaneous leukocytoclastic vasculitis	?	Polyclonal	?
Connective tissue disease	Multiple autoantigens	Polyclonal	+ (e.g., complement deficiencies)
Henoch-Schonlein purpura	?	IgA	+ (decreased clearance of IgA)
Mixed cryoglobulinemia vasculitis (Hepatitis C)	IgG	Monoclonal IgM	−
Hepatitis B-associated panarteritis nodosa	HBs	Polyclonal	−

↓

Subendothelial deposition of immune complexes

↓

Complement activation / Production of C5a

↓

Neutrophil recruitment and activation

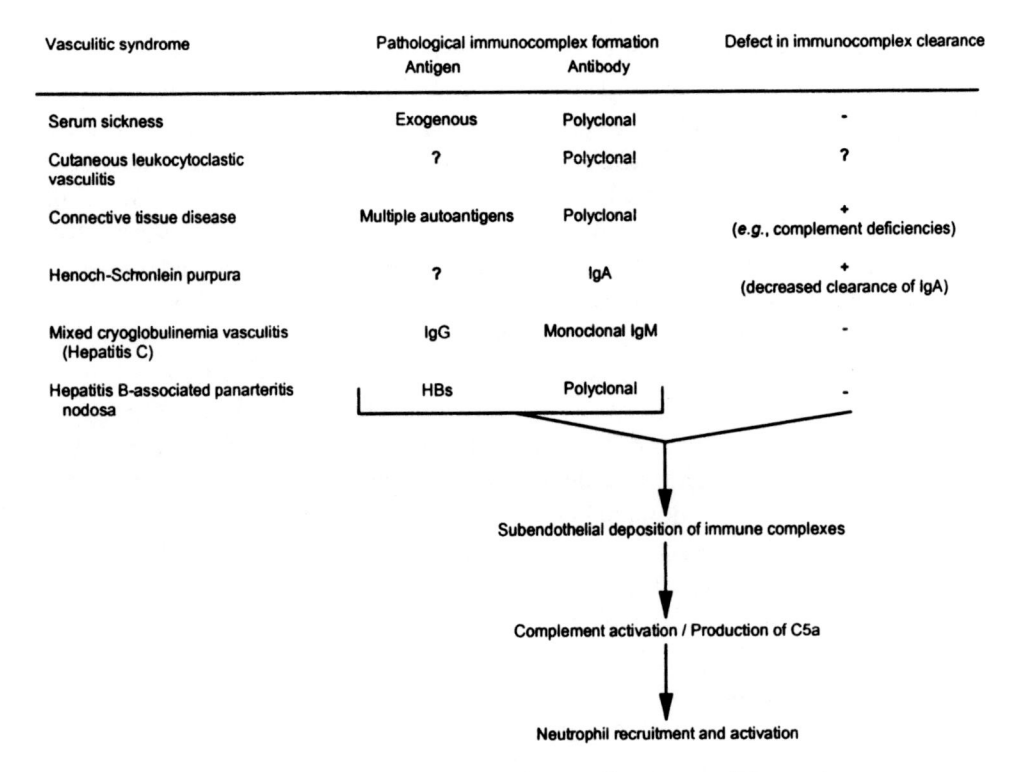

Fig. 2. Mechanisms in immune-complex-mediated vasculitic syndromes.

initiating the vessel-wall-destructive inflammation. However, regardless of whether leukocyte extravasation has a primary or secondary role in vasculitis, these pathways represent promising targets for therapeutic intervention.

3. Immune Complex Deposition, Endothelial Cell Activation, and Vascular Injury in Small Vessel Vasculitis

Deposition of immune complexes has long been recognized as a mechanism inducing vessel wall inflammation (6). Studies in models of acute serum sickness have demonstrated that circulating immune complexes can induce vasculitic lesions in small arteries. These observations have been confirmed in human serum sickness. Patients treated with antithymocyte globulin frequently develop serum sickness, coincident with an increase in circulating immune complexes, decreased serum complement, and deposition of globulin and complement in affected small cutaneous blood vessels. The mere presence of circulating immune complexes is not sufficient to produce vasculitis; additional factors must be present to elicit a vasculitic response (Fig. 2). Formation of immune complexes is a regular feature of any antibody-mediated immune response. However, these complexes are usually rapidly cleared from the circulation. Clearance of immune complexes requires the activation of the classical complement pathway, resulting in deposition of C3b on the antigen–antibody complexes. Immobilized C3b binds to complement receptors on erythrocytes and monocytes that capture and remove immune complexes from the circulation. Reduced clearance of immune complexes is an important factor in their subendothelial deposition in the vascular wall. Other factors include hemodynamic changes, activation of platelets, and the size and nature of immune complexes, all of which contribute to the pathological subendothelial deposition.

To induce vasculitic lesions, deposited immune complexes need to recruit polymorphonuclear leukocytes into the vessel wall. One important factor that can provide a homing signal is the complement factor C5a. C5a is generated inside the vessel wall after complement activation on the deposited immune complexes. It has been shown to possess chemoattractant capability, mainly targeting neutrophils, and thus may be partially responsible for the predominantly neutrophilic nature of the infiltrate in small-vessel vasculitides. Tissue-infiltrating neutrophils can be activated by at least one of two mechanisms, binding of C5a or binding of immune complexes to Fc receptors. Activated neutrophils produce oxygen radicals and secrete proteases that inflict damage to the vessel wall. In leukocytoclastic vasculitis, this response appears to be rather rapid, not allowing time for endothelial cell activation and formation of a mononuclear infiltrate. Cells undergo apoptosis in the vessel wall and macrophages and monocytes are relatively absent from the infiltrate. The apoptotic cells are, therefore, not readily phagocytosed, which may lead to the typical presentation of leukocytoclastic vasculitis. The resulting structural damage to the vessel wall is severe and allows red blood cells to enter the vessel wall.

Immunoglobulin and complement depositions in human vasculitic lesions have been mostly demonstrated for cutaneous leukocytoclastic vasculitis and are less consistently found in systemic vasculitis (Table 1). Among the vasculitic syndromes that appear to be primarily immunocomplex related are Henoch–Schönlein purpura and vasculitis associated with cryoglobulinemia, as suggested by special features of the immune complexes isolated from affected patients. In Henoch–Schönlein purpura, immunocomplexes in the circulation as well as in the vasculitic lesions are rich in IgA. The IgA isotype is not effective in triggering the classical complement pathway and in fixing C3b. IgA-containing immunocomplexes are, therefore, poorly targeted by complement receptors on erythrocytes and are primarily cleared by the lungs and kidneys, and not the spleen. In the inflamed blood vessel wall, these IgA-containing complexes may, however, activate the alternative complement pathway and form C5a as well as the membrane attack complex. A different mechanism appears to apply to vasculitides associated with cryoglobulins. Mixed cryoglobulinemia is typically associated with hepatitis C infection *(7,8)*. In these patients, monoclonal IgM antibodies emerge that have rheumatoid factor (RF) activity and, therefore, bind IgG and form large immunocomplexes. The resulting cryoglobulins may have pathogenic relevance by slowing down the blood flow, favoring platelet and leukocyte binding to endothelial cells.

4. Neutrophil Activation and Anti-neutrophil Cytoplasmic Antibodies

Circumstantial evidence supports the notion that antibody-mediated mechanisms have a role in blood vessel wall inflammation. Antiendothelial antibodies have been described, as well as antibodies to matrix proteins; however, the antigens recognized by these antibodies have not been well characterized, and the association with vasculitis is not established. In contrast, evidence has accumulated that anti-neutrophil cytoplasmic antibodies (ANCA) have a pathogenic contribution in some of the vasculitic syndromes *(9–11)*. Several antigens have been identified that are recognized by ANCAs, proteinase 3 and myeloperoxidase being the most important ones. Both anti-

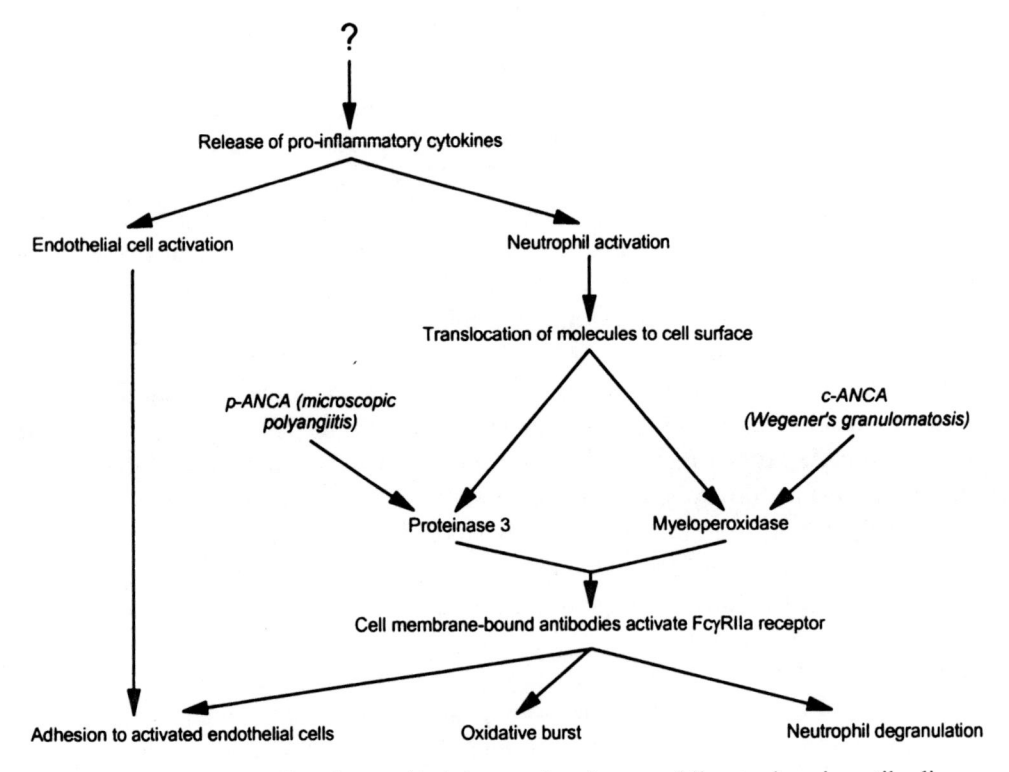

Fig. 3. Neutrophil-mediated vascular injury and antineutrophil cytoplasmic antibodies.

gens are contained in neutrophil primary granules. Antibodies to proteinase 3 are characteristic in patients with Wegener's granulomatosis. They are expressed in the majority of, but not all, patients with this disease, and their titer has been correlated to disease activity, suggesting that they are not absolutely required in pathogenesis but play an important role. Antibodies to myeloperoxidase are predominantly found in patients with microscopic polyangiitis, but they are considered to be less diagnostic for any particular vasculitic entity.

The current paradigm holds that anti-proteinase-3 and antimyeloperoxidase antibodies recognize their antigen on the cell surface of neutrophils and that this recognition event provides neutrophil-activating stimuli (Fig. 3). In resting neutrophils, neither myeloperoxidase nor proteinase 3 is detected on the cell surface. However, after exposure to TNF-α, both antigens can be found on the cell surface, where they may interact with ANCA. It has been demonstrated that ANCAs induce respiratory burst and degranulation in neutrophils and that ANCA-activated neutrophils adhere to and kill endothelial cells in vitro *(12)*. It is therefore possible that ANCAs contribute to the recruitment of neutrophils into vasculitic lesions. Whether these antibodies have a primary role in inducing vasculitis or enhance the vasculitic response remains to be investigated. The excellent specificity of the anti-proteinase-3 antibodies for Wegener's granulomatosis suggests that this antibody plays a central role in this syndrome. However, attempts to establish an animal model in which anti-proteinase-3 antibodies induce vasculitis have not been successful.

Additional evidence for a possible role of antibodies in blood vessel wall inflammation has come from studies associating vasculitic complications with polymorphisms in Fc receptors. Fc receptors modulate immune reactions by controlling the binding of antigen–antibody complexes to neutrophils, monocytes, and natural-killer (NK) cells. Allelic polymorphisms of the FcγRIIa receptor have been described that influence the binding affinity to immunoglobulin isotypes. This allelic polymorphism has been found to be associated with glomerulonephritis in patients with systemic lupus erythematosus (SLE) *(13)*. Similarly, a polymorphism of the FcγRIIIa receptor expressed on NK cells appears to be a risk factor for nephritis in SLE. It is possible that these polymorphisms not only play a role in the immunocomplex-mediated renal complications of SLE but also in small-vessel vasculitides.

5. T-Cell-Mediated Immune Responses in ANCA-Associated Vasculitides, PAN, and Rheumatoid Vasculitis

Although cellular immune responses do not appear to have a major role in the vasculitides such as leukocytoclastic vasculitis, Henoch–Schönlein purpura, and mixed cryoglobulinemia that predominantly affect small-sized blood vessels, they do contribute to the ANCA-associated vasculitides. Wegener's granulomatosis and Churg–Strauss syndrome are granulomatous diseases. Granuloma formation is a T-cell-dependent process that requires the activation of T-cells as well as macrophages. Dependent on the type of T-cell involved, the cellular composition of the granuloma varies. T-cells preferentially producing IL-4 and IL-5, so-called Th2 T-cells, support the formation of granulomatous lesions containing eosinophils, as seen in parasitic diseases. Eosinophils are essentially absent in granulomas formed by T-cells preferentially producing IFN-γ, so-called Th1 T-cells. Both types of granulomatous inflammation are encountered in vasculitic syndromes. It has been proposed that a Th1 response is characteristic of Wegener's granulomatosis, whereas a Th2 response is found in Churg–Strauss vasculitis. Lymphocytes accumulated in the tissue lesions have been described to express activation markers. Data indicate that the involvement of T-lymphocytes is not limited to the vasculitic inflammation. Both syndromes characteristically form areas of necrosis and granulomatous inflammation in the tissue that are unrelated to the blood vessel wall (Table 1). This finding implies systemic abnormalities, and it emphasizes that the injurious inflammatory response displays preference for blood vessels but is not restricted to them.

Cellular immune responses mediated by T-lymphocytes also play a role in PAN and in rheumatoid vasculitis. PAN is characterized by an inflammation of the entire vessel wall of mid-sized arteries with an infiltrate consisting of a mixture of lymphomononuclear cells and varying numbers of neutrophils and eosinophils. PAN has been associated with pre-existing hepatitis B infection. This association raises the question of whether the arterial wall inflammation is a downstream effect of antiviral immunity. However, the nature of the T-cell response and its relation to potentially initiating antigens has not been elucidated. Several lines of evidence support a critical involvement of T-cells in rheumatoid vasculitis *(14,15)*. Rheumatoid vasculitis is a complication of rheumatoid arthritis. Histomorphologically, it can resemble PAN. It preferentially affects male patients with production of high titers of rheumatoid factors. Homozygosity for HLA-DRB1*0401 has been identified as a risk factor, suggesting a role for antigen presentation and T-cell recognition. Patients with rheumatoid vasculitis display a striking abnormality in their T-cell repertoire. They express monoclonal populations of CD4⁺ T-cells. Clonally expanded CD4 T-cells have been found to be phenotypically (CD28 deficient) and functionally distinct from classical helper T-cells. Monoclonality suggests, as one possibility, the chronic stimulation with antigen, but the perturbations in the T-cell repertoire may reflect more fundamental abnormalities in T-cell homeostasis. Expanded CD4$^+$CD28^{null} clonotypes isolated from patients with rheumatoid vasculitis have been described to exhibit autoreactivity, providing an explanation for their systemic representation and their possible involvement in vascular pathology.

6. The Interplay of T-Cells, Macrophages, and Arterial-Resident Cells in GCA and TA

Large arteries, such as the aorta and its major branches, are the preferred target for two vasculitic syndromes, GCA and TA. In both diseases, the blood vessel wall is the site of an immune response, and T-cells and macrophages represent the major players. GCA and TA share pathogenetic features that separate them from the other vasculitides, but differences in pathogenesis and clinical presentation between the two forms of arteritis prevail. TA targets the large elastic arteries, whereas GCA primarily affects the medium-sized muscular arteries that have well-defined internal and external elastic laminae. GCA affects Caucasians with the highest risk for individuals of Scandinavian descent, whereas TA is more frequent in patients with an Asian background or in native Mexicans, suggesting a major contribution of genetic factors in the pathogenesis of both diseases. Age appears to be a second important variable in disease expression. The diagnosis of TA requires an age at onset of younger than 40 yr, whereas GCA is a disease of the elderly. The precise role of age in the pathogenesis of these arteritides remains unclear.

Both TA and GCA are HLA-associated diseases, supporting the model that T-cell-mediated immune responses are important in the pathogenesis. In the Japanese population, TA is associated with the major histocompatibility complex (MHC) class I B52 allele *(16)*. For GCA, increased frequencies of the MHC class II HLA-DRB1*04 alleles are generally found. These HLA associations allow conclusions to be drawn on the nature of the cellular immune response in those diseases. MHC class I molecules function as antigen-presenting molecules for CD8 T-cells, and MHC class II molecules present antigenic peptides to CD4 T-cells, suggesting that different subsets of T-cells have dominant roles in the pathogenesis of these two vasculitides. Sequence comparisons of HLA-DRB1 alleles in patients with GCA have provided further support for the hypothesis that binding of antigenic peptide and presentation to CD4 T-cells is relevant in the disease process. MHC molecules have binding pockets to accommodate antigenic peptides. Studies in GCA patients have demonstrated that one of these binding pockets is conserved. It has, therefore, been proposed that CD4⁺ T-cells recognize an antigen in the arterial wall that initiates a cascade of events, ultimately resulting in structural damage *(17)*. This concept has been explored in GCA in great detail (Fig. 4). T-cells that accumulate in the arterial wall of GCA patients are not a random representation of the peripheral blood repertoire, but are highly selected, as one would expect in an antigen-specific immune response. A small proportion of tissue-infiltrating T-cells from temporal artery biopsies have undergone clonal expansion. T-cells with identical T-cell receptor sequences can be detected in different biopsy specimens from the same patient,

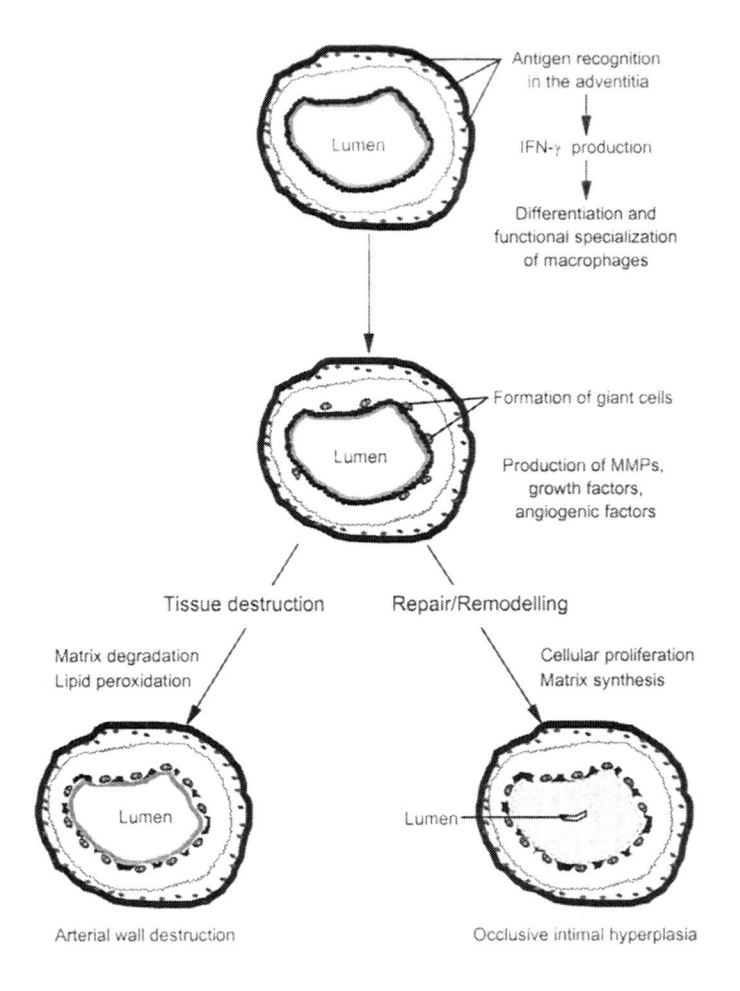

Fig. 4. Schematic diagram of pathogenic pathways in GCA. (Reprinted, with permission, from Weyand, C. M. and Goronzy, J. J. Arterial wall injury in giant cell arteritis. *Arthritis Rheum.* **42**, 844–853. Copyright 1999, Lippincott Williams & Wilkins.)

suggesting that the same antigen is recognized at different inflammatory sites. T-cell lines derived from the vascular lesions respond to arterial wall extracts from GCA patients but not to extracts from control temporal artery specimens. Histological studies for the T-cell-derived cytokine IFN-γ and for additional T-cell activation markers have shown that only T-cells in the adventitia, but not T-cells in the media, are activated. Taken together, these data suggest that T-cells enter mid-size arteries from the vasa vasorum, recognize an antigen in the adventitial tissue, and initiate an inflammatory cascade. The major effector function of these T-cells is the secretion of IFN-γ, assigning a critical role of this cytokine to disease pathogenesis. Formal proof for this model has been developed in adoptive transfer experiments using a severe combined immunodeficiency (SCID) mouse chimera model. In these experiments, inflamed temporal artery biopsy specimens were engrafted into SCID mice. Adoptive transfer of tissue-derived CD4 T-cell clones, but not of control clones, into human tissue–SCID mouse chimeras induced increased expression of the T-cell-derived cytokine IFN-γ and of the macrophage-derived cytokines, IL-1 and IL-6, in the engrafted tissue.

How does IFN-γ production in the adventitia translate into the structural damage of vessel wall integrity in GCA patients? Vessel wall destruction and aneurysm formation develops late in a small subset of patients and is limited to the aortic arch. Classically, GCA patients develop ischemic symptoms of large and mid-size muscular arteries. Structural changes in these arteries are characterized by a varying degree of intimal hyperplasia. Studies in GCA patients have shown that the degree of intimal hyperplasia and the concomitant clinical ischemic symptoms directly correlate with the amount of IFN-γ produced in the adventitia, linking the IFN-γ production to the chain of events leading to intimal proliferation *(18)*. Intimal hyperplasia is the result of an interplay between tissue-infiltrating macrophages and resident cells. Macrophages in the infiltrate display diverse functions, depending on their topographical location. Macrophages in the adventitial layer preferentially produce the proinflammatory monokines, IL-1 and IL-6, and interact with the tissue-infiltrating T-cells. Macrophages in the media are characterized by metalloproteinase production and the formation of oxygen radicals. These medial macrophages tend to fuse and form giant cells that are arranged along the internal and external elastic laminae. Interestingly, the number of giant cells in the tissue correlates with the amount of IFN-γ produced in the adventitia. Formation of the oxygen radicals results in lipid peroxidation, thereby destroying the structural integrity of the media. In addition, matrix components, including the elastic laminae, are digested by locally secreted metalloproteinases. Smooth-muscle cells are mobilized and are able to migrate to the intima. Migration and proliferation of these smooth-muscle cells is under the control of platelet-derived growth factor (PDGF) that is secreted by medial macrophages and giant cells. Vascular endothelial growth factor (VEGF), mainly produced by giant cells, allows for neoangiogenesis in the media as well as in the hyperplastic intima. Finally, intimal macrophages produce transforming growth factor (TGF)-β and inducible nitric oxide synthase. The role of TGF-β in the intima may lie in the formation of a neomatrix. Inducible nitric oxide synthase results in the formation of nitric oxide, which can mediate tissue injury as well as act compensatory to the hyperplastic intima via its vasodilatory properties.

In conclusion, macrophages and giant cells are the major effector cells in promoting the structural changes in the vascular wall *(18)*. The formation of giant cells as well as several of the macrophage functions are under the control of IFN-γ that is released by T-cells in the adventitia subsequent to recognizing antigen. The nature of this antigen is undetermined and there is no hint as of yet that this antigen is an exogenous pathogen. In contrast to the small-vessel vasculitides, the macroendothelium in GCA remains relatively inert and there is no evidence of thrombus formation and leukocyte extravasation into the intima.

The sequence of events has been less well studied in TA. However, the inflammatory infiltrate is also likely to be formed via the vaso vasorum in the adventitia. Histopathologically, TA is a granulomatous panarteritis with a variable number of giant cells and a predominantly lymphoplasmocytic arteritis involving the media and the adventitia. Degeneration of the internal elastic lamina and of the media, intimal hyperplasia, tissue fibrosis, and neovascularization are characteristic of later stages of the disease. Marked inflammation of the vasa vasorum is a typical feature of TA. Studies of the effector mechanisms in vascular damage have mainly focused on cytotoxic T-cells

(19). It has been shown that perforin-secreting cells in the inflammatory infiltrate deposit perforin on vascular resident cells. Perforin is a pore-forming protein that is secreted by CD8 T-cells as well as cytotoxic γδ T-cells and NK cells and that allows for the induction of apoptosis of target cells by granzyme B. Thus, the extracellular finding of perforin suggests a cytotoxic mechanism that may be involved in the vessel wall injury in TA. CD4 T-cells and macrophages have been less well studied in TA than in GCA; however, similar effector mechanisms may be functioning in TA that result in the formation of a lumen-obstructing neointima.

6. Infection and Vasculitis

The concept that infection of resident cells of the vessel walls is the primary cause of the inflammatory response in vasculitis has been vigorously pursued over many years. A recent murine model has renewed the interest in a viral pathogenesis of vasculitides *(20)*. In this model, certain family members of the herpes family can persistently infect medial smooth-muscle cells of large arteries and induce a chronic vasculitic inflammatory response. This animal model made use of an immunodeficient mouse that lacked the expression of the IFN-γ receptor. Establishment of a virus latency with viral antigen expression in the vascular wall was dependent on the defective IFN-γ response and, therefore, quite different from human vasculitides that generally occur in patients who do not show any evidence of immunodeficiency. Certain herpes viruses have also been associated with rare vasculitic entities in humans. Varicella zoster has been suspected to be involved in a segmentally distributed inflammatory vasculopathy. Also, HTLV-1 can infect endothelial cells, which may be responsible for the cutaneous vasculitis associated with HTLV-1-induced T-cell leukemia. Obviously, virally induced vasculitides are rare exceptions and vessel wall infection by a viral pathogen has not been demonstrated for any of the more common syndromes.

As already alluded to, chronic viral infection can, however, be associated with vessel wall inflammation. The mechanism appears to be more indirect and not related to a direct infection of vascular resident cells. The viruses most frequently implicated are hepatitis B and hepatitis C. Hepatitis B infection has been linked to cases of PAN and essential mixed cryoglobulinemia. Hepatitis B surface antigen, immunoglobulin, and complement have been found in lesions of the small muscular artery as well as cutaneous vessels, and deposition of immunocomplexes in the vessel wall has been proposed as the underlying pathomechanism. It is important to stress that only a small proportion of hepatitis-B-infected patients develop vasculitic complications. Risk factors predisposing to this progression of disease have not been identified. Hepatitis C infection is strongly associated with mixed cryoglobulinemia. It is likely that the initial observations of cryoglobulinemia in hepatitis-B-infected individuals was secondary to a coinfection with hepatitis C. Between 70% and 100% of all patients with mixed cryoglobulinemia have been shown to be chronically infected with hepatitis C. Immune complexes are characterized by polyclonal IgG and monoclonal IgM with RF activity. Immune complexes with mixed cryoglobulinemic activities have a high propensity to induce leukocytoclastic vasculitis as well as occasional vasculitis in small and medium-sized vessels *(7,8)*. How hepatitis C induces a monoclonal proliferation of B-cells with secretion of IgM RF is unclear. However, there is evidence that hepatitis C is a lymphotropic virus that may be able to induce B-cell proliferation and transformation. Thus, these viral infections primarily induce aberrations in the immune system that may, at times, clinically present as vasculitis.

References

1. Jennette, J. C., Falk, R. J., Andrassy, K., Bacon, P. A., Churg, J., Gross, W. L., et al. (1994) Nomenclature of systemic vasculitides. Proposal of an international consensus conference. *Arthritis Rheum.* **37**, 187–192.
2. Sneller, M. C. and Fauci, A. S. (1997) Pathogenesis of vasculitis syndromes. *Med. Clin. North Am.* **81**, 221–242.
3. Sundy, J. S. and Haynes, B. F. (1995) Pathogenic mechanisms of vessel damage in vasculitis syndromes. *Rheum. Dis. Clin. North Am.* **21**, 861–881.
4. Springer, T. A. (1994) Traffic signals for lymphocyte recirculation and leukocyte emigration: the multistep paradigm. *Cell* **76**, 301–314.
5. Salmi, M. and Jalkanen, S. (1997) How do lymphocytes know where to go: current concepts and enigmas of lymphocyte homing. *Adv. Immunol.* **64**, 139–218.
6. Cochrane, C. G. and Koffler, D. (1973) Immune complex disease in experimental animals and man. *Adv. Immunol.* **16**, 185–264.
7. Agnello, V., Knight, G., and Abel, G. (1994) Interferon alfa-2a for cryoglobulinemia associated with hepatitis C virus. *N. Engl. J. Med.* **331**, 400.
8. Misiani, R., Bellavita, P., Fenili, D., Vicari, O., Marchesi, D., Sironi, P. L., et al. (1994) Interferon alfa-2a therapy in cryoglobulinemia associated with hepatitis C virus. *N. Engl. J. Med.* **330**, 751–756.
9. Kallenberg, C. G. M., Cohen-Tarvaert, J. W., van der Woude, F. J., Goldschmeding, R., von dem Borne, A. E., and Weening, J. J. (1991) Autoimmunity to lysosomal enzymes: new clues to vasculitis and glomerulonephritis. *Immunol. Today* **12**, 61–64.
10. Gross, W. (1995) Antineutrophil cytoplasmic autoantibody testing in vasculitides. *Rheum. Dis. Clin. North Am.* **21**, 987–1011.
11. Hoffman, G. S. and Specks, U. (1998) Antineutrophil cytoplasmic antibodies. *Arthritis Rheum.* **41**, 1521–1537.
12. Falk, R. J., Terrell, R. S., Charles, L. A., and Jennette, J. C. (1990) Anti-neutrophil cytoplasmic autoantibodies induce neutrophils to degranulate and produce oxygen radicals in vitro. *Proc. Natl. Acad. Sci. USA* **87**, 4115–4119.
13. Salmon, J. E., Millard, S., Schachter, L. A., Arnett, F. C., Ginzler, E. M., Gourley, M. F., et al. (1996) Fc gamma RIIA alleles are heritable risk factors for lupus nephritis in African Americans. *J. Clin. Invest.* **97**, 1348–1354.
14. Weyand, C. M. and Goronzy, J. J. (1997) Pathogenesis of rheumatoid arthritis. *Med. Clin. North Am.* **81**, 29–55.
15. Weyand, C. M., Klimiuk, P. A., and Goronzy, J. J. (1998) Heterogeneity of rheumatoid arthritis: from phenotypes to genotypes. *Springer Semin. Immunopathol.* **20**, 5–22.
16. Kerr, G. S. (1995) Takayasu's arteritis. *Rheum. Dis. Clin. North Am.* **21**, 1041–1058.
17. Weyand, C. M. and Goronzy, J. J. (1995) Giant cell arteritis as an antigen driven disease. *Rheum. Dis. Clin. North Am.* **21**, 1027–1039.
18. Weyand, C. M. and Goronzy, J. J. (1999) Arterial wall injury in giant cell arteritis. *Arthritis Rheum.* **42**, 844–853.
19. Seko, Y., Minota, S., Kawasaki, A., Shinkai, Y., Maeda, K., Yagita, H., et al. (1994) Perforin-secreting killer cell infiltration and expression of a 65-kD heat-shock protein in aortic tissue of patients with Takayasu's arteritis. *J. Clin. Invest.* **93**, 750–758.

20. Weck, K. E., Dal Canto, A. J., Gould, J. D., O'Guin, A. K., Roth, K. A., Saffitz, J. E., et al. (1997) Murine gamma-herpesvirus 68 causes severe large-vessel arteritis in mice lacking interferon-gamma responsiveness: a new model for virus-induced vascular disease. *Nature Med.* **3,** 1346–1353.

25
Osteoarthritis

A. Robin Poole and Ginette Webb

1. Introduction

Osteoarthritis (OA) represents a clinical collection of conditions involving a progressive pathological alteration of joint structure that involves the degeneration of articular cartilage, a remodeling of subchondral bone, and limited synovitis. OA may be described as a part of a process of age-related change or as a disease. It is twice as prevalent in women than men and increases in incidence with age, there being a major rise in incidence after 60 yr *(1)*. Changes that lead to the development of OA are slow. In idiopathic OA, clinical presentation may result from change over a period of up to 30 yr. The disease can involve one or two large joints or may be generalized and involve multiple joints, as in postmenopausal OA. Following joint trauma, there is an increased incidence *(1)*, which probably results from accelerated degeneration over a period of up to 15 yr. Degeneration may also be accelerated by synovitis. In contrast, familial OA presents very early, resulting from a genetic defect causing changes in cartilage matrix and physiology, leading to the manifestation of joint degeneration following natural cessation of growth. Such a condition is seen for example in patients with a mutation in the type II collagen gene and is usually accompanied by skeletal dysplasia.

2. Skeletal Changes in Osteoarthritis
2.1. Bone

Osteoarthritis involves not only the progressive degeneration of articular cartilage, leading to eburnation of bone, but also a little studied extensive remodeling of subchondral bone, resulting in the so-called sclerosis of this tissue observed radiographically. These changes in bone are often accompanied by the formation of subchondral cysts by a process of apparent focal resorption. These cysts are particularly noticeable by magnetic resonance imaging. The bone changes may also be systemic as suggested, for example, by the work of Dequeker and his colleagues *(2)*. They have produced evidence of changes in bone in remote extra-articular sites such as the iliac crest. Analyses of the molecular composition of OA bone reveal fundamental changes in metabolism. Deoxypyridinoline crosslinks, resulting from bone resorption, are elevated in urine, as is osteocalcin (a bone turnover marker) elevated in serum *(3)*. Femoral neck bone is less stiff and less dense in hip OA than normal, but not as reduced in density as in osteoporosis. Remote bone mineral density in the arms and spine is higher. In generalized OA, there is hypermineralization. Yet in women with hand OA, there is evidence that with increasing grade of OA, there is decreased bone mass. In hip OA, subchondral bone is less mineralized and has more osteoid indicative of incomplete mineralization (4). The elevated content of osteoid is accompanied by increased type I collagen content and its synthesis and increased alkaline phosphatase content. Transforming growth factor-β TGF-β, a bone growth factor, is also increased. Thus, bone changes may vary according to the type of OA.

Dieppe and his colleagues have shown that scintigraphy reveals changes in bone metabolism several years prior to intra-articular evidence of disease onset, as revealed by joint-space narrowing with loss of articular cartilage (5). Whether these bone changes precede those in cartilage remains to be determined once comparable analyses can be made of changes in cartilage metabolism. Also, increased bone turnover detected by scintigraphy is associated with disease progression. Studies in animals, such as the aging Guinea pig, using histology and magnetic resonance imaging, suggest that degenerative changes in articular cartilages accompany local changes in subchondral bone, which involve cyst formation and altered trabecular and osteoid thickness and bone formation rates.

Changes in one tissue may influence the other and thus determine the development of OA. This interplay is most strikingly observed in osteoporosis, where bone density is reduced by excessive osteoclastic resorption of bone. Patients with osteoporosis usually show little or no evidence of OA. Moreover, patients with OA do not usually develop osteoporosis (6). These observations may be explainable in part at the level of biomechanical interactions in that reduced bone density may protect against degeneration caused by excessive loading of articular cartilage during articulation.

A principle anatomical feature of OA is the development of peripheral osteophytes. The osteophytes, which have a cap of healthy articular cartilage over bone, may serve to reintroduce some stability into an otherwise unstable joint. These form from an endochondral process in sites at the edges of the damaged articular cartilage. They also reflect enhanced bone turnover. Addition of TGF-β to periosteum in culture, or injection in vivo, results in induction of endochondral bone formation, which is characterized by expression of the hypertrophic phenotype by newly formed chondrocytes in periosteal tissue and subsequent mineralization of extracellular matrix and bone formation in vivo. Intra-articular injection of TGF-$β_1$ also induces osteophyte formation. Thus, TGF-β, which is upregulated in bone in OA and probably other members of the bone morphogenetic protein superfamily, likely plays an important role in osteophyte formation.

2.2. Cartilage Degeneration

2.2.1. General Changes

The loss of articular cartilage may be initiated as a focal process, as is seen in early experimentally induced OA in animals, such as rabbits, where OA was induced following sectioning of the anterior cruciate ligament and/or partial medial meniscectomy. Focal lesions may progressively enlarge to involve specific joint compartments, inducing alterations in articulating surfaces by producing changes in loading. Usually, degeneration of the medial tibial plateau of the knee is first observed in developing animal and human intra-articular degeneration for reasons that are unclear. Degenerative changes may involve the whole articular cartilage in posttraumatic OA, where alterations in cartilage matrix turnover are detectable within days or weeks following joint injury *(7)*.

In idiopathic OA, degeneration is first observed at the articular surface in the form of fibrillation. This initially involves splits more or less parallel to the articular surface. Later splits penetrate the damaged and weakened cartilage. Cell division is observed early on, but, again, is confined to more superficial sites. Progressive loss of cartilage then occurs. Apoptosis is enhanced in OA, particularly (when measured *in situ*) at and close to the articular surface *(8)*.

Superficial fibrillation at and close to the articular surface is associated with increased denaturation and loss of type II collagen as collagen fibrils are degraded *(9,10)*. This leads to a loss of tensile properties, particularly in OA-susceptible joints such as the hip and knee *(11)*. These tensile properties are normally much higher at the articular surface than elsewhere in the cartilage. Damage to the cartilage characterized by increased denaturation and cleavage of type II collagen is seen especially around chondrocytes, but it extends into interterritorial sites remote from these cells in OA, unlike what is seen in aging. Thus, the chondrocyte is implicated as the mediator of this damage to the "resident" matrix, which was originally synthesized by this cell. Damage to the fibrils leads to a loss of the small proteoglycans decorin and biglycan (which are usually closely associated with these structures at the articular surface and, in the case of decorin, play a key role in regulating fibril diameter) and is accompanied by a loss of the large proteoglycan aggrecan.

These collagen molecules are degraded primarily as a result of the increased cleavage of type II collagen by collagenase, particularly collagenase-3 *(12)*, the cleavage of small proteoglycans on collagen fibrils and aggrecan cleavage *(13)* (Fig. 1). This is usually associated with increased expression and activity of metalloproteinases (MMP), starting at the articular surface early in the degenerative process, these include stromelysin-1 (MMP-3), gelatinases A (MMP-2) and B (MMP-9), collagenase-1 (MMP-1), collagenase-2 (neutrophil collagenase or MMP-8), collagenase-3 (MMP-13), and MT1-MMP (membrane type 1- MMP or MMP-14). Matrilysin expression is also upregulated. MMPs are very much involved in the excessive matrix degradation that characterizes cartilage degeneration in OA. They are secreted as latent proenzymes, which are then activated in the extracellular matrix (Fig. 2). Activators of prometalloproteinases, which are increased in OA, include MT1-MMP, which can activate gelatinase A and collagenase-3. Gelatinase A can also superactivate collagenase-3. Stromelysin-1, a superactivator of collagenases, and plasminogen activator activates plasminogen to produce plasmin, which is a general MMP activator. The cysteine proteinase cathepsin B is also upregulated in OA and may also be an important activator of MMPs. Many of these changes are reviewed elsewhere *(15,16)*.

Analyses of the proteoglycan aggrecan have revealed excessive cleavage in the core protein in OA cartilage. The best characterized sites are between the G1 and G2 domains: the MMP site, where multiple MMPs, including stromelysin-1 can cleave, and the aggrecanase site where cleavage can also be produced by a number of proteinases *(15)*, including membrane proteinases with characteristics of the ADAMTS fam-

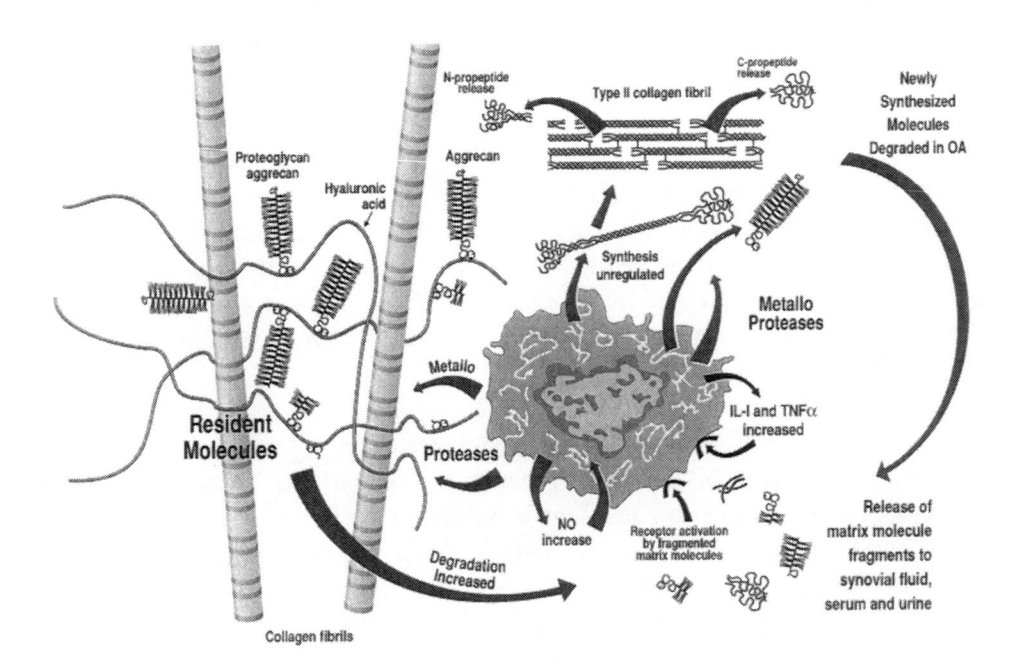

Fig. 1. Representation of a chondrocyte in articular cartilage which normally assembles and maintains an extensive extracellular matrix composed of collagen fibrils, the large proteoglycan aggrecan bound to hyaluronic acid, as well as many other molecules. This matrix is normally remodeled in a very controlled manner, especially in pericellular sites, involving metalloproteinases (MMPs) and limited synthesis of matrix molecules. In OA, there is excessive proteolysis, which leads to excessive damage to "resident" molecules and newly synthesized matrix molecules. Synthesis of matrix is increased, but net degradation and loss of both the new and resident matrix results. This degradation involves increased generation of paracrine and autocrine acting cytokines such as TNF-α and IL-1, increased receptor-mediated stimulation of chondrocytes by these cytokines and by matrix degradation products and upregulation of nitric oxide (NO). The matrix degradation products, that include degraded type II collagen, the c-propeptide of this molecule (synthetic marker) and aggrecan are released into body fluids where they can be detected, offering the potential to monitor these events in vivo (*see* Fig. 4). (Modified from ref. *14* with permission.)

ily *(17)*. Such cleavages are much enhanced in OA cartilage *(13)*. It is still unclear as to the relative contributions of different proteinases in aggrecan degradation because quantitative assays to measure both cleavage sites have not been used.

In OA, there is a deficiency of the tissue inhibitors of MMP (TIMPs) *(15)* (Fig. 2). This clearly favors the excessive proteolysis that is observed in the diseased articular cartilage.

The early damage to, and loss, of these molecules in OA is accompanied by an increased content and synthesis of biglycan and decorin and aggrecan in the mid-zone and deep zone, presumably to compensate for the increased loading on the chondrocytes as a consequence of the damage to, and loss, of the more superficial cartilage. Synthesis of other proteoglycans such as versican, fibromodulin, and lumican, as well as link protein and cartilage oligomeric protein are also increased. Other matrix molecules change in distribution in OA and the contents of molecules rich in developing tissues

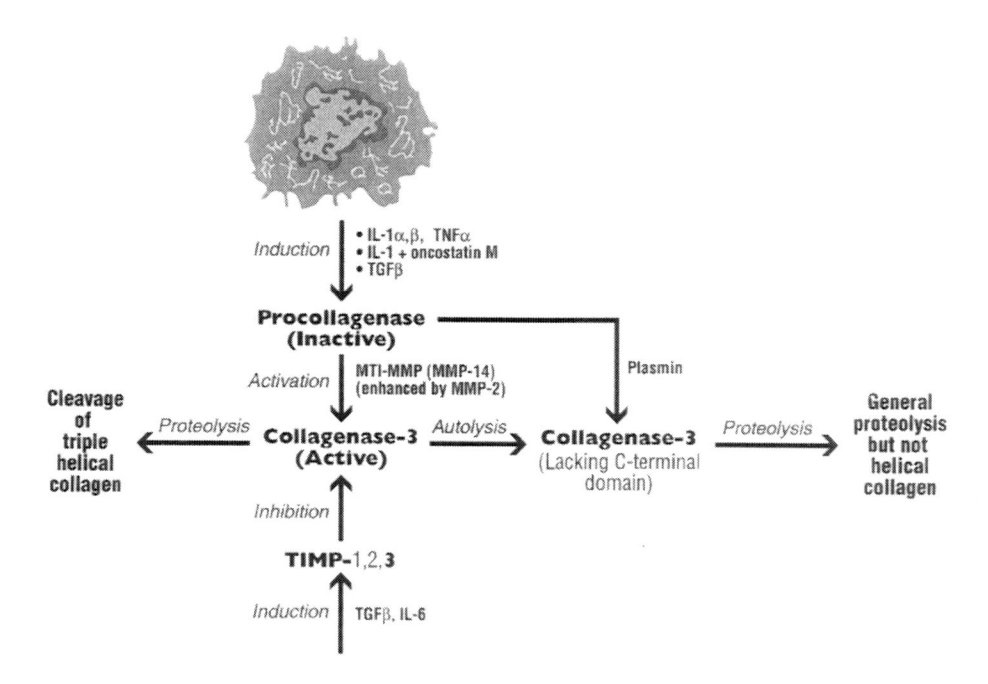

Fig. 2. Example of the increased secretion by a chondrocyte of an important degradative MMP, collagenase-3, and the regulation of its activity. Synthesis and secretion of latent proenzyme is stimulated by various cytokines/growth factors. Activation of the MMP is by other extracellular proteinases. Activity is regulated both by activation and inhibition of the MMP (and/or activator) by tissue inhibitors of MMPs (TIMPs), which can also be synthesized and released by chondrocytes. There is upregulation of MMPs and a deficiency of TIMPs in OA favoring excessive proteolysis.

such as fibronectin, tenascin, and osteonectin increase in content. There is a striking increase in the synthesis of type II collagen in these sites *(18)* (Fig. 1), mainly type IIB as revealed by experimental studies but also some type IIA, normally only observed prior to chondroblast differentiation early in development. Limited expression and synthesis of type III collagen is also seen. Type VI content (normally pericellular in location) is also increased. There is evidence that these and other newly synthesized matrix molecules are also degraded as part of the pathology (Fig. 1).

In OA, type X collagen expression and synthesis are activated. This may occur in developing articular cartilage but is usually only observed in calcifying cartilage in endochondral ossification *(19)*. In degenerate OA cartilage, it is found in association with increased expression of the cell-surface type II collagen receptor annexin V and parathyroid-hormone-related peptide and its receptor, which are normally highly expressed by early or mature hypertrophic chondrocytes. This expression of hypertrophy in OA is associated with apoptosis (another feature of terminal hypertrophic cells) and partial calcification of the matrix. These changes are first observed in the more superficial zones and mid-zones and could represent a cellular response to a degraded matrix. The increased expression of type II procollagen and collagenase-3 as described is also a feature of hypertrophy in the physics of the growth plate.

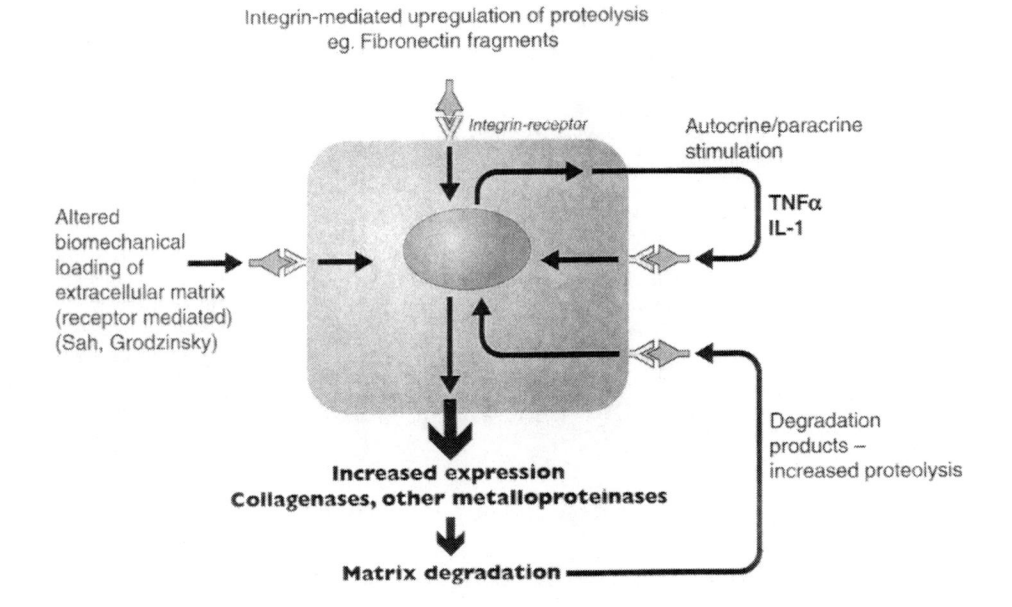

Fig. 3. Mechanisms involving cell–matrix interactions that can alter and regulate expression and activities of MMPs in chondrocytes in articular cartilage. These involve both integrin-mediated signaling responses to fibronectin fragments, biomechanical loading, and paracrine/autocrine production of cytokines such as IL-1 and/or TNF-α.

In the partially calcified cartilage (delimited by the tide mark), there is also reactivation of endochondral ossification. Here, upregulation of type X collagen is often seen with duplication or replication of the tide mark separating this zone from uncalcified cartilage. Vascular invasion reappears that resembles that seen in the growth plate.

2.2.2. Mechanisms

The reasons for the increased synthesis and activation of these MMPs at the cellular level are becoming more apparent. For example, there is evidence that some fragments of fibronectin, which are present in elevated levels in OA, can stimulate chondrocyte-mediated cartilage resorption via cell-surface receptor activation. This was originally shown in fibroblasts where MMP-1 is upregulated through an arganine, glycine, asparatate (RGD)-integrin receptor activation *(20)*. These degradation products could play an important role in establishing a positive-feedback mechanism for the generation and maintenance of proteolysis. These cell–matrix responses involve the production of cytokines such as IL-1, which play an autocrine/paracrine role (Fig. 3).

Receptors on chondrocytes for interleukin-1 are upregulated in OA, even more than in rheumatoid arthritis (RA). Tumor necrosis factor-α (TNF-α) in particular is upregulated compared to articular cartilage in RA. The receptor for TNF-α also shows increased expression when compared to normal cartilage, and expression of the TNF-α p55 receptor (but not the p75) on OA chondrocytes correlates with susceptibility of cartilage to TNF-α-induced proteoglycan loss *(21)*.

Interleukin-1 (IL-1) and TNF-α are both potent activators of cartilage degradation in vitro *(15,16)*. For example they can stimulate collagenase-3 production (Fig. 2).

However, in combination with oncostatin M, IL-1 is even more potent in causing cartilage resorption. Yet, this cytokine, a member of the IL-6 family, is not normally elevated in OA synovial fluid. Thus, oncostatin may be of more importance when synovitis is more pronounced in the OA joint and this is associated with accelerated degeneration (see Subheading 3). Other cytokines that are upregulated in OA include macrophage inflammatory protein-1β.

Nitric oxide (NO) synthase (iNOS) is associated with increased generation of NO. Il-1 and TNF-α are potent stimulators of NO production in cartilage, which is upregulated in OA chondrocytes compared to normal and to RA cartilage. There is a linkage in the expression of iNOS with TNF-α and IL-1β gene expression in OA chondrocytes. NO induced by IL-1 can inhibit aggrecan synthesis. However, protease activity and proteoglycan degradation are enhanced when NO production is blocked, suggesting that it may also have a protective role. Increased cell death seen in OA may also be due, in part the result, of NO because it can induce apoptosis in chondrocytes.

Changes in matrix loading can also alter matrix degradation as well as altering the synthesis of extra cellular matrix (ECM) macromolecules *(16)*. The pathological changes in cartilage matrix in OA likely result in a disturbance of the normal balance between mechanical loading and direct cytokine/growth factor signalling changing gene expression. Insulin-like growth factor-1, which is upregulated in OA, may be responsible for the increased matrix synthesis *(22)*. Some of these changes that influence chondrocyte-mediated matrix turnover are summarized in Fig. 3.

3. Synovitis and Systemic Inflammation

Osteoarthritis is characterized by some synovitis (inflammation of the synovium), albeit much less than is ordinarily observed in rheumatoid arthritis. Inflammation may be of early onset. In posttraumatic OA, the early increase in MMP-3 (stromelysin-1) in synovial fluid is likely to come mainly from activated synovial cells.

Fas ligand, which induces apoptosis, is also present in synovial fluid in OA and may induce chondrocyte apoptosis by engagement of its receptor on chondrocytes.

Synovial cells actively synthesize and secrete hyaluronic acid (HA, hyaluronan), as well as many other cells in the body. However, studies of RA reveal a close correlation between serum HA and joint inflammation and disease progression (joint damage) *(4)*. In OA, persistent elevation of serum HA is associated with accelerated progression of joint damage *(3)*. Serum HA also inversely correlates with knee joint-space width in OA, suggesting a link between synovitis and joint damage. Similarly, cartilage oligomeric protein, which is synthesized by synovial cells and chondrocytes (particularly when exposed to TGF-β), is increased in patients who exhibit accelerated large-joint degeneration *(3)*. Thus, joint inflammation may accelerate joint damage. This likely results from local pro-inflammatory cytokine generation by the synovium.

The C-reactive protein is also elevated in serum in patients with OA, as is the eosinophil cationic protein and myeloperoxidase. Together, these changes provide evidence for systemic and local inflammation in OA. Recently, evidence for T-cell immunity to the cartilage proteoglycan aggrecan and link protein has been reported for OA. T-Cell immunity to type II collagen has previously been seen in experimental OA induced by partial meniscectomy. Thus, joint inflammation in OA may share some of the features of inflammation found in RA joints.

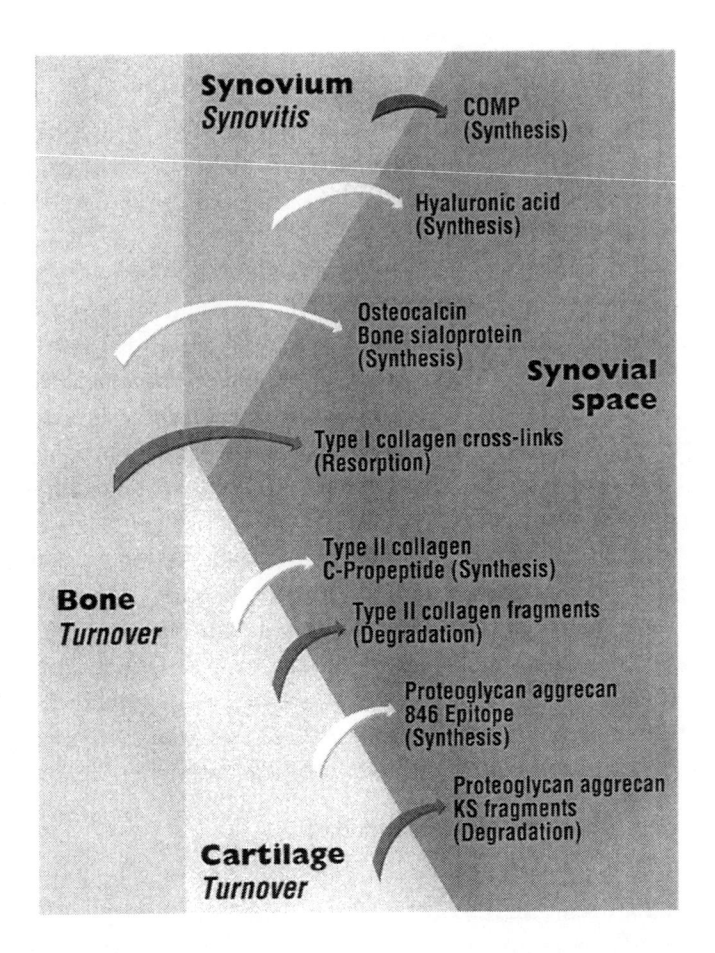

Fig. 4. Summary of some of the potential surrogate molecular (biochemical) markers that are released from synovium, cartilage, and bone into body fluids, where their measurement may reflect synovitis, cartilage, and bone damage and/or repair in arthritis.

3.1. Molecular Changes in Body Fluids Reflect Skeletal Change

Cartilage degradation can now be detected using antibodies to the collagenase-generated cleavage site in type II collagen (Fig. 4). This is increased in joint fluids of rabbits and dog following sectioning of the anterior cruciate ligament. Other assays to detect type II collagen-degradation products involving the carboxy telopeptide–crosslink complex are under development. Synthesis of type II procollagen can be detected by measurement of the c-propeptide of this molecule *(18)*. This is increased in OA synovial fluid and following traumatic injury that can lead to OA. However, serum c-propeptide content is decreased in idiopathic OA, suggesting systemic changes in cartilage matrix synthesis. In familial OA, serum c-propeptide content is clearly increased in most patients, reflecting the degeneration of the articular cartilage.

Proteoglycan aggrecan degradation products bearing an antigenic KS epitope may be increased or decreased in serum in OA patients *(3)*. An epitope (termed 846) present on some of the chondroitin sulfate chains of the proteoglycan aggrecan is released from cartilage and correlates with synthesis of aggrecan. This is markedly increased in content in OA synovial fluid *(3)*. Development or progression of OA from knee joint pain to joint-space narrowing is reflected by an increase in serum cartilage oligomeric protein *(3)*. Increased bone turnover in OA is reflected by increases in the bone-specific deoxypyridinoline crosslinks in urine *(3)*. Serum osteocalcin and bone sialoprotein may also be increased *(3)*.

These potential surrogate markers, which are summarized in Fig. 4, are proving useful in assessing disease progression and activity and responses to therapy designed to control inflammation, arrest cartilage degradation, and promote cartilage synthesis and repair. They are being introduced into clinical trials to both investigate chondroprotection and determine whether these markers may be prognostic of longer-term outcome of therapy.

4. The Management of OA: Key Therapeutic Targets and Strategies
4.1. Identification of the Problem

One of the most fundamental problems that is encountered in the management of this condition is the fact that joint degeneration ordinarily presents as joint pain and disability. By the time it has reached a level that proves difficult to manage by the patient, joint cartilage degeneration is often very advanced and it is almost too late to achieve effective arrest and reversal of the degenerative changes, even if effective treatment was available, which it is not. Thus, for future therapy to stand some chance of success, earlier detection and treatment of these degenerative changes is recommended.

At present, screening for early loss of joint space cannot usually be achieved radiographically. Yet, earlier changes, leading to loss of joint space, may be detectable by magnetic resonance (MRI) imaging and scintigraphy. However, more work needs to be done to improve access to imaging and to reduce the financial burden of MRI. Clearly, new technology needs to be developed and clinical trials need to incorporate and compare different imaging technologies so they can be more effectively assessed.

The identification and use of biological "surrogate" markers may offer us the opportunity to identify patients "at risk" for OA and to identify patient populations that can then be investigated by imaging. However, before this approach can be instigated, careful blinded assessments of these old and new technologies are required in aging populations and phase III clinical trials. Hopefully this will be forthcoming.

4.2. Therapeutic Targets

At the present time, MMPs present a prime target for intervention. Collagenase-3 in particular is upregulated in OA in articular cartilage and there is now evidence in support of its involvement in OA in the destruction of type II collagen in articular cartilages. MMPs such as "aggrecanases" are also prime targets. Whether inhibition of cleavage of both collagen and proteoglycans is required remains to be seen. An obvious approach would be to inhibit sets of cleavages. However, as in 'knockout' technology we may find that as one "key" proteinase is inhibited, others take over. However, from recent in vitro studies, this will probably prove less likely with careful target selection. At least the degenerative process should be slowed.

Clearly, there is good evidence for an attempt at increased matrix synthesis in OA cartilage. Whether this can be enhanced and maximized depends on how well we can protect newly synthesized molecules from degradation and promote synthesis even further over degradation. The formation of healthy new cartilage on osteophytes reveals that the potential is there!

The cytokines and growth factors produced as part of the changes that occur in OA cartilage can have profound effects on cartilage metabolism. The pro-degradative cytokines IL-1 and/or TNF-α are prime candidates for intervention. How important they are in cartilage pathology remains to be more clearly established in human studies, although a mouse "knockout" approach points to the importance of Il-1α, and IL-β in cartilage and bone damage.

Concluding Remarks

A much clearer understanding of the pathogenesis of OA has resulted from increased research in recent years. The application of very major advances in analytical techniques to study cells and tissues has provided important new insights into the pathophysiology of OA in a way which would not have been possible a few years ago. This has led to the identification of new therapeutic targets for intervention and regulation of this degenerative process.

Acknowledgments

The authors' work is funded by the Shriners Hospitals for Children, Medical Research Council of Canada, The Canadian Arthritis Network, The Riva Foundation, the National Institute of Aging, and the National Institutes of Health (USA).

References

1. Felson, D. T. (1997) Epidemiology of the rheumatic diseases, in Arthritis and Allied Conditions: A Textbook of Rheumatology, 13th ed. (Koopman, W. J., ed.), Williams & Wilkins, Baltimore.
2. Dequeker, J., Mokassa, L., Aerssens, J., and Boonen, S. (1997) Bone density and local growth factors in generalized osteoarthritis. *Microsc. Res. Tech.* **37,** 358–371.
3. Poole, A. R. (1997) Skeletal and inflammation markers in aging and osteoarthritis. Implications for "early" diagnosis and monitoring of the effects of therapy, in Osteoarthritis and the Ageing Population (Hamerman, D. ed.), Johns Hopkins University Press, Baltimore.
4. Mansell, J. P. and Bailey, A. J. (1998) Abnormal cancellous bone collagen metabolism in osteoarthritis. *J. Clin. Invest.* **101,** 1596–1603.
5. McCarthy, C., Cushnaghan, J., and Dieppe, P. (1994) The predictive role of scintigraphy in radiographic osteoarthritis of the hand. *Osteoarthritis Cart.* **2,** 25–28.
6. Dequeker, J. (1997) Inverse relationship of interface between osteoporosis and osteoarthritis. *J. Rheumatol.* **24,** 795–798.
7. Lohmander, L. S., Lark, M. W., Dahlberg, L., Walakovitz, L. A., and Roos, H. (1992) Cartilage matrix metabolism in osteoarthritis: markers in synovial fluid, serum and urine. *Clin. Biochem.* **25,** 167–174.
8. Hashimoto, S., Ochs, R. L., Komiya, S., and Lotz, M. (1998) Linkage of chondrocyte apoptosis and cartilage degradation in human osteoarthritis. *Arthritis Rheum.* **41,** 1632–1638.
9. Hollander, A. P., Heathfield, T. F., Webber, C., Iwata, Y., Bourne, R., Rorabeck, C., et al. (1994) Increased damage to type II collagen in osteoarthritic articular cartilage detected by a new immunoassay. *J. Clin. Invest.* **93,** 1722–1732.

10. Hollander, A. P., Pidoux, I., Reiner, A., Rorabeck, C., Bourne, R., and Poole, A. R. (1995) Damage to type II collagen in ageing and osteoarthritis starts at the articular surface, originates around chondrocytes and extends into the cartilage with progressive degeneration. *J. Clin. Invest.* **96**, 2859–2869.
11. Kempson, G. E., Muir, H., Pollard, C., and Tuke, M. (1973) The tensile properties of the cartilage of human femoral condyles related to the content of collagen and glycosaminoglycans. *Biochim. Biophys. Acta* **297**, 465–472.
12. Billinghurst, R. C., Dahlberg, L., Ionescu, M., Reiner, A., Bourne, R., Rorabeck, C., et al. (1997) Enhanced cleavage of type II collagen by collagenases in osteoarthritic articular cartilage. *J. Clin. Invest.* **99**, 1534–1545.
13. Lark, M. W., Bayner, E. K., Flanagan, J., Harper, C. F., Hoerrner, L. A., Hutchinson, N. I., et al. (1997) Aggrecan degradation in human cartilage: evidence for both matrix metalloproteinase and aggrecanase activity in normal, osteoarthritic, and rheumatoid joints. *J. Clin. Invest.* **100**, 93–106.
14. Poole, A. R., Rizkalla, G., Ionescu, M., Reiner, A., Brooke, E., Rorabeck, C., et al. (1993) Osteoarthritis in the human knee: dynamic process of cartilage matrix degradation, synthesis and reorganization, in *Joint Destruction in Arthritis and Osteoarthritis*, Birkhaeuser, Basel, pp. 3–13.
15. Poole, A. R., Alini, M., and Hollander, A. H. (1995) Cellular biology of cartilage degradation, in *Mechanisms and Models in Rheumatoid Arthritis* (Henderson, B., Edwards, J. C. W., and Pettipher, E. R., eds.), Academic, London.
16. Poole, A. R. (1997) Cartilage in health and disease, in *Arthritis and Allied Conditions. A Textbook of Rheumatology*, 13th ed. (Koopman, W. J., ed.), Williams & Wilkins, Baltimore.
17. Tortorella, M. D., Burn, T. C., Pratta, M. A., et al. (1999) Purification and cloning of aggrecanase-1. A member of the ADAMTS family of proteins. *Science* **284**, 1664–1666.
18. Nelson, F., Dahlberg, L., Reiner, A., Pidoux, I., Fraser, G., Brooks, E., et al. (1998) The synthesis of type II procollagen is markedly increased in osteoarthritic cartilage *in vivo*. *J. Clin. Invest.* **102**, 2115–2125.
19. von der Mark, K., Kirsch, T., Nerlich, A., Kuss, A., Weseloh, G., Glückert, K., et al. (1992) Type X collagen synthesis in human osteoarthritic cartilage. Indication of chondrocyte hypertrophy. *Arthritis Rheum.* **35**, 806–811.
20. Werb, Z., Tremble, P. M., Behrendtsen, O., Crowley, E., and Damsky, C. H. (1989) Signal transduction through the fibronectin receptor induces collagenase and stromelysin gene expression. *J. Cell. Biol.* **109**, 877–889.
21. Webb, G. R., Westacott, C. I., and Elson, C. (1997) Chondrocyte tumor necrosis factor receptors and focal loss of cartilage in osteoarthritis. *Osteoarthritis Cart.* **5**, 427–437.
22. Schneiderman, R., Rosenberg, N., Hiss, J., Lee, P., Liu, F., Hintz, R. L., et al. (1995) Concentration and size distribution of insulin-like growth factor-1 in human normal and osteoarthritic synovial fluid and cartilage. *Arch. Biochem. Biophys.* **324**, 173–188.

26
Osteoporosis

Stavros C. Manolagas

1. Introduction

Osteoporosis (thin bones) is a disease caused by loss of bone mass and microarchitectural deterioration of the skeleton, leading to enhanced bone fragility and increased risk for fractures with minimal or no trauma at all. Conventionally, the disease is diagnosed when the bone mineral density is 2.5 standard deviations below the young adult mean. A bone mineral density between 1 and 2.5 standard deviations below the young adult mean is termed "osteopenia." Osteoporosis is the most common disease of the musculoskeletal system. Fifty-four percent of postmenopausal women in the United States have osteopenia and another 30% have osteoporosis. Up to 20% of patients with osteoporosis die after hip fractures and 40% can no longer live independently. Although not a rheumatic disorder, osteoporosis is of major interest to rheumatologists, as the arthritic processes that affect the cartilage surfaces and the synovial lining may also involve the subchondral bone and the joint capsule. Moreover, rheumatic diseases such as osteoarthritis, rheumatoid arthritis, systemic lupus erythematosus, and the spondyloarthropathies may involve not only skeletal tissues at juxtaarticular and subchondral sites but also produce generalized effects on bone remodeling that affect the entire skeleton.

As discussed in Chapter 18, the normal adult skeleton undergoes continuous regeneration in the form of a periodic replacement of old bone with new at the same location. This so-called remodeling is carried out not by individual osteoclasts and osteoblasts, but rather by temporary anatomical structures (basic multicellular units [BMUs]), comprised of teams of osteoclasts in the front and osteoblasts in the rear. Both men and women start losing bone around the age of 50. However, women experience a rapid phase of loss during the first 5–10 yr after menopause, because of the precipitous loss of estrogen. In men, of course, this phase is obscure, as there is only a slow and progressive decline in sex steroid production; hence, the loss of bone in men is linear and slower. Besides losing bone faster at the early postmenopausal years, women also accumulate less skeletal mass than men during growth, particularly in puberty, resulting in smaller bones with thinner cortices and shorter diameter. Consequently, the incidence of bone fractures is twofold to threefold higher in women as compared to men.

In addition to sex steroid deficiency and the aging process itself, loss of bone mass is accentuated when several other conditions are present. The most prominent are chronic

Table 1
Histologic and Clinical Features of Different Types of Bone Loss

	Remodeling (turnover) rate	Histomorphometric characteristics	Fractures
Postmenopausal	High	Removal of trabeculae	Vertebral, coles
Senescence	Low (variable)	Thinning of cortices and residual trabeculae (in women)	Hip, vertebral
Glucocorticoid induced	Low	Thinning of trabeculae and aseptic necrosis	Vertebral, ribs, hips

glucocorticoid excess—the iatrogenic form of which is particularly relevant to those receiving steroid therapy for chronic arthritides, hyperthyroidism—often the result of inappropriately high thyroxin replacement, alcoholism, prolonged immobilization, gastrectomy and other gastrointestinal disorders, hypercalciuria, some types of malignancy, and cigaret smoking.

2. The Features of Bone Loss Are Different Depending on the Underlying Cause

Even though bone loss and eventually fractures are the end result of all the forms of osteoporosis, the clinical presentation and the pathogenetic mechanisms are quite distinct. Indeed, the two phases of bone loss associated with normal aging—the rapid one that affects women and is the result of menopause, and the slow one that affects both women and men after the age of 50—have distinct features (Table 1). In women, of course, these two phases eventually overlap, making it difficult to distinguish the effect of sex steroid deficiency from the effect of the aging process itself. The effect of the aging process itself is also frequently obscured because of overlapping secondary hyperparathyroidism—resulting from impaired calcium absorption from the intestine with advancing age (>75 yr old). The bone loss that is the result of glucocorticoid excess shares several features with the bone loss resulting from senescence, but it also has unique features of its own (Table 1). Nonetheless, as it is the case with the other types of bone loss, the heterogeneity of the underlying conditions—some of which (e.g., postmenopausal state, rheumatoid arthritis, etc.) independently contribute to skeletal deterioration—can distort the clinical and histologic picture.

Even though the specific features of bone loss are different depending on the underlying cause, the fundamental problem in all forms of osteoporosis seems to be aberrant bone cell number (1), which depends both on the birth rate reflecting the frequency of division of the appropriate precursors, and the life-span, reflecting the timing of death by apoptosis (Table 2). Appreciation of this general concept has greatly advanced our understanding of the pathogenesis of osteoporosis and is likely to lead in the near future to improved therapies for this condition.

3. The Pathogenesis of the Bone Loss Caused by Sex Steroid Deficiency

At menopause (or after castration in men), the rate of bone loss in the spine increases by as much as 10-fold. These clinical observations can be explained by evidence that sex steroids exert bone protective effects, at least in part, by regulating the develop-

Table 2
Cellular Changes and Their Culprits
in the Three Most Common Types of Osteoporosis

	Cellular changes	Probable culprits
Sex steroid deficiency	↑Osteoblastogenesis ↑Osteoclastogenesis[a] ↑Life-span of osteoclasts ↓Life-span of osteoblasts ↓Life-span of osteocytes	Increased IL-6, TNF, IL-1RI/IL-RII MCSF; decreased TGF-β; OPG Loss of proapoptotic and antiapoptotic effects of sex steroids, respectively
Senescence	↓Osteoblastogenesis[b] ↓Osteoclastogenesis ↑Adipogenesis ↓Life-span of osteocytes	Increased PPARγ2, pgJ2, noggin; decreased IL-11, IGFs
Glucocorticoid excess	↓Osteoblastogenesis ↑↓Osteoclastogenesis[c] ↑Adipogenesis ↓Life-span of osteoblasts ↓Life-span of osteocytes	Decreased Cbfa1 and TGF-β R1; and BMP-2 and IGF1 action Increased PPARγ2 Decreased Bcl-2/BAX ratio

[a]Oversupply of osteoclasts relative to the need for remodeling.
[b]Undersupply of osteoblasts relative to the needs for cavity repair.
[c]Osteoclastogenesis may increase transiently at the early stages of steroid therapy, but decreases subsequently.

ment of bone cells in the bone marrow, via their ability to alter the production of cytokines and the responsiveness of bone marrow cell progenitors to cytokines *(2)*, as well as by regulating the rate of death of mature cells (apoptosis) *(3)*.

The best documented paradigm of a cytokine playing a critical pathogenetic role in the osteoporosis caused by loss of sex steroids is interleukin-6 (IL-6). IL-6 exerts its effects on target cells via a bipartite cell surface receptor. Binding of the ligand to the α-subunit of the IL-6 receptor, a glycoprotein with molecular weight of 80 kDa (gp80), causes the homodimerization of the signal transducing β-subunit (gp130). The production of IL-6 by cells of the stromal/osteoblastic lineage is inhibited in vitro by estrogen and androgen as well as selective estrogen-receptor modulators (SERMs), such as raloxifene, through receptor-mediated actions on the transcriptional activity of the IL-6 gene promoter *(4)*. This effect does not require direct binding of the estrogen receptor to DNA *(5,6)*. Instead, it is the result of protein–protein interaction between the estrogen receptor and transcription factors such as nuclear factor-κb (NF-κb) and C/EBP. This mechanism provides a model that best fits current understanding of the molecular pharmacology of estrogen and SERMs.

Estrogen, as well as androgen, also suppress the expression of both gp80 and gp130 in cells of the bone marrow stromal/osteoblastic lineage *(7)*. Moreover, loss of sex steroids causes an increase in the expression of the IL-6 gene, as well as gp80 and gp130, in cells of the bone marrow, indicating that sex hormones not only regulate the production of IL-6 but also control the sensitivity of bone marrow cells to this cytokine. In agreement with this evidence, the levels of IL-6 in the bone marrow (and in the peripheral blood) are elevated in estrogen-deficient mice and rats as well as in humans, albeit not all studies have shown this. Nonetheless, in direct support of the contention that IL-6 is responsible for the increased bone resorption that ensues following loss of sex steroids, injections of an IL-6-neutralizing antibody to gonadectomized female or male mice prevented the increase in osteoclastogenesis in the bone marrow and the increase in the number of osteoclasts in sections of trabecular bone *(2)*. Furthermore, unlike wild-type controls, IL-6 knockout mice did not exhibit the expected cellular changes in the marrow and trabecular bone sections and were protected from the loss of bone following loss of sex steroids *(6,8)*.

In support of the evidence for a critical role of IL-6 in the bone loss caused by loss of gonadal function, IL-6 seems to play a similar role in several other conditions associated with increased bone resorption, as evidenced by increased local or systemic production of IL-6 and the IL-6 receptor in patients with multiple myeloma, Paget's disease, rheumatoid arthritis, Gorham–Stout or disappearing bone disease, hyperthyroidism, primary and secondary hyperparathyroidism, as well as McCune–Albright syndrome.

Besides upregulating osteoclastogenesis, loss of sex steroids increases the number of osteoblast progenitors in the murine bone marrow. This cellular change is temporally associated with increased bone formation, and parallels the increased osteoclastogenesis and bone resorption *(9)*. Overproduction of IL-6 and increased sensitivity to IL-6 and other members of this cytokine's family may explain also the increased osteoblast formation that follows the loss of gonadal function. Evidence that IL-6-type cytokines promote differentiation of osteoblastic progenitors and also stimulate osteoclastogenesis via their effects on the former cell type, taken together with the evidence that mesenchymal cell differentiation and osteoclastogenesis are tightly linked, raises the possibility that the stimulation of mesenchymal cell differentiation toward the osteoblastic lineage following estrogen loss may be the first event that ensues following the hormonal change, and that increased osteoclastogenesis and bone loss are downstream consequences *(10)*.

Interleukin-1 (IL-1) and tumor necrosis factor (TNF) are strong stimulators of osteoclast formation and bone resorption. Unlike IL-6 that is produced at high levels by stromal/osteoblastic cells, IL-1 and TNF are produced at very low levels, if at all, by these cells. Instead, the main cellular source of IL-1 and TNF in bone is probably bone marrow monocytes and macrophages. These two genes, as well as M-CSF, may be also regulated by estrogen *(11)*. Moreover, estrogen loss may increase the sensitivity of osteoclasts to IL-1 by increasing the ratio of the IL-1RI over the IL-1 receptor antagonist (IL-RII) *(12)*. In support of the contention that IL-1 and TNF play an important role in the bone loss caused by loss of estrogen, IL-1 and TNF stimulate the expression of M-CSF, a cytokine that it is essential for osteoclastogenesis, and administration of IL-1RA and/or TNF-BP ameliorates the bone loss caused by ovariectomy in both rats and mice. However, in contrast to IL-6, which stimulates osteoblast differentiation, IL-1 and TNF inhibit the expression of the osteoblast phenotype. In addition, IL-1 and TNF suppress the production of pro-osteoblastogenic cytokines such as IGF and platelet-derived growth factor (PDGF), and stimulate the expression IGFBP-4, which inhibits osteoblastogenesis. Therefore, these properties distinguish them from IL-6 and make them unlikely mediators of the increased osteoblastogenesis and thus the increased rate of bone remodeling that follows loss of sex steroids. Nonetheless, it is possible that IL-1 and TNF may arrest the differentiation of stromal/osteoblastic cells at a stage where

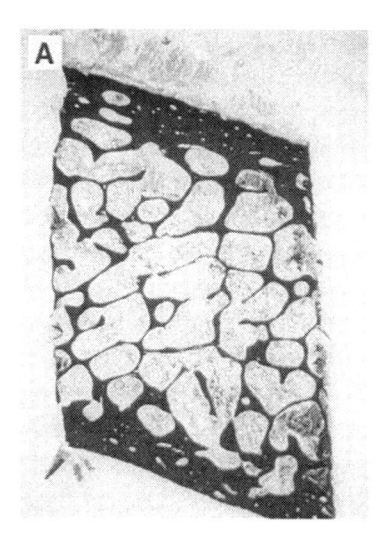

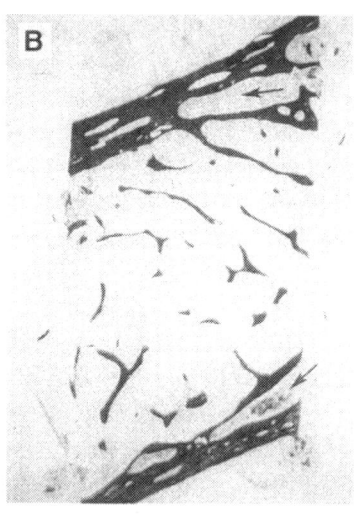

Fig. 1. Low-power panoramic views of transiliac bone biopsies taken from a 20-yr-old (**A**) and 70-yr-old (**B**) subject. The closely spaced and connected trabecular plates of the youth have been transformed to a disconnected, gossamer array typical of the elderly. Note the deep and coalescent endocortical erosions in the specimen obtained from the older subject (arrows). Modified Masson stain, original magnification ×10. (Courtesy of R. S. Weinstein.)

these cells can stimulate osteoclastogenesis, thereby accounting for the evidence that IL-1RA and TNF-BP prevent loss of bone in estrogen deficiency. Several earlier lines of evidence have implicated transforming growth factor-β (TGF-β) as another mediator of the effects of estrogen loss on bone; however, this contention remains tenuous.

In addition to increases in osteoclastogenesis and osteoblastogenesis, a qualitative abnormality also occurs following loss of sex steroids; osteoclasts erode deeper than normal cavities. Increased remodeling alone can cause a transient loss of bone mineral density because bone resorption is faster than bone formation and new BMUs are less dense than older ones. Additionally, if resorption penetrates through a trabecular structure, the substrate for the coupled bone formation is lost forever. In this manner, sex steroid deficiency leads to the removal of some cancellous elements entirely; the remainder are more widely separated and less well connected. An equivalent amount of cancellous bone distributed as widely separated, disconnected, thick trabeculae is biomechanically less competent than when arranged as more numerous, connected, thin trabeculae (Fig. 1). Concurrent loss of cortical bone occurs by enlargement and coalescence of subendocortical spaces, a process resulting from deeper penetration of endocortical osteoclasts.

This deeper erosion can be now explained by evidence that estrogen acts on mature osteoclasts to promote their apoptosis; consequently, loss of estrogen leads to prolongation of the life-span of osteoclasts *(3)*. Specifically, estrogen promote osteoclast apoptosis in vitro and in vivo by twofold to threefold—an effect seemingly mediated by TGF-β and IL-6. In direct contrast to their proapoptotic effects on osteoclasts, estrogen (as well as androgen) exert antiapoptotic effects on osteoblasts and osteocytes; consequently, loss of estrogen or androgen leads to the shorter life-span of osteoblasts and osteocytes *(13)*. Extension of the working life of the bone resorbing cells and simultaneous shortening of the working life of the bone forming cells, can explain the imbalance between bone resorption and formation that ensues following loss of sex steroids. Furthermore, the increase in osteocyte apoptosis could further weaken the skeleton by impairment of the osteocyte—canalicular mechanosensory network. The increase in bone remodeling that occurs with estrogen deficiency would partly replace some of the nonviable osteocytes in cancellous bone, but cortical apoptotic osteocytes might accumulate because of their anatomic isolation from scavenger cells and the need for extensive degradation to small molecules to dispose of the osteocytes through the narrow canaliculi. Hence, the accumulation of apoptotic osteocytes caused by loss of estrogen could increase bone fragility even before significant loss of bone mass, because of the impaired detection of microdamage and repair of substandard bone.

In conclusion, the increased rate of bone remodeling in estrogen deficiency is the result of increased production of both osteoclasts and osteoblasts, and the imbalance between bone resorption and formation is the result of an extension of the working life-span of the osteoclast and shortening of the working life-span of the osteoblast. Moreover, a delay of osteoclast apoptosis seem responsible for the deeper resorption cavities and thereby the trabecular perforation associated with estrogen deficiency.

Some observations have raised the possibility that estrogen derived by peripheral aromatization of androgens are critical for the maintenance of bone mass in men as well as in women. However, evidence that individuals that lack functional androgen receptors have decreased bone mass, in spite of elevated estrogen levels, and that androgen (including nonaromatizable ones) regulate the birth as well as the death of bone cells in vitro and in vivo make it unnecessary to invoke a unifying role of estrogen in male and female osteoporosis.

4. The Pathogenesis of Bone Loss Resulting from Senescence

The bone loss that follows the acute loss of estrogen is followed by a slower rate of bone loss, similar to that seen just before menopause in women or in elderly eugonadal men. The amount of bone formed during each remodeling cycle decreases with age in both sexes. This is indicated by a consistent histologic feature of the osteopenia that occurs during aging, namely a decrease in wall thickness, especially in trabecular bone. Wall thickness is a measure of the amount of bone formed in a remodeling packet of cells and is determined by the number and activity of osteoblasts at the remodeling site.

Changes in the differentiation of bone cell progenitors of the bone marrow provides a potential mechanism for the development of senile osteoporosis as well. Indeed, studies with animal models of early senescence or plain old age have elucidated decreased osteoblastogenesis in the bone marrow. This change is temporally linked with a low rate of bone formation and decreased bone mineral density *(14)*. The decreased osteoblastogenesis in these models is associated with increased adipogenesis in the bone marrow, suggesting that in aging there must be changes in the expression of genes that favor the differentiation of multipotent mesenchymal stem cells toward adipocytes at the expense of osteoblasts *(15)*. The factors responsible for the reciprocal changes in osteoblastogenesis and adipogenesis in the aging bone marrow remain unknown. However, IL-11, the transcription factor PPARγ2 and its ligand (the prostaglandin J2), and growth factors such as IGFs are potential culprits *(16)*. Irrespective of the identity of the precise mediator, the reciprocal change between adipogenesis and osteoblastogenesis can explain the association of decreased bone formation and the resulting osteopenia with the increased adiposity of the marrow seen with advancing age in animals and humans.

In addition to defective osteoblastogenesis and estrogen deficiency, many other factors have been implicated in the bone loss associated with aging, including secondary hyperparathyroidism caused by vitamin D deficiency or decrements in creatinine clearance, decreases in gastrointestinal calcium absorption and renal calcium conservation, a sedentary lifestyle, genetic and racial factors, peak adult bone mass, concurrent diseases and treatment with glucocorticoids, anticonvulsant drugs, and immunosuppressive agents. Because of these factors, bone turnover in involutional osteoporosis is highly variable and the frequency of activation may be diminished, normal, or accelerated, although bone formation always remains less than adequate to counterbalance bone resorption.

Today, little is known about the effects of aging on apoptosis of osteoblasts and osteoclasts, but a loss of viable osteocytes with increasing age was recognized 40 yr ago (17). Osteocyte death in cancellous bone, indicated by absence of lactic dehydrogenase activity, increases in prevalence with age in the femur but not in lumbar vertebrae, probably because of the higher rate of bone remodeling in the spine. Empty lacunae and enzyme absence can reveal the fact but not the mode of osteocyte death; however, osteocyte apoptosis was identified in osteophytes obtained from patients with osteoarthritis. Moreover, in patients with hip fractures, osteocyte viability was occasionally less than 25% and little or no fracture callus was observed if osteocyte viability was low, suggesting that dead osteocytes compromise repair of fatigue damage and bone strength.

5. The Pathogenesis of Bone Loss Caused by Glucocorticoid Excess

The cardinal histologic features of glucocorticoid-induced osteoporosis are decreased bone formation rate, decreased wall thickness of trabeculae (a strong indication of decreased work output by osteoblasts), and *in situ* death of portions of bone. The decreased bone formation and osteonecrosis can now be explained by evidence that glucocorticoid excess has a suppressive effect on osteoblastogenesis in the bone marrow and also promotes the apoptosis of osteoblasts and osteocytes (18). Indeed, mice receiving glucocorticoids for 4 wk (a period equivalent to approx 3–4 yr in humans) exhibit decreased bone mineral density associated with a decrease in the number of osteoblast (as well as osteoclast) progenitors in the bone marrow and a dramatic reduction in cancellous bone area and in trabecular width compared to placebo controls. These changes are associated with a significant reduction in osteoid area and a decrease in the rates of mineral apposition and bone formation. More strikingly, glucocorticoid administration to mice causes a threefold increase in the prevalence osteoblast apoptosis in vertebrae and induced apoptosis in 28% of the osteocytes in metaphyseal cortical bone. Albeit, even though there is a significant correlation between the severity of the bone loss and the extent of reduction in bone formation, some of the bone loss may be the result of an early increase in bone resorption, as evidenced by an early increase in osteoclast perimeter of vertebral cancellous bone after 7 d of steroid treatment.

The same histomorphometric changes have been confirmed in biopsies from patients receiving long-term glucocorticoid therapy. Moreover, as in mice, an increase in osteoblast and osteocyte apoptosis was found in human biopsies. Compared to osteoblast apoptosis, osteocyte apoptosis was far more prevalent, probably because of the anatomical isolation of osteocytes from scavenger cells. Consistent with these findings, glucocorticoids promote osteoblast and osteocyte apoptosis in vitro. Decreased production of osteoclasts can explain the reduction in bone turnover with chronic glucocorticoid excess, whereas decreased production and apoptosis of osteoblasts can explain the decline in bone formation and trabecular width.

Accumulation of apoptotic osteocytes may also explain osteonecrosis. This contention is supported by evidence that whole femoral heads obtained from patients with glucocorticoid-induced osteoporosis exhibit abundant apoptotic osteocytes adjacent to the subchondral fracture crescent. Glucocorticoid-induced osteocyte apoptosis, a cumulative and unrepairable defect, could uniquely disrupt the proposed mechanosensory role of the osteocyte network and thus promote collapse of the femoral head. It is possible that changes in the regulation of osteocyte programmed cell death contribute to the bone loss associated with other forms of osteoporosis. Indeed, as it was mentioned earlier, osteocyte apoptosis is increased in estrogen-deficient women; furthermore, a significant proportion of osteocytes gradually die with age.

The mediators of the cellular changes caused by glucocorticoid excess are a matter of conjecture. Nonetheless, there is evidence that glucocorticoids directly suppress BMP-2 and OSF-2 (two critical factors for osteoblastogenesis) and that may also decrease the production of IGFs. In addition, glucocorticoids increase the production of PPARγ2, favoring adipogenesis in the bone marrow. The proapoptotic effect of glucocorticoids on osteoblasts can be prevented by overexpression of the Bcl-2 gene, suggesting that suppression of Bcl-2 is a key mechanism.

6. Current Concepts of Osteoporosis Treatment

Estrogen replacement therapy, SERMs (raloxifene), bisphosphonates (fosomax), calcitonin, sodium fluoride, as well as calcium and vitamin D have been used to prevent and treat bone loss, irrespective of its cause, with different measures of success. Recent in vitro studies raise the possibility that the antiresorptive agents among them may exert part of their antifracture efficacy and may prevent osteocyte apoptosis. Be that as it may, our understanding of the pathogenesis of the various forms of osteoporosis clearly points out that the ideal therapy for patients who already have advanced bone loss should be an anabolic agent that will increase bone mass by rebuilding bone.

Sodium fluoride does have anabolic properties, but the therapeutic range is very narrow. Intermittent parathyroid hormone (PTH) administration increases bone mass in animals and humans. Recent studies show that prevention of osteoblast apoptosis is the principal mechanism for the anabolic effect of PTH on bone. Thus, in mice, PTH increased the life-span of mature osteoblasts by preventing apoptosis—an effect readily reproduced in vitro—rather than by changing the rate of generation of new osteoblasts. Moreover, PTH prevents glucocorticoid-induced osteoblast and osteocyte apoptosis in vitro *(19)*. Consistent with this evidence, in a recent clinical trial, daily subcutaneous injections of PTH were shown to be a safe and effective treatment for corticosteroid-induced osteoporosis (20).

The elucidation of the importance of osteoblast and osteocyte apoptosis in the mechanism of glucocorticoid-induced osteoporosis and the elucidation of the mechanism of the anabolic effects of PTH on bone readily explain how PTH can be such an effective therapy in this condition. Hence, PTH and perhaps future PTH mimetics and nonpeptide inhibitors of apoptosis pathways in osteoblasts represent, for the first time, pathophysiology-based (i.e., rational as opposed to empirical) pharmacotherapies for osteopenias; in particular, those in which osteoblast progenitor formation is suppressed, like the osteoporoses associated with old age and glucocorticoid excess.

References

1. Manolagas, S. C. and Jilka, R. L. (1995) Bone marrow, cytokines, and bone remodeling: emerging insights into the pathophysiology of osteoporosis. *N. Engl. J. Med.* **332**, 305–311.
2. Jilka, R. L., Hangoc, G., Girasole, G., Passeri, G., Williams, D., Abrams, J., et al. (1992) Increased osteoclast development after estrogen loss: mediation by interleukin-6. *Science* **257**, 88–91.
3. Hughes, D. E., Dai, A., Tiffee, J. C., Li, H. H., Mundy, G. R., and Boyce, B. F. (1996) Estrogen promotes apoptosis of murine osteoclasts mediated by TGF-β. *Nature Med.* **2**, 1132–1136.
4. Girasole, G., Jilka, R. L., Passeri, G., Boswell, H. S., Boder, G., Williams, D. C., et al. (1992) 17β-Estradiol inhibits Interleukin-6 production by murine bone marrow stromal cells and human osteoblasts in-vitro: a potential mechanism for the antiosteoporotic effects of estrogens. *J. Clin. Invest.* **89**, 883–891.
5. Pottratz, S., Bellido, T., Mocharla, H., Crabb, D., and Manolagas, S. C. (1994) 17β-Estradiol inhibits transcription from the human interleukin-6 promoter. *J. Clin. Invest.* **93**, 944–950.
6. Bellido, T., Jilka, R. L., Boyce, B., Girasole, G., Broxmeyer, H., Dalrymple, S. A., et al. (1995) Regulation of interleukin-6, osteoclastogenesis and bone mass by androgens: the role of the androgen receptor. *J. Clin. Invest.* **95**, 2886–2895.
7. Lin, S.-C., Yamate, T., Taguchi, Y., Borba, V. Z. C., Girasole, G., O'Brien, C. A., et al. (1997) Regulation of the gp80 and gp130 subunits of the IL-6 receptor by sex steroids in the murine bone marrow. *J. Clin. Invest.* **100**, 1980–1990.
8. Poli, V., Balena, R., Fattori, E., Markatos, A., Yamamoto, A., Tanaka, H., et al. (1994) Interleukin-6 deficient mice are protected from bone loss caused by estrogen depletion. *EMBO J.* **13**, 1189-1196.
9. Jilka, R. L., Takahashi, K., Munshi, M., Williams, D. C., Roberson, P. K., Parfitt, A. M., et al. (1998) Loss of estrogen upregulates osteoblastogenesis in the murine bone marrow: evidence for autonomy from factors released during bone resorption. *J. Clin. Invest.* **101**, 1942–1950.
10. Weinstein, R. S., Jilka, R. L., Parfitt, A. M., and Manolagas, S. C. (1997) The effects of androgen deficiency on murine bone remodeling and bone mineral density are mediated via cells of the osteoblastic lineage. *Endocrinology* **138**, 4013–4021.
11. Pacifici, R. (1998) Cytokines, estrogen, and postmenopausal osteoporosis: the second decade. *Endocrinology* **139**, 2659–2661.
12. Sunyer, T., Lewis, J., Collin-Osdoby, P., and Osdoby, P. (1999) Estrogen's bone-protective effects may involve differential IL-1 receptor regulation in human osteoclast-like cells. *J. Clin. Invest.* **103**, 1409–1418.
13. Manolagas, S. C., Weinstein, R. S., Bellido, T., and Bodenner, D. L. Opposite effects of estrogen on the life span of osteoblasts/osteocytes versus osteoclasts in vivo and in vitro: an expla-

nation of the imbalance between formation and resorption in estrogen deficiency. *J. Bone Miner. Res.* (abstract), in press.
14. Jilka, R. L., Weinstein, R. S., Takahashi, K., Parfitt, A. M., and Manolagas, S. C. (1996) Linkage of decreased bone mass with impaired osteoblastogenesis in a murine model of accelerated senescence. *J. Clin. Invest.* **97,** 1732–1740.
15. Kajkenova, O., Lecka-Czernik, B., Gubrij, I., Hauser, S. P., Takahashi, K., Parfitt, A. M., et al. (1997) Increase adipogenesis and myelopoiesis in the bone marrow of SAMP6, a murine model of defective osteoblastogenesis and low turnover osteopenia. *J. Bone Miner. Res.* **12,** 1772–1779.
16. Lecka-Cznernik, B., Gubrij, I., Moerman, E. A., Kajkenova, O., Lipschitz, D. A., Manolagas, S. C., et al. (1999) Inhibition of Osf2/Cbfa1 expression and terminal osteoblast differentiation by PPAR-gamma 2. *J. Cell. Biochem.* **74,** 357–371.
17. Frost, H. M. (1960) In vivo osteocyte death. *J. Bone Joint Surg. [Am.]* **42,** 138–143.
18. Weinstein, R. S., Jilka, R. L., Parfitt, A. M., and Manolagas, S. C. (1998) Inhibition of osteoblastogenesis and promotion of apoptosis of osteoblasts and osteocytes by glucocorticoids: potential mechanisms of their deleterious effects on bone. *J. Clin. Invest.* **102,** 274–282.
19. Jilka, R. L., Weinstein, R. S., Bellido, T., Roberson, P., Parfitt, A. M., and Manolagas, S. C. (1999) Increased bone formation by prevention of osteoblast apoptosis with parathyroid hormone. *J. Clin. Invest.,* **104,** 439–446.
20. Lane, N. E., Sanchez, S., Modin, G. W., Genant, H. K., Pierini, E., and Arnaud, C. D. (1998) Parathyroid hormone treatment can reverse corticosteroid-induced osteoporosis. *J. Clin. Invest.* **102,** 1627–1633.

27
Heritable Disorders of Connective Tissue

Petros Tsipouras

1. Introduction

The Marfan syndrome, Ehlers–Danlos syndrome, and osteogenesis imperfecta are systemic genetic disorders of connective tissue. The wide variability of expression has led to the delineation of distinct phenotypic types within each of the three disorders. The Mendelian nature of all three disorders was established earlier this century, and their molecular basis and pathogenesis have been studied extensively during the past 20 yr. Mutations in genes encoding structural molecules present in the extracellular matrix of the connective tissue and their modifying enzymes have been identified. In the Marfan syndrome, mutations have been found in the FBN1 gene encoding a large glycoprotein, fibrillin-1. In osteogenesis imperfecta, mutations have been found in the COL1A1 and COL1A2 genes encoding the two constituent protein chains of collagen type I. A variety of mutations in the genes encoding collagen type I, collagen type III, collagen type V, and certain collagen-modifying enzymes have been causally linked to the different types of the Ehlers–Danlos syndrome. Despite the dizzying variety of genes and mutations described, at least one common mechanism underlies the pathogenesis of each disorder. The abnormal protein chain appears to exert a dominant negative effect that impairs the structure and function of the collagen fibers or the elastin-associated microfibrils.

2. Marfan Syndrome
2.1. Clinical Manifestations

Marfan syndrome is an autosomal dominant systemic disorder of connective tissue whose diagnosis is based on defined diagnostic criteria. The distribution of the Marfan syndrome is panethnic and its prevalence has been estimated to be 4–6 per 100,000 population. The Marfan syndrome is associated with a high new mutation rate, as positive family history can be found in approximately 70% of affected individuals. The Marfan syndrome presents with manifestations from the musculoskeletal, cardiovascular, ocular, pulmonary, skin, and central nervous system. Clinical variability between affected relatives is one of the hallmarks of this disorder *(1)*. The presence of major and minor diagnostic criteria correlated with family history and genotypic information are required for the diagnosis of the Marfan syndrome *(2)*.

From: *Current Molecular Medicine: Principles of Molecular Rheumatology*
Edited by: G. C. Tsokos © Humana Press Inc., Totowa, NJ

A characteristic body habitus, described as dolichostenomelia, decreased upper to lower segment ratio, highly arched palate, pectus deformities, kyphoscoliosis, limitation of extension of the elbows, pes planus, decreased muscle mass, aortic root dilatation, aortic regurgitation, aortic dissection, ectopia lentis, pneumothorax, striae distensae, and dural ectasia are the clinical manifestations typically associated with the Marfan syndrome *(2)*. Several other distinct nosological entities present with manifestations overlapping to those observed in the Marfan syndrome and must be considered in the differential diagnosis. Among those are homocystinuria, the MASS phenotype, congenital contractural arachnodactyly, familial thoracic aortic aneurysm, and the mitral valve prolapse syndrome *(2)*. These conditions form a phenotypic continuum with the Marfan syndrome and might share similar pathogenesis. The term *fibrillinopathies* has been coined to describe the nosologic group of Marfan syndrome and related disorders. The molecular basis of the Marfan syndrome has been defined *(3)*. Mutations in the FBN1 gene, encoding fibrillin-1, have been described in many individuals affected with the Marfan syndrome *(4)*.

2.2 Elastin-Associated Microfibrils

The term "microfibrils" was originally used to identify morphologically similar matrix structures displaying a diameter of less than 20 nm and lacking the characteristic 67-nm banding periodicity of interstitial collagen fibers. Currently, microfibrils are divided into two classes according to their average diameter. The larger of the two classes has an average diameter of 10 nm and is commonly referred to as the elastin-associated microfibril. Microfibrils, either associated with or devoid of elastin, give rise to a variety of extracellular networks in elastic and nonelastic tissues. Immunohistochemical studies have identified microfibrils in the suspensory ligament of the lens, pleura, perichondrium, periosteum, meninges, aorta, cartilage, tendon, muscle, and many other tissues. It is thought that microfibrils regulate elastic fiber formation by guiding tropo-elastin deposition during embryogenesis and early postnatal life. The complete macromolecular composition of the microfibril is as yet unclear, because its elucidation is made difficult by the highly insoluble nature of the matrix aggregate. The major protein component of the microfibril, however, appears to be fibrillin-1 *(5)*.

2.3. Fibrillin and the FBN1 Gene

Fibrillin-1 is an acidic glycoprotein with an estimated molecular mass of 350 kDa. A closely related protein, fibrillin-2, has also been identified and characterized. Fibrillin-1 has an unusually high cysteine content (14%). One-third of the cysteine residues has the potential to form disulfide bonding. In vitro studies suggest that fibrillin-1 is synthesized as the precursor profibrillin and is converted to the mature form following secretion into the extracellular matrix. Study of the biosynthesis of fibrillin has shown that molecules are rapidly incorporated into a high-molecular-weight aggregate, supporting the notion that fibrillin-1 does not exist as an extracellular monomer. The structure of fibrillin-1 is complex and redundant. Much of the molecule is comprised of a series of epidermal growth factor (EGF)-like sequences, 46 of which are tandemly repeated and irregularly interspersed among eight cysteine transforming growth factor-β (TGF-β)-binding proteinlike domains *(6)*. The size of the FBN1 gene is approxi-

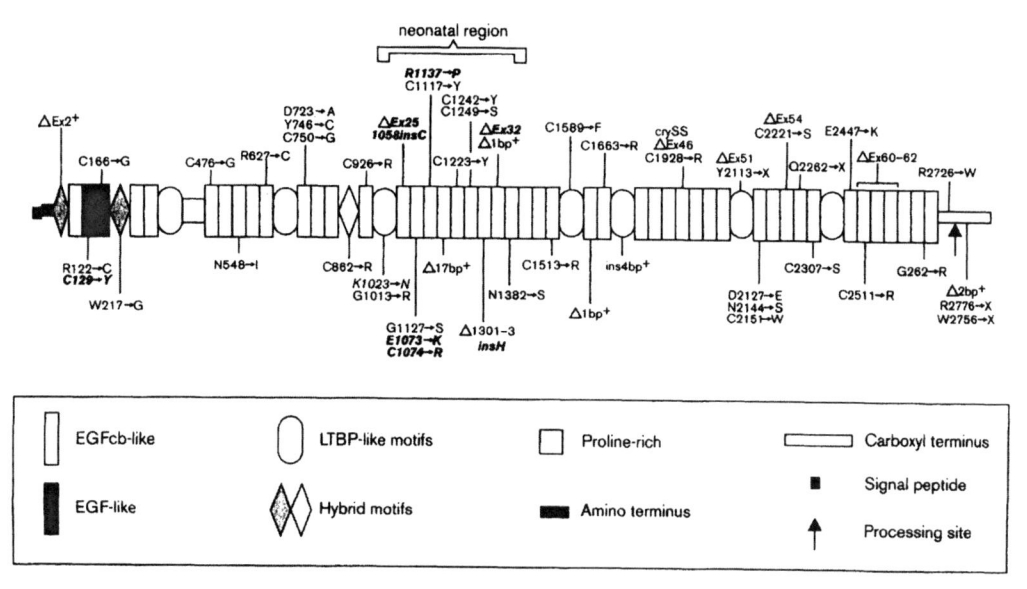

Fig. 1. Schematic representation of fibrillin-1 structure with the location and nature of mutations causing Marfan syndrome and related phenotypes superimposed. Mutations associated with severe presentation of the disorder are in bold and are italicized, whereas those creating premature stop codons are denoted by +. Deletions of exons (ex) or of specific base pairs (bp) are denoted by open triangles (e.g., Ex); aminoacids are listed using single-letter abbreviations. (The cluster of mutations in the center of the molecule leading to a severe neonatal Marfan syndrome is also marked.) [Reprinted with permission from Ramirez, F. (1996) Fibrillin mutations in Marfan syndrome and related phenotypes. *Curr. Opin. Genet. Dev.* **6**, 309–315.

mately 110 kb in length and the coding information is distributed in 65 exons. The FBN1 gene has been localized on chromosome 15 (15q21).

2.4. Etiology and Pathogenesis

More than 100 different FBN1 gene mutations have been identified in individuals affected with the Marfan syndrome, the MASS phenotype, and ectopia lentis *(4)* (Fig. 1). Almost all of the mutations are specific to a particular individual or family and they are distributed throughout the gene with no obvious correlation between location and phenotypic severity, apart from an apparent clustering of mutations causing neonatal Marfan syndrome in the middle of the molecule. The majority of mutations are missense point mutations, but small, in-frame deletions or insertions, premature termination codons, and larger deletions have also been detected. Protein studies using cultured skin fibroblasts have shown that the FBN1 gene mutations cause abnormalities in the synthesis and extracellular matrix deposition of fibrillin; however, the results of these studies are not sufficient to fully explain the pathogenesis of the Marfan syndrome.

Recently, two transgenic mouse models have been generated *(7,8)*. In the first, the mouse was homozygous for a 6-kb interstitial in-frame deletion (mgΔ, encompassing exons 19–24 of the Fbn1 gene). In the second (mgR/mgR), the synthesis of fibrillin-1 is greatly reduced and homozygosity for the mutation leads to early death. Homozygous (mgΔ/mgΔ) mice synthesized reduced steady-state levels of the mutant truncated fibrillin-1 mRNA and protein. Immunohistochemical analysis of (mgΔ/mgΔ) tissues documented a substantial reduction of extracellular fibrillin-1 but normal elastin staining. Immunohistochemical comparison of extracellular fibrillin-1 deposition by cultured dermal fibroblasts from homozygous mice and control littermates showed only scant amounts of immunoreactive material 72 h after plating. Mutant cells had the ability to accumulate extracellular fibrillin over time; however, the architecture of immunoreactive material remained primitive when compared to the multilayered meshwork of wild-type cultures. These results are remarkably similar to those observed in tissues from individuals affected with Marfan syndrome, in which seemingly normal microfibrils are shown by electron microscopy despite severely reduced microfibrillar immunostaining. Taken together, the data suggest that mutant fibrillin-1 monomers can polymerize and that elastic fibers can assemble in the absence of normal fibrillin-1 macroaggregates.

The homozygous (mgΔ/mgΔ) mice appear to be normal at birth. However, they all die suddenly of cardiovascular complications at approximately 3 wk after birth. Necropsy findings included hemothorax, hemopericardium, and significant thinning of the wall of the ascending aorta, suggesting aneurysmal dilatation; however, skeletal manifestations were absent. Histopathological findings included focal fragmentation of elastic fibers, accumulation of amorphous matrix, and dissection of blood into the aortic media (7). The abundance and architecture of the elastic fibers appeared preserved between focal lesions and in unaffected tissues. Heterozygous (mgΔ/+) mice are morphologically and histologically indistinguishable from wild-type littermates and have a normal life-span.

Under the current model of pathogenesis, high levels of abnormal fibrillin-1 exert dominant negative activity. In that respect, the biochemical and immunohistochemical findings from the mgΔ/mgΔ transgenic mouse are compatible with the observation that patients expressing high levels of mutant protein fail to efficiently utilize wild-type protein, resulting in a sparse and disorganized network of microfibrils (9). This group of patients, overall, presents with more severe cardiac complications and requires aortic surgery at an earlier age. In contrast, patients heterozygous for nonsense FBN1 alleles that are associated with low levels of mutant transcripts exhibit, overall, a mild phenotype and show preserved matrix deposition of proteins derived from the normal allele.

The study of the homozygous mgΔ/mgΔ mouse suggests the following model explaining the genesis and progressive failure of the ascending aorta to fulfill its fundamental mechanical function as an auxiliary pump. Because the adventitial layer is thought to sustain the bulk of hemodynamic stress, aortic dilatation in Marfan syndrome results primarily from loss of tensile strength by the adventitia, in which fibrillin-1 microfibrils are required to properly organize the primarily collagenous connective tissue (7). This mechanical collapse, in turn, leads to overstretching and fracturing of the elastic laminae of the media, a process that is facilitated by the failure of fibrillin-1 microfibrils to weave the elastic lamellae in the media and to anchor the endothelial layer of the intima. Furthermore, these studies suggest that the functional role of fibrillin-1 is tissue homeostasis and not microfibril formation.

2.5 Therapy

A direct relationship has been observed between aortic root dimension and life-threatening complications of the Marfan syndrome. In light of the findings from the

Table 1
Classification of Ehlers–Danlos Syndromes

New	Former	OMIM	Inheritance
Classical type	Gravis (EDS type I)	130000	AD
	Mitis (EDS type II)	130010	AD
Hypermobility type	Hypermobile (EDS type III)	130020	AD
Vascular type	Arterial-ecchymotic (EDS type IV)	130050 (225350) 225360	AD
Kyphoscoliosis type	Ocular-scoliotic (EDS type VI)	225400 (229200)	AR
Arthrochalasia type	Arthrochalasis multiplex congenita (EDS types VIIA and VIIB)	130060	AD
Dermatosparaxis type	Human dermatosparaxis (EDS type VIIC)	225410	AR
Other forms	X-Linked EDS (EDS type V)	305200	XL
	Periodontitis type (EDS type VIII)	130080	AD
	Fibronectin-deficient EDS (EDS type X)	225310	?
	Familial hypermobility syndrome (EDS type XI)	147900	AD
	Progeroid EDS	130070	?
	Unspecified forms	—	—

Source: From ref. *12*.

homozygous mgΔ/mgΔ mouse, therapeutic interventions directed to the aorta should aim either at reducing the hemodynamic stress or correcting the fundamental genetic defect, thus rescuing the aortic wall with relatively preserved structure and function. Reduction of hemodynamic stress is achieved by the use of β-adrenergic receptor antagonists. These therapeutic agents have been shown to reduce the rate of aortic dilatation and improve aortic compliance in individuals affected with the Marfan syndrome *(10)*. Defined most simply as the rate of change in aortic dimension with increasing aortic pressure, aortic compliance can be measured noninvasively by both echocardiography and magnetic resonance imaging. Aortic wall stiffness, pulse-wave velocity, and aortic distensibility, all of which reflect compliance, are increased in patients with the Marfan syndrome compared to controls. Although the treatment with β-adrenergic receptor antagonists reduces the rate of aortic dilatation, it does not eliminate the prospect of aortic surgery. Strategies directed to strengthening the mechanical properties of the ascending aorta might be successful in providing normal structure and function. One such strategy could involve selective targeting and cleavage of mutant FBN1 mRNA species by hammerhead ribozymes *(11)*. This approach could succeed in eliminating the synthesis of mutant fibrillin-1 protein and, potentially, the dominant negative effects exerted on fibrillin macroaggregates.

3. Ehlers–Danlos Syndrome

This eponym describes a group of Mendelian disorders whose protean manifestations include joint laxity, skin abnormalities, and tissue fragility. Six different types have been delineated on the basis of clinical manifestations, mode of inheritance, and laboratory findings (Table 1). A list of diagnostic criteria, classified as major and minor, provides the basis for distinguishing between the different types and differentiating the Ehlers–Danlos syndrome from phenotypically similar conditions *(12)*. Analogous phenotypes have been identified in several domesticated and wild animal species, one of them being dermatosparaxis in cattle and sheep.

3.1. Clinical Manifestations

Joint hypermobility is the most specific manifestation observed in the Ehlers–Danlos syndrome. Evaluation of joint hypermobility should follow a consistent and rigorous pattern. Age-related changes in joint hypermobility are common. The degree of hypermobility does not correlate with the frequency of joint dislocations. Congenital dislocations and hip dysplasia are the hallmark of the arthrochalasia type. Chronic musculoskeletal pain is one of the most common complaints. Joint instability is frequently observed in the hypermobility type and its most common side effect is loss of ambulation *(13)*.

The skin manifestations are the most readily recognized signs of the Ehlers–Danlos syndrome. Abnormalities of the skin texture (described as soft and doughy) and elasticity (increased), redundant skinfolds in the extensor areas of the knee and elbow joints, and wide atrophic scars are clinical manifestations present in most types of the Ehlers–Danlos syndrome. In the dermatosparaxis type, the skin is particularly fragile and it forms excessive skinfolds. The propensity to develop deep skin wounds even after minimal injury is characteristic. One of the earliest clinical observations in Ehlers–Danlos syndrome was the delay in wound healing involving the skin and internal organs. Wound dehiscence following abdominal surgery frequently poses a serious therapeutic challenge in individuals affected with the vascular type *(13)*.

Tissue fragility is extreme in the vascular type. Arterial, intestinal, or uterine ruptures are potentially fatal complications. Although rupture of the thoracic and abdominal aorta occurs in approximately 10% of all arterial episodes, it is primarily the medium size arteries that are particularly susceptible. The sigmoid is the segment of the gastrointestinal tract that most frequently perforates. Rupture of the gravid uterus is a life-threatening situation for both the mother and the unborn fetus *(13)*.

Easy bruising, another manifestation of tissue fragility is observed in all types of the Ehlers–Danlos syndrome. The bruising is particularly severe in the vascular type. A characteristic facies and acrogeria are frequently observed in the vascular type. Severe hypotonia, kyphoscoliosis, joint hypermobility, and ocular abnormalities are observed in the kyphoscoliosis type. Congenital joint dislocations and hip dysplasia are pathognomonic manifestations of the athrochalasia type *(13)*.

3.2. Etiology and Pathogenesis

The molecular delineation of the Ehlers–Danlos syndrome is evolving. Heterozygous mutations in several collagen genes have been identified in most of the dominantly inherited types of the condition. Homozygosity or compound heterozygosity for mutations in the genes encoding lysyl hydroxylase-1 and procollagen I *N*-proteinase has been found in individuals affected with the kyphoscoliosis and dermatosparaxis types, respectively.

Historically, collagen type III, a homotrimer, was the first molecule associated with the Ehlers–Danlos syndrome. To date, well over 100 different COL3A1 gene mutations have been identified *(13)*. These are primarily missense or splice junction mutations. The latter cause missplicing involving either a single or multiple exons. Overall, very few COL3A1 null mutations have been identified and all are associated with a severe phenotype. No biochemical defects have been identified, to date, in the carboxy-propeptide segment of collagen type III. The effects of the COL3A1 gene mutations on the protein synthesized by cultured skin fibroblasts could be categorized as follows: (1) decreased secretion associated with increased collagen chain glycosylation and intracellular retention; (2) interference with triple helix nucleation; and (3) premature termination codons leading to the synthesis of unstable transcripts and resulting in functional haplo-insufficiency. Despite the wide topological distribution of defects across the collagen type III molecule, there are no discernible phenotypic differences indicative of a clinical–molecular correlation.

Collagen type V is also a triple helical type of collagen with a tissue distribution similar to that of collagen type I. Collagen type V is composed of three different chains and its stoichiometry varies in different tissues. Several missense and exon-splicing mutations have been identified in the COL5A1 and COL5A2 genes in the classical type of the Ehlers–Danlos syndrome *(14)*. A substantial fraction (approximately 25%) of affected individuals have been found to carry a COL5A1 null mutation, which leads to functional haplo-insufficiency and an $\alpha 1(V)/\alpha 2(V)$ chain ratio of <0.6. The presence of haplo-insufficiency was demonstrated by single nucleatide polymorphisms (SNPs) at the 3' end of the COL5A1 gene.

The arthrochalasia type of the Ehlers–Danlos syndrome is associated with a specific biochemical defect consisting of the retention of either the pNα1(I)- or pNα2(I)-propeptide *(13)*. In contrast, mutations in the gene encoding the enzyme catalyzing the conversion of pN-collagen to triple helical collagen have been identified in the dermatosparaxis type. The retention of the pN-propeptide is the result of the elimination of the procollagen I *N*-proteinase recognition site contained within the sequence encoded by exon 6 of the COL1A1 and/or the COL1A2 gene. Point mutations in either the donor or acceptor site of exon 6 cause aberrant splicing. Of the 20 arthrochalasia mutations studied to date, 17 involve the COL1A1 gene and the remaining 3 involve the COL1A2 gene. There are no phenotypic differences between individuals carrying either the COL1A1 or the COL1A2 mutations.

Procollagen I *N*-proteinase, a collagen-modifying enzyme, contains a Zn^{2+}-binding site, a Met turn, and four properdin-like repeats *(15)*. It is still unknown whether the enzyme is active in a monomeric or polymeric form. Two different point mutations have been identified and both result in stop codons. The first predicts the synthesis of a polypeptide lacking the Zn^{2+}-binding domain and all four properdin-like repeat domains, whereas the second predicts the synthesis of a protein chain lacking the last three properdin-like repeat domains. In the calf, a 17-bp deletion alters the reading frame and predicts a premature termination codon. It appears that the absence of properdin-like domains renders the enzyme inactive in the two species.

Mutations in the PLOD gene encoding lysyl hydroxylase-1, another collagen-modifying enzyme, have been identified in individuals affected with the kyphoscoliosis type of Ehlers–Danlos syndrome *(16)*. Lysyl hydroxylase-1 is one of four, possibly five, enzymes with a similar catalytic function. The different hydroxylases are not molecule (collagen type)-specific, but rather cell-type-specific. The active form of the enzyme is a homodimer. The enzyme deficiency typically results in a significant reduction of the hydroxylation of collagen type I primarily in the skin and less in the bone and tendons. A sensitive indicator of the hydroxylation of collagen is the measurement, in the urine, of the total hydroxylysyl pyridinoline and lysyl pyridinoline crosslinks by high performance liquid chromatography (HPLC) after hydrolysis. Eighteen different mutations have been detected in affected individuals, three of which have been found in several unrelated individuals. Duplications of exons 10–16, splice-site deletions of exons 16, 17, and 19, and missense mutations have been described.

The previous enumeration of mutations identified in individuals affected with Ehlers–Danlos syndrome is by no means complete. This should not be surprising given the clinical and genetic heterogeneity of the disorder. Recently, missplicing of exon 9 of the COL1A2 gene has been detected in at least three unrelated individuals presenting with joint hypermobility, joint dislocations, skin extensibility, atrophic scars, easy bruising, and bone fractures. Other mutations in the genes encoding collagen type I have been found in individuals presenting with an Ehlers–Danlos-syndrome phenotype that could not be categorized. Although the clinical phenotype in most instances has been linked to defects in a particular collagen type or collagen-modifying enzyme, several exceptions to that rule suggest that these associations are not absolute and that should be kept in mind when counseling the individual patient.

It is reasonable to assume that a variety of pathogenetic mechanisms are operative in a condition as heterogeneous as the Ehlers–Danlos syndrome. The various mutations described in the different dominantly inherited types involve fibrillar collagens that exhibit significant similarity in structure and, in general, function. General principles are discussed in Subheading 4.3. The pathogenesis of the recessively inherited types, although affecting ultimately the structure and function of collagen type I, might be different because abnormalities in enzyme activity might affect the function of substrates other than collagen type I. More light into the pathogenesis of the Ehlers–Danlos syndrome will be shed from the combined in-depth study of human mutations and transgenic animal models.

4. Osteogenesis Imperfecta
4.1. Clinical Manifestations

Osteogenesis imperfecta (OI) is a systemic disorder of connective tissue involving the bone, skin, ligaments, tendons, fascia, sclera, and ear *(17)*. Osteogenesis imperfecta is clinically and genetically heterogeneous, and four types have been defined based on clinical, radiologic, and genetic criteria. OI type I is inherited as an autosomal dominant trait and presents with postnatal onset of fractures, mild skeletal deformity, blue sclerae, loose jointedness, and hearing loss. OI type II (lethal perinatal type) is incompatible with life. Almost all affected infants die within the neonatal period. The onset of fractures in OI type II is intrauterine. The long bones are shortened and angulated, a characteristic facies is present, the chest is small and frequently pear shaped, and the hue of the sclerae is slate gray. Radiographically, short and undermineralized femora whose appearance has been described as concertina-like, multiple rib fractures, and severely undermineralized calvarium are characteristically observed. OI type II results primarily from *de novo* dominant mutations in the collagen type I genes. Individuals affected with OI type III are born with fractures in their long bones. The frequency of fractures continues unabated into childhood and adolescence. Significant skeletal deformity and short stature are present. Most individuals affected with OI type III are unable to walk. Blue sclerae, a characteristic triangular facies, dentinogenesis imperfecta, and hearing loss are frequent manifestations in OI type III. The mode of inheritance is autosomal dominant. OI type IV is characterized by short stature, moderate to occasionally severe skeletal deformity, hearing loss, dentinogenesis imperfecta, and joint laxity. Individuals affected with OI type IV are frequently born with fractures of the long bones. OI type IV is also inherited as an autosomal dominant trait.

4.2. Etiology

Null alleles are the most common cause of OI type I. Biochemically, collagen type I synthesized by cultured skin fibroblasts is about half the normal level. The structure of the secreted procollagen type I is normal, and the decrease in procollagen type I production resulted from the synthesis of only half the usual amount of the proα1(I) chains. The most completely characterized mutation in the COL1A1 gene that results in abnormal production of procollagen type I is a 5-bp deletion near the 3' end of one COL1A1 allele. The mutation shifts the reading frame and predicts an extension of 84 amino acids beyond the normal termination site. Although the abnormal mRNA can be translated in vitro, it has proved extremely difficult to identify the abnormal chains in cells; it appears that although the mRNA is present in near-normal quantities, the protein product is unstable. This mutation provides a model of how many different mutations in the COL1A1 gene could produce the OI type I phenotype by resulting in the synthesis of half the normal amount of functional proα1(I) chain. In each instance, the synthesis of proα2(I) chains would be expected to be normal, but about half of them could not be incorporated into intact molecules [because the proα2(I) chains cannot associate into trimeric molecules] and, thus, would be degraded *(17)*. Although less common than null allele mutations, point mutations resulting in amino acid substitutions or missplicing in the COL1A1 and COL1A2 genes can also produce OI type I (Table 2).

Osteogenesis imperfecta type II is the most extensively studied variant of OI *(17)*. The OI type II phenotype is caused by a wide array of mutations, including point mutations in the triple helical domain that result in substitutions for glycine (mostly in the COL1A1 gene), multiexon rearrangements, small deletions (usually the result of splicing defects) in the triple helical domain of either chain, and mutations in the carboxyl-terminal propeptides interfering with molecular assembly. In almost all instances, the affected individual is heterozygous for the mutations (Table 2). The OI type III phenotype usually results from mutations in the COL1A1 or COL1A2 genes *(17)*. The gamut of detected mutations is similar to that observed in OI type II with substitutions of glycine in the triple helical domain being by far the most numerous group. Similar types of mutations have been identified in OI type IV (Table 2) *(17)*.

Table 2
Biochemical and Genetic Abnormalities in Osteogenesis Imperfecta

OI type I	
Common	"Nonfunctional" COL1A1 alleles
	Frameshift with long extension of carboxyl-terminal propeptides
	Exon-skipping mutations with very unstable mRNA
Rare	Substitution for glycine residue in carboxyl-terminal telopeptide of the α1(I) chain
	Substitution of glycine at position 94 of the triple helix in the proα1(I) chain
	Exon deletion (skipping) in the proα1(I) chain triple helical domain
OI type II	
Common	Substitutions for glycyl residues in the triple helical domains of the α1(I) and α2(I) chains
Rare	Rearrangement in the COL1A1 and COL1A2 genes
	Exon deletions in the triple helical domain of COL1A1 and COL1A2
	Substitutions and small deletions in the non-triple-helical carboxyl-terminal propeptide
	Tripeptide deletion in the proα1(I) chain triple helical domain
(Rare)	Exon-skipping mutation in the α2(I) chain on the background of a null allele
OI type III	
Common	Substitutions for glycyl residues in the triple helical domains of the α1(I) and α2(I) chains
Uncommon	Single amino acid deletion in the triple helical domain of the α1(I) chain
(Rare)	Frameshift (4-bp deletion) in COL1A2 that prevents incorporation of proα2(I) chains into molecules
OI type IV	
Common	Substitutions for glycyl residues in the triple helical domains of the α1(I) and α2(I) chains
	Exon-skipping mutations in COL1A2
Rare	Triplet deletion in the triple helical domain of the proα2(I) chain

Source: From ref. *17*.

4.3. Pathogenesis

4.3.1. Mechanisms

For several reasons, collagen genes appear to be good reporters of mutations. First, there is a high density of invariant and required glycine residues in the triple helical domain (one-third of all amino acids). Substitution of either of the first two nucleotides of the glycine codon (GGN) changes the encoded amino acid to one which has a side chain that does not fit in the central core of the triple helix. Thus, the alteration of any of 22% (two out of nine) of the nucleotides encoding the triple helical domain will probably give rise to a phenotypic change in the heterozygote. Second, the large exon number, and sensitivity to exon loss regardless of position in the protein, provides more than 200 additional mutation-sensitive sites in each gene (consensus donor and acceptor sites). Third, the need to maintain structure in the globular carboxyl-terminal domain to allow for interactions that generate a triple helical molecule provides an additional number of additional targets. Finally, because collagen type I forms fibrils from identical subunits, the presence of any abnormal molecules in the matrix presumably interferes with the production of normal fibrillar structure.

Most characterized mutations that produce recognizable forms of OI are single nucleotide substitutions that change a glycine codon to that for another amino acid. Few of the cataloged mutations have occurred independently in unrelated individuals. Two recurrent mutations appeared at CpG dinucleotides and are consistent with the deamidation of a methyl cytosine to produce thymidine on the antisense DNA strand. Although mutations at CpG dinucleotides are not overrepresented, those sites may present sequences where recurrent mutations are more likely to appear. The majority of point mutations that have been characterized do not arise at CpG dinucleotides and, thus, other mechanisms must be invoked.

It is surprising, given the repetitive structure of the collagen type I genes and the apparently higher proportion of multiexon rearrangement in other fibrillar collagen genes (e.g., the COL3A1 gene that encodes the chains of procollagen type III) that large deletions within collagen type I genes are uncommon. The multiexon deletions that have been identified in collagen type I genes occurred as results of intron–intron events, and only a single instance of recombination through exon exchange in the COL1A1 gene has been recognized. Although the structure of the genes themselves may be sufficient to limit recombination, it is possible that there are other explanations for the paucity of total gene deletion events.

Exon-skipping mutations most often occur as the result of point mutations in the consensus splice donor and acceptor domains. However, small deletions within the intron and exon may produce similar results. The mechanism by which small deletions occur is unclear, whether they result in exon-skipping events or simply in shorter amino acid deletions.

4.3.2. Translation of Mutation to Phenotype

The phenotypic consequences of mutations in collagen type I genes reflect the gene in which the mutation occurred, the nature and location of mutation, and its effect on the behavior of both the abnormal chain and molecules that contain it. It has been proposed that mutations could be considered in two major categories: those that resulted in the exclusion of the product of the mutant allele from the mature molecule (i.e., "excluded mutations") and those that permitted the incorporation of a structurally abnormal chain, or "included mutations." Heterozygosity for such mutations would be expected to have different consequences than homozygosity.

Excluded mutations can be thought of in two ways: as failure to synthesize the product of an allele and as failure of the synthesized chain to be incorporated into the protein. Both appear to result in mild phenotypes in the heterozygote and are generally found in individuals with the OI type I phenotype. In the homozygote, such mutations appear to be lethal in the case of COL1A1 but only moderately severe in the case of COL1A2. Very few "excluded" mutations have yet been identified or have been characterized at the molecular level. Because the expression of the abnormal allele may be low, the mutations must be identified at the genomic level, a formidable task with genes that encompass 18 kb and 38 kb, respectively, and have more than 50 exons apiece. Nonetheless, the phenotypic effects of having too little collagen in bone are apparently far milder than those resulting from the presence of molecules containing abnormal chains.

The effects on tissue strength of decreased production of procollagen type I is not well understood. It has been demonstrated that in the mouse, there is a marked decrease in bone strength, compatible with a tissue that has decreased amounts of collagen type I. It is not clear, however, that a decreased mass of collagen is the only factor. The striking morphology of collagen fibrils in the skin of individuals with OI type I, similar to that seen in skin from people with Ehlers–Danlos syndrome classical type, suggests that altered ratios of the major components of the matrix may contribute to abnormal tensile strength. Thus, even the simplest mutations are likely to have complex effects on extracellular matrix, forcing us to recognize the interrelationships of the numerous macromolecules in the tissue.

On the whole, the phenotypic effects of mutations that result in the generation of abnormal procollagen type I molecules are more deleterious compared to those of null mutations. There is, however, an enormous range in the clinical presentation of these mutations that appears to reflect the gene in which the mutation occurs, the nature of the mutation, the location of the abnormal sequence in the protein, and the effects of the mutation on the behavior of the chain and of the mature molecule into which it is incorporated.

If the abnormal chain leads to very rapid intracellular degradation of molecules that incorporate the chain, the clinical consequences should differ depending on the gene in which the mutation occurs. Mutations in the COL1A1 gene may be highly deleterious and even lethal, because they compromise three-quarters of all procollagen type I molecules synthesized. In contrast, a similar mutation in the COL1A2 gene would result in the loss of only half the molecules made and so might be similar in effect to a null COL1A1 allele (i.e., only half the normal amount of procollagen type I molecules would be completed in each case). If none of the abnormal protein is secreted but is not rapidly degraded, the effects of intracellular accumulation cannot be overlooked.

The effects of mutations reflect the domain of the procollagen molecule in which they occur and, within that domain, the way in which the specific mutation alters function. For point mutations in the COL1A1 gene that result in the substitution of glycine residues within the triple helical domain of the chain, there is a broad "phenotypic gradient" such that defects near the caboxyl-terminal end of the chain are generally more severe than those near the amino-terminal end of the chain. This gradient is modified by the nature of the substituting amino acid, so that some may be lethal along the entire domain (e.g., aspartic acid), whereas others may have a lethal to nonlethal transition in the carboxyl-terminal half of the chain (e.g., cysteine).

Point mutations that substitute for glycine residues have several effects on the protein. First, almost all molecules that contain chains with mutations in the triple helical domain are less stable than their normal counterparts (i.e., they display a reduced thermal stability). Second, the molecules that result are asymmetric in that they fold normally to the site of the mutant sequence and then appear either to fold slowly or to form a subtly different triple-helical-structure amino-terminal to it. Third, as a result of the change in structure or in the rate of propagation of the triple helix, the chains in the molecules remain accessible to the posttranslationally modifying enzymes and undergo additional hydroxylation of lysyl residues in the triple helix and additional hydroxylysyl glycosylation, further accentuating the asymmetric character of the molecules. Fourth, these molecules often have a long residence time in the rough endoplasmic reticulum where increased posttranslational modification occurs. The dilatation of the rough endoplasmic reticulum, which in some instances may be striking, could alter the architecture of the cell to distort its other functions, including the secretion of other proteins and activation of the intracellular response to stress. Fifth, the amino-terminal propeptides of the abnormal molecules that are secreted may not be cleaved as efficiently as those from the normal molecules, with the result that partially processed molecules can interfere with normal fibril nucleation and growth. Sixth, abnormal fibrils are probably poor substrates for mineralization. Finally, the relative tissue specificity of the effects of these mutations in collagen type I genes may reflect more stringent requirements of bone than skin and other soft tissues for aspects of molecular structure that can be altered by helix-altering mutations.

Point mutations and deletions (large or small) affect the processing of molecules in much the same way. In the amino-terminal of the mutant sequence, all the chains of molecules that contain a shortened abnormal chain are overmodified. This finding provided some of the most convincing evidence that the triple helix must be stabilized by forces beyond those conventionally considered to be important, and that large interactions, and possibly hydrophobic interactions, might be significant. Also, such findings suggested that a registration shift in the triple helical domain of molecules with, for example, chains that have substitutions of single glycine residues could explain the apparently slower propagation of the abnormal structure along the full length of the triple helix. Rotary-shadowing electron microscopic studies of procollagen resistant to procollagen I N-proteinase produced by cultured fibroblasts from a patient with OI type II, showing a cysteine for glycine substitution at position 748 of the $\alpha1(I)$ chain have shown the presence of a kink in the molecule at the site of the substitution, as predicted in model-building studies incorporating a phase shift of one tripeptide unit N-terminal to the defect in one or both $\alpha1(I)$ chains. A similar kink has been observed in collagen from another OI mutant cell strain in which there is a cysteine for glycine substitution at position 718 of the $\alpha1(I)$ chain. This is probably not, however, a general phenomenon, as far as amino acid substitutions are concerned. Other models that propose a more local disturbance in structure would be more compatible with a situation in which the mutation produces a delay in folding the triple helix to account for prolonged accessibility of modifying enzymes. It is likely that different mutations have different effects on molecular assembly that can only be identified by more detailed experimental study.

References

1. Pyeritz, R. E. and McKusick, V. A (1979) The Marfan syndrome: diagnosis and management. *N. Engl. J. Med.* **300,** 772–777.
2. De Paepe, A., Devereux, R. B., Dietz, H. C., Hennekam, R. C. M., and Pyeritz, R. E. (1996) Revised diagnostic criteria for the Marfan syndrome. *Am. J. Med. Genet.* **62,** 417–426.
3. Lee, B., Godfrey, M., Vitale, E., Hori, H., Mattei, M.-G., Sarfarazi, M., et al. (1991) Linkage of Marfan syndrome and a phenotypically related disorder to two different fibrillin genes. *Nature* **352,** 330–334.
4. Dietz, H. C. and Pyeritz, R. E. (1995) Mutations in the human gene for fibrillin-1 (FBN1) in the Marfan syndrome and related disorders. *Hum. Mol. Genet.* **4,** 1799–1809.

5. Sakai, L. Y., Keene, D. R., and Engvall, E. (1986) Fibrillin, a new 350-kD glycoprotein, is a component of extracellular microfibrils. *J. Cell Biol.* **103,** 2499–2509.
6. Pepeira, L., D'Alessio, M., Ramirez, F., Lynch, J. R., Sykes, B., Pangilinan, T., et al. (1993) Genomic organization of the sequence coding for fibrillin the defective gene product in Marfan syndrome. *Hum. Mol. Genet.* **2,** 961–968.
7. Pereira, L., Lee, Y.-L., Gayraud, B., Andrikopoulos, K., Shapiro, S. D., Bunton, T., et al. (1999) Pathogenetic sequence for aneurysm revealed in mice underexpressing fibrillin-1. *Proc. Natl. Acad. Sci. USA* **96,** 3819–3823.
8. Pereira, L., Andrikopoulos, K., Tian, J., Lee. S-Y., Keene. D. R., Ono, R., et al. (1997) Targeting of the gene encoding fibrillin-1 recapitulates the vascular aspect of Marfan syndrome. *Nature Genet.* **17,** 218–222.
9. Aoyama, T., Francke, U., Dietz, H. C., and Furthmayr, H. (1994) Quantitative differences in biosynthesis of cultured fibroblasts distinguish five groups of Marfan syndrome patients and suggest distinct pathogenetic mechanisms. *J. Clin. Invest.* **94,** 13–17.
10. Shores, J., Berger, K. R., Murphy, E. A., and Pyeritz, R. E. (1994) Progression of aortic dilatation and the benefit of long-term b-adrenergic blockade in Marfan's syndrome. *N. Engl. J. Med.* **330,** 1335–1341.
11. Kilpatrick, M. W., Phylactou, L. A., Godfrey, M., Wu, C. H., Wu, G. Y., and Tsipouras, P. (1996) Delivery of a hammerhead ribozyme specifically down-regulates the production of fibrillin-1 by cultured dermal fibroblasts. *Hum. Mol. Genet.* **5,** 1939–1944.
12. Beighton, P., De Paepe, A., Steinmann, B., Tsipouras, P., and Wenstrup, R. J. (1998) Ehlers–Danlos syndromes: revised nosology, Villefranche, 1997. *Am. J. Med. Genet.* **77,** 31–37.
13. Steinmann, B., Royce, P. M., and Superti-Furga, A. (1993) The Ehlers–Danlos syndrome, in *Connective Tissue and Its Heritable Disorders* (Royce, P. M. and Steinmann, B., eds.), Wiley-Liss, New York, pp. 351–407.
14. Wenstrup. R. J., Langland, G. T., Willing, M. C., D'Souza, V. N., and Cole, W. G. (1996) A splice-junction mutation in the region of COL5A1 that codes for the carboxyl propeptide of proα1(V) chains results in the gravis form of the Ehlers–Danlos syndrome (type I). *Hum. Mol. Genet.* **5,** 1733–1736.
15. Colige, A., Beschin, A., Samyn, B., Goebels, Y., Van Beeumen, J., Nusgens, B. V., et al. (1995) Characterization and partial amino acid sequencing of a 107-kDa procollagen I N-proteinase purified by affinity chromatography on immobilized type XIV collagen. *J. Biol. Chem.* **270,** 16,724–16,730.
16. Ha, V. T., Marshall, M. K., Elsas, L. J., Pinnell, S. R., and Yeowell, H. N. (1994) A patient with Ehlers–Danlos syndrome type VI is a compound heterozygote for mutations in the lysyl hydroxylase gene. *J. Clin. Invest.* **93,** 1716–1721.
17. Byers, P. H. (1993) Osteogenesis imperfecta, in *Connective Tissue and Its Heritable Disorders* (Royce, P. M. and Steinmann, B., eds.), Wiley–Liss, New York, pp. 317–350.

IV

Molecular Aspects of Treatment of Rheumatic Diseases

28
Corticosteroids

Henry K. Wong and George C. Tsokos

1. Introduction

Corticosteroids remain as one of the most reliable drugs used for the rapid palliation of autoimmune rheumatic diseases. Although this drug is not curative, there is a uniform clinical response to steroids in patients with rheumatoid arthritis (RA), systemic lupus erythematosus (SLE), polymyositis, dermatomyositis, inflammatory bowel disease, and other autoimmune inflammatory diseases (reviewed in ref. *1*). At times, long-term remission can be achieved with steroids. In acute disease flares, pulse doses of steroids offer dramatic and often life-saving improvement in symptoms. Steroids when used appropriately in low doses with other disease modifying medications can offer long-term relief and control of exacerbation of clinical symptoms. Unfortunately, corticosteroids, once started, have undesirable side effects. Long-term use has been associated with immune suppression, adrenal suppression, myopathy, peptic ulcer disease, osteoporosis, growth retardation, cataracts, diabetes, ischemic bone necrosis, atrophy of skin, increases in telangiectasia, striae, and impaired wound healing.

The structure of the therapeutic glucocorticoids is the C-21 steroid molecule, which is modified at different carbon residues as shown (Fig. 1). The different modifications of the natural dominant steroid cortisone at different sites lead to the more potent and longer acting synthetic hormones, such as prednisone, dexamethasone, and hydrocortisone. Cortisol is the predominant naturally produced steroid required for basic metabolic function and is secreted in the range of 15–30 mg/d. The hormone molecules are 90% protein bound and metabolism of steroids occurs in the liver. The physiologic effects are extensive and include protein catabolism, increase gluconeogenesis, and immunoregulation.

2. Mechanism of Action

There are over 30 natural steroid molecules produce by the body, primarily by the adrenal glands. The different hormones impact on the metabolism of every cell in a different manner and act principally by altering gene regulation. Glucocorticoids have an important role in the homeostasis of normal metabolic function and affect the immune response. The mechanism by which the steroid family of hormone function became clear after the human glucocorticoid receptor (GR) was cloned in 1985 *(2,3)*. Characterization by subcellular localization studies showed that the receptor of these

From: *Current Molecular Medicine: Principles of Molecular Rheumatology*
Edited by: G. C. Tsokos © Humana Press Inc., Totowa, NJ

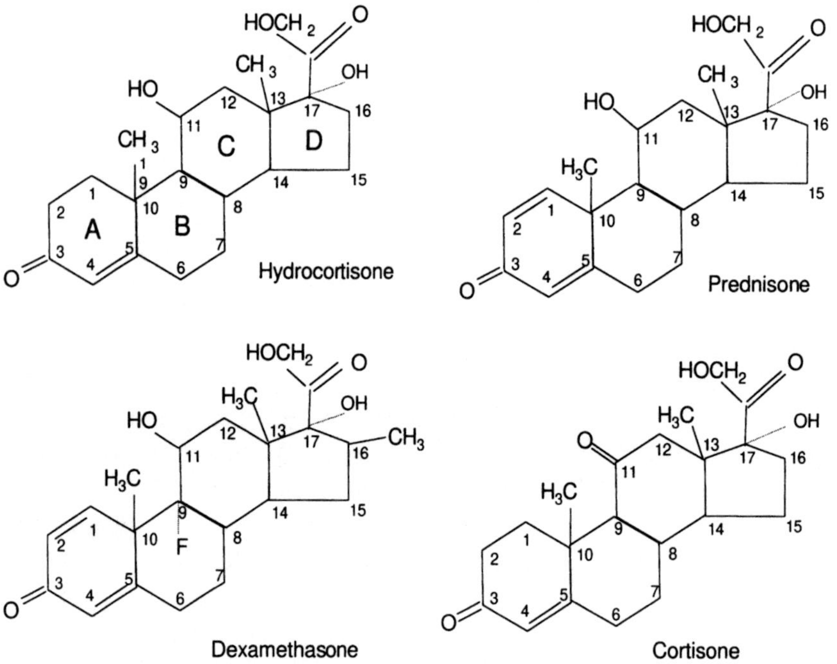

Fig. 1. Chemical structure of therapeutic steroid molecules. Cortisone and hydrocortisone are natural steroids. Prednisone and dexamethasone are synthetic steroids.

lipophilic hormone molecules bind to the intracellular receptors. Unlike surface receptors, such as protein tyrosine kinases or cyclic nucleotide binding proteins, which require intermediate proteins to transmit the signal to the nucleus after ligand binding, steroid hormone receptors transmit signal to the nucleus directly. At present, there are numerous steroid hormone molecules that constitute a large family and each member binds a specific receptor. There are receptors for different classes of hormones and these receptors make up a superfamily that includes thyroid hormone (TR), retinoic acid receptor (RAR), steroid receptors, vitamin D receptor (VDR), and orphan hormone receptors (Fig. 2). The receptors can be divided into two subfamilies, based on the amino acid homologies: the steroid and thyroid hormone subfamilies. When the receptors are not bound to the ligand, it is in an inactive complex that is bound to immunophilins or heat-shock proteins of various sizes, from 56 to 90 kDa. The heat-shock protein complexes prevent the unoccupied receptor from entering the nucleus. The primary sequence of the different hormone receptors show structural similarity and amino acid homology. These molecules show the presence of three functional domains that are modular in nature in that these regions retain their respective function when separated from the native molecule and fused onto another molecule to form a chimera. The three regions are the DNA-binding domain, the steroid or ligand-binding domain (LBD) and the variable amino terminus transactivation domain.

The DNA-binding domain is a 66–68 amino acid region located in the central region of the protein. This domain is highly conserved evolutionarily and the amino acid sequence varies among the different receptors by 42–94% (reviewed in ref. *4*). Among the different steroid hormone receptors such as the progesterone receptor, mineralocor-

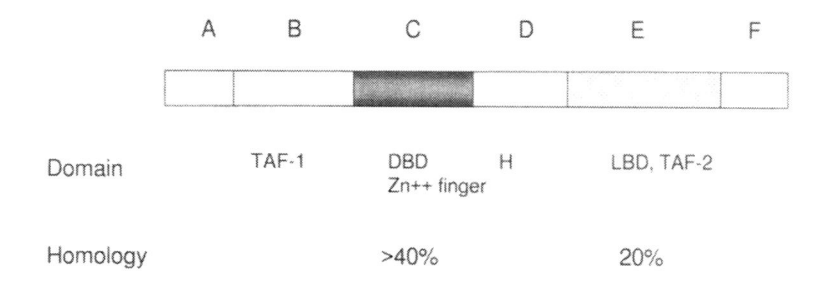

```
     A      B        C       D        E         F
  ┌─────┬────────┬────████████┬────────┬──────────┬──────┐
  └─────┴────────┴────████████┴────────┴──────────┴──────┘

Domain           TAF-1      DBD      H      LBD, TAF-2
                          Zn++ finger

Homology                   >40%             20%
```

Fig. 2. Linear organization of steroid hormone receptor. The conserved domains found in the steroid receptor super family are shown (A–F). The degree of homology for the two domains are shown. A and B contain regions required for transactivation. C contains two zinc fingers and is required for dimerization. E contains multiple functions and is also the region bound by HSP70. H = hinge region. DBD = DNA-binding domain. LBD = Ligand-binding domain. TAF = transactivating factor binding region.

ticoid receptor, and glucocorticoid receptor, the homology is 90%. The structure of this region is defined by a constant invariant 20 amino acid region with conserved cysteine residues that form two "fingerlike" structures that coordinate zinc for DNA binding. Although two zinc-finger structures are predicted by amino acid sequence, only one is required for DNA binding. Each zinc-finger domain has four conserved cysteine residues that coordinate zinc. In the absence of the ligand, the DNA-binding function of this region is repressed by the carboxyl terminus.

The DNA sequence recognized by these receptors have a particular common motif consisting of two repeating sets of hexanucleotides (half-sites) separated by 0–4 random nucleotides (5). Each half-site can be oriented as a palindrome or as a direct repeat relative to the other site. This organization allows different combinations of receptors to associate and bind DNA to increase the diversity of complexes forming at the promoter. The type of DNA sequences recognized by the glucocorticoid receptor family members are half-sites of the sequence 5'-TGTTCT-3' that are arranged as palindromes. The spacing separating the palindrome determines whether the sequence is recognized by the glucocorticoid receptor (GR), the androgen receptor (AR), the progesterone receptor (PR), or the mineralocorticoid receptor (MR). Other members of the receptor superfamily such as the thyroid hormone receptors and the retinoic acid receptor family recognized half-sites 5'-TGACCT–3' that is oriented as direct repeats.

When the LBD is unoccupied by the respective ligand, this domain prevents dimerization and activation of the receptors. Upon binding of the hormone ligand, the receptor undergoes an allosteric structural conformational change to expose the domain that mediates dimerization and DNA binding (Fig. 3). Ligand-bound LBD mediates dimerization and allows the complex to translocate into the nucleus where it can affect gene expression. The inhibitory role of the LBD was elucidated when deletion of the LBD created a constitutively active DNA-binding protein. The LBD is also important for the dissociation of heat-shock proteins, to which the receptor is bound when it is in the cytoplasm.

There are several mechanisms by which steroid hormone receptors affect gene expression. One is by directly binding-specific regulatory sequences. Once bound to DNA, steroid receptors act by recruiting general transcription factors to the promoters

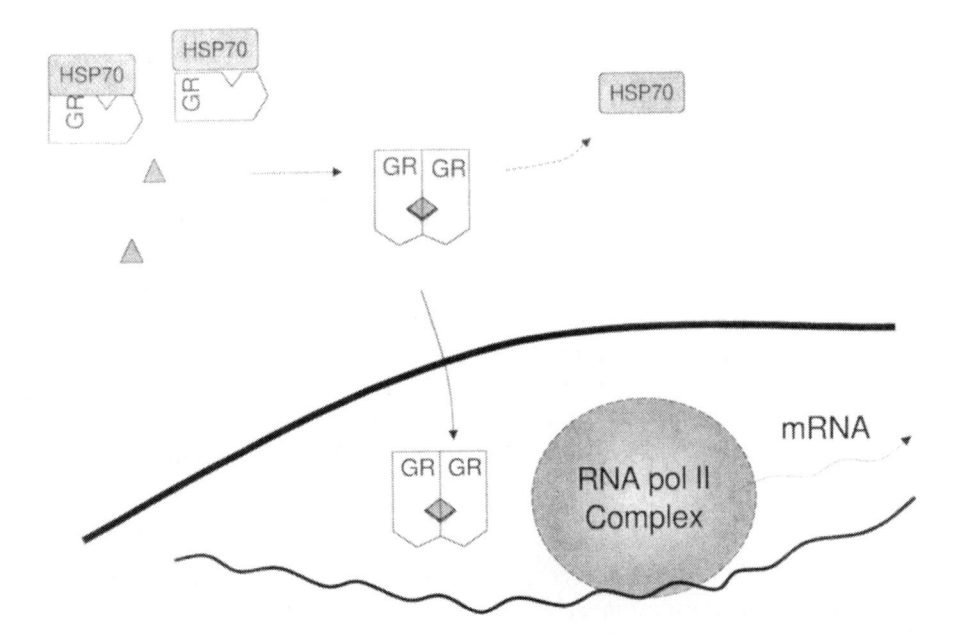

Fig. 3. Activation of steroid hormone receptor. Schematic for activation of steroid hormone receptors. The first step is ligand binding followed by nuclear translocation. In the nucleus, the receptor complex can bind DNA to affect gene expression at the promoter.

of specific genes or by interacting with other DNA-binding proteins. The type of interaction is dependent on the promoter of the gene, which can lead to an increase or decrease in transcription. Another mechanism is to inhibit transcription by interfering with the function of transcription factors.

The amino terminus of the receptor is the domain that has the most variability in amino acid sequence among the different receptors and is necessary for transactivation. There are also regions in the C-terminus that contribute to transactivation function. These regions are required for recruitment of general transcription factors that assist in the initiation of transcription by RNA polymerase II once the receptor is stably bound to DNA. The transactivating region interacts with a coactivator complex, Creb-binding protein (CBP/p300), or steroid receptor coactivator 1 (SRC1) *(6)*. Transcription coactivators function to recruit a class of enzymes called histone acetylase that modifies the chromatin structure of DNA to decondense the DNA molecule. Once histones that inhibit access to transcription machinery are removed, a stable interaction between the general transcription factors and sequence-specific transcription factors form to initiate mRNA synthesis.

3. Molecular Mechanism of Anti-inflammatory Effect

Inflammatory diseases lead to extensive activation and mobilization of immune cells to cause disruption of normal homeostasis and pathology. During inflammation, there is a profound activation of gene expression for cytokines, chemokines, cell adhesion molecules, proteases, and other inflammatory mediators. Glucocorticoids intervene in the pathology and permit a restoration of balance of cytokines to the noninflammatory level (7). The efficacy of glucocorticoids as an anti-inflammatory agent, on a physiologic level, can be appreciated by the rapid vasoconstriction that leads to blanching when potent topical steroids are applied to the skin. There is a decrease vascular permeability and local blood flow. At the cellular and molecular level (e.g., in endothelial cells), there is decreased swelling and leakage of immune complexes across the basement membrane. There is decreased leukocyte traffic and decreased lymphokine gene expression. The sum of these effects all lead to a decrease in inflammation and swelling.

Possible mechanisms have been proposed for the effects of glucocorticoids at different doses (8). Low doses near physiologic levels can be administered in certain diseases with dramatic clinical effects, such as in temporal arteritis and polymyalgia rheumatica where 5 mg is sufficient for clinical response. Intermediate dosages from 20 to 80 mg is often used in maintaining control of disease activity, and pulse intravenous doses of several grams per day are used in acute organ-threatening flares of autoimmune inflammatory disorders. From the dose-dependent effects of steroids, there are likely different targets affected at different dosage levels. At low levels, high-affinity target sites on the genome may be affected. Additional genes are affected at increasing concentrations of glucocorticoid in the intermediate range. At pulse steroid doses, nonspecific effects, which are immediate, may occur that affect general gene expression through disruption of transcription via squelching, which would overwhelm the transcription system. A pulse steroid dose could also cause physicochemical actions through the disruption of ionic flow of calcium and other salts by affecting cell-membrane function. In some cells, glucocorticoids can affect up to 1% of the total genes being expressed.

4. Cellular Targets of Glucocorticoids

In asthma, steroids lead to inhibition of lung macrophage production of interleukin (IL-1). Leukocyte migration is profoundly inhibited by affecting cell adhesion molecule expression, which prevents the influx of inflammatory cells that lead to tissue damage (9). Eosinophils are directly inhibited from releasing mediators, and there is a corresponding decrease in the cell number in the circulation. Steroids can induce apoptosis in dendritic cells, eosinophils, T-cells, and other cells of the immune system (7). Surprisingly, certain T-cell populations are activated, such as the Th2 cells, whereas the Th1 cells are suppressed. However not all cells are affected equally and specific T-cell types such as the NK1.1, a T-cell that produces IL-4, do not undergo apoptosis in the presence of steroids. The preferential survival of this T-cell subset may contribute to the Th2-type cytokines switch. There is an effect on the balance of cytokines with a decrease of type 1 cytokine (interferon-γ [IFN-γ], IL-2, IL-12) and an increase in type 2 cytokine (IL-4, IL-5, IL-6, IL-10, IL-13) (10). The pro-inflammatory cytokine IL-1 and transforming growth factor-β (TGF-β) are also decreased.

Both B- and T-cells are affected by steroids; however, each type of cell is affected to a different degree. T-Cells are depleted from the vascular spaces more rapidly more than B-cells. B-Cell function is not rapidly affected by steroids and the synthesis of antibodies is not decreased significantly. Thus, steroids do not have immediate effects on the circulatory level of antibodies and antibody levels remain unchanged in the short term. In the treatment of autoimmune diseases whose pathology is a direct conse-

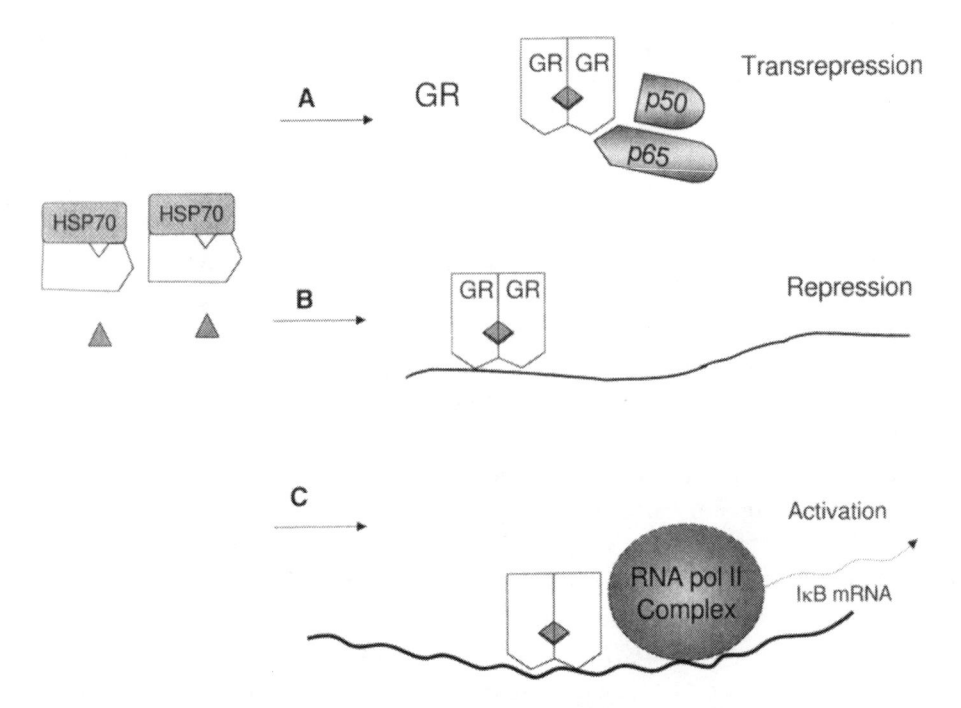

Fig. 4. Mechanisms for the regulation of gene expression by activated GR. (A) Transrepression of inflammatory genes by targeting essential transcription factors. (B) Repression of pro-inflammatory genes at the promoter by blocking the formation of a functional transcription initiation complex. (C) Activation of anti-inflammatory genes, such as upregulation of IκB.

quence of autoantibodies, such as the blistering skin disease, pemphigus, response to steroids may take several days. Over a period of days, the level of autoantibody decreases and this may be secondary from increased catabolism. Another possible mechanism is the inhibition of T-cell help to B-cells by downregulation of T-cell activation.

There are many genes modulated by glucocorticoids. The expression of numerous pro-inflammatory cytokine genes is directly inhibited, whereas the expression of inhibitory cytokines is stimulated. Nitric oxide synthase (NOS), a molecule induced during inflammation by cytokines and potentiates inflammation, is a target for glucocorticoid suppression *(11)*. Other molecules involved in amplifying the inflammatory response, such as adhesion molecules, are also inhibited. Steroids antagonize these inflammatory mediators at the molecular level by affecting gene expression. The anti-inflammatory action of glucocorticoids can potentially act through targeting different steps in transcription activation. Once activated by the glucocorticoid ligand, the receptors dimerize and expose the functional regions of the molecule that are necessary for nuclear translocation, interaction with other nuclear transcription factors, and DNA binding. Based on the current understanding of how the GR is regulated, there are three mechanisms through which GR could potentially mediate anti-inflammatory action at the molecular level: (1) block the function of essential transcription factors that activate transcription of pro-inflammatory genes; (2) block gene expression by directly binding to promoters of pro-inflammatory genes and preventing transcription, and (3) the activated GR binds to promoters of genes that have anti-inflammatory properties and increase transcription (Fig. 4) *(12,13)*.

Table 1
Genes Inhibited by Glucocorticoid

Gene	Target cell	Mechanism of inhibition
IL-1α	Macrophage	Block promoter at GRE
IL-1β	Monocyte	Destabilize mRNA and block GRE
IL-2	T-Cells	Block promoter by transrepression
IL-3	Mast cells, T cells	Inhibit transcription
IL-4	T-Cells, PBMC, mast cells	Transrepression of AP-1
IL-5	PBMC, mast cells	Inhibit transcription
IL-6	T-Cells, accessory cells	Transrepression
IL-8	Fibroblasts, epithelial cells	GRE binding
IL-12	T-Cells, monocytes, dendritic cells	?
IFN-γ	T-Cells, fibroblasts	GRE binding
TNF-α	Monocytes, macrophage, fibroblasts	GRE binding and transrepression
ICAM-1		Transrepression
E-selectin	Endothelial cells	Transrepression
Cyclooxygenase-2	PBMC, pulmonary epithelial cells	Transrepression
PGE2	Lung epithelial cells	
INOS	Endothelial cells	
POMC	Neuronal cells	
Granzyme B	CTL, NK cells	Transrepression
c-kit	Mast cells	?

Supporting the first mechanism is the group of genes stimulated by GR (summarized in Table 1). This class of genes have sequences in the promoter that are recognized by GR. These genes, in general, downregulate inflammation. GR induces the expression of IκB, an inhibitor of nuclear factor-κb (NF-κB), by increasing the transcription of the gene *(14,15)*. This, in turn, leads to retention of NF-κB, a pro-inflammatory transcription factor, in the cytoplasm where it can no longer affect gene expression. Because NF-κB acts in many pro-inflammatory responses, an increase in the IκB level would prevent the function of NF-κB and counteract inflammation.

A gene product that is increased in some cell types by glucocorticoids is lipocortin-1, which is thought to have anti-inflammatory properties through its ability to inhibit phospholipase A2. Another group of genes regulated by steroids is certain cytokine receptors, one of which is a decoy receptor, IL-1RII, that does not signal and essentially sequesters the function of the pro-inflammatory ligand. Another receptor is the B2-adrenergic receptor. A summary of upregulated receptors is presented in Table 2 *(16)*.

The glucocorticoid receptor can also cooperate with transcription factors to increase gene expression *(17)*. One family that GR interacts with together to stimulate gene expression is the STAT family. GR interacts with Stat3 to stimulate the α2-macroglobulin promoter activity *(18)*. In the prolactin promoter, GR cooperates with Stat5 to increase expression of target genes *(19)*.

In the second mechanism, GR inhibits gene expression through specific negative GR sequence elements (nGRE) that have been identified in the promoter of several different genes. A promoter involved intimately in the control of inflammation is that of the IL-1β gene, which contains a nGRE and is inhibited by GR *(20)*. Another class

Table 2
Genes Stimulated by Glucocorticoids

Lipocortin-1	IL-6R
B adrenoceptors	IFN-γR
IL-10	CSF-1R
IL-1R	GM-CSFR
IL-2Rα	CEBP

Table 3
Transcription Factor Affected by Glucocorticoids

AP-1	Repressed
NF-κB	Repressed
NF-AT	Repressed
Nur77/Egr1	Repressed
CREB	Repressed
Ikaros	Repressed
Stat3, Stat6	Activated
Pbx	Repressed
Oct-1	Repressed

of genes that is negatively regulated by GR participates in the regulation of the hypothalamic–pituitary–adrenal axis. The human pro-opiomelanocortin (POMC) gene, prolactin gene, and the corticotropin-releasing hormone (CRH) gene also contain, within their respective promoters, nGREs that are functional and regulate cortisol level *(21)*. Human osteocalcin, a gene expressed by osteoblasts, has a nGRE within the promoter, and this sequence may be responsible for the osteoporosis that follows long-term steroid use *(22)*.

Finally and most commonly, GR exerts its anti-inflammatory effect by inhibiting the normal function of other transcription factors needed for the expression of pro-inflammatory genes. This mechanism has been called trans-repression and requires the DNA-binding domain of GR to interact with the targeted transcription factor *(17)*. This complex of transcription factor with GR can no longer bind DNA, and pro-inflammatory genes that depend on these GR-targeted factors are inhibited. GR can interact with diverse transcription factors, including NF-κB, AP-1, CREB, and Nur77, which regulate inflammatory gene expression (Table 3).

Because NF-κB activates numerous proinflammatory cytokines and cell-surface markers, inhibiting the activity of NF-κB by glucocorticoids can lead to effective antagonism of the inflammatory process *(23)*. NF-κB is important in the regulation of adhesion molecules such as ICAM, ELAM, and cytokines. In addition to the regulation of NF-κB signaling by stimulating IκB gene expression, GR can directly target the p65-RelA component of NF-κB, prevent NF-κB from binding DNA, and, thus, lead to inhibition of gene expression. Cyclooxygenase, which is responsible for the synthesis of prostaglandin E_2 (PGE_2) and PGI_2 from arachidonic acid, is a target of anti-inflammatory drugs such as aspirin and glucocorticoids. Corticosteroids inhibit the synthesis of this enzyme at the transcriptional level by blocking activation of NF-κB. In addition, the stability of the cyclooxygenase mRNA is decreased by steroids.

AP-1, which is composed of two subunits, the leucine zipper proteins c-fos and c-jun, as discussed in Chapter 7, is critical in the regulation of cytokines and inflammatory genes *(24)*. The expression of IL-2 in T-cells is profoundly inhibited by glucocorticoids because this gene is dependent on AP-1 and NF-κB, transcription factors that are inhibited by glucocorticoids. The IFN-γ gene is inhibited through suppression of AP-1 function and CREB function. The human granzyme B expression is inhibited through the AP-1 site in cooperation with the Ikaros binding site *(25)*.

Another mechanism for the action of steroids in repressing inflammation is that both steroid receptors and NF-κB can interact with a coactivator such as CBP *(26)*. This competition for coactivators by the steroids receptors can lead to inhibition of NF-κB-dependent gene expression because the coactivators are limiting. Because these coactivators interact with other transcription factors such as STAT and CREB, the expression of genes regulated by these transcription factors will also be affected. Thus, competition of coactivators is a mechanism for disruption of genes that potentiate inflammation.

5. Conclusion

The mechanism of glucocorticoid action has been analyzed extensively at the molecular level. This chapter reviews our understanding of how glucocorticoids act in an isolated system, which has increased substantially since the cloning of the gene for the steroid hormone receptor. This newfound knowledge on corticosteroids provides a glimpse into the diverse clinical effects. Presently, we have an understanding of the structure of the glucocorticoid receptor and many of the molecular targets. Although we can extrapolate the effects of GR action in model systems where cytokine expression is inhibited to explain some of the effects at the cellular level, many questions concerning the clinical action of glucocorticoids remain to be answered. We should not be content with the superficial understanding that permits rationalization of chemical effects based on few in vitro molecular studies. A deeper insight and understanding that can explain consistently how steroids act in different cells in organs at various doses is important in guiding appropriate treatment and developing better therapeutic steroid molecules. Importantly, studies need to be designed at the organ system level that permits analysis at the molecular level so that confirmation of our previous cellular studies is made. At that time, better treatment regiments for rheumatic diseases may be developed.

Reference

1. Boumpas, D. T., Chrousos, G. P., Wilder, R. L., Cupps, T. R., and Balow, J. E. (1993) Glucocorticoid therapy for immune-mediated diseases: basic and clinical correlates. *Ann. Intern. Med.* **119**, 1198–1208.
2. Ribeiro, R. C., Kushner, P. J., and Baxter, J. D. (1995) The nuclear hormone receptor gene superfamily. *Annu. Rev. Med.* **46**, 443–453.
3. Beato, M., Herrlich, P., and Schutz, G. (1995) Steroid hormone receptors: many actors in search of a plot. *Cell* **83**, 851–857.
4. Funder, J. W. (1997) Glucocorticoid and mineralocorticoid receptors: biology and clinical relevance. *Annu. Rev. Med.* **48**, 231–240.

5. Forman, B. M. and Evans, R. M. (1995) Nuclear hormone receptors activate direct, inverted, and everted repeats. *Ann. NY Acad. Sci.* **761,** 29–37.
6. Chen, J. D. and Li, H. (1998) Coactivation and corepression in transcriptional regulation by steroid/nuclear hormone receptors. *Crit. Rev. Eukaryote Gene Express* **8,** 169–190.
7. Ramdas, J. and Harmon, J. M. (1998) Glucocorticoid-induced apoptosis and regulation of NF-kappaB activity in human leukemic T cells. *Endocrinology* **139,** 3813–3821.
8. Buttgereit, F., Wehling, M., and Burmester, G. R. (1998) A new hypothesis of modular glucocorticoid actions: steroid treatment of rheumatic diseases revisited. *Arthritis Rheum.* **41,** 761–767.
9. Cronstein, B. N., Kimmel, S. C., Levin, R. I., Martiniuk, F., and Weissmann, G. (1992) A mechanism for the antiinflammatory effects of corticosteroids: the glucocorticoid receptor regulates leukocyte adhesion to endothelial cells and expression of endothelial-leukocyte adhesion molecule 1 and intercellular adhesion molecule 1. *Proc. Natl. Acad. Sci. USA* **89,** 9991–9995.
10. Visser, J., van Boxel-Dezaire, A., Methorst, D., Brunt, T., de Kloet, E. R., and Nagelkerken, L. (1998) Differential regulation of interleukin-10 (IL-10) and IL-12 by glucocorticoids in vitro. *Blood* **91,** 4255–4264.
11. Brack, A., Rittner, H. L., Younge, B. R., Kaltschmidt, C., Weyand, C. M., and Goronzy, J. J. (1997) Glucocorticoid-mediated repression of cytokine gene transcription in human arteritis-SCID chimeras. *J. Clin. Invest.* **99,** 2842–2850.
12. Schule, R. and Evans, R. M. (1991) Cross-coupling of signal transduction pathways: zinc finger meets leucine zipper. *Trends Genet.* **7,** 377–381.
13. Cato, A. C., Wade, E., Northrop, J. P., Crabtree, G. R., and Mattila, P. S. (1996) Molecular mechanisms of anti-inflammatory action of glucocorticoids Negative regulation of interleukin 2 transcription by the glucocorticoid receptor. *BioEssays* **18,** 371–378.
14. Auphan, N., DiDonato, J. A., Rosette, C., Helmberg, A., and Karin, M. (1995) Immunosuppression by glucocorticoids: inhibition of NF-kappa B activity through induction of I kappa B synthesis. *Science* **270,** 286–290.
15. Scheinman, R. I., Cogswell, P. C., Lofquist, A. K., and Baldwin, A. S., Jr. (1995) Role of transcriptional activation of I kappa B alpha in mediation of immunosuppression by glucocorticoids [see comments]. *Science* **270,** 283–286.
16. Almawi, W. Y., Beyhum, H. N., Rahme, A. A., and Rieder, M. J. (1996) Regulation of cytokine and cytokine receptor expression by glucocorticoids. *J. Leukocyte Biol.* **60,** 563–572.
17. Gottlicher, M., Heck, S., and Herrlich, P. (1998) Transcriptional cross-talk, the second mode of steroid hormone receptor action. *J. Mol. Med.* **76,** 480–489.
18. Takeda, T., Kurachi, H., Yamamoto, T., Nishio, Y., Nakatsuji, Y., Morishige, K., et al. (1998) Crosstalk between the interleukin-6 (IL-6)-JAK-STAT and the glucocorticoid-nuclear receptor pathway: synergistic activation of IL-6 response element by IL-6 and glucocorticoid. *J. Endocrinol.* **159,** 323–330.
19. Pfitzner, E., Jahne, R., Wissler, M., Stoecklin, E., and Groner, B. (1998) p300/CREB-binding protein enhances the prolactin-mediated transcriptional induction through direct interaction with the transactivation domain of Stat5, but does not participate in the Stat5- mediated suppression of the glucocorticoid response. *Mol. Endocrinol.* **12,** 1582–1593.
20. Zhang, G., Zhang, L., and Duff, G. W. (1997) A negative regulatory region containing a glucocorticosteroid response element (nGRE) in the human interleukin-1beta gene. *DNA Cell Biol.* **16,** 145–152.
21. Drouin, J., Trifiro, M. A., Plante, R. K., Nemer, M., Eriksson, P., and Wrange, O. (1989) Glucocorticoid receptor binding to a specific DNA sequence is required for hormone-dependent repression of pro-opiomelanocortin gene transcription. *Mol. Cell Biol.* **9,** 5305–5314.
22. Morrison, N. and Eisman, J. (1993) Role of the negative glucocorticoid regulatory element in glucocorticoid repression of the human osteocalcin promoter. *J. Bone Miner. Res.* **8,** 969–975.

23. Barnes, P. J. and Karin, M. (1997) Nuclear factor-kappaB: a pivotal transcription factor in chronic inflammatory diseases. *N. Engl. J. Med.* **336,** 1066–1071.
24. Karin, M., Liu, Z., and Zandi, E. (1997) AP-1 function and regulation. *Curr. Opin. Cell Biol.* **9,** 240–246.
25. Wargnier, A., Lafaurie, C., Legros-Maida, S., Bourge, J. F., Sigaux, F., Sasportes, M., et al. (1998) Down-regulation of human granzyme B expression by glucocorticoids. Dexamethasone inhibits binding to the Ikaros and AP-1 regulatory elements of the granzyme B promoter. *J. Biol. Chem.* **273,** 35,326–35,331.
26. Sheppard, K. A., Phelps, K. M., Williams, A. J., Thanos, D., Glass, C. K., Rosenfeld, M. G., et al. (1998) Nuclear integration of glucocorticoid receptor and nuclear factor- kappaB signaling by CREB-binding protein and steroid receptor coactivator-1. *J. Biol. Chem.* **273,** 29,291–29,294.

29
Cytotoxic Drugs

David A. Fox and W. Joseph McCune

1. Introduction

Cytotoxic and immunosuppressive medications are of great value in the treatment of a variety of severe systemic rheumatologic and autoimmune diseases, as well as various forms of inflammatory arthritis. This chapter will review information on mechanisms of action and clinical usage of cyclophosphamide, azathioprine, methotrexate, and cyclosporine, for which the chemical structures are shown in Fig. 1. It should be remembered that use of these medications in the most effective and appropriate manner differs from one disease to another. This likely reflects the fact that the pathogenesis of autoimmune and systemic inflammatory diseases is complex, with many features distinct between different diseases (such as rheumatoid arthritis and systemic lupus erythematosus). It also reflects the complex and multiple mechanisms of action of these agents, which may include both immunomodulating and anti-inflammatory effects *(1)*. Drug metabolism and distinct biological effects of various drug metabolites must also be considered when explaining efficacy, toxicity, and changes in immunologic parameters. In this regard, it is clear that the dosing intervals and routes of administration are important parameters for some drugs, especially cyclophosphamide, with which biological and clinical effects may be very different with intermittent parenteral dosing compared to daily oral dosing.

2. Effects of Cytotoxic and Immunosuppressive Agents

2.1. T-Lymphocyte Numbers and Function

Cyclophosphamide, whether administered orally or parentally, produces a dose-dependent reduction in lymphocyte numbers in both animals and human patients. This effect is evident in patients with rheumatoid arthritis (RA), Wegener's granulomatosis, or systemic lupus erythematosus (SLE). In SLE, the lymphocyte count is frequently low at baseline because of the effects of anti-lymphocyte antibodies present in such patients, as well as systemic corticosteroid treatment. With daily oral cyclophosphamide treatment for RA or vasculitis, peripheral blood T-lymphocyte counts often dip to 50% of pretreatment levels by 2 mo and 25% by 6 mo. Presumably, this reflects depletion of T-lymphocytes in lymphoid organs as well, as has been observed in rodents exposed to this agent *(2)*.

From: *Current Molecular Medicine: Principles of Molecular Rheumatology*
Edited by: G. C. Tsokos © Humana Press Inc., Totowa, NJ

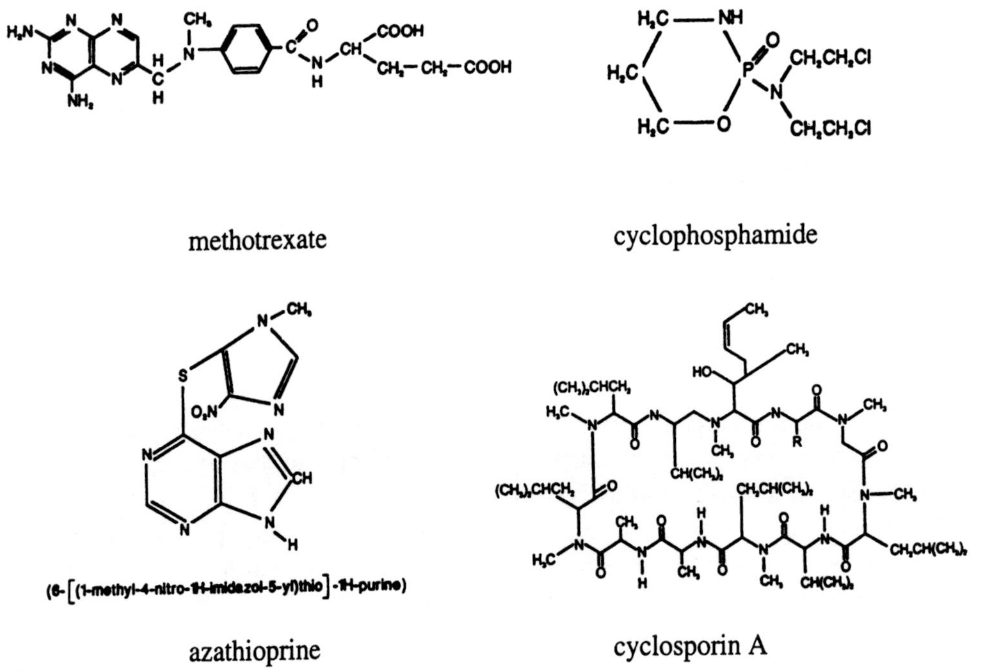

methotrexate

cyclophosphamide

(6-[(1-methyl-4-nitro-1H-imidazol-5-yl)thio]-1H-purine)

azathioprine

cyclosporin A

Fig. 1. Immunosuppressive and cytotoxic drugs.

At lower doses, cyclophosphamide can have interesting differential effects on lymphocyte subsets. In various rodent systems, administration of low-dose cyclophosphamide can actually augment a variety of immune responses, both antibody mediated and cell mediated. This has been thought to result from greater sensitivity of regulatory T-cell subsets versus effector lymphocyte subsets to cyclophosphamide (2). Even at somewhat higher doses, cyclophosphamide can actually enhance the immune response to tumors, both in rodents and in humans, possibly by selective activation of specific effector T-cell subsets in the recovery phase after cytotoxic depletion of lymphoid cells (3). Furthermore, cyclophosphamide is capable, under some circumstances, of triggering autoimmune disease, at least in certain rodent strains such as the NOD diabetic mouse. Other reports indicate that in humans treated with cyclophosphamide, certain T-lymphocyte functions and expression of cell-surface markers can be selectively affected. The overall implication of this information would suggest the use of very low-dose cyclophosphamide or a very brief course of higher-dose cyclophosphamide, as an initial treatment for any autoimmune disease should be discouraged. At currently used doses (1–2 mg/kg orally) or 500–750 mg/m^2 intravenously, there is no evidence that cyclophosphamide exacerbates autoimmunity or undesirably augments lymphocyte effector functions in man (1,2).

Azathioprine has less profound effects on lymphocyte numbers, but a dose-dependent lymphopenia can be produced after 6 mo or more of treatment. Various T-cell responses, such as mixed lymphocyte reactions and proliferation to mitogens, are reduced by azathioprine. There are also striking effects on natural-killer cell functional activity, although the relevance of this to the treatment of rheumatologic disease is not known. Like cyclophosphamide, azathioprine seems to have the ability to affect

Table 1
**Possible Mechanisms of Action
of Low-Dose Methotrexate in Rheumatologic Diseases**

Effects on lymphocytes and immune responses
    Cytotoxic killing of proliferating lymphocytes
    Enhanced apoptosis and clonal deletion of activated T-cells
    Decreased production of rheumatoid factor and other autoantibodies
    Alteration of lymphocyte subset distribution
Anti-inflammatory effects
    Inhibition of leukotriene synthesis
    Interference with production or action of cytokines, particularly interleukin-1
    Stimulation of production of cytokine inhibitors, such as the interleukin-1 receptor antagonist
    Inhibition of polyamine synthesis by inhibition of transmethylation reactions
    Stimulation of adenosine release at sites of inflammation
    Inhibition of leukocyte migration into inflammatory lesions
    Inhibition of angiogenesis
    Inhibition of neutrophil chemotaxis

surface expression of various markers on T-cells and other cells of the immune system *(1,2)*.

The target of action of methotrexate is not clear, and notable lymphopenia or impairment of T-cell function is not generally seen with low-dose methotrexate treatment of rheumatoid arthritis. However, the ability of methotrexate to augment levels of free adenosine could potentially lead to an environment toxic for activated lymphocytes in inflammatory lesions *(4)*. Furthermore, recent data suggest that methotrexate can cause apoptosis and clonal deletion of activated peripheral T-cells *(5)*. Some of the numerous possible mechanisms of action of methotrexate in rheumatologic disease are listed in Table 1.

Cyclosporine (cyclosporin A) has immunosuppressive properties based on its ability to impair T-lymphocyte activation, particularly transcription of cytokine genes *(6)*. This occurs by the binding of cyclosporin A to intracellular receptors (termed immunophilins) which can, in turn, bind to and regulate the function of the phosphatase calcineurin. Calcineurin is normally required for activation of transcription factors essential for IL-2 production. Cyclosporin A can impair most T-cell responses in vivo and in vitro. This effect is readily reversible, such that lymphocytes from patients treated with cyclosporine can be washed free of the drug and function normally in culture. Such observations correlate with the clinical experience that therapeutic control of inflammatory disease by cyclosporine is rapidly lost if the drug is discontinued.

2.2. B-Lymphocyte Function and Autoantibody Production

In therapeutic doses, cyclophosphamide is toxic for B-lymphocytes, particularly activated B-cells. The selective sensitivity of activated cells can lead to the favorable outcome of profound reduction of autoantibody titers with less notable changes in total immunoglobulin levels. Following completion of a course of pulse iv cyclophosphamide, B-lymphocyte numbers recover more rapidly, at least in the peripheral blood of SLE patients, than do the numbers of CD4+ helper T-cells. Cyclophosphamide and azathioprine can both affect antibody production through impairment of helper T-cell function, not only by direct effects on B-cells.

In patients with RA treated with methotrexate, the titers of rheumatoid factor tend to fall. However, it is not clear whether this represents a direct action of methotrexate on rheumatoid factor producing B-cells or is a consequence of a reduction in disease activity brought about by other mechanisms. Although it is possible that increased adenosine release in lymphoid and inflammatory tissues, brought about by biochemical effects of methotrexate, could impair B-cell function, this issue has not been extensively studied. Cyclosporine A may have effects on transcription of specific genes in B-cells, but this is likely to be less important than indirect effects on antibody production mediated by inhibition of T-cell function.

2.3. Anti-inflammatory Effects

All of the cytotoxic agents used in the treatment of rheumatologic disease are likely to have important anti-inflammatory effects that not only help to explain long-term efficacy but that may also be of primary importance to the rapid onset of action of such agents in active, severe systemic disease *(1,2)*. Such anti-inflammatory properties have been most extensively studied in the case of methotrexate *(4,7)*. Methotrexate has been found to reduce neutrophil production of leukotriene B4, inhibit production and biological effects of interleukin-1 (IL-1), reduce synovial fluid concentration of tumor necrosis factor-α (TNF-α), reduce levels of IL-6 in RA, and stimulate production of a cytokine inhibitor. Such responses are the result of effects of methotrexate on inflammatory cells such as macrophages and neutrophils. The complexity of the biochemical mechanisms of action of methotrexate is still not fully understood. Traditionally viewed as a folate antagonist, it is nevertheless clear that it remains effective in patients with rheumatoid arthritis, even if folic acid is supplemented at doses as high as 28 mg per week.

Cyclosporin A has been shown to exert anti-inflammatory effects by altering signal transduction in a wide variety of cell types, in addition to its primary effect on T-cells *(8)*. Cyclophosphamide and azathioprine also have important anti-inflammatory effects, but these are even less well understood than for methotrexate. Available information, however, is sufficient to allow the conclusion that a strict distinction between immunosuppressive/cytotoxic and anti-inflammatory medications is not realistic. Alteration of cytokine production by nonlymphoid cells can, for example, lead to important changes in the pathogenicity of an immune response. It has been proposed that, in cyclophosphamide treatment of multiple sclerosis, normalization of elevated macrophage IL-12 synthesis by cyclophosphamide may be of special importance in curbing undesirable TH$_1$ immune responses, which are dependent on IL-12 *(9)*.

3. Use of Immunosuppressive and Cytotoxic Drugs in Rheumatic Diseases

3.1. Alkylators

Alkylating agents are the most potent immunosuppressive drugs currently used for the treatment of rheumatic diseases. As noted earlier, clinical effects differ depending on the dose, route of administration, and frequency of administration. For example, both daily oral cyclophosphamide and nitrogen mustard are highly effective in treatment of rheumatoid arthritis, but intravenous pulse cyclophosphamide is not. Cyclophosphamide, the most frequently used agent, will be reviewed in detail with additional comments regarding chlorambucil and nitrogen mustard.

3.1.1. Cyclophosphamide

Cyclophosphamide, a merchlorethamine derivitive, is inactive as administered and is metabolized in the liver to multiple active compounds with varying half-lives, immunosuppressive properties, and toxicities. There is, therefore, little quantitative data about the effect of renal and/or hepatic dysfunction on its metabolism, although the dose should be reduced in renal failure. It is readily absorbed orally, and oral and intravenous doses are considered to be equivalent in effect. Because metabolites appear sequentially over a 12-h period, allergic reactions may be delayed. Toxic metabolites such as acrolein may continue to appear in the urine for up to 24 h *(1,2,10)*.

Daily cyclophosphamide has been the mainstay of treatment for rheumatic diseases such as systemic vasculitis and Wegener's granulomatosis *(11)*. Its major disadvantage is high cumulative doses (i.e., 166 g after 3 yr of 150 mg/day!). Hence, in diseases traditionally treated with daily oral cyclophosphamide, such as Wegener's, alternate regimens, such as prednisone plus methotrexate, or sequential regimens such as prednisone plus cyclophosphamide followed by a substitution of methotrexate for cyclophosphamide, are being used *(12,13)*. If rapid onset of action is desired during the initiation of daily cyclophosphamide, it may be helpful either to begin with a dose of 4 mg/kg/d for 3 or 4 d and then reduce it to 1–2 mg/kg as a maintenance dose or give a single pulse of 500–750 mg/m^2 body surface area on d 1. In contrast to bolus cyclophosphamide, daily oral cyclophosphamide regimens appear to vary significantly in the incidence of infectious complications depending on the degree of leukopenia achieved. Specifically, those regimens in which the white blood cell count is kept above 3500 cells/mm^3 but *not* intentionally lowered to that level appear to have fewer complications than those in which leukopenia is deliberately induced *(12,14)*.

Monthly bolus cyclophosphamide is widely used in the treatment of rheumatic diseases, particularly systemic lupus. It is arguably the current standard of care in severe lupus nephritis *(11,15)*. Boluses usually are administered intravenously, although oral boluses are well absorbed if somewhat poorly tolerated. Vigorous hydration prior to and 24 h after drug administration may be supplemented by the use of MESNA (sodium 2-mercaptoethane sulfate) to avoid hemorrhagic cystitis and subsequent bladder cancer. Monthly administration results in approximately one-third the cumulative dose of drug compared to daily oral administration. The "maintenance" phase of treatment, using pulses every 3 mo, equals approximately one-tenth of the cumulative daily oral dose.

3.1.1.1. COMPLICATIONS OF CYCLOPHOSPHAMIDE

3.1.1.1.1. Infections

Infectious complications are frequent, although usually treatable. The occurrence of pneumocystis carinii pneumonia (PCP) is emphasized in recent studies *(14)*, the highest risk obtaining when administration of daily oral cyclophosphamide sufficient to produce leukopenia and lymphopenia is combined with high daily doses of prednisone. Prophylaxis for PCP is becoming widely accepted (i.e., with trimethoprim-sulfamethoxisole three times weekly or [in patients with sulfa allergy] with dapsone). Administration of greater than 20 mg daily of prednisone concomitantly with monthly pulse cyclophosphamide results in a substantial increase in infections compared with lower daily doses of prednisone *(10)*. With the availability of granulocyte colony stimulating factor, drug-induced leukopenias are less worrisome.

3.1.1.1.2. Gonadal Toxicity

Gonadal toxicity is a particular concern in patients treated with alkylating agents. The mean cumulative dose of cyclophosphamide required to cause gonadal failure in women of different ages is approximately 6 g over the age of 40, 10 g in women between the ages of 30 and 40; and 20 g in women between the ages of 20 and 30. Hence, even short courses of cyclophosphamide are a serious issue in some groups of patients, such as women over 30 who wish to bear children. Strategies for gonadal protection include use of estrogen-containing contraceptives or ovarian suppression with a gonadotropin-releasing hormone analog [e.g., "depot-Lupron" *(17)*]. Fetal malformations are frequently encountered when cyclophosphamide is administered during pregnancy, particularly during the first 10 wk of gestation. There are occasional reports of use of cyclophosphamide in critically ill women during the latter half of pregnancy without fetal malformation, although there may be other risks. Flawless contraception (ideally not reliance on condoms alone) is mandatory until 3–6 mo after cessation of the drug. Skilled gynecologic care, including at the very minimum, annual Papanicolaou (Pap) smears is required, because cyclophosphamide, like azathioprine, accelerates the development of human papilloma-virus (HPV)-related lesions. Patients with recent cervical dysplasia are at particularly high risk for developing worsening cervical atypia, and colposcopy should be considered at the time treatment is instituted. These patients should probably be followed with Pap smears every 6 mo *(11)*.

3.1.1.1.3. Bladder Toxicity

Hemorrhagic cystitis is a well-known complication of therapy with alkylating agents. It is attributed in part to the generation of acrolein during metabolism of cyclophosphamide. Other mechanisms, however, may also be involved. We have recently observed two patients with anuric renal failure who had been treated in intensive care units with standard boluses of cyclophosphamide for rheumatic disease and developed clinically significant hemorrhagic cystitis. Such patients should have bladder irrigation with a triple lumen catheter for at least 24 h after drug administration. The occurrence of hemorrhagic cystitis mandates discontinuation of cyclophosphamide and annual evaluation by a urologist, including cystoscopy and urine cytologic examination *(2)*. Cancers of the genitourinary tract are increased for decades after cyclophosphamide administration *(18)*.

3.1.1.1.4. Oncogenicity

With the exception of HPV-related malignancies, development of neoplasia in cyclophosphamide-treated patients is usually delayed 5 yr or more. The incidence of cancers of the urinary tract, particularly transitional cell carcinoma of the bladder, is increased for up to 20 yr after treatment and is particularly high in patients with prior hemorrhagic cystitis. Myelodysplastic syndromes, including monosomy-5 and monosomy-7, occur with high frequency in patients with cumulative doses of cyclophosphamide of 50–100 g or more. There is a substantial increase of cutaneous malignancies.

3.1.1.1.5. Other Toxicities

An important short-term complication is hyponatremia. This may result from a combination of the syndrome of inappropriate antidiuretic hormone resulting from cyclophosphamide administration and hydration with hypotonic fluids. Patients may develop significant central nervous system toxicity, including seizures, as a result. Cyclophosphamide is an antibiotic and its administration may trigger development of *clostridium difficile* colitis.

3.1.1.2. MANAGEMENT GUIDELINES: CYCLOPHOSPHAMIDE

Although highly toxic, cyclophosphamide is currently essential for the management of some rheumatic diseases. As a general rule, pauci-immune forms of vasculitis, such as Wegener's granulomatosis and microscopic polyarteritis nodosa, as well as polyarteritis nodosa have been treated with daily cyclophosphamide with or without an initial bolus. It is controversial whether or not pulse cyclophosphamide given monthly, or perhaps more frequently, can be as effective. Series in which monthly administration of cyclophosphamide yields satisfactory results tend, in the authors' opinion, to include patients who are less "sick." The authors have had several patients with Wegener's who have failed monthly bolus cyclophosphamide only to respond to daily oral cyclophosphamide. At the present time, treatment of the "sickest" patients who have active life-threatening disease is best initiated with daily therapy. Subsequent disease management, after control is established, is evolving. It is likely that for each disease, a specific "maintenance" regimen will be developed that is effective but less toxic. For example, substitution of methotrexate for cyclophosphamide when Wegener's granulomatosis is under good control is becoming widely accepted. Methotrexate is also becoming accepted as first-line therapy in milder Wegener's *(13,14)*. Rheumatoid vasculitis appears to respond well to daily cyclophosphamide but not to monthly bolus cyclophosphamide. There are no series establishing cyclophosphamide as effective therapy for Takayasu disease or giant-cell arteritis, nor have the authors been able to achieve substantial corticosteroid tapers with addition of cyclophosphamide.

Monthly bolus cyclophosphamide appears to be particularly effective in patients with autoantibody-mediated diseases, such as systemic lupus *(15)*. Administration of monthly bolus cyclophosphamide, in combination with initially high doses of corticosteroids (0.5–1 mg/kg/d), results in control of most cases of systemic lupus. Improved control of recalcitrant disease can sometimes be achieved with the addition of monthly boluses of methylprednisolone *(16)*. Other cyclophosphamide bolus regimens, such as every 2 wk, or every week, have been proposed. Because the mean time for recovery of circulating granulocytes and lymphocytes to normal levels is approximately 3 wk, the effects on circulating leukocyte populations and their precursors would clearly be different with more frequent administrations.

3.1.2. Chlorambucil

Chlorambucil, which like cyclophosphamide is derived from merchlorethamine, exerts its immunosuppressive effects by mechanisms that are poorly characterized but presumably similar to cyclophosphamide. It is administered orally in doses of 2–12 mg/d and has been used as intravenous pulse therapy in doses of 0.4–1.5 mg/kg, given as a single dose or two divided doses monthly.

From a practical standpoint, the two major features of chlorambucil are its slower onset of action than cyclophosphamide, which may expose patients to risk of a longer period of uncontrolled disease and its toxicity. Because it is not metabolized to acrolein, which is at least partially responsible for development of hemorrhagic cystitis and bladder cancer, it can be substituted for cyclophosphamide in patients who develop hemorrhagic cystitis. However, administration is probably associated with an even greater likelihood of developing other malignancies, particularly hematologic and cutaneous neoplasms *(11)*. Prolonged administration may result in myelodysplastic syndromes. A larger number of patients will develop insidious marrow suppression, characterized by the appearance of myelodysplastic changes and cytopenias.

There are considerable specialty-specific or even regional variations in the therapeutic use of chlorambucil for nonmalignant conditions. Historically, it has been extensively used in autoimmune ophthalmologic disease, although its advantages over daily or monthly cyclophosphamide in this regard are not established. In idiopathic membranous nephritis, daily administration of chlorambucil may be comparably effective to daily cyclophosphamide and superior to monthly bolus cyclophosphamide. Another protocol that has been used in membranous nephritis involves alternating months of chlorambucil with months of administration of corticosteroids.

In the treatment of rheumatic diseases, it is the authors' opinion that the current indications for chlorambucil are primarily those situations in which an alkylating agent is clearly needed, but the patient has developed hemorrhagic cystitis because of cyclophosphamide. Like cyclophosphamide, chlorambucil can potentially be used sequentially or in combination with methotrexate.

Chlorambucil is highly effective in treating both adult and juvenile rheumatoid arthritis. Series in both patient populations have amply demonstrated both clinical efficacy and a highly unsatisfactory rate of development of cutaneous and systemic malignancies *(11)*. The introduction of anti-tumor necrosis factor (TNF) therapies may further reduce indications for use of alkylating agents in adults or children with rheumatoid arthritis, except in the presence of severe vasculitis or associated complications such as corneal melting syndromes.

3.1.3. Nitrogen Mustard

Nitrogen mustard is an extremely potent alkylating agent that is active as administered, and therefore extremely locally toxic, capable of creating extensive tissue damage in the skin. Extensive tissue damage may result from extravasation. In addition, it directly suppresses autoimmune processes in the skin when applied topically. Patients with systemic disease usually receive only one or two "courses" of nitrogen mustard, consisting of one or two intravenous infusions totaling 0.2–0.4 mg/kg/d. The drug is profoundly and rapidly immunosuppressive in lupus nephritis and, before the days of potent diuretics, was reported to bring about a diuresis in patients with nephrotic syndrome within 3 or 4 d. It has recently been used in lupus nephritis unresponsive to intravenous cyclophosphamide treatment, with apparent success *(10)*.

3.2. Azathioprine

Azathioprine is administered orally in doses of 1–3 mg/kg/d, not to exceed 250 mg/d. It has occasionally been used intravenously (i.e., in patients with Crohn's disease) in an attempt to improve on its usual snail-like onset of action over weeks or months. The dose does not need to be adjusted in renal failure. The well-known interaction with allopurinol requires the dose of each to be reduced to one-third, if a decision is made to administer them together. Toxicity is increased in patients with thiopurine methyltransferase deficiency (0.3% of the population is homozygous, 11% heterozygous). Such patients are at increased risk for azathioprine-induced aplastic anemia *(11)*.

A major practical problem is bone marrow suppression, which usually occurs gradually in the setting of macrocytosis. This is particularly irksome in patients with lupus who may already have cytopenias. In such patients, a further decline of cell counts may require bone marrow biopsy to sort out peripheral consumption versus marrow suppression. In addition to frequently encountered gastrointestinal toxicities, including nausea, vomiting, and diarrhea, often encountered on initial administration, some patients will develop hepatic venoocclusive disease.

Although azathioprine has traditionally been viewed as a "steroid-sparing" agent (i.e., an agent that allows tapering of corticosteroids after clinical improvement has been achieved), it may have additional beneficial properties. It has most widely been used in systemic lupus, a disease in which it is less effective but also less toxic than cyclophosphamide. Initial "head-to-head" studies of azathioprine versus cyclophosphamide in severe lupus, particularly nephritis, demonstrated that azathioprine was less effective *(10)*. Clinical experience confirms that lupus patients who develop severe progressive disease while on full-dose azathioprine often rapidly improve when cyclophosphamide is substituted. However, there may be additional roles for this agent. The elegant studies by Esdaile et al. of immunosuppression of lupus nephritis showed that early addition of azathioprine probably helped avoid later use of cyclophosphamide *(19)*. Use of azathioprine combined with a low dose of cyclophosphamide, both administered daily orally, provided slightly better efficacy and markedly reduced side effects than a higher dose of daily oral cyclophosphamide in lupus nephritis patients in the long-term NIH study *(12)*. Recently, attention has been focused on using monthly bolus cyclophosphamide as "induction" therapy in lupus nephritis, followed by substitution of azathioprine for long-term maintenance *(20)*. Azathioprine is also a useful adjunct to corticosteroids in controlling recalcitrant "minor" manifestations of lupus such as pleurisy, arthritis, and skin disease.

Azathioprine and methotrexate are being used earlier in treating patients with inflammatory myositis. Exclusive use of corticosteroids predisposes to extensive complications, including steroid myopathies that interfere with evaluation of the therapeutic response. Azathioprine is also an effective disease-modifying antirheumatic drug (DMARD) in rheumatoid arthritis and may be safer than methotrexate in the elderly. However, the expanding list of newer DMARDs, particularly tumor necrosis factor (TNF) inhibitors, is likely to prompt a further reduction in the use of azathioprine in RA. Historically, azathioprine has been used as a second-line agent in treating systemic vasculitides, although it is rarely used at the present time. An exception is Behçet's disease in which azathioprine improved the control of severe disease manifestations, particularly ocular manifestations.

3.3. Methotrexate

The administration, monitoring and toxicity of methotrexate, particularly the evolving approach to hepatotoxicity, are the subject of numerous reviews *(11,21)* emphasizing a greater effort to maintain transaminases close to the normal range and correspondingly reduced inclination to perform surveillance liver biopsies. It is likely that the reader has extensive experience with this compound. Therefore, the discussion will focus on recent trends in administration and use that are of particular interest. It is increasingly evident that all patients on methotrexate for prolonged periods of time should be placed on folic acid. Administration of methotrexate without folic acid increases circulating levels of homocysteine, correspondingly increasing the risk of cardiovascular disease. In addition, as noted, the therapeutic effects of methotrexate appear to not directly relate to folate inhibition, and folate supplementation appears to reduce toxicity to a much greater degree than efficacy. In some cases, such as patients who develop nausea after methotrexate administration, folinic acid has also been employed. However, large doses of folinic acid (i.e., 5 mg daily) may reduce therapeutic efficacy. Folinic acid is, therefore, recommended for use only 1 or 2 d after each weekly administration of methotrexate *(22,23)*.

Until recently, the maximum dose of methotrexate employed in routine clinical practice as well as in clinical trials was 15 mg/wk. There is now ample evidence that increasing the dose to 20 or even 25 mg weekly in appropriately selected patients with rheumatoid arthritis may result in significantly improved efficacy. Doses of >15 mg/wk may be much better tolerated when the drug is administered subcutaneously, rather than orally. Subcutaneous administration not only improves tolerance but also can sometimes increase bioavailability. Therefore, unexpected toxicity may occur if oral methotrexate is switched to parenteral methotrexate at the same time that the dose is increased.

Methotrexate pneumonitis remains a rare but potentially catastrophic complication. Affected patients may present with cough, dyspnea, and bilateral or unilateral pulmonary infiltrates. Because physicians who do not routinely use methotrexate are frequently unaware of this complication, patients must, therefore, be educated to specifically raise the issue of methotrexate pneumonitis in appropriate circumstances. The small number of patients in the literature who have been rechallenged with methotrexate after methotrexate-induced pneumonitis have fared particularly badly, with some deaths reported *(10,24,25)*.

The most widely studied application of methotrexate is the treatment of rheumatoid arthritis, for which it remains the cornerstone of modern therapy. Use of higher doses, parenteral administration, and awareness that incremental increases in methotrexate dosage in patients who are initially controlled but lose control may be efficacious have contributed to its success. Because remissions are extraordinarily rare in rheumatoid arthritis patients treated with any therapeutic regimen, there is almost always a need for improved disease control even in patients on full-dose methotrexate. The two major strategies employed are (1) the addition of hydroxychloroquine and sulfasalazine to methotrexate (triple therapy) and *(2)* the addition of TNF inhibitors. These two strategies have not been compared head to head.

Methotrexate is emerging as an important agent in the treatment of systemic vasculitides, particularly, as noted, for Wegener's granulomatosis. It may have steroid-sparing properties in Takayasu disease. It is clearly effective in a variety of inflammatory arthropathies such as psoriatic arthritis. It is the authors' opinion that in systemic lupus, conventional doses of methotrexate are particularly helpful in individuals with inflammatory synovitis, with more limited benefits in other manifestations.

3.4. Cyclosporine

Cyclosporine is administered orally, twice daily, and monitored with trough levels exactly 12 h after administration. Absorption (about 30%) varies with different preparations and even with the concomitant use of grapefruit juice. Maintenance requirements fall as tissues are saturated, mandating dose reduction. Numerous disparate factors alter drug levels, resulting in at least 10-fold variation in levels achieved in individual patients receiving comparable doses. These factors, which have been reviewed elsewhere *(11)*, include levels of serum low-density lipoproteins and magnesium, hepatic dysfunction, cystic fibrosis, and drugs that increase excretion (rifampin, phenytoin, phenobarbital) or decrease excretion (calcium channel blockers, macrolide antibiotics, progesterone). Hence, this compound is a leading contender for the dubious distinction of being the most inconvenient of immunosuppressive drugs to administer. Although monitoring of drug levels is not specified in the product information for treatment of RA, it is prudent to monitor levels in patients with RA *(11)*.

Renal insufficiency is the side effect of greatest import in management of patients with rheumatic diseases on cyclosporine. The occurrence of renal insufficiency, as assessed by the notoriously insensitive criterion of rising creatinine levels, is almost uniform at doses of 8 mg/kg/d and gradually falls, along with therapeutic efficacy, as the dose is reduced. Toxicity has been reported to be related to the dose administered and/or blood levels attained. Studies of cyclosporine-treated patients with no underlying renal disease (e.g., uveitis) include examples of dramatic bandlike scarring in a vascular distribution in renal biopsies from patients who have relatively modest changes in renal function *(11)*. This agent, therefore, should not be used as a first-line drug in rheumatic diseases that may produce renal dysfunction, in the absence of controlled clinical trials. Particular caution is required in the presence of concomitant hypertension, a complication reported in up to 50–80% of transplant patients and 11–50% of nontransplant patients receiving cyclosporine. Hypertension, even of mild degree, is regarded as a major risk factor for eventual development of renal insufficiency in patients with nephritis.

Other adverse effects of cyclosporine, such as gout, infection, lymphoproliferative disorders, central nervous system toxicity, tremor, paresthesias, hirsutism, gingival hypertrophy and other cosmetic changes, and hemolytic uremic syndrome have been reviewed elsewhere *(11)*. The resemblance of vaso-occlusive changes (e.g., in the kidney) to scleroderma-induced vascular pathology leads one to seriously question the use of cyclosporine in patients with scleroderma and related illnesses.

In addition to its mechanisms of action that differ from other immunosuppressives, potential advantages of cyclosporine include lack of bone marrow suppression, relative safety in pregnancy *(26)*, and compatibility with other agents, such as methotrexate and azathioprine. The ability of cyclosporine to nonspecifically inhibit renal protein excretion, a potentially important consideration in the management of nephrotic syndrome, is controversial.

Therapeutic use of cyclosporine in the rheumatic diseases in the past has focused on rheumatoid arthritis *(2)*. In sufficient doses (e.g., 5 mg/kg), cyclosporine appears to be capable of retarding radiographic progression and producing significant responses, in association with unacceptable nephrotoxicity. Used in combination with methotrexate at lower doses, cyclosporine produces better results than methotrexate alone with less toxicity than higher-dose cyclosporine. We have used this regimen with success in refractory cases of RA, but only rarely. As with azathioprine, the availability of TNF inhibitors will limit use of cyclosporine in RA. Patients with systemic lupus appear to respond modestly to cyclosporine in controlled trials, although the mechanism of action is unclear (2). Clinical improvement is not, in general, accompanied by serologic improvement. Studies in nephritis have suggested stabilization of serum creatinine levels and reduction of proteinuria. We recently treated a women with onset of severe diffuse proliferative nephritis and approximately 15–20 g/d proteinuria during pregnancy with bolus steroids, azathioprine, cyclosporine, and daily steroids without benefit. After the end of pregnancy, disease activity was easily controlled with bolus cyclophosphamide. Anecdotal reports and uncontrolled series suggest that cyclosporine may be effective in some patients with other rheumatic diseases.

3.5. Mycophenolate Mofetil

Mycophenolate appears to be superior to azathioprine for many applications in transplantation and is reported to combine immunosuppressive effects similar to those of azathioprine with increased suppression of autoantibody formation (27). A variety of inflammatory diseases ranging from psoriasis to Takayasu disease have been reported to respond to this agent, and initial abstracts and anecdotal reports suggest that it may be particularly effective in severe systemic lupus.

4. Summary

Use of cytotoxic drugs in rheumatic diseases has been largely empiric, with understanding of the mechanism of action of some of the most widely employed agents, such as methotrexate, lagging behind proof of efficacy. Improved understanding of the mechanisms by which these agents are effective, as well as toxic, has been associated with more rational and successful approaches to therapy and better control of toxicity. Using agents that are not new, such as methotrexate, cyclophosphamide, and azathioprine, we are able to achieve clinical outcomes in illnesses such as lupus or RA that are clearly superior to those achieved two or three decades ago. Most rheumatic diseases can be well controlled over the short term; long-term control with acceptable toxicity remains a challenge in many cases.

References

1. McCune, W. J. and Fox, D. A. (1999) Immunosuppressive agents—biologic effects *in vivo* and *in vitro*, in *Lupus: Molecular and Cellular Pathogenesis* (Tsokos, G. C. and Kammer, G., eds.), Humana, Totowa, NJ, pp. 612–641.
2. Fox, D. A. and McCune, W. J. (1989) Immunologic and clinical effects of cytotoxic drugs used in the treatment of rheumatoid arthritis and systemic lupus erythematosus, in *Therapy of Autoimmune Diseases, Concepts Immunopathology 7* (Cruse, J. M. and Lewis, R. E., eds.), Karger, Basel, pp. 20–78.
3. Proietti, E., Greco, G., Garrone, B., Baccarini, S., Mauri, C., Venditti, M., et al. (1998) Importance of cyclophosphamide-induced bystander effect on T cells for a successful tumor eradication in response to adoptive immunotherapy in mice. *J. Clin. Invest.* **101,** 429–441.
4. Cronstein, B. N. (1996) Molecular therapeutics—methotrexate and its mechanism of action. *Arthritis Rheum.* **39(12),** 1951–1960.

5. Genestier, L., Paillot, R., Fournel, S., Ferraro, C., Miossec, P., and Revillard, J.-P. (1998) Immunosuppressive properties of methotrexate: Apoptosis and clonal deletion of activated peripheral T cells. *J. Clin. Invest.* **102,** 322–328.
6. Schreiber, S. L. and Crabtree, G. R. (1992) The mechanism of action of cyclosporin A and FK506. *Immunol. Today* **13,** 136.
7. Seitz, M., Zwicker, M., and Loetscher, P. (1998) Effects of methotrexate on differentiation of monocytes and production of cytokine inhibitors by monocytes. *Arthritis Rheum.* **41,** 2032–2038.
8. Misra, U. K., Gawdi, G., and Pizzo, S. V. (1998) Cyclosporin A inhibits inositol 1,4,5-triphosphate binding to its receptors and release of calcium from intracellular stores in peritoneal macrophages. *Immunology* **161,** 6122–6127.
9. Comabella, M., Balashov, K., Issazadeh, S., Smith, D., Weiner, H. L., and Khoury, S. J. (1998) Elevated interleukin-12 in progressive multiple sclerosis correlates with disease activity and is normalized by pulse cyclophosphamide therapy. *J. Clin. Invest.* **102,** 671–678.
10. McCune, W. J. (1997) Cytotoxic drugs, in *Dubois' Lupus Erythematosus,* 5th ed. (Wallace, D. J. and Hahn, B. H., eds.), Williams & Wilkins, Baltimore, pp. 1163–1180.
11. Lynch, J. P. and McCune, W. J. (1997) State of the art: immunosuppressive and cytotoxic pharmacotherapy for pulmonary disorders. *Am. J. Respir. Crit. Care Med.* **155,** 395–420.
12. Lynch, J. P., III and Hoffman, G. S. (1998) Wegener's granulomatosis: controversies and current concepts. Comprehens. Ther. **24,** 421–440.
13. Langford, C. A., Sneller, M. C., and Hoffman, G. S. (1997) Methotrexate use in systemic vasculitis. *Rheum. Dis. Clin. North Am.* **23,** 841–853.
14. Ognibene, F. P., Shelhamer, J. H., Hoffman, G. S., Kerr, G. S., Reda, D., Fauci, A. S., et al. (1995) Pneumocystis carinii pneumonia: a major complication of immunosuppressive therapy in patients with Wegener's granulomatosis. *Am. J. Respir. Crit. Care Med.* **151,** 795–799.
15. Austin, H. A., Klippel, J. H., Balow, J. E., le Rice, N. G., Steinberg, A. D., Plotz, P. H., et al. (1986) Therapy of lupus nephritis: controlled trial of prednisone and cytotoxic drugs. *N. Engl. J. Med.* **314,** 614–619.
16. Gourley, M. F., Austin, H. A., III, Scott, D., Yarboro, C. H., Vaughan, E. M., Muir, J., et al. (1996) Methylprednisolone and cyclophosphamide, alone or in combination, in patients with lupus nephritis. A randomized, controlled trial. *Ann. Int. Med.* **125,** 549–557.
17. Slater, C. A., Liang, M. H., McCune, W. J., Christman, G. M., and Laufer, M. R. (1999) Preserving ovarian function in patients receiving cyclophosphamide. *Lupus* **8,** 3–10.
18. Talar-Williams, C., Hijazi, Y. M., Walther, M. M., Linehan, M. W., Hallahan, C. W., Lubensky, I., et al. (1996) Cyclophosphamide-induced cystitis and bladder cancer in patients with Wegener granulomatosis. *Ann. Intern. Med.* **124,** 477–484.
19. Esdaile, J. M., Joesph, L., MacKenzie, T., Kashgarian, M., and Hayslett, J. P. (1994) The benefit of early treatment with immunosuppressive agents in lupus nephritis. *J. Rheum.* **21,** 2046–2051.
20. Chan, T., Li, F., Wong, R. W. S., Wong, K., Chan, K., and Cheng, I. K. P. Sequential therapy for diffuse proliferative and membranous lupus nephritis: cyclophosphamide and prednisolone followed by azathioprine and prednisolone. *Nephron* **71,** 321–327.
21. Weinblatt, M. E., Maier, A. L., Fraser, P. A., and Coblyn, J. S. (1998) Longterm prospective study of methotrexate in rheumatoid arthritis: conclusion after 132 months of therapy. *J. Rheum.* **25,** 238–242.
22. van Ede, A. E., Laan, R. F., Blom, H. J., De Abreu, R. A., and van de Putte, L. B. (1998) Methotrexate in rheumatoid arthritis: an update with focus on mechanisms involved in toxicity. *Semi. Arthritis Rheum.* **27,** 277–292.

23. Morgan, S. L., Baggott, J. E., Lee, J. Y., and Alarcon, G. S. (1998) Folic acid supplementation prevents deficient blood folate levels and hyperhomocysteinemia during longterm, low dose methotrexate therapy for rheumatoid arthritis: implications for cardiovascular disease prevention. *J. Rheum.* **25,** 441–446.
24. Kremer, J. M., Alarcon, G. S., Weinblatt. M. E., Kaymakcian, M. V., Macaluso, M., Cannon, G. W., et al. Clinical, laboratory, radiographic, and histopathologic features of methotrexate-associated lung injury in patients with rheumatoid arthritis: a multicenter study with literature review. *Arthritis Rheum.* **40,** 1829–1837.
25. Alarcon, G. S., Kremer, J. M., Macaluso, M., Weinblatt, M. E., Cannon, G. W., Palmer, W. R., et al. (1997) Risk factors for methotrexate-induced lung injury in patients with rheumatoid arthritis. A multicenter, case-control study. Methotrexate–Lung Study Group. *Ann. Int. Med.* **127,** 356–364.
26. Gaughan, W. J., Morita, M. J., Radomski, J. S., Burke, J. F. Jr., and Armenti, V. T. (1994) National Transplantation Pregnancy Registry: report on outcomes in cyclosporine-treated female kidney transplant recipients with an interval from transplant to pregnancy of greater than five years. *Transplantation* **57,** 502–506.
27. Sievers, T. M., Rossi, S. J., Ghobrial, R. M., Arriola, E., Nishimura, P., Kawano, M., et al. (1997) Mycophenolate Mofetil. *Pharmacotherapy* **17,** 1178–1197.

30

Complement Inhibitors

Savvas C. Makrides

1. Introduction

The inappropriate activation of the complement system is at the core of a long list of disease pathologies that affect the immune, renal, cardiovascular, neurological, and other systems in the body *(1)*. During the last two decades, the molecular cloning of the many components of the complement pathway has led to a detailed understanding of the mechanisms of complement activation in inflammation. This, in turn, has allowed for the potential for drug development based on the genetic engineering of receptors and other components of the complement pathway, as well as the expression of human transgenes in animal organs. These developments hold promise for the therapeutic management of complement-mediated injury in certain diseases.

The objective here is to review published studies on the use of inhibitors (Table 1) for the therapeutic abrogation of pathologic complement activation. Many original references are regrettably not cited because of editorial limits on the bibliography, and the reader is referred to recent reviews on specific topics, including an overview of the complement system *(2)*, clinical complementology *(1)*, and the use of complement inhibitors for therapy *(3)*.

2. Regulation of the Complement System

The complement system consists of three linked biochemical cascades, the classical, alternative, and lectin pathways (Fig. 1). The system is regulated at multiple levels temporally as well as spatially. This regulation facilitates recognition of self from foreign tissue and, therefore, allows for control over the potent tissue-damaging capabilities of complement activation. What follows is a brief description of the complement system, as this topic has been covered in detail in this volume (Chapter 9) and elsewhere *(2)*.

2.1. The Classical Pathway

The classical pathway is usually initiated when a complex of antigen and IgM or IgG antibody binds to the first component of complement, C1. Activation of this step of complement is regulated by the C1 inhibitor, which binds to C1r and C1s and dissociates them from C1q. Activated C1 cleaves both C4 and C2 to generate C4a and C4b, as well as C2a and C2b. The C4b and C2a fragments combine to form the C3 convertase, which, in turn, cleaves the third component of complement, C3, to form

Table 1
Protein Inhibitors of Complement Activation

Protein	Identity	Site/mode of action
TP10 (sCR1)	Soluble CR1	C3/C5 convertases, classical/alternative
sCR1-SLe^x	sCR1 glycosylated with SLe^x	C3/C5 convertases, classical/alternative selectin-mediated
sCR1(desLHR-A)	sCR1 minus LHR-A	C3/C5 convertases, alternative
sCR1(desLHR-A)-SLe^x	sCR1 minus LHR-A glycosylated with SLe^x	C3/C5 convertases, alternative, selectin-mediated
sCD59	Soluble CD59	MAC assembly
sDAF	Soluble DAF	C3/C5 convertases, classical/alternative
sMCP	Soluble MCP	Factor I cofactor activity
C1-INH	C1 esterase inhibitor	C1 inactivation, classical
CAB-2	Soluble chimeric MCP-DAF	C3/C5 convertases, classical/alternative
DC	Membrane-bound chimeric NH$_2$–DAF–CD59–GPI	C3/C5 convertases, classical/alternative, MAC assembly
5G1.1-SC	Anti-human C5 humanized scFv	C5, MAC assembly
C1qR	66-kDa C1qR, detergent solubilized	Classical
C5aR antagonists	C5a oligopeptide analogs	C5aR
Factor H	SCR 1-4	C3/C5 convertases, alternative
Factor J	Glycoprotein	Classical/alternative

Source: Modified from ref. *3* with permission from the publisher.

C3a and C3b. The binding of C3b to the C3 convertase yields the C5 convertase, which cleaves C5 into C5a and C5b, the latter becoming part of the membrane attack complex (MAC) (*see* Subheading 2.4.). Activators other than antibodies are also capable of initiating the classical pathway. For example, β-amyloid activates complement in the brain, raising the possibility of therapeutic intervention in Alzheimer's disease.

The three peptides released during these steps, C3a, C4a, and C5a, are known as anaphylatoxins, C5a being the most potent one. The anaphylatoxins mediate multiple reactions in the acute inflammatory response, including smooth-muscle contraction, changes in vascular permeability, histamine release from mast cells, and neutrophil chemotaxis, platelet activation and aggregation, as well as upregulation of adhesion molecules, which can also play key roles in neutrophil recruitment. The anaphylatoxins are rapidly inactivated by carboxypeptidase N, which cleaves the carboxyl-terminal arginyl residue from each anaphylatoxin, thus converting them into their des-Arg forms.

The C3 and C5 convertases of the classical pathway (Fig. 1) are controlled by members of the regulators of complement activation (RCA) family. This protein family includes the membrane-bound regulators complement receptor type 1 (CR1; C3b/C4b receptor; CD35), complement receptor type 2 (CR2; CD21; Epstein–Barr virus receptor), mem-

Complement Inhibitors

[Diagram of complement pathways: Classical, Lectin, and Alternative pathways showing cascade from activation through C3/C5 convertases to Membrane Attack Complex, with regulators C1-INH, C4-bp, CR1, DAF, MCP, Factor H, Anaphylatoxin inactivator (Carboxypeptidase N), Vitronectin, CD59, Clusterin]

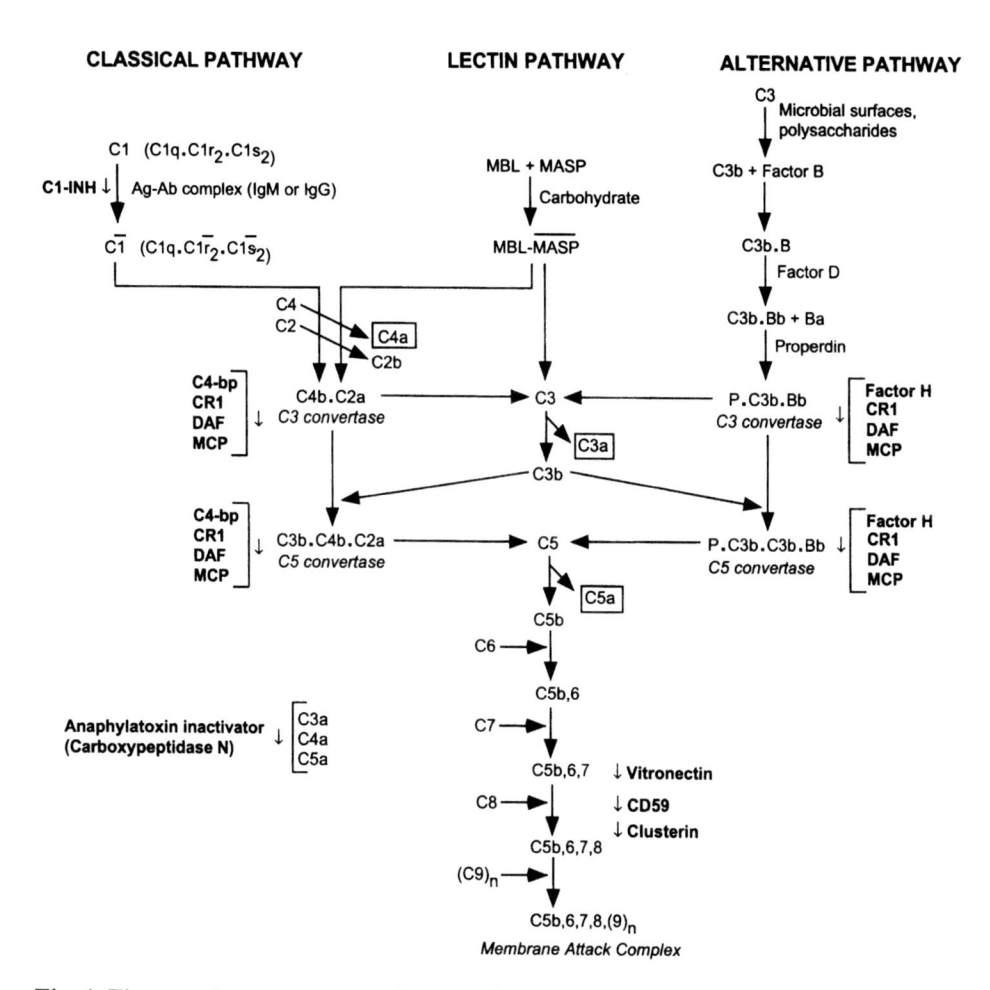

Fig. 1. The complement system and its regulators. The classical pathway is usually activated by complexes of antigen and IgM or IgG antibody classes. The alternative pathway is activated by microbial surfaces and complex polysaccharides (e.g., yeast cell walls, endotoxins, viral particles). The lectin pathway is effected in an antibody- and C1q-independent mechanism through the binding of mannose-binding lectin (MBL) and its associated MASP to carbohydrates. In all three pathways, C3 is converted into C3b by the C3 convertases. In addition, in the lectin pathway, C3 can be cleaved directly by MASP. C5 is converted into C5b by the C5 convertases. The three anaphylatoxins, C3a, C4a, and C5a, are released during the various enzymatic reactions of the cascade. The membrane attack complex is formed by the sequential binding of C5b to C6, C7, C8, and C9. The various activation reactions are subject to fine regulation by soluble (C1 inhibitor, C4bp, factor H, vitronectin, clusterin) as well as membrane-bound (CR1, DAF, MCP, CD59) proteins. The anaphylatoxins are inactivated by carboxypeptidase N.

brane cofactor protein (MCP; CD46; measles virus receptor), decay-accelerating factor (DAF; CD55), as well as the serum proteins factor H and C4b-binding protein (C4bp).

2.2. The Alternative Pathway

This arm of the complement system is triggered by microbial surfaces and a variety of complex polysaccharides. C3b, formed by the spontaneous low-level cleavage of

C3, can bind to nucleophilic targets on cell surfaces and form a complex with factor B that is subsequently cleaved by factor D (Fig. 1). The resulting C3 convertase is stabilized by the binding of properdin (P) which increases the half-life of this convertase. Cleavage of C3 and binding of an additional C3b to the C3 convertase give rise to the C5 convertase of the alternative pathway (Fig. 1). Subsequent reactions are common to both pathways and lead to the formation of the MAC. The C3 and C5 convertases of the alternative pathway are controlled by CR1, DAF, MCP, and factor H. These regulators differ in their mode of action, that is, their decay-accelerating activity (ability to dissociate convertases) and ability to serve as required cofactors in the degradation of C3b or C4b by factor I.

2.3. The Lectin PathM

An additional antibody- and C1q-independent mechanism for activation of the complement pathway involves the binding of mannose-binding lectin (MBL) to carbohydrates. Although MBL was initially termed mannan-binding protein by its discoverers *(4)*, persuasive arguments have been presented in favor of the MBL nomenclature *(5)*. MBL is a member of the collectins, a group of C-type (Ca^{2+} dependent) lectins, and it recognizes mannose or *N*-acetylglucosamine on the surface of microorganisms. Although this mechanism of complement activation is known as the lectin pathway, MBL is the only serum lectin known to date to activate complement. MBL is associated with a serine protease termed MASP (MBL-associated serine protease). MASP can cleave both C4 and C2 to generate the C3 convertase C4bC2a, and it can also cleave C3 (Fig. 1). The lectin pathway has been recently reviewed in detail *(5,6)*.

2.4. The Membrane Attack Complex

The C5 convertases in both the classical and alternative pathways cleave C5 to produce C5a and C5b. Thereafter, C5b sequentially binds to C6, C7, and C8 to form C5b-8 which catalyzes the polymerization of C9 to form the MAC. This structure inserts into target membranes and causes cell lysis. However, deposition of small amounts of MAC on cell membranes of nucleated cells may mediate a range of cellular processes without causing cell death *(7)*.

Three different molecules are known to be involved in the control of MAC formation *(2)*. Vitronectin controls fluid-phase MAC by binding to the C5b-7 complex, preventing its insertion into membranes. Similarly, clusterin blocks fluid-phase MAC by binding to the C5b-7 complex. CD59 blocks MAC formation by binding to C8 and C9 and inhibiting the incorporation and subsequent polymerization of C9.

3. Inhibitors of Complement Activation

3.1. Modified Native Complement Components

3.1.1. sCR1

The molecular properties of CR1 have been reviewed (3). Among the members of the RCA family, CR1 is the only one that possesses decay-accelerating activity for both C3 and C5 convertases in both the classical and alternative pathways, as well as factor I cofactor activity for the degradation of both C3b and C4b. Recent data indicate that C1q binds specifically to human CR1 *(8)*. Thus, CR1 recognizes all three complement opsonins, namely C3b, C4b, and C1q.

A soluble version of recombinant human CR1 (sCR1) lacking the transmembrane and cytoplasmic domains was produced and shown to retain all the known functions of the native CR1 *(9)*. Although thrombolytic agents have been used effectively in ischemic myocardium to induce reperfusion, blood reflow into ischemic tissue may induce necrosis resulting from complement activation, neutrophil accumulation in the microvasculature, and consequent damage to the endothelium *(10)*. Administration of sCR1 in a rat model of ischemia–reperfusion injury reduced myocardial infarct size by 44% assessed at 7 d postdosing and minimized the accumulation of neutrophils within the infarcted area, probably because of a decreased generation of the anaphylatoxin C5a *(9)*. In addition, sCR1 attenuated the deposition of the C5b-9 membrane attack complex. This was the first demonstration that a recombinant-soluble form of a member of the RCA family might provide a potential therapeutic agent in inflammation. sCR1 has since been shown to reduce complement-mediated tissue injury in animal models of a wide range of human acute and chronic inflammatory diseases. These include dermal vascular reactions, lung injury, trauma, myasthenia gravis, glomerulonephritis, multiple sclerosis, allergic reactions, and asthma. Moreover, sCR1 protects against vascular injury in allografts and attenuates hyperacute rejection in xenografts (reviewed in ref. *3*). The ability of sCR1 to block activation of both the classical as well as the alternative pathways has been thought to potentially reduce its therapeutic value because it inhibits generation of C3b, a C3 opsonic product that is critical for antibacterial defenses. To date, however, there is no credible evidence that sCR1 compromises bacterial defenses in animal models of inflammation.

3.1.2. sCR1(desLHR-A)

A mutant version of sCR1 lacking LHR-A was constructed with the objective of generating a selective inhibitor of the alternative pathway *(11)*. Indeed, sCR1(desLHR-A) was shown to be quantitatively equivalent to sCR1 in its ability to inhibit the alternative pathway in vitro *(11)*. On the other hand, as expected, sCR1(desLHR-A) was less effective than sCR1 in blocking activation of the classical pathway in vitro. Both sCR1(desLHR-A) and sCR1 exhibited equal capacities to serve as a cofactor in the degradation of fluid-phase C3b by factor I *(11)*.

The availability of sCR1(desLHR-A) facilitated examination of the relative contributions of the classical and alternative pathways in a model of discordant xenotransplantation in which an isolated perfused heart from a rabbit is exposed to human plasma that serves as a complement source. The interaction of rabbit heart tissue with plasma activates complement, leading to the production of anaphylatoxins and the generation of the C5b-9 membrane attack complex. Both sCR1 and sCR1(desLHR-A) had a cardioprotective effect in the rabbit heart perfused with human plasma. Complement activation was also shown to attenuate endothelium-dependent relaxation in rabbit tissue *(12)*. This attenuation was dependent on the formation of C5b-9 via the classical and alternative pathways, as demonstrated through the use of human serum depleted in factor B, C2 or C8. Murohara et al. *(13)* examined the relative contribution of the classical and alternative pathways in a rat model of ischemia and reperfusion injury using either C1 esterase inhibitor (*see* Subheading 3.1.7.), a classical pathway inhibitor, or sCR1(desLHR-A). These authors concluded that both the classical and alternative pathways contribute to reperfusion injury in myocardial ischemia by a neutrophil-dependent mechanism.

3.1.3. sCR1-SLe^x

This compound is aimed at the simultaneous inhibition of both complement activation and neutrophil recruitment at sites of inflammation (Charles Rittershaus, personal communication). The rationale behind the development of this complement inhibitor is based on the current understanding of the interaction between complement and selectins in inflammation, and the demonstration that C5a upregulates P-selectin. The migration of leukocytes to sites of inflammation is orchestrated by chemoattractants and a large number of adhesion molecules that are involved in cell–cell and cell–matrix interactions *(14)*. The selectins, L-, P-, and E-selectins, participate in the initial "rolling" adhesions, bringing the circulating leukocytes into close proximity to chemoattractants released from endothelial cells of the vessel wall. Chemoattractants bind to G-protein-coupled receptors on leukocytes, signaling the activation of integrins, which, together with members of the Ig superfamily, effect the arrest and subsequent migration of leukocytes into the tissue *(14)*.

Selectin function, unlike that of most other adhesion molecules, appears to be restricted to interactions between leukocytes and the vascular endothelium. The selectins bind carbohydrate ligands containing fucose, including sialyl Lewis^x (SLe^x) [Neu5Acα2-3Galβ1-4(Fucα1-3)GlcNAc–]. Other proteins, including PSGL-1, CD34, and GlyCAM-1, have been identified as high-affinity ligands for selectins, and there is diversity of opinions as to the identities of the physiologically relevant ligands for selectins. Nevertheless, the observation that SLe^x can inhibit neutrophil adhesion mediated by both E- and P-selectins led to vigorous efforts to develop compounds for the therapeutic disruption of the selectin–SLe^x interaction in inflammation (reviewed in ref. *3*). The biological effects of many of these compounds in selectin-dependent animal models of inflammation have been critically examined *(15)*. Conflicting results obtained in animal models using SLe^x synthetic analogs may in part be explained by the dosing regimes employed by the different investigators and the relatively short half-life of the SLe^x analog. Of key importance is the high molar concentration of compound required to inhibit reaction by 50% (IC$_{50}$), 0.5–1.0 mM of the monovalent SLe^x tetrasaccharide in inhibiting E- and P-selectin-dependent adhesion of leukocytes, as determined in static adhesion assays. SLe^x multivalency appears to enhance its binding to L-selectin *(16)*.

In order to control the damaging effects of both complement and neutrophil activation during inflammation, sCR1 was produced in a mammalian cell line capable of SLe^x glycosylation *(17)*. It was shown that sCR1 purified from conditioned media possessed SLe^x moieties on the N-linked oligosaccharides. sCR1 potentially has 25 *N*-glycosylation sites and, although not every Asn-X-Ser(Thr) sequon is an efficient oligosaccharide acceptor, it is expected that sCR1-SLe^x would be extensively decorated with SLe^x moieties. Thus, in addition to blocking complement activation, the potential multivalent interactions between sCR1-SLe^x and its selectin counterligands might render this molecule particularly effective at inhibiting neutrophil activation and recruitment to sites of inflammation on the endothelial surface. It is important to determine the half-life of sCR1-SLe^x and, especially, whether it localizes to sites of inflammation.

3.1.4. sDAF

Soluble versions of decay-accelerating factor (DAF), (sDAF) have been shown to inhibit complement activation in vitro as well as in the reversed passive Arthus reaction in guinea pigs. The clinical usefulness of a complement blocker may be enhanced by several properties. These include the ability to inhibit the C5 convertases of both classical and alternative pathways, a high affinity for the C3b and C4b components of the convertases, the irreversible inactivation of the convertases, and the ability to recycle in order to block multiple convertases. The modest inhibitory activity of sDAF and its lack of factor I cofactor activity limit its therapeutic potential as a complement blocker.

3.1.5. sMCP

Membrane cofactor protein (MCP) has factor I cofactor activity but no decay-accelerating activity. It acts jointly with DAF, which has decay-accelerating activity but no cofactor activity to block C3b/C4b deposition on cell membranes *(2)*. A recombinant soluble form of MCP (sMCP) was shown to inhibit immune-complex-mediated inflammation in the reverse passive Arthus reaction model in rats. As in the case of sDAF, the single activity of sMCP limits its potential as an effective therapeutic reagent. However, sMCP may prove to be a valuable reagent in combination with other complement inhibitors (*see* Subheading 3.2.).

3.1.6. sCD59

CD59 is a single-chain glycoprotein which is GPI-anchored to cell membranes. CD59 functions as an inhibitor of the formation of the MAC on cells by binding to C8 and C9, thereby blocking the addition of polymerized C9 molecules. Soluble forms of recombinant CD59 (sCD59) have been shown to possess complement inhibitory activity in vitro. The potential usefulness of sCD59 as a therapeutic complement blocker may be limited by its lack of certain functional properties, as discussed earlier. Moreover, the late stage in the complement cascade at which CD59 acts (Fig. 1) leaves unaffected the generation of anaphylatoxins and their pathological sequelae. Nevertheless, blocking formation of the terminal components of the complement cascade has been shown to be beneficial in several animal models of complement-mediated diseases.

3.1.7. C1 Inhibitor

C1 inhibitor, a member of the "serpin" family of serine protease inhibitors, is a glycosylated plasma protein that prevents fluid-phase C1 activation *(18)*. C1 inhibitor regulates the classical pathway of complement activation (Fig. 1) by blocking the active site of C1r and C1s and dissociating them from C1q. Studies of the role of complement activation in myocardial ischemia and reperfusion injury have utilized C1 inhibitor in feline, rat, and pig models *(3)*. All these studies have demonstrated that blocking the classical pathway of complement activation by C1 inhibitor is an effective means of protecting ischemic myocardial tissue from reperfusion injury.

3.1.8. C1q Receptor

Several types of human C1q receptors (C1qR) have been described. These include the 60- to 67-kDa receptor (calreticulin), referred to as cC1qR because it binds the collagen like domain of C1q, a 126-kDa receptor that modulates monocyte phagocytosis, designated C1qR$_p$, and a 28- to 33-kDa protein isolated and cloned from Raji cells, termed gC1qR because it interacts preferentially with the globular domains of C1q. A recent study showed that CR1 also acts as a receptor for C1q *(8)*. Evidence indicates that gC1qR may not be a membrane-bound molecule but, rather, a secreted soluble protein with affinity for the globular regions of C1q *(19)*. Thus, it may act as a fluid-phase regulator of complement activation. Furthermore, other data are consistent with the molecular properties of gC1qR. Thus, the cDNA sequence encodes a protein that lacks a membrane-spanning domain or a consensus sequence for GPI-anchoring. It is possible, however, that under certain conditions, gC1qR may be surface expressed at low level or it may bind to cell membranes as a complex with other fluid-phase molecules *(19)*. The ability of C1qR (66 kDa) to inhibit the classical pathway of complement has been demonstrated in vitro. Membrane-associated C1qR as well as detergent-solubilized C1qR, purified from polymorphonuclear leukocytes and endothelial cells, blocked complement-mediated lysis of C1q-sensitized erythrocytes.

The mechanisms by which the different types of C1qR regulate complement activation in vivo, and the physiological significance of the putative fluid-phase C1qR remain unclear. However, the studies cited here and the demonstration that C1q is required for immune complexes to stimulate endothelial cells to express adhesion molecules suggest a potential therapeutic use in preventing vascular injury.

3.2. Chimeric Molecules

3.2.1. DAF-CD59

The molecular fusion of different complement regulatory proteins has been used to create chimeric molecules endowed with novel functions. Fodor and colleagues *(20)* constructed two such chimeric complement inhibitors for cell-surface expression using a GPI anchor: CD (NH2-CD59-DAF-GPI) and DC (NH2-DAF-CD59-GPI). The rationale behind this work was to create a single protein that blocks C3 and C5 convertase activity as well as the assembly of the MAC. Of the two molecules, DC exhibited both DAF and CD59 activity. The DC chimera may have utility in the production of transgenic organs for the inhibition of hyperacute rejection in xenotransplantation.

3.2.2. MCP–DAF

The molecular fusion of MCP and DAF brings together the complementary activities of these two regulatory molecules to create a single protein that has both factor I cofactor activity and decay-accelerating activity. A membrane-bound chimeric MCP–DAF was expressed in Chinese hamster ovary cells and its activity was compared with that of transfectants expressing MCP or DAF or MCP plus DAF *(21)*. Thus, in this in vitro system, the hybrid surface-bound protein appeared to have greater potency at blocking alternative rather than classical pathway activation. Similar studies were performed in vitro in stably transfected swine endothelial cells exposed to human complement. In this model of xenograft hyperacute rejection, mediated mainly by the classical pathway, the surface-expressed MCP–DAF hybrid inhibited cell lysis more effectively than MCP alone, and apparently as effectively as DAF. Differences in lysis, however, were rather small, and the quantitative differences in the levels of surface expression of the molecules make it difficult to draw firm conclusions regarding their relative effectiveness *(21)*. Nevertheless, these studies demonstrate the dual functionality and complement-inhibitory activity of the MCP–DAF hybrid.

A soluble version of chimeric MCP–DAF, referred to as complement activation blocker-2 (CAB-2), possessed factor I cofactor activity and decay-accelerating activity and inactivated both classical and alternative C3 and C5 convertases in vitro as measured by assays of inhibition of cytotoxicity and anaphylatoxin generation *(22)*. CAB-2 had inhibitory activity against cell-bound convertases that was greater than that of either sMCP or sDAF or both factors combined. This hybrid was shown to inhibit complement activation in vivo, in the reversed passive Arthus reaction and in the direct passive Arthus reaction, as well as in the Forssman shock model in guinea pigs. The $t_{1/2}\beta$ of CAB-2 in rats was 8 h *(22)*, which is suitable for human therapy. It is possible that the half-life of CAB-2 may be longer in humans than in rats, as has been the case for sCR1 *(3)*. One potential limitation of CAB-2 as a therapeutic is its potential immunogenicity. The molecular fusion of two otherwise natural proteins is likely to create novel epitopes, which might trigger an immune response. In this case, CAB-2 might be useful in acute indications, depending on the severity of the anti-CAB-2 response.

3.3. Antibodies

3.3.1. Anti-C5 mAb

Inhibition of C5 activation using high-affinity ($K_d < 100$ pM) anti-C5 monoclonal antibodies (mAbs) represents another therapeutic approach for blocking complement activation *(23,24)*. This strategy is aimed at inhibiting the formation of C5a and C5b-9 via both the classical and alternative pathways (Fig. 1), without affecting the generation of C3b, a C3 opsonic product that is critical for antibacterial defenses.

The efficacy of a mAb specific for murine C5 was demonstrated in the treatment of collagen-induced arthritis, an animal model for human rheumatoid arthritis. It was shown that the systemic administration of the anti-C5 mAb in mice blocked complement activation, prevented the onset of arthritis in immunized animals, and ameliorated established disease *(25)*. The same anti-C5 mAb was tested in mice that develop an autoimmune disorder similar to human systemic lupus erythematosus. Continuous treatment with the antibody resulted in significant reduction in glomerulonephritis and in increased survival *(26)*.

The anti-human C5 mAb N19/8 which does not inhibit formation of C3a, was tested in an in vitro model of extracorporeal blood flow that activates complement, platelets, and neutrophils (24). This mAb inhibited the generation of C5a and soluble C5b-9 and blocked serum complement hemolytic activity, without affecting the production of C3a. In addition, the anti-C5 mAb inhibited neutrophil CD11b upregulation, abolished the increase in P-selectin-positive platelets, and reduced the formation of leukocyte–platelet aggregates *(24)*. Thus, it appears that C5a and C5b-9, but not C3a, contribute to platelet and neutrophil activation during extracorporeal procedures. More recently, the use of an anti-C5 mAb in a rat model of myocardial ischemia and reperfusion significantly inhibited cell apoptosis, necrosis, and neutrophil infiltration despite C3 deposition *(27)*, indicating that C5a and C5b-9 mediate tissue injury in this model.

Although murine, chimeric, or humanized mAbs could be used in human therapy, it is recognized that chronic application of such mAbs is likely to elicit human anti-mouse antibody (HAMA) responses. Recent advances in transgenic animal technology now make it possible to produce completely human mAbs that are devoid of mouse or other nonhuman sequences *(28)*.

3.3.2. Anti-C5 scFv

A recombinant single-chain Fv antibody (scFv), constructed from the variable region of the N19-8 mAb, was shown to inhibit human C5b-9-mediated hemolysis of chicken erythrocytes and to partially inhibit C5a generation *(29)*. The ability of this scFv to protect against complement-mediated myocardial injury was demonstrated in isolated mouse hearts perfused with 6% human plasma. Pharmacokinetic analysis in rhesus monkeys revealed a $t_{1/2}\alpha$ of 28 min and a $t_{1/2}\beta$ of 17 h *(29)*.

3.4. Other Inhibitors of Complement

Compared with conventional drugs, recombinant proteins for therapy remain attractive to date, for reasons having to do both with the biological properties of proteins and the economics of drug development. The time required to develop protein drugs is shorter than that for conventional drugs partly because of the lower toxicity of proteins compared with chemical compounds. However, the high cost of therapeutic proteins is increasingly becoming a problem. For these reasons, efforts are being channeled toward the discovery of "small molecule" complement inhibitors. These can be synthetic compounds, peptides and their analogs, organic molecules, as well as naturally occurring compounds *(3)*.

4. Summary

During the last two decades, impressive progress has been made in our understanding of the mechanisms of complement activation and its role as either a protective or pathogenic factor in human disease. With respect to disease pathogenesis, the complexity of the complement cascade provides opportunities for several different therapeutic targets within the complement pathways. More than a century after complement was first described, we are about to witness in the near future the availability of a variety of complement inhibitors for specific therapies.

References

1. Morgan, B. P. (1994) Clinical complementology: recent progress and future trends. *Eur. J. Clin. Invest.* **24,** 219–228.
2. Liszewski, M. K., Farries, T. C., Lublin, D. M., Rooney, I. A., and Atkinson, J. P. (1996) Control of the complement system. *Adv. Immunol.* **61,** 201–283.
3. Makrides, S. C. (1998) Therapeutic inhibition of the complement system. *Pharmacol. Rev.* **50,** 59–87.
4. Kawasaki, N., Kawasaki, T., and Yamashina, I. (1983) Isolation and characterization of a mannan-binding protein from human serum. *J. Biochem.* **94,** 937–947.
5. Turner, M. W. (1996) Mannose-binding lectin: the pluripotent molecule of the innate immune system. *Immunol. Today* **17,** 532–540.
6. Matsushita, M. (1996) The lectin pathway of the complement system. *Microbiol. Immunol.* **40,** 887–893.
7. Nicholson-Weller, A. and Halperin, J. A. (1993) Membrane signalling by complement C5b-9, the membrane attack complex. *Immunol. Res.* **12,** 244–257.
8. Klickstein, L. B., Barbashov, S. F., Liu, T., Jack, R. M., and Nicholson-Weller, A. (1997) Complement receptor type 1 (CR1, CD35) is a receptor for C1q. *Immunity* **7,** 345–355.
9. Weisman, H. F., Bartow, T., Leppo, M. K., Marsh, H. C., Jr., Carson, G. R., Concino, M. F., et al. (1990) Soluble human complement receptor type 1: in vivo inhibitor of complement suppressing post-ischemic myocardial inflammation and necrosis. *Science* **249,** 146–151.

10. Homeister, J. W. and Lucchesi, B. R. (1994) Complement activation and inhibition in myocardial ischemia and reperfusion injury. *Annu. Rev. Pharmacol. Toxicol.* **34,** 17–40.
11. Scesney, S. M., Makrides, S. C., Gosselin, M. L., Ford, P. J., Andrews, B. M., Hayman, E. G., et al. (1996) A soluble deletion mutant of the human complement receptor type 1, which lacks the C4b binding site, is a selective inhibitor of the alternative complement pathway. *Eur. J. Immunol.* **26,** 1729–1735.
12. Lennon, P. F., Collard, C. D., Morrissey, M. A., and Stahl, G. L. (1996) Complement-induced endothelial dysfunction in rabbits: mechanisms, recovery, and gender differences. *Am. J. Physiol.* **270,** H1924–H1932.
13. Murohara, T., Guo, J., Delyani, J. A., and Lefer, A. M. (1995) Cardioprotective effects of selective inhibition of the two complement activation pathways in myocardial ischemia and reperfusion injury. *Methods Find. Exp. Clin. Pharmacol.* **17,** 499–507.
14. Springer, T. A. (1994) Traffic signals for lymphocyte recirculation and leukocyte emigration: the multistep paradigm. *Cell* **76,** 301–314.
15. Lowe, J. B. and Ward, P. A. (1997) Therapeutic inhibition of carbohydrate-protein interactions in vivo. *J. Clin. Invest.* **99,** 822–826.
16. Maaheimo, H., Renkonen, R., Turunen, J. P., Penttila, L., and Renkonen, O. (1995) Synthesis of a divalent sialyl Lewis[x] O-glycan, a potent inhibitor of lymphocyte–endothelium adhesion. Evidence that multivalency enhances the saccharide binding to L-selectin. *Eur. J. Biochem.* **234,** 616–625.
17. Bertino, A., Rittershaus, C., Miller, D., Guy, D., Mealey, R., Henry, L., et al. (1996) Soluble complement receptor type 1 in Lec11 cells is decorated with the carbohydrate ligand, sialyl Lewis[x]. *Mol. Biol. Cell* **7(Suppl.)** (abstract) No. 449.
18. Davis, A. E., III, Aulak, K. S., Zahedi, K., Bissler, J. J., and Harrison, R. A. (1993) C1 inhibitor. *Methods Enzymol.* **223,** 97–120.
19. van den Berg, R. H., Prins, F., Faber-Krol, M. C., Lynch, N. J., Schwaeble, W., van Es, L. A., et al. (1997) Intracellular localization of the human receptor for the globular domains of C1q. *J. Immunology* **158,** 3909–3916.
20. Fodor, W. L., Rollins, S. A., Guilmette, E. R., Setter, E., and Squinto, S. P. (1995) A novel bifunctional chimeric complement inhibitor that regulates C3 convertase and formation of the membrane attack complex. *J. Immunol.* **155,** 4135–4138.
21. Iwata, K., Seya, T., Ariga, H., and Nagasawa, S. (1994) Expression of a hybrid complement regulatory protein, membrane cofactor protein decay accelerating factor on Chinese hamster ovary. Comparison of its regulatory effect with those of decay accelerating factor and membrane cofactor protein. *J. Immunol.* **152,** 3436–3444.
22. Higgins, P. J., Ko, J. L., Lobell, R., Sardonini, C., Alessi, M. K., and Yeh, C. G. (1997) A soluble chimeric complement inhibitory protein that possesses both decay-accelerating and factor I cofactor activities. *J. Immunol.* **158,** 2872–2881.
23. Matis, L. A. and Rollins, S. A. (1995) Complement-specific antibodies: designing novel anti-inflammatories. *Nat. Med.* **1,** 839–842.
24. Rinder, C. S., Rinder, H. M., Smith, B. R., Fitch, J. C., Smith, M. J., Tracey, J. B., et al. (1995) Blockade of C5a and C5b-9 generation inhibits leukocyte and platelet activation during extracorporeal circulation. *J. Clin. Invest.* **96,** 1564–1572.
25. Wang, Y., Rollins, S. A., Madri, J. A., and Matis, L. A. (1995) Anti-C5 monoclonal antibody therapy prevents collagen-induced arthritis and ameliorates established disease. *Proc. Natl. Acad. Sci. USA* **92,** 8955–8959.
26. Wang, Y., Hu, Q. L., Madri, J. A., Rollins, S. A., Chodera, A., and Matis, L. A. (1996) Amelioration of lupus-like autoimmune disease in NZB/WF$_1$ mice after treatment with a blocking monoclonal antibody specific for complement component C5. *Proc. Natl. Acad. Sci. USA* **93,** 8563–8568.

27. Väkevä, A. P., Agah, A., Rollins, S. A., Matis, L. A., Li, L., and Stahl, G. L. (1998) Myocardial infarction and apoptosis after myocardial ischemia and reperfusion. Role of the terminal complement components and inhibition by anti-C5 therapy. *Circulation* **97,** 2259–2267.
28. Brüggemann, M. and Taussig, M. J. (1997) Production of human antibody repertoires in transgenic mice. *Curr. Opin. Biotechnol.* **8,** 455–458.
29. Evans, M. J., Rollins, S. A., Wolff, D. W., Rother, R. P., Norin, A. J., Therrien, D. M., et al. (1995) *In vitro* and *in vivo* inhibition of complement activity by a single-chain Fv fragment recognizing human C5. *Mol. Immunol.* **32,** 1183–1195.

31
Cytokine Response Modifiers

Richard E. Jones and Larry W. Moreland

1. Introduction

The development of cytokine-based therapies (supplementation or antagonism) for treatment of connective tissue diseases such as rheumatoid arthritis (RA) has been an area of intense investigation for over 10 yr. This interest stems from four general observations: (1) Cytokine secretion (along with cell–cell cognate interaction) is a method of regulation and information exchange among the cellular constituents of the immune system *(1)*, (2) abnormal immunologic regulation forms the milieu in which such diseases become manifest; *(3)* the relative lack of efficacy, along with significant toxicity, displayed by currently available therapies *(2)*, and (4) developments in molecular biology that have advanced the questions that may be asked from a basic research standpoint as well as potential clinical interventions arising from those investigations *(3)*.

To date, there are three ways to approach the problem of inappropriate cytokine secretion in rheumatic diseases. One is to render the cellular source(s) of such molecules inactive. Another is to alter the intracellular pathways affecting transcription, translation, or posttranslational modification of a given cytokine. Third, cytokine activity may be inhibited after synthesis and secretion.

2. Inhibition of Cytokine-Secreting Cells

T-Helper-cells express the surface molecule CD4 in physical proximity to the antigen receptor (reviewed in Chapters 5 and 12). The presence of CD4 enables the cell to recognize antigen on an antigen-presenting cell (APC) provided that APC expresses the appropriate class II major histocompatibility complex (MHC) molecules. Such CD4+ T-cells either initiate a cascade leading to or are the primary sources of several cytokines implicated in the pathogenesis of various rheumatic diseases (Fig. 1). Therefore, inhibition of CD4+ T-cell function theoretically may attenuate or eliminate abnormal immune responses seen in these diseases. Evidence for such a role of CD4+ cells in RA, for example, is provided by the following: (1) predominance of CD4+ T-cells infiltrating the synovium in patients with RA, (2) predominance of CD4+ T-cells in the peripheral blood of patients with RA, (3) the association of certain class II MHC molecules with susceptibility to RA, and (4) improvement in RA after thoracic duct drainage, total lymphoid irradiation, lymphapheresis, and treatment with cyclosporin and leflunomide (reviewed in ref. *3*).

From: *Current Molecular Medicine: Principles of Molecular Rheumatology*
Edited by: G. C. Tsokos © Humana Press Inc., Totowa, NJ

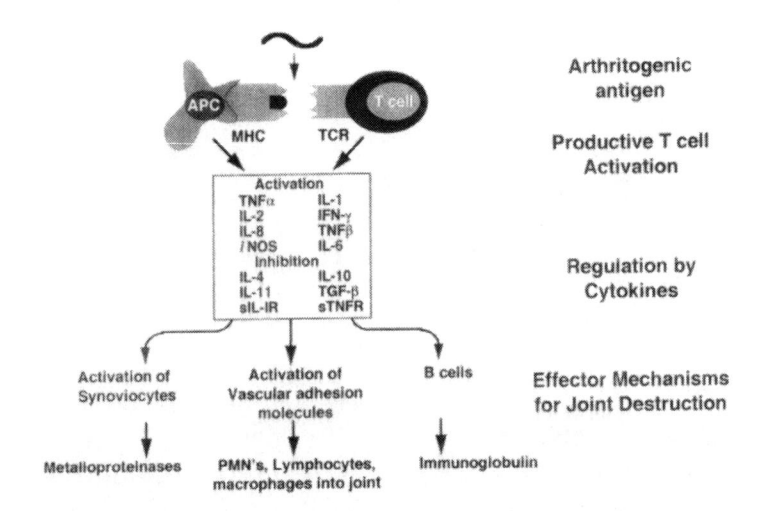

Fig. 1. Cells and cellular products implicated in the immune response of rheumatoid arthritis. (Adapted from ref. *4*.)

A potential therapeutic approach to accomplishing inhibition of CD4 T-cell function has been the use of monoclonal antibodies (mAbs) directed against the CD4 molecule (reviewed in ref. *3*). A mAb directed against the murine equivalent of CD4, L3T4, has been shown to be effective in abolishing both humoral and cellular immune responses in mice. The mechanism(s) of this inhibition are not known but may include blockage of CD4+ cell interaction with APC, direct cytotoxicity to the CD4+ cell, or transmission of a negative signal to the CD4+ cell. Interestingly, F(ab') fragments of anti-L3T4 are able to suppress immune responses as well as the intact mAb, indicating that destruction of the cell is not required for inhibition.

In view of the apparent effectiveness displayed by anti-CD4 therapy in suppressing immune responses, several studies have been completed in humans with RA to determine the safety and efficacy of such therapy. A depleting, chimeric mAb to CD4, cM-T412, has been studied in both open-label and placebo-controlled trials in patients with refractory rheumatoid arthritis (RA). This mAb produced a rapid and sustained decrease in the number of circulating CD4+ cells in all studies, but otherwise appeared safe. Although encouraging clinical results were noted in the open-label trials, in placebo-controlled trials, no therapeutic benefit was noted (reviewed in ref. *3*).

As noted, anti-CD4 mAbs need not be depleting in order to be effective. In fact, cM-T412 may lack efficacy because not all CD4+ cells are accessible for destruction. In animal models of arthritis, unless virtually all CD4+ cells are depleted by this mAb (in excess of 99%), then enough residual T-cell function remains to sustain the ongoing inflammatory response. Several anti-CD4 mAbs that are nondepleting are currently undergoing clinical trials to determine their therapeutic potential. Other T-cell antigens (CD7, CD5, CD52, CD25) have been targeted using biologic agents; however, no significant clinical benefit has been noted in placebo-controlled trials (reviewed in ref. *4*). More specific approaches to T-cell-directed immunotherapy of autoimmune diseases include identification of T-cell receptor (TCR) gene products expressed by activated T-cell clones. Recent clinical trials treating patients with RA with Vβ3, Vβ14, and Vβ17

Table 1
Cytokine Targets for Biologic Agents

Biologic agent	Target antigen/cytokine
IL-1 receptor antagonist	IL-1
Soluble IL-1 receptor	IL-1
Chimeric anti-TNF mAb	TNF
Humanized anti-TNF mAb	TNF
Soluble TNF receptor fusion proteins	TNF
Anti-IL-6 mAb	IL-6
Recombinant IL-4	Multiple
Recombinant IL-10	Multiple
Recombinant IL-11	Multiple

Source: Adapted from ref. *4*.

TCR peptides demonstrated positive improvements in some patients *(5)*. Further studies are needed to better understand the mechanisms and the doses of peptides to be used clinically.

3. Transcription, Translation, and Posttranslational Alteration

Another strategy is to intervene pharmacologically with the intracellular events leading to cytokine gene transcription, mRNA translation, and posttranslational fate of the cytokine protein. Counterregulatory cytokines such as interleukin (IL-4) and IL-10 probably work by inhibiting cytokine synthesis by their cellular targets at either the transcriptional or translational level *(1)*. Antimalarials (chloroquine and hydroxychloroquine), on the other hand, may exert their actions by posttranslational mechanisms *(2)*. A potential therapeutic target for intervention is the nuclear transcription factor NF-κB, which seems to have particular importance in the regulation of genes encoding various proteins of the inflammatory cascade.

4. Cytokine Antagonism

A third approach is inhibition of cytokine activity after synthesis and secretion. Typically, this is accomplished by competitive or noncompetitive inhibition at the level of the surface receptor(s) or administration of specific cytokine binding molecules, which also prevent access of the cytokine ligand to its cellular targets. Current experimental therapies utilizing these approaches are summarized in Table 1.

5. Biologic Therapies

Interleukin 1 (IL-1) and tumor necrosis factor (TNF) have been implicated as major contributors to the inflammatory process seen in a variety of rheumatic diseases, including both RA and osteoarthritis (OA) *(6)*. Mice transgenic for the TNF gene spontaneously develop inflammatory arthritis. Treatment of such animals with mAb to TNF or soluble TNF receptor fusion proteins attenuates this inflammatory response *(7)*. Animal models of collagen-induced arthritis have been shown to be responsive to antagonists of IL-1 and TNF *(8)*.

Although both IL-1 and TNF are members of an overlapping inflammatory cascade, they may play different roles in the components of inflammatory arthritis. In animal models, inhibition of TNF suppressed the inflammatory response, whereas IL-1 antagonism prevented joint destruction *(9)*. The clear implication of these results is that combination therapy providing inhibition of both IL-1 and TNF-α might be the most efficacious approach. Finally, combining such biologic therapy with the use of currently available disease modifying antirheumatic drugs (DMARDs) may prove more effective yet than any currently available therapy.

5.1. Interleukin-1

Interleukin-1 is secreted in two forms, α and β, predominantly by monocytes/macrophages and produces a variety of inflammatory changes by actions on various cell types *(1)*. These actions are mediated through two distinct cell-surface receptors, designated as types I and II. Several naturally occurring inhibitors of IL-1 have been described. These include IL-1 receptor antagonist (IL-1RA) and soluble IL-1 receptors (sIL-1 types I and II) derived from shedding of the extracellular portion of the two types of IL-1Rs. These IL-1 antagonists have been shown to be increased in both sera and sites of inflammation in patients with RA; however, the abundance of IL-1 in these areas occurs in great surplus to the available antagonist, leading to excessive availability of IL-1 and chronic inflammation.

IL-1RA is an acute-phase reactant, derived from a variety of cell types, which works by competitive inhibition of IL-1 at the level of its cellular receptor. However, because IL-1RA and IL-1 have similar affinity constants for the IL-1 receptor and only a few molecules of IL-1 are required to exert physiologic effects, up to 100-fold excess of IL-1RA over IL-1 is required to maintain IL-1 antagonism in vitro.

The human gene for IL-1RA has been cloned, sequenced, and expressed in a recombinant vector. Recombinant human IL-1RA (rhuIL-1RA) has been evaluated in clinical trials in patients with RA. In a 4-wk clinical trial in patients with RA a beneficial effect was noted on C-reactive protein (CRP) levels *(10)*. A large, placebo-controlled multicenter trial in Europe lasting 6 mo *(11)* demonstrated that rhuIL-1RA produced statistically significant improvements in levels of disease activity as measured by American College of Rheumatology (ACR) clinical response criteria *(12)*. Moreover, there was evidence suggesting a slowing of radiographic progression. Further, placebo-controlled trials are in progress at this writing, including continuous infusion of rhuIL-1RA by subcutaneous pump and in patients who are receiving concomitant treatment with methotrexate (MTX). Additionally, placement of the constitutively expressed gene for rhuIL-1RA in patients with RA is under investigation (*see* Chapter 34). These studies should clarify the therapeutic efficacy and safety of rhuIL-1RA.

sIL-1R functions by binding circulating IL-1 in competition with cellular-based receptors. sIL-1R derived from the type I receptor has greater in vitro affinity for IL-1RA than for IL-1α or IL-1β; conversely, the type II sIL-1R binds IL-1α and IL-1β more efficiently than IL-1RA. Theoretically, type I sIL-1R might promote the inflammatory cascade by producing a net increase in the amount of IL-1 available for binding to cellular receptors. In a phase I study evaluating type I sIL-1R in patients with RA, no disease worsening was noted, but neither was any significant clinical improvement obtained. A larger double-blind placebo-controlled trial of type I sIL-1R in RA patients also failed to demonstrate improvement in disease activity (unpublished, data on file at Immunex). Because type II sIL-1R preferentially binds the isoforms of IL-1 and not IL-1RA, this form of the soluble receptor may have anti-inflammatory properties apparently lacking in type I sIL-1R.

5.2. Tumor Necrosis Factor

Tumor necrosis factor is secreted in three isoforms, with mononuclear cells, synovial cells, and T-lymphocytes being the primary sources. TNF has a regulatory function in cell proliferation and apoptosis (see Chapter 3) and therefore is felt to be an important mediator of a variety of inflammatory conditions, including RA (13). Like IL-1, TNF has two distinct cell-surface receptors designated type I or p60 (p55) and type II or p80 (p75) (reviewed in Chapters 3 and 5). All types of TNF utilize these receptors to mediate their physiologic actions. Both types of membrane-bound TNF receptors gives rise to a corresponding soluble TNF receptor (sTNFR) by proteolytic cleavage of the extracellular ligand-binding portion of each molecule. Production of sTNFR is felt to be a regulatory step in attenuating the biologic activities of TNF. For example, neutrophils undergoing diapedesis release both types of sTNFRs, correlating to a decrease in TNF activity (reviewed in ref. 5). These same sTNFRs are able to limit the in vitro respiratory burst of neutrophils stimulated by exogenous TNF. sTNFR derived from either p60 or p80 can inhibit the cytolytic activity of TNF in vitro (14). Patients undergoing immunotherapy with IL-2 can have the IL-2-stimulated production of IL-8 inhibited by administration of IL-1RA or sTNFR. IL-4 is able to oppose many of the physiologic actions of TNF and at least one of the mechanisms involved is IL-4-stimulated release of sTNFRs. At sites of ongoing inflammation, TNF exists in large excess to sTNFR.

Evidence for utility of TNF inhibitors as therapeutic agents for human disease came first from clinical trials involving a chimeric (the murine portion makes up the TNF-binding region) anti-TNF mAb, cA2 or infliximab (reviewed in ref. 3). Both open-label and placebo-controlled trials using infliximab in patients with RA produced improvements in swollen joint counts as well as decreased levels of CRP. A problem encountered with this mAb has been the development of an antibody response against the murine portion of the molecule. Although no loss of efficacy has been seen with retreatment utilizing infliximab, the immunogenicity of infliximab may prove limiting to treatment duration. Concomitant treatment with MTX and infliximab may attenuate the anti-infliximab antibody response (15). Additionally, treatment synergy between MTX and infliximab was noted in these RA patients when compared to use of MTX alone. A subsequent phase III trial has continued the efficacy of this agent in RA patients (16).

One of the mechanisms through which infliximab probably exerts its actions in RA is the inhibition of production of vascular endothelial growth factor, thus preventing angiogenesis and pannus proliferation (17). Additionally, infliximab may downregulate TNF-induced expression of adhesion molecules on vascular endothelium, leading to decreased migration of inflammatory cells into involved joints. This is supported by decreases in serum levels of E-selectin and intracellular adhesion molecule-1 (ICAM-1) noted after administration of infliximab. Synovial biopsies confirmed reduced T-cell infiltration of synovium, as well as diminished E-selectin and vascular cell adhesion molecule-1 (VCAM-1) expression on associated endothelium. Furthermore, treatment reduced serum levels of IL-6 as well as IL-1β, indicating a regulatory role for TNF in the inflammatory cascade.

A human anti-TNF mAb, CPD571, has also shown promise in treating refractory RA. When utilized at the highest dose prescribed in a double-blind study, CDP571 produced significant clinical and biochemical reductions in disease activity. Further studies are ongoing with this anti-TNF mAb (reviewed in ref. 5).

Another approach to counteract the in vivo effects of TNF in autoimmune disease is to supply sTNFR exogenously. One agent designed for this purpose is etanercept, a soluble tumor necrosis factor receptor (TNFR) fusion protein *(18–24)*. This molecule was created by linking the DNA encoding the soluble portion of human p75 TNFR to the DNA template for the Fc portion of human IgG and then inserted into a mammalian expression vector (reviewed in ref. *14*). The resultant protein binds two TNF molecules and has increased circulating half-life due to the Fc moiety. When utilized in the murine model of collagen-induced arthritis, etanercept significantly reduced the incidence (85% of controls versus 25% of treated animals) of arthritis when given prior to collagen exposure and produced a 40% improvement in the arthritis score of mice given etanercept with already existing disease.

The initial clinical trial of etanercept in normal human volunteers had no reported adverse side effects with intravenous administration *(19)*. A phase I, dose-escalating trial in 22 patients with refractory RA also proved safe except for mild injection-site reactions *(18)*. After 31 d of therapy, 45% of patients had improvement in measures of pain and joint scores versus 22% of those receiving placebo. Treated patients also had decreases in Westergren erythrocyte sedimentation rates (ESR) as well as CRP levels, especially in the groups receiving the highest dose. These results have been subsequently verified in two multicenter placebo-controlled trials.

A phase II, double-blind, placebo-controlled trial *(20)* of etanercept evaluated the clinical efficacy and safety of 3 mo of therapy. Changes in symptoms of arthritis were evaluated per ACR criteria *(12)*. The drug was administered subcutaneously twice weekly. Etanercept produced significant improvements in all measures of disease activity, particularly at the highest dose given (16 mg/m^2, which defined a range of 23–30 mg) (*see* Fig. 2). Clinical improvement was noted within 2 wk of starting therapy. This improvement was associated with significant reductions in pain and morning stiffness as well as biochemical markers (ESR and CRP) of disease activity. Adverse reactions, again, consisted entirely of mild injection-site reactions. No antibodies against etanercept were detected.

In the subsequent phase III study evaluating etanercept *(21)*, using a dosing schedule established in the phase II study (0, 10, and 25 mg subcutaneously biweekly), this study verified the safety of etanercept as well as sustained clinical efficacy over this period of time. The 25-mg dose was superior to the 10 mg dose in terms of effectiveness. No adverse events other than injection-site discomfort were noted with either dosage. Withdrawal of the drug produced a return of arthritis activity within 3 mo of cessation.

Results of an open-label long-term treatment study of etanercept in refractory RA when given over 60 wk have also been submitted *(22)*. Given at a dose of 25 mg subcutaneously biweekly, efficacy was similar to those seen in previous studies, including

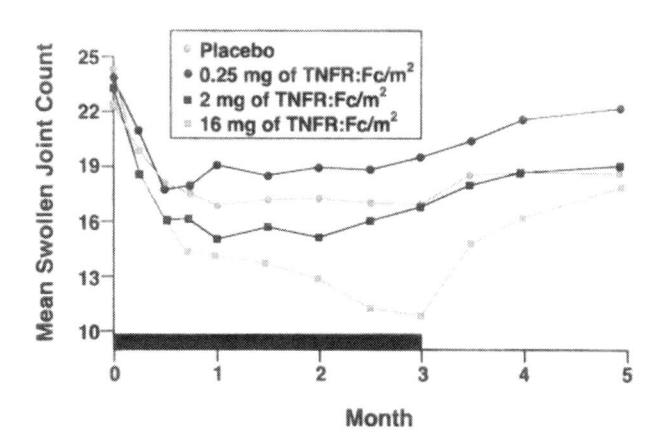

Fig. 2. Improvement in joint scores in patients treated with TNFR : Fc (etanercept). Mean swollen-joint count. The shaded bar represents the treatment period. For each patient, missing values were replaced by the last available value. [Adapted with permission from Moreland, L. W., Baumgartner, S. W., Schiff, M. H., et al. (1997) Treatment of rheumatoid arthritis with a recombinant human tumor necrosis factor receptor (p75)–Fc fusion protein. *N. Engl. J. Med.* **337**, 141–147. Copyright ©1997 Massachusetts Medical Society. All rights reserved.]

clinical improvements in ACR criteria and reductions in ESR and CRP. No increased incidence of infection was noted and mild injection-site reactions remained the most common side effect, a problem that diminished after the first month of therapy.

It is also of interest to determine the utility of etanercept and other TNF antagonists in combination with currently available pharmacologic therapy for various connective-tissue diseases. A phase II/III study of etanercept in combination with methotrexate has recently been completed in patients with RA and demonstrated a clear benefit of combined therapy with TNFR : Fc and MTX over MTX alone *(23)*. As with studies utilizing etanercept as a single agent, the only adverse side effects reported were mild injection-site reactions.

The clinical role of TNF antagonists has been studied primarily in patients with RA to date. However, etanercept has recently been reported to show efficacy in the treatment of juvenile RA *(24)*. There are several other disorders in which TNF antagonists may prove useful, including psoriatic arthritis and inflammatory bowel disease.

5.3. Interleukin-6

Interleukin-6 (IL-6) is a cytokine secreted by multiple cell types that functions along with IL-1 and TNF in sustaining a variety of inflammatory responses *(1)*. Although IL-6 is increased in synovial fluid in patients with RA, the role played by this cytokine in the disorder is unclear. For example, IL-6 clearly has anti-inflammatory properties as well. This is evidenced by IL-6-induced IL-1RA production, IL-6-induced sTNFR production, inhibition of TNF and IL-1β production in lipopolysaccharide (LPS)-stimulated monocytes, and inhibition of adjuvant arthritis in mice (reviewed in ref. *3*).

An open-label trial of anti-IL-6 mAb was performed on five patients with RA who also received anti-CD4 therapy. Although CRP levels were decreased by this therapy, four of five patients had unexpected increases in serum IL-6 levels, and no clinical improvement in these patients was noted. Clinical trials in RA patients of a mAb directed against the IL-6 receptor are currently ongoing in Europe. The multifunctional nature of IL-6 may make this cytokine a less attractive target for anticytokine therapy.

5.4. Interleukin-4, Interleukin-10, and Interleukin-11

These cytokines have immunoregulatory functions that make them potential agents for treatment of RA. Both IL-4 and IL-10 inhibit the release and function of IL-1, TNF, IL-6, and IL-8, and production of matrix metalloproteinases (MMPs), and stimulate the release of natural inhibitors such as IL-1RA and sTNFR (reviewed in ref. 4). IL-11 suppresses the production of IL-1, IL-6, IL-12, TNF, and nitric oxide. IL-10, IL-11, and IL-13 have been shown to inhibit activity of NF-κB. Trials of recombinant IL-4, IL-10, and IL-11 used in animal models of arthritis have been shown to be effective. IL-4 was particularly effective in suppressing the chronic destructive phase of streptococcal-cell-wall-induced arthritis in mice. There are clinical trials underway utilizing recombinant IL-4, IL-10, and IL-11 in patients with RA.

Interestingly, IL-10 may play a deleterious role in systemic lupus erythematosus (SLE) (reviewed in ref. 3 and Chapter 20). NZB/NZW F1 mice, which spontaneously develop features suggestive of SLE, can have the appearance of disease delayed by continuous administration of mAb to IL-10. Conversely, when given continuous infusion of IL-10, these mice develop clinical autoimmune disease in a more accelerated fashion than untreated controls. These mice have very low-baseline-level production of TNF and supplementation with TNF delays the appearance of nephritis. Therefore, the beneficial effect of anti-IL-10 mAb in these mice may stem from release of inhibition of TNF production by IL-10.

6. Future Considerations

The era of biologic therapies for rheumatic diseases has just begun. However, clear paths of future progress already exist. As alluded to previously, combination therapy providing antagonism to both IL-1 and TNF theoretically may be the most efficacious approach yet in therapy of RA as well as other autoimmune diseases. Conceptually, this could be accomplished by coadministration of separate agents or development of a single multivalent protein capable of binding multiple targets. Development of such agents are currently in progress.

Development of novel agents to interfere with the synthesis and processing of TNF, IL-1, or other molecules will become possible as pathways of gene activation/deactivation are uncovered. The specificity as well as concurrent toxicity of such agents will be crucial.

Cytokine supplementation therapy for immunologic conterregulation is a logical target of gene therapy (Chapter 34). Candidate genes for implantation include those for rhuIL-1RA, soluble TNF receptors, IL-4, IL-11, and IL-10.

7. Conclusions

Not since the time of Hench, with the development of cortisone as a therapy for RA, has such progress been made in the treatment of RA and, in all likelihood, other rheumatic diseases as well. Diverse forms of inflammation have common pathways (e.g., the importance of IL-1 and TNF in several connective-tissue diseases) and many of the agents now under development are likely to have multiple applications.

References

1. Lotz, M. (1997). Cytokines and their receptors, in *Arthritis and Allied Conditions: A Textbook of Rheumatology*, 13th ed. (Koopman, W. J., ed.), Williams & Wilkins, Baltimore, pp. 439–478.
2. Jain, R. and Lipsky, P. E. (1997) Treatment of rheumatoid arthritis. *Med Clin. North Am.* **81**, 57–84.
3. Moreland, L. M. and Koopman, W. J. (1997) Biologic agents as potential therapies for autoimmune diseases, in *Arthritis and Allied Conditions: A Textbook of Rheumatology*, 13th ed. (Koopman, W. J., ed.), Williams & Wilkins, Baltimore pp. 777–809.
4. Moreland, L. W., Heck, L. W., and Koopman, W. J. (1997) Biologic agents for treating rheumatoid arthritis: concepts and progress. *Arthritis Rheum.* **40**, 397–409.
5. Moreland, L. M., Morgan, E. E., Adamson, T. C, et al. (1998) T Cell receptor peptide vaccination in rheumatoid arthritis: a placebo controlled trial using a combination of Vb3, Vβ14, and Vβ17 peptides. *Arthritis Rheum.* **41**, 1919–1929.
6. Webb, G. R., Westacott, C. I., and Elson, C. J. (1998) Osteoarthritic synovial fluid and synovium supernatants upregulate tumor necrosis factor receptors on human articular chondrocytes. *Osteoarthritis Cart.* **6**, 167–176.
7. Joosten, L. A. B., Helsen, M. M. A., van de Loo, F. A. J., and van den Berg, W. B. (1996) Anticytokine treatment of established type II collagen-induced arthritis in DBA/1 mice: a comparative study using anti-TNFalpha, anti-IL-1alpha.beta and IL-1RA. *Arthritis Rheum.* **39**, 797–809.
8. van de Loo, F. A., Joosten, L. A., van Lent, P. L., et al. (1995) Role of interleukin-1, tumor necrosis factor alpha, and interleukin-6 in cartilage proteoglycan metabolism and destruction. Effect of in situ blocking in murine antigen- and zymosan-induced arthritis. *Arthritis Rheum.* **38**, 164–172.
9. Eliaz, R., Wallach, D., and Korst, J. (1995) Long-term protection against the effects of tumor necrosis factor by controlled delivery of the soluble p55 TNF receptor. *Cytokine* **9**, 482–487.
10. Campion, G. V., Lebsack, M. E., Lookabaugh, J., et al. (1996) Dose-range and frequency study of recombinant human interleukin-1 receptor antagonist in patients with rheumatoid arthritis. *Arthritis Rheum.* **39**, 1092–1101.
11. Bresnihan, B. (on behalf of the collaborating investigators), Lookbaugh, J., Witt, K., and Musikic, P. (1996) Treatment with recombinant human interleukin-1 receptor antagonist (rhuIL-1RA) in rheumatoid arthritis (RA): results of a randomized double-blind, placebo controlled multicenter trial. *Arthritis Rheum.* **39**, S73 (abstract).
12. Felson, D. T., Anderson, J. J., Boers, M., et al. (1993) The American College of Rheumatology preliminary core set of disease activity measures for rheumatoid arthritis clinical trials. *Arthritis Rheum.* **36**, 729–740.
13. Brennan, F. M., Maini, R. N., and Feldmann, M. (1992) TNF alpha—a pivotal role in rheumatoid arthritis? *Br. J. Rheum.* **31**, 293–298.
14. Gatanaga, T., Hwang, C. D., Kohr, W., et al. (1990) Purification and characterization of an inhibitor (soluble tumor necrosis factor receptor) for tumor necrosis factor and lymphotoxin obtained from the serum ultrafiltrates of human cancer patients. *Proc. Natl. Acad. Sci. USA* **87**, 8781–8784.
15. Maini, R. N., Breedveld, F. C., Kalden, J. R., et al. (1998) Therapeutic efficacy of multiple intravenous infusions of anti-tumor necrosis factor alpha monoclonal antibody combined with low-dose weekly methotrexate in rheumatoid arthritis. *Arthritis Rheum.* **41**, 1552–1563.
16. Main, R., St. Clair, E. W., Breedveld, F., et al. (1999) Infliximab (chimeric anti-tumour necrosis factor α monoclonal antibody) versus placebo in rheumatoid arthritis patients receiving concomitant methotrexate: a randomised phase III trial. *Lancet* **354**, 1932–1939.

17. Paleolog, E. M., Young, S., Stark, A. C., McCloskey, R. V., Feldmann, M., and Maini, R. N. (1998) Modulation of angiogenic vascular endothelial growth factor by tumor necrosis factor alpha and interleukin-1 in rheumatoid arthritis. *Arthritis Rheum.* **41,** 1258–1265.
18. Moreland, L. M. (1998) Soluble tumor necrosis factor receptor (p75) fusion protein (Enbrel™) as a therapy for rheumatoid arthritis. *Rheum. Dis. Clin. North Am.* **24,** 579–591.
19. Moreland, L. W., Margolies, G. R., Heck, L. W., et al. (1996) Recombinant soluble tumor necrosis factor receptor (p80) fusion protein: toxicity and dose finding trial in refractory rheumatoid arthritis. *J. Rheumatol.* **23,** 1849–1855.
20. Moreland, L. W., Baumgartner, S. W., Schiff, M. H., et al. (1997) Treatment of rheumatoid arthritis with a recombinant human tumor necrosis factor receptor(p75)–Fc fusion protein. *N. Engl. J. Med.* **337,** 141–147.
21. Moreland, L. W., Schiff, M. H., Baumgartner, S. W., et al. (1999) Recombinant human tumor necrosis factor receptor (p75) : Fc fusion protein in rheumatoid arthritis: a multicenter, randomized, double-blind, placebo-controlled trial. *Ann. Int. Med.* **130,** 478–486.
22. Moreland, L. W., Baumgartner, S. W., Tindall, E., et al. (1998) Long term treatment of rheumatoid arthritis with the receptor p75 Fc fusion protein (TNFR : Fc; Enbrel™). *Arthritis Rheum.* **41(Suppl.),** S364.
23. Weinblatt, M. E., Kremer, J. M., Bankhurst, A. D., et al. (1998) A controlled trial of etanercept, a recombinant human tumor necrosis factor receptor (p75)-Fc fusion protein in patients with rheumatoid arthritis receiving methotrexate. *N. Engl. J. Med.* **340,** 253–257.
24. Lovell, D. J., Giannini, E. H., Reiff, A., et al. (2000) Etanercept in children with polyarticular juvenile rheumatoid arthritis. *N. Engl. J. Med.* **342,** 763–769.

32
Restoration of Immune Tolerance

Woodruff Emlen

1. Introduction

The function of the immune response is to protect an organism from foreign material by first recognizing the material as foreign and then activating a cascade of events that leads to its removal. To perform this function without damaging the host, the immune system must distinguish between self and nonself, and target removal mechanisms only toward nonself antigens. The ability of the immune system to *not* respond to certain antigens (particularly self antigens) is an active process that is called tolerance. Tolerance is maintained by at least two processes: a system of lymphocyte "education" in the thymus and ongoing regulation of immune activation throughout life. When tolerance is lost or "broken," the immune system recognizes self antigens as foreign and tries to remove them by initiating the inflammatory cascade. It is this inflammatory process, directed against self, that causes the tissue damage and clinical features of autoimmune disease.

Although our understanding of the triggers that break tolerance and initiate autoimmune disease is still incomplete, recent understanding of the normal maintenance of tolerance has provided us with the tools to design therapies to restore tolerance. This chapter focuses on therapeutic attempts to restore tolerance to self in autoimmune disease. Although none of these therapeutic approaches have yet been approved for use in the clinic, they represent attempts to treat autoimmunity at its source, rather than merely blocking effector mechanisms of inflammation.

2. Mechanisms of Tolerance

The ability to distinguish between self and nonself (self tolerance) is established in embryonic life (central tolerance) and is actively maintained throughout adulthood (peripheral tolerance). Thymic lymphocytes, which recognize and bind to self antigens, are triggered to undergo apoptosis, resulting in clonal deletion of these autoreactive cells (negative selection). However, even in normal individuals, central tolerance is "leaky," such that some autoreactive cells escape negative selection in the thymus and are released into the periphery. In addition, some self antigens may not be expressed in the thymus (sequestered antigens) and cells reactive with these antigens are never deleted during development. Hence, autoreactive lymphocytes are present in the periphery of all normal individuals.

In addition to autoreactive cells that escape from the thymus, autoreactive cells continuously emerge in the adult as a by-product of the immunologic diversity generated during the normal immune response to foreign antigens. Thus, constant downregulation and "pruning" of autoreactive cells are needed throughout adulthood to prevent the emergence of autoreactive clones, a process referred to as peripheral tolerance. Although our understanding of peripheral tolerance is still incomplete, data indicate that it is maintained by at least several mechanisms: (1) deletion (apoptosis) of autoreactive clones, (2) induction of anergy, a state in which the cell is not deleted but remains unresponsive to antigen, (3) induction of regulatory cells and release of regulatory cytokines, and (4) immune deviation, in which the T-cell phenotype is shifted from a pro-inflammatory TH1 cytokine response to a noninflammatory TH2 cytokine response.

A failure to establish or maintain tolerance to self results in the initiation of an inflammatory response directed toward self and subsequent autoimmune disease. In animal models of autoimmunity, central tolerance appears to be intact, suggesting that autoimmunity most often arises as a result of the loss of the regulatory mechanisms that collectively constitute peripheral tolerance. Thus, restoration of these regulatory mechanisms should have the potential to restore some degree of self tolerance and thereby provide therapeutic approaches to autoimmune disease. This chapter will give a brief overview of therapies for autoimmune diseases within the context of restoring tolerance and will focus in depth on therapies aimed at restoration of specific tolerance.

3. Therapeutic Approaches to Restoring Tolerance

In the broadest sense, restoring tolerance can be defined as suppressing immunoreactivity to self. Autoreactive lymphocytes have a high probability of encountering self-antigen and, therefore, also have a high probability of being activated. Thus, any therapy directed at rapidly dividing cells or at activated cells will preferentially target autoreactive cells. This is the basis for treatment of autoimmune diseases such as systemic lupus erythematosus (SLE) and rheumatoid arthritis (RA) with nonspecific cytotoxic drugs such as cyclophosphamide and azathioprine. However, as their side-effect profiles attest, immune suppression with these drugs is clearly not limited to autoreactive cells.

As our understanding of the mechanisms of immunologic activation and tolerance has improved, our ability to specifically suppress reactivity to self antigens relative to nonspecific suppression of all immune responses is improving. Table 1 gives an overview of therapies directed at restoring tolerance, moving from the broadest, least specific immunosuppression to the most specific restoration of tolerance to specific self antigens. Many of the more general approaches are the topics of other chapters in this volume and will only be mentioned here briefly. The major focus of this chapter is the cutting-edge therapies directed at the restoration of specific tolerance to one antigen or to a set of antigens.

3.1. Nonspecific Restoration of Tolerance

Between the non-specific immunosuppressive "sledgehammer" of cytotoxic drugs and the restoration of antigen-specific tolerance, there are a number of approaches that attempt to suppress the autoimmune response to a greater extent than they suppress the immune response to foreign antigens. These include targeting activated T-cells or CD4-

Table 1
Therapeutic Strategies to "Restore Tolerance"

Therapies[a]	Mechanism of action	Disease targets
Cyclophosphamide, azathioprine	Death of rapidly dividing cells	Almost all autoimmune diseases
Autologous bone marrow transplantation	Replacing immune system with "naive" progenitor cells	Scleroderma, SLE, RA, MS, JRA
Blockade/deletion of activated T-cells	Preferential depletion of autoreactive (activated) cells	RA
Blockade/deletion of specific cell subsets	Blockade of CD4, CD5, or other cell subsets	SLE, RA
Blockade of costimulatory molecules[b]	Blockade of CD40–CD40 ligand or B7–CD28 interactions	SLE, psoriasis
Blockade of components of the MHC–peptide–TCR complex	Disruption of T-cell response to specific antigens or induction of regulatory phenotype	RA, SLE, MS, psoriasis, myasthenia gravis

[a]Therapies listed from least specific to most specific form of restoring tolerance.

positive T-cells (Chapter 31) or blockade of costimulatory molecules (Chapter 6) such as CD40 or CTLA4. One recent, unique approach has been to "reset" immunologic tolerance with bone marrow transplantation.

3.1.1. Autologous Bone Marrow Transplantation

If autoimmunity is defined as immunologic reactivity to self caused by the loss of self tolerance, the ideal way to treat autoimmunity would be to replace the entire immune system. In animal models, it has long been recognized that allogeneic bone marrow transplantation (marrow derived from a nonself donor) can transmit or lead to the resolution of a variety of autoimmune diseases, including SLE, diabetes, experimental allergic encephalomyelitis (EAE), and adjuvant arthritis. In humans, transfer of autoimmune disease from the bone marrow donor to the recipient has been reported *(1)*. Sporadic case reports have also described resolution of coincident autoimmune disease when patients were treated with bone marrow transplantation (BMT) for conventional indications such as aplastic anemia, leukemias and lymphomas. These reports have generated significant interest in the use of BMT to treat severe, intractable autoimmune diseases such as scleroderma, multiple sclerosis (MS), and resistant SLE and RA.

Despite major improvements in the safety of bone marrow transplantation, allogeneic transplantation results in chronic graft versus host disease (GVHD) in up to 40% of patients, with severe GVHD occurring in 10% of cases. Thus, treatment of autoimmune diseases has focused on the use of autologous BMT (ABMT), in which the patient is transplanted with cells derived from his/her own marrow. If autoimmunity is a disease of the immune system, however, how can transplanting autologous marrow solve the problem of loss of tolerance? Should not the disease simply recur as the same genetic cells reconstitute the immune system?

Although disease recurrences have been reported after ABMT, many patients remain disease-free. Part of the explanation for the lack of disease recurrence may lie in the fact that human autoimmune disease, unlike many murine disease models, requires both a genetic disposition and an environmental event to trigger the loss of tolerance. The rate of disease concordance in monozygotic twins is relatively low (25% in SLE, 20% in RA, 20–25% in MS), suggesting a significant contribution of environmental factors. Furthermore, the onset of most autoimmune diseases is in adulthood, and disease is frequently triggered by an infectious event. These observations suggest that loss of self tolerance occurs in the "adult" fully developed immune system. Thus, if the mature immune system is replaced with new "naive" stem cells, self tolerance should be restored (assuming the same environmental trigger is no longer present). In support of this concept is the observation that failure to adequately remove mature lymphocytes during the transplantation protocol results in disease recurrence. Therefore, protocols are designed to aggressively ablate the mature immune system and reconstitute with T-cell-depleted progenitor cells (CD34-positive cells).

Autologus BMT for autoimmune disease has now been carried out in over 100 patients, and a consortium has been formed to standardize and coordinate the use of this treatment modality *(1,2)*. By providing some degree of standardization, it is hoped that experiences from different centers can be compared and pooled to allow adequate analysis of this therapy. To date, treatment has included patients with scleroderma, MS, RA, SLE, and juvenile RA (JRA). In general, results are encouraging, with some reports of dramatic improvement in severe patients. However, there have also been some disease recurrences and the maximum duration of follow-up is still only 2–3 yr. Although this therapeutic approach is exciting, it remains extremely expensive and mortality is quite high (7–8%). Therefore, this therapy should be reserved for only the most severe, refractory cases. Nevertheless, the prospect of prolonged disease remission without maintenance medications is especially exciting when one considers the morbidity and mortality of our current therapies with chronic steroids and cytotoxic drugs.

3.2. Restoration of Specific Tolerance Through the MHC–Peptide–TCR Complex

Specificity of the immune response is determined at three steps: (1) the uptake of antigen and processing of antigen into specific peptides by antigen-presenting cells (APC), (2) the binding of these peptides to specific major histocompatibility complex (MHC) molecules and the presentation of the MHC–peptide complex on the surface of the APC, and (3) the interaction of the MHC–peptide complex with the T-cell receptor (TCR) specific for that complex. To restore immunologic nonresponsiveness to specific self antigens, therapies have been directed at each of these three levels: the antigen, the MHC, and the TCR (*see* Table 2).

3.2.1. Antigen-Directed Therapy

In most autoimmune diseases, the autoantigen(s) initiating and driving the autoimmune response has not yet been identified, making therapies directed at suppression of antigen-specific cells difficult. However, during the evolution of autoimmune disease, the pattern of autoreactivity changes. At disease initiation, autoreactivity develops to (presumably) one or a small number of antigens. Over time, previously sequestered antigens may be released as a result of inflammation, leading to the activation of new autoimmune clones. Additionally, proliferation of autoreactive cells will generate cells with slightly different antigenic specificities, allowing the autoimmune response to

Table 2
Therapeutic Strategies to Induce Specific Tolerance

Therapeutic target	Therapy	Mechanism of action	Disease targets
Antigen	Oral tolerance	Bystander suppression	RA, MS
	Altered peptide ligands	Bystander suppression	MS
	B-cell tolerance	Anergize antigen-specific B-cells	SLE, MG
MHC Class II	Anti-DR	Block antigen presentation	RA
	DR–peptide complexes	Block antigen presentation	RA
TCR	Anti TCR		MS
	TCR Vaccines	Bystander suppression	RA, MS, psoriasis

spread to new epitopes on the same antigen. This phenomenon, known as epitope spreading (3), results in a widening spectrum of autoimmune responses as disease progresses. By the time disease is clinically evident, the autoimmune response has moved well beyond the antigens that may have initiated the process. For example, in animal models of experimental allergic encephalomyelitis (a model for human MS), which are induced by immunization with myelin basic protein (MBP), reactivity to other unrelated central nervous system (CNS) antigens develops over time. In models of arthritis, reactivity to collagen proteins frequently develops after joint inflammation occurs, even in models in which the inciting stimulus is not collagen.

Whereas at first glance this phenomenon appears to make the task of antigen-specific blockade more daunting, epitope spreading may actually be of benefit in developing antigen-based therapeutics. Thus, antigens from target tissues, such as cartilage in RA or the myelin sheath in MS, may provide potential targets for therapeutic intervention even though they might not be the inciting antigens driving the disease. This principle provides the basis for some current antigen-directed therapies, including oral tolerance and administration of altered peptide ligands (APL).

3.2.1.1. Oral Tolerance

Oral tolerance is defined as a state of antigen-specific immunologic hyporesponsiveness that develops after oral administration of that antigen (4,5). After oral administration, antigens are taken up by the gut mucosa into the gut-associated lymphoid tissue (GALT), an immunologic network designed to protect the host from ingested pathogens but also to prevent the host from reacting to ingested proteins. Depending on the nature and dose of the administered antigen, presentation of antigen via the GALT can result in either active immunity (similar to the response elicited with systemic administration of antigen) or tolerance. Tolerance to orally administered antigens occurs through three potential mechanisms: clonal deletion, clonal anergy, or active suppression. High doses of administered antigen lead to deletion or anergy, whereas low doses of antigen result in active suppression.

Active suppression is mediated by the release of cytokines that act to downregulate TH1 responses. Suppression was originally thought to occur through the induction of TH2 cells in the GALT, with resultant production of IL-4 and IL10, which act to suppress TH1 responses. However, oral tolerance has been demonstrated in IL-4 knockout

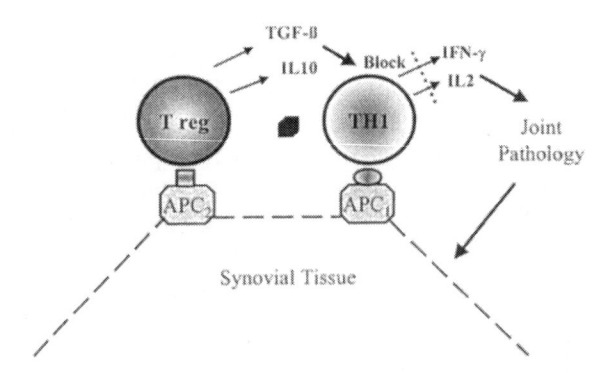

Fig. 1. Bystander suppression. Schematic diagram showing immunosuppression of a pathogenic TH1 cell in the joint. APC$_1$ and APC$_2$ take up and present two distinct antigens, both present in the synovium. APC$_1$ presents peptide to an autoimmune TH1 cell, which becomes activated, releasing pro-inflammatory cytokines IFN-γ and IL-2, which help to drive the inflammatory process. APC$_2$ presents a second antigen, also present in the synovium, to a second T-cell that has been induced to be of the regulatory phenotype (e.g., by oral tolerance). Upon stimulation of this T$_{reg}$-cell, suppressive cytokines such as IL-10 and TGF-β are released, which downregulate the "bystander" TH1 cell and, hence, decrease the inflammatory process.

mice, and antibody-mediated blockade of IL10 does not alter oral tolerance. Transforming growth factor-β (TGF-β) is produced by T cells in the GALT and is a potent immunosuppressive and anti-inflammatory cytokine and TGF-β knockout mice develop widespread inflammation in multiple organs. It has been suggested that subsets of regulatory T-cells, designated TH3 and Tr1, are induced in the GALT and actively suppress the immune response by the production of TGF-β, interleukin-4 (IL-4), and IL-10.

Because the pathology of many autoimmune diseases is driven by a predominantly TH1 response, the concept of suppression of TH1 responses with oral tolerance appears to be applicable to the treatment of autoimmunity. Furthermore, antigen-specific release of suppressive cytokines by tolerized T-cells into the local microenvironment may downregulate ongoing immune responses to an unrelated but anatomically colocalized antigen (5,6). This phenomenon, known as bystander suppression, is critical to oral tolerance and some other therapeutic approaches discussed in this chapter (see Fig. 1). Through bystander suppression, therapies do not need to be specifically directed to the antigens that incite or sustain the disease. If suppressor T-cells can be induced that target antigens expressed in diseased tissue, such as the brain or the joint, these T-cells may be able to suppress inflammation in that tissue even if the antigens inciting and sustaining the immune response are unknown.

The therapeutic efficacy of oral tolerance induction has been shown in a number of animal models. Feeding MBP upregulates TGF-β production, downregulates interferon-γ (IFN-γ) and tumor necrosis factor-α (TNF-α) production and suppresses disease in the rat EAE model. Furthermore, oral administration of MBP after disease induction in a relapsing model of EAE decreases disease severity and frequency of relapses. Feeding of collagen type II suppresses collagen-induced arthritis, adjuvant arthritis, and pristane-induced arthritis in animals.

These data in animal models have led to the initiation of human trials in multiple sclerosis and RA. A large 515-patient phase III trial examining the effects of feeding bovine myelin to patients with relapsing–remitting MS showed no significant difference in frequency of relapses compared to placebo, although the placebo response was so high in this study that it may have obscured a therapeutic effect *(4)*.

In RA, three double-blind, placebo-controlled clinical trials of oral tolerance in rheumatoid arthritis have been published to date. These trials have utilized several sources of type II collagen (CII) (chicken and bovine) at widely varying doses (20 µg to 10 mg per day) and have yielded mixed results *(6–8)*. The first trial examined the effects of 0.1 mg/d of chicken CII for 1 mo, followed by 2 mo therapy at 0.5 mg/d, in patients with long-standing RA (mean disease duration 10 yr). There was marginal benefit in the treated group in swollen and tender joints, but the differences were not statistically significant. A second trial looked at the effects of higher doses of bovine CII (10 mg/d) administered to 90 patients with early disease (<3 yr). No significant improvement was noted in individual disease parameters, although by responder analysis there was a trend (not statistically significant) toward improvement in the treated groups.

The largest study examined the effects of four doses of chicken CII (20 µg/d and 0.1, 0.5, and 2.5 mg/d) over 6 mo in 274 patients with long-standing disease (>10 yr disease duration). Results showed that the low-dose group (20 µg/d) had significant improvement compared to placebo by Paulus criteria, but not by ACR responder criteria. A placebo-controlled, 6-mo study of the effects of 60 µg of chicken CII in 900 patients with RA is currently underway. Results from this study should be available by the end of 1999.

Although studies to date have shown only modest therapeutic effects and appear to be conflicting at first analysis, several conclusions from this work are important:

1. Administration of collagen type II for the induction of oral tolerance is safe.
2. The optimal CII dose for therapeutic effect has not yet been determined, but there is a trend toward efficacy in the lower doses, as one would expect from the hypothesis discussed above that low doses lead to the generation of regulatory T-cells, which can lead to bystander suppression.
3. Data in animal models suggest that administration of antigen via other mucosal routes (nasal) may have similar effects as oral administration of antigen. This extends the potential of the "oral tolerance" approach to include nasal antigen administration, which may lend itself to reproducible delivery of a defined antigen dose more easily than oral administration.
4. The subset of RA patients who might benefit most from this therapy has not yet been defined.
5. Considering its safety and low cost, oral tolerance should not be discarded as a potential option in the rheumatologist's armamentarium. However, before the public and physicians embrace this concept, additional well-controlled trials carefully examining the effects of antigen source, antigen dose, and patient subsets need to be undertaken.

3.2.1.2. Altered Peptide Ligands

When a TCR is engaged with its cognate peptide–MHC complex, signals are initiated that lead to cytokine production and T-cell proliferation. Recently, however, it has been recognized that T-cell activation is not a simple all or none phenomenon. Modifications in the nature of the peptide presented to a given TCR, sometimes as subtle as changes in a single amino acid, can dramatically modify the nature of the T-cell response *(9)*. The modified peptides, known as altered peptide ligands (APL), do not appear to simply compete for MHC and TCR binding with native peptide, because they generally bind to the TCR with decreased avidity compared to native peptide. Binding of APL to T-cells may activate different signaling pathways within the cell and may change the phenotype of the cell from a pro-inflammatory TH1 cell to a regulatory cell, producing anti-inflammatory cytokines such as TGF-β and IL-10.

Support for the concept that APL may be useful therapeutically in autoimmune disease comes from animal models. For example, in Lewis rats, EAE can be induced by immunization with a specific peptide of MBP spanning amino acids 87–99 (MBP 87–99). Treatment of these rats with slightly modified forms of MBP 87–99 prevents the initiation of disease and reverses paralysis in established disease. The mechanism for this phenomenon is postulated to be via induction of regulatory T-cells that release suppressive cytokines and exert a bystander suppression effect, similar to that previously described for oral tolerance. Detailed work has delineated the requirements necessary for modification of MBP 87–99 to generate suppressive APL *(9)*.

Although the inciting antigen in human MS is unknown, there is a major T-cell response directed towards MBP 87-99. Thus, administration of APL based on MBP 87-99 APL may be capable of decreasing disease in human MS, analogous to the rat EAE model. Development of this therapeutic approach is underway. The principal of using APL to modify the T-cell phenotype in RA and other autoimmune diseases has not yet been applied. However, as we begin to identify the antigens involved in driving the autoimmune process in these diseases, generating APL based on these antigens may prove to be an extremely powerful therapeutic approach.

3.2.1.3. INDUCTION OF B-CELL TOLERANCE

In some autoimmune diseases, including myasthenia gravis, autoimmune thyroiditis and possibly SLE, tissue damage is mediated primarily by autoantibodies directed to known antigens. Thus, if specific B-cell tolerance to these antigens can be restored, autoantibody production should cease and antibody-mediated tissue damage should decrease. As with the T-cell, B-cell activation requires two signals: one delivered through the antigen-specific surface immunoglobulin (sIg) and the other through costimulation. Generation of one of these signals in the absence of the other renders the B-cell anergic or induces apoptosis. Alternatively, specific B-cells could be tolerized by binding their sIg in the absence of costimulation.

This approach is currently under investigation in SLE, where antibodies to double-stranded DNA have long been thought to play a major role in the pathogenesis of lupus glomerulonephritis. Administration of a molecule (LJP394), which presents a multivalent array of DNA oligonucleotides, results in binding of the sIg of DNA specific B-cells. However, because no protein is present in the LJP394, no peptide is available for presentation by the T-cell and hence no costimulatory signal is delivered to the DNA-specific B-cell. The result is anergy or apoptosis of DNA-specific B-cells and a reduction of DNA antibody levels.

Preliminary data in the BXSB murine model of SLE has shown that LJP394 decreases DNA antibody levels, reduces clinical nephritis, and improves survival. Human trials to date have shown a modest decrease in DNA antibody levels that persist for up to 2 mo after discontinuation of the agent. A large phase III clinical trial looking at the ability of LJP394 to increase the time between flares of lupus nephritis is now underway *(10)*.

3.2.2. MHC-Directed Therapy

Many autoimmune diseases have been shown to be associated with MHC class II alleles, including RA with HLA-DR4 and DR1, MS with HLA-DR2, and diabetes with HLA-DR3 and DR4. Because the function of the MHC class II molecule is to present antigen to the TCR, the association of a specific class II allele with a given autoimmune disease suggests that a specific class II molecule is involved in presenting antigens that are important in driving the disease process. Thus, blockade of class II molecules might disrupt presentation of critical antigens and ameliorate disease.

The administration of antibodies to disease-associated class II molecules has shown beneficial effects in animal models of EAE, myasthenia gravis, and collagen-induced arthritis. Primate studies with antibodies to class II molecules resulted in significant toxicity, most likely as a result of the immune response to the antibodies themselves, rather than as a result of DR blockade. Nonetheless, because of this experience, anti-DR antibody therapy in humans is no longer under active investigation.

An alternative approach has been to immunize animals with peptides derived from disease-associated class II molecules. In an SJL mouse model of EAE, immunization with an 18 amino acid peptide derived from the disease-associated class II molecule induced antibodies that blocked antigen presentation and abrogated disease. Although the mechanism of disease suppression is not known with certainty, there is some evidence to suggest that the number of MHC class II molecules on the surface of APC is decreased by this treatment, resulting in decreased antigen presentation *(11)*.

Up to 90% of patients with RA express at least one DR allele containing a specific five amino acid sequence (QKRAA) known as the shared epitope. This sequence is located in the peptide-binding groove of the MHC molecule, suggesting that this epitope is involved in binding and/or presenting peptide to the TCR. Thus, blockade of this shared epitope might be expected to block antigen presentation and, in particular, block the presentation of antigens important in the pathogenesis of RA. Because DR is involved in presenting many antigens, however, there is also concern that blockade of DR could result in generalized immunosuppression, an effect that has been seen in some animals homozygous at the DR locus. A phase II clinical trial has examined the effects of immunizing RA patients who are heterozygous for the shared epitope with a 20 amino acid peptide that contains the shared epitope. Results indicate that this strategy generates antibodies to the shared epitope in approximately 25% of patients and does not result in generalized immunosuppression. In these early studies, there was modest improvement in clinical disease; larger trials are underway to determine if this approach will lead to significant clinical improvement in RA.

As an alternative approach, the same investigators are administering DR peptides containing the shared epitope coupled to peptides from a cartilage-derived antigen that has been implicated in arthritis pathogenesis in animal models (gp39). Clinical results from these novel therapies should be available within the next few years.

3.2.3. T-Cell Receptor-Directed Therapy

Once antigen is processed and bound in the MHC groove, this complex is presented to the T-cell receptor, and if appropriate costimulatory signals are present, T-cell proliferation is triggered. Thus, therapeutic targeting of the TCR should result in disruption of this signal. However, like immunoglobulins, TCR are extremely diverse and each TCR binds with a high degree of specificity to only a small group of closely related MHC–peptide complexes. Therefore, unless the specific TCR present on each autoreactive clone of cells is known, such specific blockade does not appear to be feasible. Furthermore, epitope spreading suggests that an increasing number of T-cell clones, each expressing a unique TCR, are recruited over time during the development of autoimmune disease. Thus, by the time clinical disease is evident, TCR-directed therapies would have the Herculean task of impacting multiple unique TCR targets.

Nonetheless, many investigators have examined T-cells in autoimmune disease in an attempt to define TCR usage at sites of inflammation such as the joint in RA or the central nervous system (CNS) in MS. Evidence indicates that multiple clones of T-cells are involved in tissue damage and that T-cell involvement varies from individual to individual and over time within the same individual. However, several investigators have shown that certain T-cell families, defined by similarities in their non-peptide-binding Vβ region, are overrepresented in inflammatory lesions. For example, samples from the CNS or cerebrospinal fluid (CSF) from patients with MS show an increased frequency of T-cells of the Vβ5.2 or Vβ6 families relative to T-cells in peripheral blood of the same patients. In RA, synovial fluid and synovial tissue have been reported to show an increased frequency of Vβ3, Vβ12, Vβ14, and Vβ17 T-cells relative to peripheral blood. Although there is some controversy on the extent to which these observations apply to different patient populations, these data raise the possibility that if specific Vβ T-cells families are overrepresented at sites of tissue damage, therapies might be directed at these T-cell subsets *(12)*. Because Vβ T-cell families may constitute 2–10% of the total T-cell population, this population provides a more feasible therapeutic target than individual T-cell clones each expressing a unique TCR.

The therapeutic efficacy of this concept has been demonstrated in the EAE animal model, in which the MBP-reactive, pathogenic T-cells are members of the Vβ8 family *(13)*. In this model, immunization with a peptide derived from the CDR2 region of Vβ8 has been shown to prevent disease induction and shorten the course of established disease. The immune response to these peptides has been shown to induce regulatory T-cells that release suppressive cytokines when they encounter their antigen (Vβ8). These regulatory T-cells localize to the site of tissue inflammation by virtue of the increased number of T-cells expressing Vβ8 (the cognate antigen of the induced regulatory cells) present at those sites. Once they encounter their target antigen, they release immunosuppressive cytokines such as TGF-β and IL-10 and decrease inflammation either directly or through bystander suppression (*see* Fig. 1). Similar efficacy of TCR vaccination has been shown in adjuvant and collagen-induced arthritis models.

The application of this concept to human disease is under development for RA, MS, and psoriasis, diseases in which there is at least some data to indicate a biased TCR Vβ usage at sites of inflammation *(14,15)*. Immunization with TCR peptides has been shown to be safe and well tolerated. A phase II trial in RA examining the effects of immunization with a combination of peptides to Vβ3, Vβ14, and Vβ17 has been completed. This study, conducted in 99 RA patients with active disease of moderate duration (mean 10.9 yr), showed that the peptides were well tolerated and demonstrated moderate efficacy *(15)*. Of patients adhering to the protocol, 50% achieved an ACR 20 response at 24 wk compared to 19% of placebo-treated patients. Although this response may not be as dramatic as some other therapies, the low cost, good safety profile, ease of administration, and potential for long-term response make this an attractive therapeutic option if the efficacy of this approach can be confirmed.

4. Summary

Since the discovery of corticosteroids nearly 50 yr ago, the pharmacopia for the treatment of autoimmune diseases has consisted almost exclusively of agents to block the inflammatory consequences of autoimmunity. Nonsteroidal anti-inflammatory drugs, gold, methotrexate, and even the new cytokine inhibitors all act primarily at the distal end of the autoimmune process. As our understanding of basic immunology and the mechanisms of normal tolerance grows, we are now beginning to obtain the knowledge and tools to treat autoimmune diseases closer to the source—the autoimmune response itself.

Restoring tolerance to just the right extent will be a difficult and complex task, however. Broad immunosuppression may "tolerize" many autoreactive cells, but at the cost of suppressing the normal immune response as well. At the other extreme, restoration of tolerance to only a few specific antigens may prove to be too little, too late, because the autoimmune response has expanded by epitope spreading by the time clinical disease is evident. Therapies to restore tolerance are clearly in their infancy, just as anti-inflammatory therapies were in the 1950s. However, if autoreactive cells can be tolerized by some of the methods described in this chapter or by other methods yet to be developed, there is a potential for the induction of long-term, drug-free disease remissions in our patients. The pace of immunology research makes one optimistic that this goal should be attainable in considerably less than 50 yr.

References

1. Tyndall, A. and Gratwohl, A. (1997) Hemopoietic blood and marrow transplants in the treatment of severe autoimmune disease. *Curr. Opin. Hematol.* **4,** 390–394.
2. Marmont, A. M. (1998) Stem cell transplantation for severe autoimmune diseases: progress and problems. *Haematologica* **83,** 733–743.
3. Craft, J. and Fatenejad, S. (1997) Self antigens and epitope spreading in systemic autoimmunity. *Arthritis Rheum.* **40,** 1374–1382.
4. Weiner, H. L. (1997) Oral tolerance: immune mechanisms and treatment of autoimmune diseases. *Immunol. Today* **18,** 335–343.
5. Strobel, S. and Mowat, A. M. (1998) Immune responses to dietary antigens: oral tolerance. *Immunol. Today* **19,** 173–181.
6. Trentham, D. E. (1998). Oral tolerization as a treatment of rheumatoid arthritis. *Rheum. Dis. Clin. North Am.* **24,** 525–536.
7. Kalden, J. R. and Sieper, J. (1998) Oral collagen in the treatment of rheumatoid arthritis. *Arthritis Rheum.* **41,** 191–194.
8. Barnett, M. L., Kremer, J. H., St. Clair, E. W., Clegg, D. O., Furst, D., Weisman, M., et al. (1998) Treatment of rheumatoid arthritis with oral type II collagen. *Arthritis Rheum.* **41,** 290–297.
9. Fairchild, P. J. (1997) Altered peptide ligands: prospects for immune intervention in autoimmune disease. *Eur. J. Immunogenet.* **24,** 155–167.
10. Weisman, M. H., Bluestein, H. G., Berner, C. M., and deHaan, H. A. (1997) Reduction in circulating dsDNA antibody titer after administration of LJP394. *J. Rheumatol.* **24,** 314–318.

11. Spack, E. G. (1997) Treatment of autoimmune diseases through manipulation of antigen presentation. *Crit. Rev. Immunol.* **17,** 529–536.
12. Kotzin, B. L. and Kappler, J. (1998) Targeting the T cell receptor in rheumatoid arthritis. *Am. Coll. Rheumatol.* **41,** 1906–1910.
13. Vandenbark, A. A., Chou, Y. K., Whitham, R., Mass, M., Buenafe, A., Liefeld, D., et al. (1996) Treatment of multiple sclerosis with T-cell receptor peptides: Results of a double-blind pilot trial. *Nature Med.* **2,** 1109–1115.
14. Vandenbark, A. A., Hashim, G., and Offner, H. (1993) TCR peptide therapy in autoimmune diseases. *Int. Rev. Immunol.* **9,** 251–276.
15. Moreland, L. W., Morgan, E. E., Adamson, T. C., III, Fronek, Z., Calabrese, L. H., Cash, J. M., et al. (1998) T cell receptor peptide vaccination in rheumatoid arthritis. *Arthritis Rheum.* **41,** 1919–1929.

33

Metalloproteases and Their Modulation as Treatment in Osteoarthritis

Johanne Martel-Pelletier, Ginette Tardif, Julio Fernandes, and Jean-Pierre Pelletier

1. Osteoarthritis

Osteoarthritis (OA) is a disease characterized by a degeneration of articular cartilage. Although the etiology of OA is not yet known and is likely multifactorial, this disease process involves a disturbance in the normal balance of degradation and repair in articular cartilage (1). The breakdown of the cartilage matrix leads to the development of fibrillation, fissures, the appearance of gross ulcerations, and the disappearance of the full thickness surface of the joint. This is accompanied by hypertrophic bone changes with osteophyte formation and subchondral plate thickening. The cartilage matrix breakdown products released into the synovial fluid are phagocytosed by the synovial membrane. Consequently, the membrane becomes hypertrophic and hyperplastic, and an inflammatory reaction is often observed. Although the remodeling of subchondral bone is associated with OA pathology, it is still under debate whether this tissue change initiates or is involved in the progression of cartilage loss.

In OA cartilage, it appears that the earliest histopathological lesions, which are a depletion of proteoglycans and a breakdown of the collagen network, result from an increased synthesis and/or activity of proteolytic enzymes. Current knowledge (1) indicates a major involvement of the metalloprotease (MMP) family in this disease process. Other enzymes from the serine- and cysteine-dependent protease families, such as the plasminogen activator/plasmin system and cathepsin B, respectively, also play a role but primarily as activators of MMPs. Another protease, the aggrecanase, an enzyme belonging to the adamalysin family (i.e. having desintegrin and metalloprotease domains (1), appears responsible for proteoglycan cleavage as found in human OA synovial fluid.

2. Identification and Regulation of Metalloproteases

2.1. Definition

Matrix MMPs are enzymes implicated in the natural turnover of the extracellular macromolecules (2). They are produced by cells of the articular joint tissues, including

From: *Current Molecular Medicine: Principles of Molecular Rheumatology*
Edited by: G. C. Tsokos © Humana Press Inc., Totowa, NJ

chondrocytes, fibroblasts, osteoclasts, osteoblasts, and inflammatory cells (macrophages, lymphocytes, neutrophils). Collectively, they can degrade all the major macromolecules of the extracellular matrix: collagens, proteoglycans, laminin, fibronectin, and other glycoproteins. MMPs are the product of different genes, but they share structural and functional features such as an optimal activity at neutral pH (with the exception of stromelysin-1 for which the optimal pH is at about 5) and require calcium and zinc for activity. Most MMP proteins are organized into three distinct and well-conserved domains: an amino-terminal propeptide consisting of about 80–90 amino acids involved in the maintenance of enzyme latency; a catalytic domain that binds zinc and calcium ions; and a hemopexin-like domain at the carboxy terminal. This last domain seems to play a role in substrate binding. MMP are synthesized as proenzymes and must be activated by proteolytic cleavage. Generally, they are present as soluble forms, but some are membrane bound. The activation of the latent secreted enzymes results from the proteolytic cleavage of the propeptide domain from the N-terminus of the enzyme. As MMP are so potent, they are carefully controlled. Synthesis, activation, and inhibition of the active enzymes are controlled by physiological and pathological factors such as pro-inflammatory cytokines, hormones, growth factors, and proteases.

2.2. Classification

Metalloproteases are broadly classified into four groups, based on substrate specificity and cellular location: the collagenases, stromelysins, gelatinases, and membrane-type MMP (MT-MMP) *(3)*. Members of the first three groups have been found at increased levels in OA tissues *(1)*. Other MMPs such as matrilysin and macrophage metalloelastase have been described but have not been assigned to any of these groups.

The collagenases are secreted as latent enzymes and, once activated, are capable of degrading native collagens. Three collagenases have been identified in human cartilage and their levels are clearly elevated in OA: collagenase-1 (MMP-1), collagenase-2 (MMP-8), and collagenase-3 (MMP-13) *(4)*. Although all three collagenases are active on collagen fibrils, they are biochemically different. The coexistence of different types of collagenase in the articular tissue points to distinct roles and regulations for each. Collagenase-3 preferentially cleaves type II collagen (the major collagen type in articular cartilage) and is five times more active on this substrate than collagenase-1; collagenase-2 has a higher specificity for type I collagen, and collagenase-1 for type III collagen. It has also been shown that a different topographical distribution exists between collagenase-1 and collagenase-3 within pathological cartilage, suggesting a selective involvement of each collagenase during the disease process. In OA, collagenase-1 and collagenase-2 are located predominantly in the superficial and upper intermediate layers of the cartilage, whereas collagenase-3 is found mostly in the lower intermediate and deep layers. Moreover, from an immunohistochemical study using an OA animal model, it was shown that the collagenase-1 chondrocyte score increased steadily in the superficial zone of the cartilage with the progression of the lesions, whereas the collagenase-3 cell reached a plateau at the moderate stage of the disease in the lower intermediate and deep layers *(5)*. All together, the data on the collagenases in OA tissues suggest an involvement of collagenase-1 during the inflammatory process and an implication of collagenase-3 in the remodeling phase of the tissue.

The gelatinases are also secreted as proenzymes. They have a substrate preference for denatured collagen, gelatin, and types IV and V collagens. Two gelatinases have been found in the articular tissues: gelatinase-B (92 kDa or MMP-9) and gelatinase-A (72 kDa or MMP-2), but only the gelatinase-B level is increased in human OA cartilage.

The stromelysins show a broader substrate specificity and include proteoglycans, fibronectin, elastin, laminin, and so forth. Stromelysin-1 (MMP-3), stromelysin-2 (MMP-10), and stromelysin-3 (MMP-11) have been described in human tissues, but of those, only stromelysin-1 has been found in elevated levels in OA. Stromelysin-2 and stromelysin-3 were detected only in the synovial fibroblasts from synovial membrane of rheumatoid arthritis patients. Histochemical studies suggested a relationship between the level of stromelysin-1 and the severity of degradation of proteoglycans. This enzyme is also implicated in the enzymatic cascade responsible for the activation of procollagenase.

For the MT-MMP, to date six members have been identified and designated MT1-MMP through MT6-MMP *(3,3a,3b)*. MT1-MMP is expressed in human articular cartilage, and possesses collagenolytic activity. MT1-MMP, MT2-MMP, MT5-MMP, and MT6-MMP activate gelatinase A, and MT1-MMP and MT2-MMP also activate collagenase-3. The relevance of these enzymes in the pathogenicity of OA has yet to be determined.

Matrilysin (PUMP-1, MMP-7) has not been assigned to any of the previous groups. This enzyme is highly active against various molecules of the extracellular matrix, especially the proteoglycans. Matrilysin was found overexpressed in human OA cartilage and its expression enhanced by treatment with the proinflammatory cytokines interleukin (IL)-1α and tumor necrosis factor-α (TNF-α).

2.3. Regulation

The synthesis, activation, and inhibition of MMP are tightly regulated at several levels in order to maintain a proper balance between the anabolism and catabolism of the articular tissue, because excessive amounts of MMP result in the overall destruction of the extracellular matrix. Regulatory pathways are found at the transcriptional (stimulation or inhibition of mRNA) and posttranslational levels (activation of the secreted latent enzymes and inhibition of activated MMP).

The mechanisms governing MMP transcription regulation are complex. The promoter regions of the MMP genes have been cloned and sequenced, and their analysis revealed the presence of several cis-acting DNA sequences, which have been implicated in both basal and modulatory transcriptional activities. Many of the proteins binding to these sequences have also been identified and an understanding of their role as either stimulators or inhibitors of transcription has emerged.

2.3.1. Transcriptional and Posttranscriptional Levels

2.3.1.1. STIMULATION OF TRANSCRIPTION

Metalloprotease genes are generally expressed in cartilage and synovial membrane cells in low levels, and their gene transcription induced by factors such as pro-inflammatory cytokines (IL-1β, TNF-α) and some growth factors including epidermal growth factor (EGF), platelet-derived growth factor (PDGF), and basic fibroblast growth factor (bFGF) *(6)*. For most of them, transcription activation of the MMP genes depends, at least in part, on the presence of an AP-1 site (activator protein-1, TGAG/CTCA), located at position –65 to –79 bp in the promoter of the MMP genes *(7,8)*, the exceptions being the gelatinase A and stromelysin-3 genes whose promoters do not possess a consensus AP-1 site. Proteins of the Jun and Fos families of transcription factors bind the AP-1 site as dimers (Jun/Jun or Jun/Fos) and contribute to both basal and induced MMP transcription. Although important, this factor is not the only regulator of transcription, but rather seems to act in concert with other cis-acting sequences. For example, in the collagenase-1 promoter, the AP-1 and PEA3 (polyomavirus enhancer A) sites have been found to act as a transcriptional unit to achieve maximal induction.

2.3.1.2. INHIBITION OF TRANSCRIPTION

Metalloprotease gene transcription can be suppressed by various factors, and those of physiological interest for articular tissues are the transforming growth factor TGF-β (depending on the cell type, the state of the cell, and the isoforms), vitamin A analogs (retinoids), and glucocorticoids. Although each of these agents has its own pathway for inhibiting MMP gene transcription, the presence of an AP-1 site in the promoter of MMP genes appears to be a key element in the inhibitory effect.

TGF-β belongs to a superfamily of sequence-related molecules involved in regulation of growth, differentiation, and development. This family presently comprises over 30 distinct molecules. In mammals, three isoforms, TGF-β1, TGF-β2, and TGF-β3, are found. In regards to MMP, TGF-β shows bifunctional properties: it can either inhibit or stimulate gene transcription. TGF-β2 was found to stimulate collagenase-1 production in keratinocytes by stimulating c-Jun; the c-Jun/c-Fos dimer efficiently binds the AP-1 site thereby upregulating transcription. In contrast, it inhibits collagenase-1 synthesis in fibroblasts by upregulating the synthesis of Jun-B; the Jun-B/c-Fos dimer does not bind the AP-1 site as efficiently as a c-Jun/c-Fos dimer, therefore preventing the synthesis of collagenase-1 *(9)*. In addition to the AP-1 site, other sites have also been implicated in the mediation of the TGF-β effect. One of these is the TIE (TGF-β inhibitory element) site present in the promoter of human collagenase-1, gelatinase B, matrilysin, and collagenase-3 (for this enzyme, it is on the opposite strand). The TIE site was found to negatively regulate stromelysin-1 gene expression.

In human OA chondrocytes, it was recently found that TGF-β1 and TGF-β2 showed differential regulatory patterns on collagenase-3, depending whether the cells had a low (upregulation) or high (no effect) basal level. Importantly, this did not occur for collagenase-1. Moreover, an opposite pattern was found between the isoforms in regard to collagenase-1—TGF-β1 upregulates collagenase-1 on these OA cells, and TGF-β2 had no effect *(10)*.

Although the precise mechanisms involved in the glucocorticoids' and retinoids' downregulation of MMP gene synthesis are still under study, data showed that in this process the AP-1 site is targeted *(7,8)*. Briefly, both factors first bind their respective hormone receptors and the ligand–receptor complexes translocate to the nucleus. One proposed pathway of repression is by the interaction of the ligand–receptor complexes with the Jun or Fos proteins, thus interfering with the transcriptional activation of

AP-1. Another pathway found for the retinoids involved the mRNA downregulation of the c-Fos protein.

2.3.2. Posttranslational Levels

The secreted MMP proenzymes are activated by a number of physiological activators. In turn, the activated MMP are regulated by inhibitors that bind the active site of the MMP and inhibit their catalytic activity.

2.3.2.1. METALLOPROTEASE ACTIVATION CASCADES

There are at least two activation processes. Extracellular activation occurs in the tissue for most of the MMP and at the cell surface for collagenase-3 and gelatinase A. In contrast, MT-MMP and stromelysin-3 are intracellularly activated in the Golgi compartment *(11)*. The extracellular activation is a stepwise process in which an activator generates an intermediate; the intermediate or partially activated MMP fully activates the MMP. This process allows for very fine regulation of the enzymatic activity.

Several enzyme families have been proposed as activators for MMP. Enzymes from the serine- and cysteine-dependent protease families, such as plasminogen activator (PA)/plasmin system and cathepsin B, respectively, have been proposed as activators *(1)*. Cathepsin B is a lysosomal enzyme, with a maximal activity at pH 6.0 and requiring thiol as an activator. This protease may play a role in cartilage degradation through direct degradative action on both the collagen and proteoglycans as well as by the activation of MMP. Although other cathepsins have been found in the synovial membrane, cathepsin B appears to be most relevant to MMP activation in cartilage. Cathepsin B levels have been found in increased levels in OA articular tissue, whereas cysteine protease inhibitory activity was decreased.

The plasminogen activators urokinase-type (uPA) and tissue-type (t-PA) are proteases which convert plasminogen to plasmin. The PA/plasmin proteases have a broad spectrum of activity. Their levels are increased in OA joints suggesting a role in cartilage destruction. Plasmin has the potential to degrade cartilage proteoglycans as well as to activate latent collagenase-1 and stromelysin-1. The PA are themselves inactivated by a glycoprotein, PAI (plasminogen activator inhibitor), which can be modulated in cartilage and cultured chondrocytes by inflammatory cytokines and growth factors. Decreased levels of PAI-1 have been reported in human OA cartilage. Moreover, a positive relationship has also been reported between levels of plasmin and active collagenase in OA cartilage.

The collagenases and gelatinases, however, can also be activated by other active MMP *(11)*. MT1-MMP activates collagenase-3 and gelatinase A potentiates the latter activation; MT1-MMP also activates gelatinase A. Collagenase-3 is itself capable of activating progelatinase B. Stromelysin-2 activates procollagenase-2, whereas stromelysin-1 has been shown to cleave the proforms of both collagenase-1 and collagenase-3, gelatinase B, and matrilysin. The activated matrilysin can itself activate collagenase-1 and gelatinase B. Examples of the enzymatic cascades described show the complexity of the interactions between MMP and the delicate balance between MMP synthesis and activation that must be maintained to preserve the integrity of the articular tissue.

In addition, some MMP activated intracellularly, such as stromelysin-3 and MT-MMP, have a 10 amino terminal insert between the propeptide and the N-terminal domain. This sequence, GLSARNRQKR in stromelysin-3, is recognized by a Golgi-associated serine protease, furin. The latter activates this MMP, which is then secreted in an active form.

2.3.2.2. INHIBITION OF ACTIVE METALLOPROTEASES

Once activated, the MMP are further regulated by several naturally occurring inhibitors, such as the tissue inhibitor of metalloproteases (TIMP) and the α_2-macroglobulin *(12)*. The α_2-macroglobulin is a large protein (750 kDa) produced by the liver and found in the serum and synovial fluids of normal and OA patients. It acts as a nonspecific inhibitor of proteases by trapping the enzyme and blocking its access to the substrate. Because of its high molecular weight, this inhibitor may not be capable of penetrating the cartilage, and its relevance to this tissue degradation appears unlikely. Its role appears restricted to the fluid or inflammatory exudates.

TIMP are the specific physiological inhibitors of MMP, and they are synthesized by the same cells that produce MMP. To date, four TIMP molecules have been identified (TIMP-1, TIMP-2, TIMP-3, and TIMP-4). Each TIMP molecule is the product of a different gene, but the proteins share several structural features: they all possess 12 conserved cysteine residues and an amino-terminal domain necessary for MMP inhibitory activity. All active MMP are inhibited by TIMP with a stoichiometric ratio of 1 : 1. Their inhibitory capacity is the result of their specific noncovalent binding to the active site of MMP and to the proforms of gelatinase A (TIMP-2, TIMP-3, and TIMP-4) and gelatinase-B (TIMP-1 and TIMP-3). These latter complexes can still be activated, but they show lower specific activities than the noncomplexed gelatinases. TIMP-1 and TIMP-2 are present in cartilage and are synthesized by chondrocytes, but only TIMP-1 has been detected in the OA synovial tissue and fluid. TIMP-3 is found exclusively in the extracellular matrix and not in conditioned media. TIMP-4 has approximately 50% sequence identity with TIMP-2 and TIMP-3, and 38% with TIMP-1. Moreover, TIMP-4 was found only in cancer cells and appears responsible for modulating the cell-surface activation of pro-gelatinase A, suggesting its importance as a tissue-specific regulator of extracellular matrix remodeling. An imbalance between the amounts of TIMP and MMP toward higher levels of active MMP, such as that seen in OA tissues, may account, at least in part, for the increased levels of active MMP in pathological tissues.

3. Treatment with Metalloprotease Inhibitors

3.1. Design of Metalloprotease Inhibitors

Conventional treatments do not affect the OA disease process. Recently, the use of protease inhibitors or factors responsible for blocking MMP activation and synthesis has been suggested as a new therapeutic approach. Inhibiting MMP synthesis/activity as a treatment for OA has been the focus of very intensive research over the last decade. A large variety of synthetic approaches have been used, and highly effective MMP inhibitors have been tested. Some of these MMP inhibitors were shown to reduce or block cartilage destruction on animal models and some were also shown to be effective in preventing the progression of certain human tumors. Figure 1 gives a summary of representative activators and inhibitors of MMP synthesis and activity.

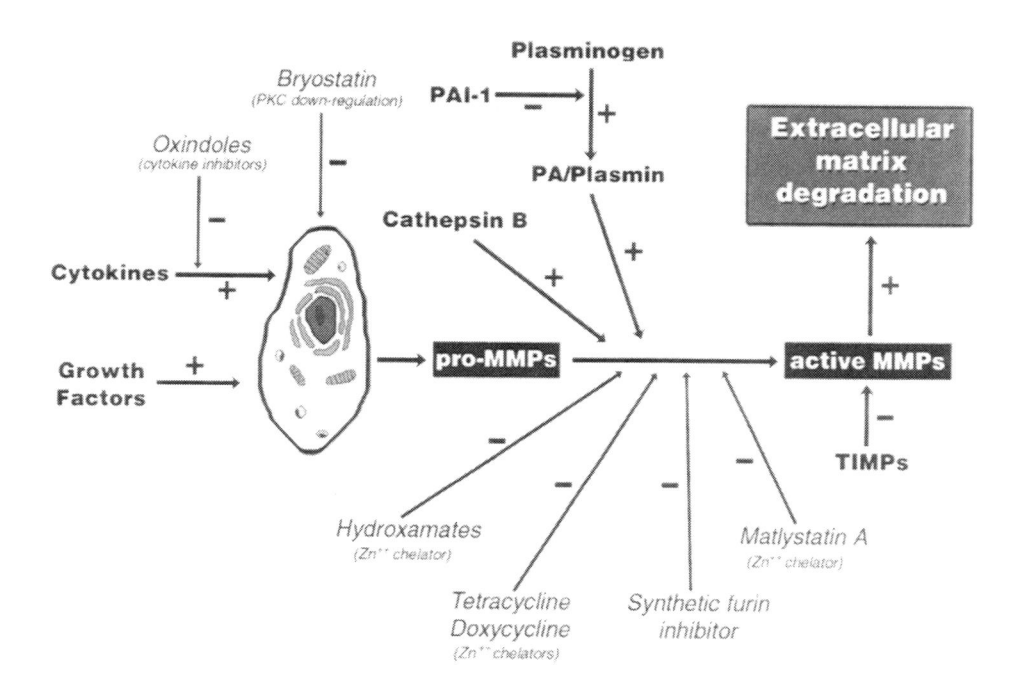

Fig. 1. Schematic diagram of representative activators (+) and inhibitors (−) of MMP synthesis and activity. Physiological compounds are shown in bold and synthetic compounds in italic.

Developing protease inhibitors that are therapeutically active is very challenging. In addition to ensuring that the molecule has the required potency, it must also be bioavailable, preferably administered orally, be specific for the targeted enzyme family, and have no significant toxicity. Encouragingly, many of these conditions have been met with the development of inhibitors of another protease family, the zinc-dependent metalloexopeptidase angiotensin-converting enzyme. These compounds form a model for the design of MMP inhibitors. This approach consists of choosing a zinc chelating ligand and attaching it to a peptide that mimics the cleavage site of the MMP target substrates *(13)*.

Importantly, if such compounds are to be used in vivo, untoward side effects will have to be tested. A possible side effect may be an imbalance in the activity of MMP involved in bone remodeling and wound healing. Another undesirable consequence is a potential overall increased deposition of connective tissue matrix. As MMPs are also involved in the implantation of the embryo, the development of the fetus, and many of the processes involved during parturition, administration of these compounds will need to be initially restricted to selected patient groups.

A primary reason for looking at MMP inhibitors was to block the degradation process of the two major cartilage macromolecules: collagens and proteoglycans. The first rational approach to the design of inhibitors was made for collagenase. Different chelating moieties were tested, and these included thiols, carboxyl-alkyls, phosphonic acids, phosphonamides, and hydroxamate groups *(14)*. Some interest has been shown in screening natural products for the presence of MMP inhibitors, and a series of gelatinase inhibitors has been recently described.

The inhibition of proteoglycan degradation in cartilage has, however, encountered a higher level of difficulty. This may be the result of tissue penetration. It is known that lower concentrations of inhibitor are required to prevent collagen release from cartilage, which takes place after the highly charged proteoglycan molecules have been removed. However, this may suggest that the enzyme responsible for proteoglycan degradation may differ substantially from the known MMP (aggrecanase?).

Another interesting new therapeutic target may be the convertase furin. Indeed, and as mentioned earlier, some MMPs (stromelysin-3 and MT-MMP) could be activated intracellularly by this enzyme. This may be an important step in the control of some MMP activation.

3.2. Inhibitors of Metalloprotease Activity

3.2.1. Physiological Inhibitors, TIMP

The balance between the level of activated MMP and the available TIMP determines the net enzyme activity and is a key determinant of extracellular matrix turnover. Increasing the local synthesis of TIMP would be an effective way to prevent connective-tissue turnover and OA progression. However, the natural TIMP has limited possible application as a therapeutic agent, mainly because of its limitation regarding the administration of proteins. Indeed, it is well known that peptides within the circulation are often rapidly removed by either the liver or the kidneys and/or rapidly hydrolyzed in the gut, in the blood, or in the tissues. Nonetheless, the use of recombinant TIMP and gene therapy has been shown to be effective in antimetastatic treatment *(15)*. Recently, the three-dimensional structure of TIMP complex with stromelysin-1 has been demonstrated *(16)*. This study revealed that TIMP fits into the active MMP domain by the TIMP N-terminal part and binds in a substrate manner. Based on current knowledge of the TIMP/MMP complex structure, researchers have begun to look at engineering the TIMP in order to be selective to a specific MMP; this can be achieved by specific point mutation of TIMP at the MMP contact site *(17)*. There might therefore be a regain of interest in TIMP as treatment in the field of OA in the near future.

3.2.2. Chemical Inhibitors (Table 1)

Although the prospects for the prevention of cartilage macromolecule breakdown using synthetic MMP inhibitors look promising, opinions differ as to the best MMP to target. One option points to the collagenases, as it was shown that loss of the collagen network leads to irreversible damage and that proteoglycans and other proteins can be readily lost from cartilage but rapidly replaced. Others suggest that the inhibitors should have a broad spectrum, the advantage being to inhibit yet undiscovered MMPs that may be involved in the disease process. For example, it was noted in initial animal studies that treatment with a MMP inhibitor, in addition to sparing cartilage and bone, also had an anti-inflammatory effect. However, one should be cautious as broad-spectrum inhibitors could also lead to unwanted side effects by preventing previously unrecognized but essential proteolytic pathways from operating. Perhaps the principle of MMP inhibition should first be tested with broad-spectrum inhibitors to establish the potential of these compounds. Then it would be possible to make highly specific inhibitors for individual MMP by exploiting unique cleavage sites for each enzyme and so begin to evaluate the contribution of the targeted enzyme to the pathology.

Table 1
Metalloprotease Inhibitors: A Nonexhaustive Listing of Chemical Agents

Metalloproteases	MMP number	Metalloprotease inhibitors
Collagenase-1	MMP-1	BB94, BB2516, Ro3555, doxycycline, bryostatin-1, Ro 31-7467, tenidap, BE-16627B
Gelatinase-A	MMP-2	BB94, BB2516, CT-1746, doxycycline, matlystatin, CT1166, synthetic furin inhibitor, N-sulfonylamino acid derivatives, leupeptin analogs
Stromelysin-1	MMP-3	BB94, BB2516, CGS27023A, bryostatin, tenidap
Matrilysin	MMP-7	BB94, BB2516,
Collagenase-2	MMP-8	Ro3555
Gelatinase B	MMP-9	BB94, BB2516, CGS27023A, CT-1746, matlystatin, GM-6001, doxycycline, bryostatin-1, N-sulfonylamino acid derivatives, CT1166
Stromelysin-2	MMP-10	CGS27023A, bryostatin
Stromelysin-3	MMP-11	CGS27023A, bryostatin
Metalloelastase	MMP-12	Doxycycline
Collagenase-3	MMP-13	Ro3555, doxycycline
MT-MMP	MMP-14	BB94, BB2516, CGS27023A, synthetic furin inhibitor

MMP inhibitors	Manufacturer
BB94, BB2516	British Biotech Inc., Oxford, UK
Ro3555, Ro31-7467	Roche Products Ltd., Herts, UK
Matlystatin	Sankyo Co. Ltd., Tokyo, Japan
CT1166, CT1746	Celltech Ltd., Slough, UK
Tenidap	Pfizer Central Research, Groton, CT, USA
Synthetic furin inhibitor	Alexis Biochemicals Corp., San Diego, CA, USA
N-Sulfonyl amino acid derivatives	Shionogi Res. Lab. Inc., Osaka, Japan
CG27023A	Ciba Geigy Corp., Summit, NJ, USA
GM6001 (galardin)	Glycomed, Alameda, CA, USA
Doxycycline	Collagenex, Newtown, PA, USA
Leupeptin analogs	Nippon Kayaku Co. Ltd., Tokyo, Japan

One approach is based on the cysteine switch mechanism of MMP, in which proforms of MMP are inhibited by a highly conserved sequence in the prosegment, which is cleaved on activation. This sequence contains a cysteine residue that is believed to coordinate the active-site zinc atom, thereby maintaining enzyme latency. This linear peptide sequence (MRKPRCGN/VPDV) has been shown to exhibit inhibitory activity against gelatinase A and stromelysin-1.

Antibiotics such as tetracycline and its semisynthetic forms (doxycycline and minocycline) have very significant inhibitory properties that impact MMP activity *(17)*. Their action is mediated by chelating the zinc present in the active site of MMP. Tetracycline is a poor inhibitor of MMP (50% inhibitory concentration [IC$_{50}$] about 350 μM), whereas semisynthetic homologs are more potent, making them more attractive. Furthermore, tetracycline and homologs are also suppressors at the transcriptional level of some MMP (such as stromelysin-1, gelatinase A). Several in vitro studies have demonstrated that tetracycline can inhibit collagenases (collagenase-1 and collagenase-3) as well as gelatinase A activities. Tetracycline and doxycycline were shown to reduce in vivo the severity of OA in animal models, whereas doxycycline reduced collagenase and gelatinase activities. A clinical trial is presently underway to explore the therapeutic efficacy of doxycycline in human knee OA.

The hydroxamate-based compounds are potent inhibitors of MMP *(13)*. They were designed originally as collagenase selective inhibitors and are believed to work by interacting with the active site of the MMP molecule, binding with the zinc molecule, thus inactivating the enzyme. Thiols and carboxylalkyls, also inhibitors of MMP, have a similar mode of action. The hydroxamate compounds are very common and some of them are orally active. Several of these compounds are currently under investigation *(18)*. Among them, CGS27023-A (Ciba-Geigy Corp, Summit, NJ, USA), an orally active stromelysin inhibitor, was shown to block cartilage matrix degradation in vivo in rabbits. Another inhibitor, Ro-3555 (Roche Products Ltd., Herts, UK), a competitive inhibitor of human collagenase-1, collagenase-2, and collagenase-3, inhibits in vitro IL-1-induced cartilage degradation. This compound was also shown in vivo to inhibit articular cartilage degradation in the rat monoarthritic model. Clinical trials are currently being conducted in both rheumatoid arthritic and OA patients. Two hydroxamate inhibitors, BB-1101 and BB-1433 (British Biotech, Oxford, UK) have broad specificity of MMP inhibition but also inhibit the TNF-α-converting enzyme. When administered orally, they inhibit the progression of arthritic lesions in rat adjuvant-induced arthritis.

3.3. Inhibitors of Metalloprotease Synthesis

3.3.1. Growth Factors

Polypeptide growth hormones play a major role in the regulation of cell metabolism, including that of chondrocytes. Therapy with growth factors remains, however, a challenging option to improve the outcome of OA lesions. Among the most influential of these factors are insulin-like growth factor-1 (IGF-1) and transforming growth factor-β (TGF-β). These and other factors interact to modulate their respective actions, creating effector cascades and feedback loops of intercellular and intracellular events. Experimental treatment of canine OA using intra-articular injections of IGF-1, both alone and in combination with intramuscular pentosan polysulfate has demonstrated that combined therapy was successful in blocking protease activity and maintaining cartilage structure and biochemistry. Moreover, although TGF-β possesses anabolism properties, including upregulation of proteoglycan synthesis, TIMP, and IL-1 receptor antagonist and downregulation of IL-1 receptors and some proteases such as stromelysin-1, this factor was recently found to increase the production of other MMP (collagenase-3, gelatinase A) and seems a pivotal mediator in osteophyte formation *(19)*. Caution should be taken for the in vivo clinical application of TGF-β because, as discussed previously, contradictory in vitro results were obtained.

3.3.2. Transcription Factors

Another means of decreasing MMP synthesis could be by acting on the transcription factors involved in the expression of MMP. As mentioned earlier, interaction of multiple elements within the promoter appears to govern the regulation of MMP gene expression. Among the various sites involved is the AP-1. However, this site is used for the expression of many other genes, making it a nonspecific site to target as therapy with several potential side effects. Nevertheless, strategies to specifically inhibit the regulation of posttranscriptional mechanisms of MMP are currently under study.

3.3.3. Inhibitors of Inflammatory Factors

An interesting approach is to reduce the pro-inflammatory cytokine production and/or activity, leading to a reduction of the MMP synthesis. In the pathophysiology of OA, IL-1 seems to be a predominant cytokine implicated in the major events that lead to cartilage destruction *(1)*. A potential role of TNF-α in the disease process cannot, however, be ruled out at this time.

A recent study using the Pond-Nuki dog model of OA has demonstrated that Tenidap (Pfizer Central Research, Groton, CT, USA), a cytokine-modulating drug, can significantly reduce cartilage damage and osteophyte formation while simultaneously inhibiting the synthesis of IL-1 and the activity of collagenase-1 and stromelysin-1. The oxyndole family could represent potentially interesting drugs for the treatment of OA.

The inhibition of cytokine synthesis by using a p38 kinase inhibitor was shown to reduce the production of IL-1, TNF-α, and MMP. Antisense oligonucleotide therapy using complementary sequence to a nontransduced 5' region of IL-1β RNA has also been shown to be effective in reducing IL-1β synthesis.

The inhibition of IL-1 activity by modulating the enzymatic conversion of the pro-cytokine (31 kDa) in active mature cytokine (17 kDa) is an attractive therapeutic target. Intracellular transformation of IL-1β is carried out via a converting enzyme called ICE or caspase-1 (IL-1β-converting enzyme) and can be well controlled by antisense therapy or ICE inhibitors. The expression and production of ICE in human OA cartilage and synovial membrane has recently been demonstrated *(19A)*. A recent in vivo study demonstrated that an ICE inhibitor effectively reduced the progression of murine type II collagen-induced arthritis.

The inhibition of IL-1 at the extracellular level can be achieved using either type I (IL-1RsI) or type II (IL-1RsII) soluble receptors. In vitro data has recently established some advantages of the latter, and some clinical assays are currently underway with rheumatoid arthritic patients. No data are yet available for OA.

There is evidence that a relative deficit in the production of IL-1Ra, the natural antagonist of the IL-1 receptor, occurs in OA tissues. This, coupled with an upregulation of the receptor level, might enhance the catabolic effect of IL-1 in OA *(1)*. A recent study developed in our laboratory has investigated the in vivo effect of human recombinant IL-1Ra (rhIL-1Ra) injected intra-articularly. We demonstrated a dose-dependent protective effect on the development of osteophytes and cartilage lesions. Importantly, injections of this protein led to a significant reduction of collagenase expression in OA cartilage *(20)*.

Many strategies designed to downregulate TNF-α synthesis and/or activity are presently underway, mostly for the rheumatoid arthritic patient. It is now well known that the extracellular portion of the two types of TNF receptors can be released from the cellular membrane to form soluble receptors (TNF-sR55 and TNF-sR75). Both are shed from the OA cells. It was shown in inflammatory diseases that decreasing the shedding of the TNF-R75 may contribute to reducing the response of these cells to stimulation by TNF-α. Although the exact role of TNF-sR in the control of TNF-α action remains ambivalent, some studies indicate that they function as an inhibitor of cytokine activity by rendering the cells less sensitive to the activity of the ligands or by scavenging ligands not bound to cell-surface receptors.

Anti-TNF-α treatment in murine collagen-induced arthritis (CIA) has been shown to significantly improve the disease. Clinical trials using an anti-TNF-α chimeric monoclonal antibody (cA2) in rheumatoid arthritis compared to a placebo group have shown that this approach is very encouraging for this disease, although TNF-α is not a prominent cytokine in terms of OA.

Another interesting means to reduce pro-inflammatory cytokine production and/or activity is through the use of certain cytokines having anti-inflammatory properties. Three such cytokines, IL-4, IL-10, and IL-13, have been identified as able to modulate various inflammatory processes. Their anti-inflammatory potential, however, appears to depend greatly on the target cell. Their inhibitory effect on MMP is indirect and occurs via the inhibition of pro-inflammatory cytokines such as IL-1 and TNF-α and/ or by the elevation of TIMP in the articular tissue. Augmenting their production in situ by gene therapy or supplementing it by injecting the recombinant protein could represent an attractive new form of treatment. A clinical trial is presently underway in which the effect of human recombinant IL-10 is tested in rheumatoid arthritic patients. IL-10 inhibits the synthesis of IL-1 and TNF-α, as well as gelatinase A and B expression. Human recombinant interleukin-4 (rhIL-4) has been tested in vitro in OA tissues and has been shown to suppress the synthesis of both TNF-α and IL-1β in the same manner as low-dose dexamethasone. Similarly, IL-13 significantly inhibits lipopolysaccharide (LPS)-induced TNF-α production by mononuclear cells from peripheral blood, but not by cells from inflamed synovial fluid. Interleukin-13 has important biological activities such as inhibition of the production of a wide range of pro-inflammatory cytokines in monocytes/macrophages, B cells, natural-killer cells and endothelial cells while increasing IL-1Ra production. In OA synovial membranes treated with LPS, IL-13 inhibited the synthesis of IL-1β, TNF-α, and stromelysin-1 while increasing IL-1Ra production.

In addition to the suggested factors that promote cartilage catabolism in OA is nitric oxide (NO) *(21)*. Compared to normal, OA cartilage produces a larger amount of NO, both under spontaneous and pro-inflammatory cytokine-stimulated conditions. This results from an enhanced expression and protein synthesis of the inducible NO synthase (iNOS) enzyme responsible for the production of NO. Among other effects, NO inhibits the synthesis of cartilage matrix macromolecules and enhances MMP activity. Moreover, the increase in NO production reduces the synthesis of IL-1Ra by chondrocytes. Recently, a selective inhibitor of the iNOS has proven in vivo to exert therapeutic effects on the progression of lesions in an experimental animal OA model, and the inhibition of NO production correlated with a reduction in MMP activity in the cartilage *(22)*.

3.4. Gene Therapy

A number of biological agents such as pro-inflammatory cytokine inhibitors, cytokine-soluble receptors, and anti-inflammatory cytokines have demonstrated potentially beneficial therapeutic properties in in vitro and some in vivo models of arthritis. The necessity of maintaining a sustained level of the agents over time is the major concern with this kind of therapy. In the last few years, much attention has been focused on the use of gene-transfer techniques as a method of delivery. Many techniques have been developed using various genes, and a great deal of work is currently devoted to these techniques to facilitate the transfer of genes into joint cells and tissues both in vitro and in vivo. The attractions of this treatment of arthritis are numerous and include the identification of a very specific target, a consistently high local concentration in the joint of the therapeutic protein, and the maintenance of a sustained delivery over time.

There is at this time no definitive information to indicate the best gene to use for the treatment of arthritis. Currently, two main systems—viral and nonviral—are used for gene transfer to cells *(23)*, with the viral system favored. Moreover, a recent study has demonstrated that a gene can successfully be transferred in vivo in rat articular cartilage by a combination of a virus (HVJ, Sendai virus) and liposomes. The selection of gene(s) that would offer the best protection against OA has yet to be determined.

4. Conclusion

In summary, in OA, MMPs are intimately involved in the degradation of cartilage matrix as well as in the structural changes occurring during the course of the disease. This provides a strong incentive for testing the efficacy of MMP inhibitors as possible structure-modifying agents. It is therefore no surprise that considerable attention has been devoted to developing strategies to reduce their levels in diseased joints. Most efforts have focused in inhibiting their activity, either by increasing the concentration of natural inhibitors such as TIMP or by using compounds that will inhibit their synthesis and/or inactivate them. Administration of the agents can be done orally or more specifically by intra-articular injections.

It will be interesting to see if blocking a single MMP is sufficient to halt the progressive and chronic destruction of connective tissue seen in the arthritides. If the release of connective-tissue fragments leads to joint inflammation, leading to a chronic cycle of damage with further destruction of connective tissue, then these compounds could be effective on their own. It may be necessary to combine protease inhibitors, either in sequence or with other agents that block specific steps in the disease process, before the chronic cycle of joint destruction found in these diseases can be broken.

Collagenase and stromelysin have a premier role in the irreversible degradation of the extracellular matrix seen in OA. As to which of the MMP should be targeted, at this time collagenase-3 seems an attractive candidate. This enzyme is present in only a few normal human cells; therefore, inhibiting it will not be harmful to normal tissues. Its role appears to be related to the remodeling process of the cartilage in the early stages of OA in addition to degradation. Moreover, it is the most potent peptidolytic enzyme of three collagenases. It hydrolyses type II collagen more efficiently (at least 5 times more) than collagenase-1 and collagenase-2, and gelatin 44 times more efficiently than collagenase-1 and 8 times better than collagenase-2.

There are other issues in the development of drugs for therapeutic purposes that include bioavailability, pharmacokinetics, and targeting the tissue of interest. However, as MMP are biologically (physiologically) important, one must also consider the consequence of systematically inhibiting those enzymes. Moreover, toxicity must be considered because of the possibility of long-term treatment for OA; therefore, monitoring the efficacy of the drug may introduce numerous challenges.

We now have promising new developments in the area of natural (TIMP) and synthetic MMP inhibitors and gene therapy. Furthermore, researchers are now beginning to study MMP-binding sites to matrix components. This research may lead to new ways to inhibit specific noncatabolic binding sites of MMP to prevent the interaction between the enzyme and the matrix macromolecules.

References

1. Pelletier, J. P., Martel-Pelletier, J., and Howell, D. S. (1997) Etiopathogenesis of osteoarthritis, in *Arthritis and Allied Conditions. A Textbook of Rheumatology* (Koopman, W. J., ed.), Williams & Wilkins, Baltimore, pp. 1969–1984.
1a. Tortorella, M. D., Burn, T. C., Pratta, M. A., Abbaszade, I., Hollis, J. M., Liu, R., et. al. (1999) Purification and cloning of aggrecanase-1: a member of the ADAMTS family of proteins. *Science* **284,** 1664–1666.
2. Birkedal-Hansen, H., Moore, W. G., Bodden, M. K., Windsor, L. J., Birkedal-Hansen, B., DeCarlo, A., et al. (1993) Matrix metalloproteinases: a review. *Crit. Rev. Oral Biol. Med.* **4,** 197–250.
3. Massova, I., Kotra, L. P., Fridman, R., and Mobashery, S. (1998) Matrix metalloproteinases: structures, evolution, and diversification. *FASEB J.* **12,** 1075–1095.
3a. Pei, D. (1999) Identification and characterization of the fifth membrane-type matrix metalloproteinase MT5-MMP. *J. Biol. Chem.* **274,** 8925–8932.
3b. Velasco, G., Cal, S., Merlos-Suarez, A., Ferrando, A. A., Alvarez, S., et al. (2000) Human MT6-matrix metalloproteinase: identification, progelatinase A activation, and expression in brain tumors. *Cancer Res.* **60,** 877–882.
4. Martel-Pelletier, J. and Pelletier, J. P. (1996) Wanted—the collagenase responsible for the destruction of the collagen network in human cartilage. *Br. J. Rheumatol.* **35,** 818–820.
5. Fernandes, J. C., Martel-Pelletier, J., Lascau-Coman, V., Moldovan, F., Jovanovic, D., Raynauld, J. P., et al. (1998) Collagenase-1 and collagenase-3 synthesis in early experimental osteoarthritic canine cartilage An immunohistochemical study. *J. Rheumatol.* **8,** 1585–1594.
6. Laiho, M. and Keski-Oja, J. (1989) Growth factors in the regulation of pericellular proteolysis: a review. *Cancer Res.* **49,** 2533–2553.
7. Vincenti, M. P., White, L. A., Schroen, D. J., Benbow, U., and Brinckerhoff, C. E. (1996) Regulating expression of the gene for matrix metalloproteinase-1 (collagenase): mechanisms that control enzyme activity, transcription, and mRNA stability. *Crit. Rev. Eukaryocyte Gene Express* **6,** 391–411.
8. Benbow, U. and Brinckerhoff, C. E. (1997) The AP-1 site and MMP gene regulation: what is all the fuss about? *Matrix Biol.* **15,** 519–526.
9. Mauviel, A., Chung, K. Y., Agarwal, A., Tamai, K., and Uitto, J. (1996) Cell-specific induction of distinct oncogenes of the Jun family is responsible for differential regulation of collagenase gene expression by transforming growth factor-beta in fibroblasts and keratinocytes. *J Biol Chem* **271,** 10,917–10,923.
10. Tardif, G., Pelletier, J. P., Dupuis, M., Geng, C. S., Cloutier, J. M., and Martel-Pelletier, J. (1999) Collagenase-3 production by human OA chondrocytes in response to growth factors and cytokines is a function of the physiological state of the cells: TGF-β preferentially upregulates collagenase-3 production. *Arthritis Rheum.* **42,** 1147–1158.
11. Nagase, H. (1997) Activation mechanisms of matrix metalloproteinases. *Biol. Chem.* **378,** 151–160.
12. Gomez, D. E., Alonso, D. F., Yoshiji, H., and Thorgeirsson, U. P. (1997) Tissue inhibitors of metalloproteinases: structure, regulation and biological functions. *Eur. J. Cell Biol.* **74,** 111–122.

13. Beckett, R. and Whittaker, M. (1998) Matrix metalloproteinase inhibitors. *Exp. Opin. Ther. Patents* **8,** 259–282.
14. Cawston, T. E. (1996) Metalloproteinase inhibitors and the prevention of connective tissue breakdown. *Pharmacol. Ther.* **70,** 163–182.
15. Wojtowicz-Praga, S. M., Dickson, R. B., and Hawkins, M. J. (1997) Matrix metalloproteinase inhibitors. *Invest. New Drugs* **15,** 61–75.
16. Gomis-Ruth, F. X., Maskos, K., Betz, M., Bergner, A., Huber, R., et al. (1997) Mechanism of inhibition of the human matrix metalloproteinase stromelysin-1 by TIMP-1. *Nature* **389,** 77–81.
17. Huang, W., Meng, Q., Suzuki, K., Nagase, H. and Brew, K. (1997) Mutational study of the amino-terminal domain of human tissue inhibitor of metalloproteinases 1 (TIMP-1) locates an inhibitory region for matrix metalloproteinases. *J. Biol. Chem.* **272,** 22,086–22,091.
18. Levy, D. and Ezrin, A. (1997) Matrix metalloproteinase inhibitor drugs. *Emerg. Drugs* **2,** 205–230.
19. van den Berg, W. B. (1995) Growth factors in experimental osteoarthritis: transforming growth factor beta pathogenic? *J. Rheumatol.* **43(Suppl.),** 143–145.
19a. Saha, N., Moldovan, F., Tardif, G., Pelletier, J. P., Cloutier, J. M., Martel-Pelletier, J. (1999) Interleukin-1β-converting enzyme/caspase-1 in human osteoarthritic tissues: localization and role in the maturation of IL-1β and IL-18. *Arthritis Rheum.* **42,** 1577–1587.
20. Caron, J. P., Fernandes, J. C., Martel-Pelletier, J., Tardif, G., Mineau, F., Geng, C., et al. (1996) Chondroprotective effect of intraarticular injections of interleukin-1 receptor antagonist in experimental osteoarthritis: suppression of collagenase-1 expression. *Arthritis Rheum.* **39,** 1535–1544.
21. Evans, C. H., Stefanovic-Racic, M., and Lancaster, J. (1995) Nitric oxide and its role in orthopaedic disease. *Clin. Orthop.* **312,** 275–294.
22. Pelletier, J. P., Jovanovic, D., Fernandes, J. C., Manning, P. T., Connor, J. R., Currie, M. G., et al. (1998) Reduced progression of experimental osteoarthritis *in vivo* by selective inhibition of inducible nitric oxide synthase. *Arthritis Rheum.* **41,** 1275–1286.
23. Evans, C. H. and Robbins, P. D. (1994) Gene therapy for arthritis, in *Gene Therapeutics: Methods and Applications of Direct Gene Transfer* (Wolff, J. A., ed.), Birkhauser, Boston, pp. 320–343.

34
Gene Therapy

Robert P. Kimberly

1. Introduction

Just as systemic lupus erythematosus (SLE) is often considered a prototype for multisystem autoimmune disease that is characterized by antigen-specific T-cell activation and autoantibody production, it can also serve as an analytical framework to consider gene therapy for a range of autoimmune diseases. Autoantibodies in SLE form immune complexes that lead to an immune-complex glomerulonephritis. Immune complexes are also be involved in the clinical manifestations of skin rashes, arthritis, vasculitis, and pleuropericarditis. Within the spectrum of autoantibodies found in lupus patients, some may be targeted to cell-surface antigens, leading to hemolytic anemia, leukopenia, thrombocytopenia, and possibly to central nervous system injury. Other autoantibodies, such as the antiphospholipid antibodies, are be targeted to cell and/or protein constituents. These antibodies may interfere with the coagulation cascade, and some evidence suggests that they may alter the uptake of apoptotic cells. In our current understanding, the development of pathogenic IgG autoantibodies depends on a break in immunologic tolerance with the generation of antigen-specific, autoreactive T-cells and B-cells. A more comprehensive understanding of the factors shaping that host immune response—the contributions of innate immune mechanisms, the determinants of Th1/Th2 balance, the development of Tr1 regulatory cells, and the characteristics of the inflammatory response—will be fundamental to advances in the pathophysiology of autoimmune disease and to opportunities for treatment based on gene transfer. Indeed, in this context, consideration of gene therapy in SLE highlights issues and challenges which apply to each of the rheumatic diseases.

2. Genetics and SLE

Family studies show that the risk for developing SLE in a sibling of a family member affected by SLE (the λ_s) is approximately 20 times that for the general population (reviewed in refs. *1–3*). Twin studies of monozygotic and dizygotic twins have shown that the concordance for SLE ranges from 24% to 50% in monozygotic twins compared to 2% to 5% for dizygotic twins and siblings. This evidence points to a strong genetic contribution to the lupus diathesis and raises the possibility that once "lupus gene(s)" have been identified, a gene therapy approach to lupus may be feasible.

Early genetic studies in human SLE focused on the class I and class II polymorphisms in the major histocompatibility complex (MHC) and these studies revealed some relationships between certain class II MHC alleles, autoantibody specificities, and disease manifestations. However, work in various murine models of autoimmune disease, including lupus-like disease, has emphasized that the autoimmune diathesis is a complex genetic trait reflecting contributions from MHC and from non-MHC background genes that may be strain-specific. Conceptually, in a complex genetic trait, each gene contributes a small amount to disease risk and no single gene is either necessary or sufficient for disease expression. In this disease model, gene therapy to replace a single defective gene product is unlikely to be effective.

The evidence in lupus favors a complex genetic trait derived from multiple contributing genes, many of which will have common polymorphisms, each with a subtle clinical phenotype. In this context, however, the strong association between hereditary complement C1q deficiency and lupus, and between C1r/C1s and complete C4 deficiency and lupus, stands out. These experiments of nature strongly support the concept that the complement system is important in pathogenesis, and experiments by man with knockout technology in mouse models provide dramatic confirmation of this inference (4). Nonetheless, the rarity of complete complement deficiencies in human populations reminds all investigators that there must be more subtle genetic variations in the complement system if complement system polymorphisms provide a genetic contribution to any more than a very small proportion of SLE cases. From a gene therapy perspective, these observations also indicate that for any given gene, its contribution to the complex trait of SLE may vary with the specific functional properties of the variant of that gene. These observations also temper our expectations for finding a universal defect that can be corrected by a single approach using gene therapy.

Strategies for gene therapy in SLE, therefore, are integrally linked to the search for lupus genes. Although it is possible that one or two genetic variants will play a dominant role in the lupus diathesis, severe functional alterations are likely to be rare in human SLE patients. Current experience suggests that it is more likely that the clinical syndrome of SLE becomes apparent when an aggregate of susceptibility alleles at different genetic loci exceeds a certain threshold. Other important factors might include environmental stimuli. Viewed in this light, understanding SLE and autoimmunity as a model of a complex genetic trait with a threshold genetic liability emphasizes several challenges in identifying contributing genes. From the perspective of gene therapy, genetic heterogeneity, or the occurrence of the same clinical syndrome (disease phenotype) in the context of different combinations of susceptibility alleles, not only slows the identification of susceptibility and/or severity alleles but also complicates the therapeutic gene transfer strategy. The occurrence of epistasis, or the interaction of different susceptibility alleles to yield a disease phenotype, has been shown in some murine models and will most likely occur in human lupus as well. These interactions will have to be clearly understood before undertaking genetic alteration. Finally, if lupus susceptibility alleles are common variants that might be functionally adaptive in some situations, the concept of replacement therapy to correct "defective" protein products—which is tenable in cystic fibrosis and other dominant single-gene-defect models—will have to be carefully considered, especially in the context of long-term gene expression.

Table 1
Therapeutic Strategies in Gene Therapy

Single-Gene-Disease
    Modify gene product or production capacity
        Quality (defective host protein)
        Quantity (insufficient host protein)
Complex, Multigenic Disease
    Modify "pivotal" gene product or production
        Quality (defective host protein)
        Quantity (insufficient host protein)
    Provide drug delivery system
        "Pharmacologic" delivery of agonist or antagonist
    Ablate specific cells or tissues
        Antigen-specific cells
        Effector cells (e.g., CD4+ T-cells)
        Pathologic tissues (e.g., inflamed synovium)

3. Autoimmunity and Gene Therapy

In addition to replacement of defective or deficient protein products, several additional strategies can harness the potential of gene transfer for therapeutic benefit (Table 1). Although certainly applicable to SLE, these strategies may be even more important in other autoimmune rheumatic diseases in which the genetic pathophysiology may be less well established. Gene therapy can be used as a drug delivery system to modify T-cell responsiveness, to alter the balance of Th1 and Th2 cells, and to modulate proinflammatory cytokines. Gene therapy can also be used to target cells for destruction in an antigen-specific, in a cell-type-specific, and in a tissue-specific fashion. Although our current understanding suggests that these strategies may be important in rheumatoid arthritis and other inflammatory diseases, it is important to recognize that a number of disorders of the immune system do reflect dominant single-gene defects that may be amenable to replacement therapy (Table 2). The recent descriptions of TNF receptor autoinflammatory periodic syndrome (TRAPS) and autoimmune lymphoproliferative syndrome (ALPS) II serve as timely reminders that new discovery often holds surprises for current conceptual frameworks (5,6).

CD4+ T-cells play an important role in the initiation and continuation of many autoimmune diseases. In model systems, such as experimental allergic encephalitis and collagen-induced arthritis, disease can be transferred to naive animals by antigen-specific CD4+ T-cells with a Th1 phenotype. Although CD4+ T-cells seems unlikely to change their phenotype once fully differentiated into Th1 or Th2 cells, the development of Th0 cells into defined phenotypes and/or the balance of phenotypes among incompletely differentiated CD4+ memory cells can most probably be influenced by their cytokine milieu. Targeting cytokines such as interleukin (IL)-4, IL-10, and/or IL-13 to such differentiating cells to facilitate the development of Th2 cells, which are often associated with recovery from disease, provides a challenging but important opportunity for drug delivery.

Of course, a critical issue in any therapeutic is one of specificity, and from an immunologist's perspective, specificity can be defined either in terms of antigen reac-

**Table 2
Some Molecular Deficiencies
in the Immune System**

Apoptosis-related genes
  ALPS Ia, Ib, II, (?III)
  TRAPS
Cell-signaling genes
  ζ Chain
  ZAP70, Btk, JAK3 deficiencies/mutations
Cytokines and receptors
  TNF-α, IL-1, IL-6, IL-10
  Cytokine receptor γc chain deficiency
Opsonins and opsonin receptors
  Complement deficiencies
  Mannose-binding lectin
  Complement receptors (CR1)
  Fcγ receptors (FcγRIIA, FcγRIIIA)

tivity or in terms of target cell or target tissue type. One can envision using antigen specificity as a means of directing a gene therapy vector to antigen-specific T-cells and B-cells. Currently, such targeting technologies are not available, but the development of antigen/MHC tetramers to define antigen-specific T-cells by flow cytometry (7) anticipates the modification of this approach to focus a gene therapy delivery system. In the adenoviral system, one possible strategy might be modification of the adenovirus knob protein to accommodate such antigen/MHC tetramers. A second possibility could utilize antigen-presenting cells (APCs), such as macrophages or dendritic cells, pulsed with antigen ex vivo. These cells could be transduced through gene transfer to express specific cytokines to modulate Th1/Th2 balance and, after infusion into the host, to cause immune deviation of antigen-specific cells that are uncommitted or plastic with regard to Th phenotype. Alternatively, these cells could be transduced through gene transfer to express Fas ligand and become antigen-specific killer cells designed to arrest T-cell-mediated attacks and to induce antigen-specific tolerance. This approach has already been used successfully in model systems (8,9).

Autoimmunity, however, represents the end result of the deviation of a immune-complex system, and opportunities for therapeutic gene transfer that extend beyond modulation or modification of the T-cell repertoire are clearly evident. Precedent established with the C1q knockout and the SAP (serum amyloid protein) knockout mice, in which aggressive immune-complex autoimmune disease develops (4,10), and in the Fc receptor knockout mice, in which immune-complex glomerulonephritis is abrogated (11), suggests that careful consideration should be given to components of the innate immune system. The handling of immune reactants and cellular debris intersects both innate and acquired immune mechanisms. In the context of lupus in which the handling of nucleosomes and the development of antinucleosome antibodies appear to be pivotal (12), this approach would most likely involve transient gene expression during flares of disease activity or following provocative insults to the immune system. In C1q or other complement-component-deficient individuals, one might envision gene transfer and transient expression of the deficient component with effects on both innate and acquired immune mechanisms *(13,14)*. Because C-reactive protein (CRP) binds nucleosomes and mediates their removal from the circulation, one might also envision gene transfer of the newly recognized receptors for CRP (human FcγRIA and FcγRIIA), with expression targeted to the fixed mononuclear phagocyte system in liver and spleen and with transient expression being an intentional therapeutic strategy. This approach is particularly appealing, given the role of genetic polymorphisms of these receptors in determining the efficiency of both CRP binding *(15,16)* and IgG binding *(17)*.

Because an actual clinical disease phenotype involves inflammation and tissue injury, targeting of these pathways by gene therapy is also highly promising. Indeed, the limitations of our current knowledge base regarding specific antigens in human disease make genetic intervention with local expression of regulatory or immunomodulatory proteins and intervention with ablation of inflamed tissue compelling therapeutic strategies. Currently, there is little basis for predicting which gene products will have the most effective therapeutic properties, and both agonists [e.g., IL-4 *(18,19)*] and antagonists [e.g., IL-1ra, IL-1 type I receptor, TNF receptor *(20–23)*] have been tested. As an experimental model, antigen-induced arthritis in New Zealand White rabbits has been used for local gene therapy. In this model, Robbins and colleagues have demonstrated a strong anti-inflammatory and chondroprotective effect when both IL-1 type I receptors and TNF type I receptors were coexpressed. Although antigen-induced arthritis in unlikely to be the best experimental model for SLE, several important lessons for rheumatic diseases in general do emerge from this experience *(20)*. First, combinations of genes may be more powerful than single genes in controlling inflammation and tissue injury. Second, even locally introduced gene therapy may have effects at more distal sites.

4. Gene Therapy Vectors

Several different approaches are available as gene delivery systems (Table 3), and they include both viral and nonviral systems (reviewed in ref. *24*). Among the viral vectors, all of which have been modified to reduce intrinsic pathogenicity, retroviruses and adeno-associated viruses (AAV) have the capacity to mediate integration of their genetic material into host cell genomic DNA. This capacity provides the theoretical potential for long-term expression of the transgene, although in practice this has been difficult to accomplish. Turnover and death of virally transduced cells contribute to this phenomenon and have led to consideration of targeting stem cells for gene therapy. Of course, in biology, anatomically restricted, tissue-specific, and appropriately regulated expression of genes is the ideal goal. In the future, this may be accomplished by using eukaryotic, tissue-specific promoters. This is an exciting prospect that will require careful understanding of the pertinent promoters, as well as an appreciation for the implications of the genetic variations that occur in such promoters.

The major limitation of retroviral vectors is their inability to transduce nondividing cells. Strategies to overcome this limitation include stimulation of cell division in the target cell population and the use of lentiviruses, which do not require division of the target cell for successful transduction. A second theoretical limitation of retroviral vectors is the random integration into the host cell genome with "insertional mutagenesis" leading to an unanticipated pathologic state. Although never seen with replication incompetent retroviruses, malignancies have been found in mice with replication competent murine

Table 3
Approaches to Gene Delivery

Retrovirus	Integrate into host cell genome
	Good prospect for long-term expression
	but Target cells must divide to allow integration
	Possibility of insertional mutagenesis
Adenovirus	High infectivity for dividing and nondividing cells
	High titers and high levels of gene expression achievable
	but Induce inflammatory host response
	Lack of genome integration
	Expression is self-limited
Adeno-associated virus	Infectivity for dividing and nondividing cells
	Nonpathogenic in humans
	Broad cellular tropism
	but Difficulty achieving high titers
	Small packaging capacity
Nonviral systems	Nonpathogenic in humans
Liposomes	*but* Lack of genome integration
DNA immunization	Typically low levels of gene expression
	Expression is self-limited

retroviruses. Conceptually, this possibility could be circumvented by incorporation of a conditional lethality gene in the vector that would allow for elimination on demand.

The appeal of adenoviral vectors is their ability to transduce both dividing and nondividing cells with high efficiency and the opportunity to modify the Knob protein on adenovirus fibers to provide more specific targeting strategies. The major limitation of adenoviral vectors is the host inflammatory response that they elicit to viral gene products and potentially to transgene products. While re-engineering of viral genes is being pursued as a strategy around this problem, incorporation of anti-inflammatory transgenes such as the soluble tumor necrosis factor-α (TNF-α) receptor appears to be an effective strategy to dampen the host immune response to the adenovirus and accompanying transgenes *(25)*. Of course, the impact of such anti-inflammatory genes on the overall therapeutic strategy must be considered, but the ability to render adenoviral vectors nonimmunogenic will be central to their use in chronic diseases, which may require repeated administration.

Nonviral vectors avoid many of these problems but have inefficiency of gene transfer and time-limited gene expression as their major limitations. Naked DNA can be incorporated into liposomes to facilitate uptake, coated on small inert particles, and injected by a "gene gun," or be included in a variety of DNA–carrier complexes. Typically these strategies are amenable to repeated administration. Their suitability, however, for gene therapy in the rheumatic diseases will depend on the adequacy of expression achieved and on the ability to target this expression to the appropriate anatomic and tissue sites.

5. Human Trials of Gene Therapy

Primum non nocere is the guiding principle for all medical therapeutics, and safety is always a concern in introducing novel therapies for human disease. No doubt many

Table 4
Model Approaches in Rheumatic Diseases

Alter induction and maintenance of the T-cell response
    Interrupt costimulatory molecules (e.g., soluble CTLA4, CD40)
Induce antigen-specific tolerance
    Antigen-specific APC expressing Fas ligand or other apoptosis-inducing ligands (e.g., TRAIL)
Alter Th balance of the immune response (Th1/2, Tr1)
    Interleukin 10
    TGF-β
Facilitate handling of immune reactants
    Complement components
    Fcγ receptors (allele-specific)
Modify the inflammatory response
    TNF-α antagonist (e.g., soluble TNF receptor)
    IL-1 antagonist (e.g., IL-1ra, soluble IL-1 receptor)
    Other cytokines (IL-6, IL-4, IL-10, IL-13)
Alter the tissue injury and repair programs
    Herpes thymidine kinase/gancyclovir (ablative synovectomy)
    Enzyme inhibitors (TIMPs, tissue inhibitors of metalloproteinases)
    Growth factors:
        Insulin-like growth factor-1 (IGF-1)
        Bone morphogenetic proteins (BMPs)
        Fibroblast growth factors (bFGF)

of the technical issues with gene therapy will be explored in clinical situations that have more life-threatening immediacy and more clear-cut strategies for gene therapy. Lessons will be learned in oncology, in acquired immunodeficiency syndrome, in single-gene disorders, including cystic fibrosis, glycogen and metabolic storage diseases, and in other conditions. Nonetheless, several human trials of gene therapy in rheumatoid arthritis as a model "autoimmune" or rheumatic disease have been initiated. The first trial, which involves ex vivo transduction of synovial fibroblasts with the IL-1ra gene and reintroduction into the metacarpophalangeal joints of the patient 1 wk before joint replacement surgery, is designed primarily to assess the expression of the transgene and secondarily to assess evidence for a local biological effect *(24)*. Although carefully circumscribed in scope, this approach is an important first step in defining the role of gene therapy in autoimmune and inflammatory diseases.

6. Opportunities in Systemic Lupus Erythematosus and Other Rheumatic Diseases

The extent to which gene therapy becomes an established part of the therapeutic armamentarium will depend on the extent to which gene transfer provides a unique therapeutic advantage relative to biologics and other competing therapies. This advantage, which must have superior efficacy and comparable safety, must also be cost-effective.

With the technical feasibility of gene transfer in the rheumatic diseases now being established, the opportunity will be open, but several critical questions will need to be addressed. The number of potential candidate genes, the products of which could influence the overall disease process, is large (Table 4). Much of the future of gene therapy, therefore, rests with advances in our understanding of the pathophysiology of each disease and with the selection of appropriate target genes. Some genes might confer unique biologies on the host *(26)*, and others may be unique drug delivery systems *(27)*. How and where to deliver these genes will be critical issues that will, no doubt, vary with the target gene. Whether to strive for transient, regulated, or sustained expression will, most probably, also vary with the target gene as well, and the technologies to achieve these goals will need to be developed. Whether one envisions a few broadly applicable gene transfer strategies or an array of genes and vectors to be tailored to the specific disease and genetic background, it is clear that the pursuit of these goals will lead to a large increase in our fundamental understanding of disease, which is certain to improve our care and management of all patients with rheumatic diseases.

References

1. Vyse, T. J. and Kotzin, B. L. (1996) Genetic basis of systemic lupus erythematosus. *Curr. Opin. Immunol.* **8,** 843–851.
2. Kimberly, R. P. (1999). The genetics of human lupus, in *Genes and Genetics of Autoimmunity, Current Directions in Autoimmunity, Volume 1* (Theofilopoulos, A. N., ed.), Karger, Basel, pp. 99–120.
3. Deapen, D., Escalante, A., Weinrib, L., Horwitz, D., Bachman, B., Roy-Burman, P., et al. (1992) A revised estimate of twin concordance in systemic lupus erythematosus. *Arthritis Rheum.* **35,** 311–318.
4. Botto, M., Dell'Agnola, C., Bygrave, A. E., Thompson, E. M., Cook, H. T., Petry, F., et al. (1998) Homozygous C1q deficiency causes glomerulonephritis associated with multiple apoptotic bodies. *Nature Genet.* **19,** 56–59.
5. McDermott, M. F., Aksentijevich, I., Galon, J., McDermott, E. M., Ogunkolade, B. W., Centola, M., et al. (1999) Germline mutations in the extracellular domains of the 55 kDa TNF receptor, TNFR1, define a family of dominantly inherited autoinflammatory syndromes. *Cell* **97,** 133–144.
6. Wang, J., Zheng, L., Lobito, A., Chan, F. K., Dale, J., Sneller, M., et al. (1999) Inherited human caspase 10 mutations underlie defective lymphocyte and dendritic cell apoptosis in autoimmune lymphoproliferative syndrome type II. *Cell* **98,** 47–58.
7. Altman, J. D., Moss, P. A. H., Goulder, P. J. R., Barouch, D. H., McHeyzer-Williams, M. G., Bell, J. I., et al. (1996) Phenotypic analysis of antigen-specific T lymphocytes. *Science* **274,** 94–96.
8. Zhang, H. G., Su, X., Liu, D., Liu, W., Yang, P., Wang, Z., et al. (1999) Induction of specific T cell tolerance by Fas ligand-expressing antigen-presenting cells. *J. Immunol.* **162,** 1423–1430.
9. Zhang, H. G., Liu, D., Heike, Y., Yang, P., Wang, Z., Wang, X., et al. (1998) Induction of specific T-cell tolerance by adenovirus-transfected, Fas ligand-producing antigen presenting cells. *Nature Biotechnol.* **16,** 1045–1049.
10. Bickerstaff, M. C., Botto, M., Hutchinson, W. L., Herbert, J., Tennent, G. A., Bybee, A., et al. (1999) Serum amyloid P component controls chromatin degradation and prevents antinuclear autoimmunity. *Nature Med.* **5,** 694–697.
11. Clynes, R., Dumitru, C., and Ravetch, J. V. (1998) Uncoupling of immune complex formation and kidney damage in autoimmune glomerulonephritis. *Science* **279,** 1052–1054.
12. Burlingame, R. W., Volzer, M. A., Harris, J., and Du Clos, T. W. (1996) The effect of acute phase proteins on clearance of chromatin from the circulation of normal mice. *J Immunol.* **156,** 4783–4788.

13. Mitchell, D. A., Taylor, P. R., Cook, H. T., Moss, J., Bygrave, A. E., Walport, M. J., et al. (1999) Cutting edge: C1q protects against the development of glomerulonephritis independently of C3 activation. *J. Immunol.* **162,** 5676–5679.
14. Cutler, A. J., Botto, M., van Essen, D., Rivi, R., Davies, K. A., Gray, D., et al. (1998) T cell-dependent immune response in C1q-deficient mice: defective interferon gamma production by antigen-specific T cells. *J. Exp. Med.* **187,** 1789–1797.
15. Bharadwaj, D., Stein, M. P., Volzer, M., Mold, C., and Du Clos, T. W. (1999) The major receptor for C-reactive protein on leukocytes is Fcγ receptor II. *J. Exp. Med.* **190,** 585–590.
16. Stein, M. P., Edberg, J. C., Kimberly, R. P., Mangan, E. K., Bharadwaj, D., Mold, C., et al. (2000) C-Reactive protein binding to FcγRIIa on human monocytes and neutrophils is allele specific. *J. Clin. Invest.*, **105,** 369–376.
17. Wu, J., Edberg, J. C., Redecha, P. B., Bansal, V., Guyre, P. M., Coleman, K., et al. (1997) A novel polymorphism of FcγRIIIa (CD16) alters receptor function and predisposes to autoimmune disease. *J. Clin. Invest.* **100,** 1059–1070.
18. Woods, J. M., Tokuhira, M., Berry, J. C., Katschke, K. J., Jr., Kurata, H., Damergis, J. A., Jr., et al. (1999) Interleukin-4 adenoviral gene therapy reduces production of inflammatory cytokines and prostaglandin E2 by rheumatoid arthritis synovium ex vivo. *J. Invest. Med.* **47,** 285–292.
19. Volpert, O. V., Fong, T., Koch, A. E., Peterson, J. D., Waltenbaugh, C., Tepper, R. I., et al. (1998) Inhibition of angiogenesis by interleukin 4. *J. Exp. Med.* **188,** 1039–1046.
20. Ghivizzani, S. C., Lechman, E. R., Kang, R., Tio, C., Kolls, J., Evans, C. H., et al. (1998) Direct adenovirus-mediated gene transfer of interleukin 1 and tumor necrosis factor alpha soluble receptors to rabbit knees with experimental arthritis has local and distal anti-arthritic effects. *Proc. Natl. Acad. Sci. USA* **95,** 4613–4618.
21. Muller-Ladner, U., Evans, C. H., Franklin, B. N., Roberts, C. R., Gay, R. E., Robbins, P. D., et al. (1999) Gene transfer of cytokine inhibitors into human synovial fibroblasts in the SCID mouse model. *Arthritis Rheum.* **42,** 490–497.
22. Muller-Ladner, U., Roberts, C. R., Franklin, B. N., Gay, R. E., Robbins, P. D., Evans, C. H., et al. (1997) Human IL-1Ra gene transfer into human synovial fibroblasts is chondroprotective. *J. Immunol.* **158,** 3492–3498.
23. Lechman, E. R., Jaffurs, D., Ghivizzani, S. C., Gambotto, A., Kovesdi, I., Mi, Z., et al. (1999) Direct adenoviral gene transfer of viral IL-10 to rabbit knees with experimental arthritis ameliorates disease in both injected and contralateral control knees. *J. Immunol.* **163,** 2202–2208.
24. Evans, C. H., Ghivizzani, S. C., Kang, R., Muzzonigro, T., Wasko, M. C., Herndon, J. H., et al. (1999). Gene therapy for rheumatic diseases. *Arthritis Rheum.* **42,** 1–16.
25. Zhang, H. G., Zhou, T., Yang, P., Edwards, C. K., III, Curiel, D. T., and Mountz, J. D. (1998) Inhibition of tumor necrosis factor alpha decreases inflammation and prolongs adenovirus gene expression in lung and liver. *Hum. Gene Ther.* **9,** 1875–1884.
26. Yuasa, T., Kubo, S., Yoshino, T., Ujike, A., Matsumura, K., Ono, M., et al. (1999) Deletion of Fcγ receptor IIB renders H-2(b) mice susceptible to collagen-induced arthritis. *J. Exp. Med.* **189,** 187–194.
27. Musgrave, D. S., Bosch, P., Ghivizzani, S., Robbins, P. D., Evans, C. H., and Huard, J. (1999) Adenovirus-mediated direct gene therapy with bone morphogenetic protein-2 produces bone. *Bone* **24,** 541–547.

Index

A

Activation-induced cell death (AICD),
  defects in human autoimmune disease, 40, 41
  function, 36
  T-cell receptor-mediated signaling, 82, 83
Adenovirus,
  apoptosis effects, 25
  gene therapy vector, 520
Adhesion molecules, *see also specific molecules*,
  angiogenesis role, 228, 229
  bone cell development and differentiation role, 285
  leukocyte functions,
    signal transduction, 230, 231
    trafficking, 228–230
  neutrophils, 245, 246
  rheumatoid arthritis role,
    expression and integrin ligation, 348
    fibroblast-like synoviocytes and synovial lining, 348, 349
    macrophages, 349
    monocytes, 349
  superfamilies, 227, 228
  vasculitis role,
    expression, 388
    posttranslational modification, 389, 390
    regulation, 389
Adjuvant-induced arthritis, features of model, 294
Affected sibling pair analysis,
  applications, 10
  overview, 9, 10
Aggrecan, features and functions, 269, 270
AICD, *see* Activation-induced cell death
ALPS, *see* Autoimmune lymphoproliferative syndrome
Alzheimer's disease, complement role, 157
ANCA, *see* Anti-neutrophil cytoplasmic antibody
Angiogenesis,
  inhibitors, 228, 229
  macrophage role in rheumatoid arthritis, 228, 229
Animal models,
  inflammatory arthritis,
    adjuvant-induced arthritis, 294
    bacterial cell-wall arthritis, 293, 294
    proteoglycan-induced arthritis, 296
    type II collagen-induced arthritis, 294, 295
  knockout mice as autoimmunity models, 303
  lupus,
    induced lupus,
      16/16 idiotype administration, 299, 300
      chronic graft-versus-host disease mouse, 300, 301
    spontaneous lupus,
      BXSB mouse, 298, 299
      MRL/*lpr/lpr* mouse, 297, 298
      New Zealand Black mouse, 297
      Palmerston North mouse, 299
  myositis, 303
  scleroderma,
    acute murine graft-versus-host disease, 302, 303
    tight skin mouse, 302
  spondyloarthritis,
    ank/ank mouse, 296
    HLA-B27 transgenic rat, 296
  vasculitis,
    ANCA-associated vasculitis, 301, 302
    mercuric chloride induction in rat, 301
    MRL/*lpr/lpr* mouse, 301
    myeloperoxidase-immunized rat, 301
Anti-neutrophil cytoplasmic antibody (ANCA), *see* Vasculitis

Antibody, *see* Autoantibody; B-cell; Humoral immune response; Immune complex; Immunoglobulin
Antigen-presenting cell (APC),
 B-cell activity, 220
 rheumatoid arthritis, 260, 261
 T-cell interactions, 87–89
 types, 87, 88
AP-1,
 autoimmune disease role, 122
 dimerization, 118, 119
 domains, 119
 expression, 119
 glucocorticoid effects, 447
 inflammation role, overview, 113, 114
 regulated processes, 119
 rheumatoid arthritis role, 342, 345
APC, *see* Antigen-presenting cell
Apoptosis, *see also* Fas,
 bone cells, 289, 290
 caspase role, 37, 38
 immune system functions, 35–37
 inflammatory myopathies, 369
 inhibitor of apoptosis genes, 38
 morphological changes, 35
 nitric oxide induction in cartilage, 274, 275
 phospholipid distribution in cells, 35
 rheumatoid arthritis,
  persistence role,
   fibroblast-like synoviocyte, 352, 353
   induction as therapeutic approach, 353, 354
   macrophage, 353
   synovial tissue, 352
   T-cell, 353
  regulation, 47
 systemic lupus erythematosus defects, 41–46
 T-cell receptor-mediated signaling in cell priming, 82, 83
 TRAIL induction, 38, 40
 viral effects in autoimmune patients, 25–27
Arachidonic acid,
 activities, 165
 cascade, 161, 162
Atherosclerosis,
 antiphospholipid antibody role, 138
 complement role, 157
Autoantibody,
 antigen-driven responses, 73
 definition, 70
 DNA as antigen, 71, 72
 rheumatoid factors, 70–72
Autoimmune lymphoproliferative syndrome (ALPS), apoptosis defects, 41, 83, 84
Azathioprine,
 anti-inflammatory effects, 454
 B-cell effects, 454
 complications, 459
 dosing for rheumatic disease, 458, 459
 indications, 459
 structure, 452
 T-cell effects, 452, 453

B

B7-1
 B7-1/B7-2:CD28/CTLA4 pathway, 92–98
 expression, 92, 93
 gene, 92
 signaling comparison with B7-2, 97
 structure, 92
B7-2
 B7-1/B7-2:CD28/CTLA4 pathway, 92–98
 expression, 92, 93
 gene, 92
 signaling comparison with B7-1, 97
 structure, 92
Bacterial cell-wall arthritis, features of model, 293, 294
B-cell,
 activation,
  itinerary of activated cells, 218–220
  overview, 214
  signal 1, 215, 216, 223
  signal 2, 216–218, 223
 antibody expression and tolerance, 66, 67
 antigens,
  interactions with B-cells, 67, 68
  presenting cell activity, 220
  T-independent versus T-dependent, 222
 azathioprine effects, 454
 comparison with T-cells, 213
 CpG activation, 222, 223
 cyclophosphamide effects, 453
 cytokine secretion, 223
 development, 213, 214
 maturation of immune response, 68, 69
 methotrexate effects, 454

population dynamics, 222
receptor,
  components, 69
  coreceptor, 69, 70
  editing, 67, 221
  isotypes, 214
  rheumatoid factor activity, 220
  signal transduction, 215, 216
  systemic lupus erythematosus,
    aberrant T-cell and B-cell receptor signaling, 319, 320
    CD28/CTLA4:CD80/CD86 costimulation, 320, 321
  repertoire and autoimmunity, 72, 73
  rheumatoid arthritis role,
    affinity maturation, 331, 332
    autoantibodies, 332
    rheumatoid factor production, 332
  tolerance, 221, 494, 495
Bcl-2
  apoptosis inhibition, 38
  systemic lupus erythematosus dysregulation, 42, 43
Bcl-x_L, CD28 costimulation effects on expression, 99
BMPs, see Bone morphogenetic proteins
Bone marrow transplantation,
  autologous bone marrow transplantation in tolerance restoration, 489, 490
  indications, 489, 490
Bone morphogenetic proteins (BMPs), bone cell development and differentiation role, 282, 283
Bone remodeling, basic multicellular units, 279, 413
BXSB mouse, lupus model, 298, 299

C

C1-INH, inhibition of complement activation, 153
C1q,
  autoantibodies and immune complexes, 136, 140
  collagenous sequences, 178
  knockout mouse, 303
  receptor in therapy, 471, 472
  receptors, 148, 149
C5, inhibition therapy,
  anti-C5 mAb, 473
  anti-C5 scFV, 474
Calcineurin, T-cell receptor signaling, 78, 79
Cartilage oligomeric matrix protein (COMP), features and functions, 272
Case control study,
  population stratification problem, 7, 8
  risk evaluation, 6, 7
Caspase, apoptosis role, 37, 38
Cathepsins, tissue destruction in rheumatoid arthritis, 346
Cbl, inhibition of T-cell receptor signaling, 81
CD2, LFA-3 interactions in T-cell activation, 91
CD6, ALCAM interactions, 230, 231
CD28
  anergy prevention and initiation of productive immune response, 98
  B7-1/B7-2:CD28/CTLA4 pathway, 92–98
  costimulation in functional outcome of immune response, 99
  expression, 93
  signaling, 96–98
  tolerance induction by interruption of costimulation, 99–101
CD40
  B-cell activation, 216, 217, 220
  CD28 signaling pathway relationship, 100, 101
  interaction with ligand in T-cell activation, 91, 100
CD45, T-cell receptor signaling, 76, 77
CD59
  decay-accelerating factor chimera in therapy, 472
  soluble factor in therapy, 471
CD95, activation-induced cell death role, 82, 83
CDP571, anti-tumor necrosis factor therapy, 482
C/EBPβ, rheumatoid arthritis role, 341, 342, 345, 346
CGD, see Chronic granulomatous disease
Chediak–Higashi syndrome, neutrophil defects, 255
Chemokines,
  chemotaxis role, 230
  rheumatoid arthritis role, 334, 335

Chemotaxis,
  complement role, 152
  leukocytes, 229, 230
Chlorambucil,
  complications, 457, 458
  dosing for rheumatic disease, 457
  indications, 458
Chloroquine, apoptosis induction, 48, 49
Chondrocalcin, features and functions, 272
Chondrocyte,
  biosynthesis and integration of cartilage extracellular matrix,
    accessory proteins, 272
    aggrecan, 269, 270
    chondroitin sulfate, 269
    collagens,
      articular cartilage, 271
      gene regulation, 271, 272
    leucine-rich repeat proteoglycans, 270, 271
    proteoglycans, 269
    versican, 270
  osteoarthritis role,
    cartilage homeostasis imbalance, 272
    extracellular matrix gene expression, 272, 273
    matrix degradation,
      matrix metalloproteinases, 273, 274
      signaling pathways, 274, 275
    phenotype regulation, transactivating proteins,
      c-fos, 269
      parathyroid-related peptide role, 268, 269
      SOX9, 268
    rheumatoid arthritis role, 275
Chondroitin sulfate, features and functions, 269
Chronic granulomatous disease (CGD), neutrophil defects, 254, 255
CMV, see Cytomegalovirus
Cohort study, risk evaluation, 5, 6
Colchicine, neutrophil effects, 254
Collagen,
  articular cartilage synthesis, 271
  basement membrane collagens,
    type IV, 184
    type VII, 184, 185
    type XVII, 185

biosynthesis of type I,
  messenger RNA processing, 187, 188
  overview, 187
  posttranslational processing, 188–190
  transcription, 187
  translation, 188
  triple helix formation, 190
defects in disease, 175, 177
  Ehlers–Danlos syndrome gene mutations,
    COL1A1, 429
    COL1A2, 429, 430
    COL3A1, 429
    COL5A1, 429
    lysyl hydroxylase-1, 428–430
    procollagen I N-proteinase, 428, 429
  fibril-associated collagens with interrupted triple helices,
    macromolecular association, 182
    type IX, 182, 183
    type XIV, 183
    type XIX, 183, 184
    type XVI, 183
    type XX, 184
  fibril-forming collagens,
    macromolecular association, 179, 180
    type I, 181
    type II, 181, 268
    type III, 181
    type V, 181
    type XI, 182
  functional diversity, 175
  genes,
    loci, 175, 176, 186
    regulation of expression, 190, 191, 193, 194, 271, 272
    structure, 186, 187
  multiplexins,
    type XV, 186
    type XVIII, 186
  osteoarthritis expression, 405
  osteogenesis imperfecta gene mutations,
    COL1A1, 431–433
    COL1A2, 431–433
    genotype-phenotype correlation, 433–435
  polymorphisms types and tissue distribution, 178, 179

Index

posttranslational regulation of synthesis, 191–193
short-chain collagens,
    type VIII, 186
    type X, 186, 268
structure, overview, 175–178
type II collagen-induced arthritis, 294, 295
type VI, 185
type XIII, 185
types, overview, 175, 176
Collagenase, matrix degradation, 264
COMP, see Cartilage oligomeric matrix protein
Complement, see also specific proteins,
    activation,
        alternative pathway, 147, 148, 467, 468
        classical pathway, 145, 146, 465–467
        inhibitors,
            membrane inhibitors, 153
            serum inhibitors, 153, 154
        lectin pathway, 147, 468
        proteins, 146
        subsequent steps, 148
    disease role,
        Alzheimer's disease, 157
        atherosclerosis, 157
        fetal loss, 157, 158
        glomerulopathy, 155, 156
        human immunodeficiency virus, 158
        innate immunity role, 155
        ischemia-reperfusion injury, 157
        leukocyte adhesion deficiency, 155
        pathogen receptor activity of complement components, 158
        protection from infection, 154, 155
        rheumatoid arthritis, 156
        self tolerance, 156, 157
        systemic lupus erythematosus, 152, 156, 157
        transplant rejection, 157
    functions,
        chemotaxis, 152
        humoral immunity regulation, 152
        inflammatory cell activation, 152
        phagocytosis, 152
    inhibitors of activation for therapy,
        anti-C5 mAb, 473
        anti-C5 scFV, 474
        C1 inhibitor, 471
        C1q receptor, 471, 472
        DAF–CD59, 472
        MCP–DAF, 472, 473
        sCD59, 471
        sCR1, 468, 469
        sCR1 (desLHR-A), 469, 470
        sCR1-SLe^x, 470
        sDAF, 471
        sMCP, 471
        types, overview, 465, 466
    membrane attack complex,
        assembly, 148, 468
        disease role, 152
        functions, 151
    overview of system, 145
    receptors,
        C1q, 148, 149
        C3a, 151
        C5a, 151
        CR1, 149, 150
        CR2, 150
        CR3, 150, 151
        table, 147
    regulatory proteins, 147, 152
    therapeutic targeting, 158
Corticosteroid, see Glucocorticoid
COX, see Cyclooxygenase
CpG, B-cell activation, 222, 223
CSK, T-cell receptor signaling, 76, 77
CTL, see Cytotoxic T lymphocyte
CTLA4,
    B7-1/B7-2:CD28/CTLA4 pathway, 92–98
    CD28 costimulation effects on expression, 99
    expression, 93
    inhibition of T-cell receptor signaling, 81
    knockout mouse phenotype, 96
    signaling, 98
    tolerance induction by interruption of costimulation, 99, 100
Cyclooxygenase (COX),
    COX-1, 165, 166
    COX-2, 165, 166, 172
    glucocorticoid effects, 446, 447
    inhibitors, 161, 166, 172, 253
    prostanoid biosynthesis, 165
    regulation of expression, 161, 162, 165, 166

Cyclophosphamide,
  anti-inflammatory effects, 454
  B-cell effects, 453
  complications,
    bladder toxicity, 456
    gonadal toxicity, 456
    hyponatremia, 456, 457
    infection, 455, 456
    oncogenicity, 456
  dosing for rheumatic disease, 454, 455, 457
  management guidelines, 457
  structure, 452
  T-cell effects, 451, 452
Cyclosporine,
  anti-inflammatory effects, 454
  complications, 461
  dosing for rheumatic disease, 460
  indications, 461, 462
  structure, 452
  T-cell effects, 453
Cytomegalovirus (CMV), arthritis induction and features, 18
Cytotoxic T lymphocyte (CTL), *see* T-cell

D

DAF, *see* Decay-accelerating factor
DAG, *see* Diacylglycerol
Decay-accelerating factor (DAF),
  CD59 chimera in therapy, 472
  inhibition of complement activation, 153
  membrane cofactor protein chimera in therapy, 472
  soluble factor in therapy, 471
Dermatomyositis (DM),
  adhesion molecule expression in muscle lesions, 365, 366
  clinical features, 363
  cytokine expression, 365, 366, 370
  histopathology, 363, 364, 371
  T-cells,
    cytotoxic effector mechanisms, 368, 369
    myoblast interactions,
      CD4+ T-cells, 370, 371
      CD8+ T-cells, 370
    phenotype and activation state, 366
    receptor repertoire of autoaggressive cells, 366–368

Diacylglycerol (DAG), T-cell receptor signaling, 78, 94
DM, *see* Dermatomyositis

E

EBV, *see* Epstein–Barr virus
ECM, *see* Extracellular matrix
Ehlers–Danlos syndrome,
  classification, 427, 428
  clinical features, 428
  gene mutations,
    COL1A1, 429
    COL1A2, 429, 430
    COL3A1, 429
    COL5A1, 429
    lysyl hydroxylase-1, 428–430
    procollagen I *N*-proteinase, 428, 429
  heredity, 423
Eicosanoids, *see also specific eicosanoids*,
  arachidonic acid cascade, 161, 162
  overview of types, 161, 162
ELISA, *see* Enzyme-linked immunosorbent assay
EMC, *see* Essential mixed cryoglobulinemia
Endogenous retroviral sequence (ERS), molecular mimicry and autoimmune disease, 22–25
Endothelin-1, scleroderma role, 377
Enzyme-linked immunosorbent assay (ELISA), diagnosis of viral infection, 21
Epstein–Barr virus (EBV),
  arthritis induction and features, 18
  molecular mimicry, 23, 24
Erg-1, rheumatoid arthritis role, 343
ERS, *see* Endogenous retroviral sequence
Essential mixed cryoglobulinemia (EMC), hepatitis C virus role, 19
Estrogen, abnormalities in systemic lupus erythematosus, 313, 314
Etanercept, anti-tumor necrosis factor therapy, 482, 483
Extracellular matrix (ECM),
  biosynthesis and integration of cartilage extracellular matrix,
    accessory proteins, 272
    aggrecan, 269, 270
    chondroitin sulfate, 269
    collagens,

articular cartilage, 271
gene regulation, 271, 272
leucine-rich repeat proteoglycans, 270, 271
proteoglycans, 269
versican, 270
degradation in arthritis, 231, 232, 235, 263, 264, 273–275, 334
synovial joint development, 267

F

Factor I, inhibition of complement activation, 154
Factor H, inhibition of complement activation, 153
Fas,
  apoptosis signal transduction, 37, 38
  CD28 costimulation effects, 99
  expression in inflammatory myopathies, 369
  mutations,
    autoimmune lymphoproliferative syndrome, 41
    loss of tolerance, 40
  systemic lupus erythematosus, soluble receptor levels, 44, 45
FBN1, see Marfan syndrome
FcγRIIa receptor, polymorphisms in vasculitis, 392, 393
FGF, see Fibroblast growth factor
Fibrillin-1, see Marfan syndrome
Fibroblast growth factor (FGF), rheumatoid arthritis role, 262
Fibronectin, features and functions, 272
Fyn, T-cell receptor signaling, 75, 76

G

γd T-cell, see T-cell
Gene therapy,
  autoimmunity strategies, 518, 519
  clinical trials, 520
  molecular deficiencies in immune disease, 517, 518
  osteoarthritis, 510, 511
  specificity, 517, 518
  systemic lupus erythematosus, 516, 521, 522
  T-helper cell balance modulation, 517, 518
  therapeutic strategies, 517
  vectors, 519, 520
Giant cell arteritis, see Vasculitis
Gla-protein, features and functions, 272
Glomerulopathy, complement role, 155, 156
Glucocorticoid,
  advantages in inflammatory disease treatment, 439
  anti-inflammatory mechanism, 442, 443
  bone loss pathogenesis, 419, 420
  cytokine modulation, 443
  gene targets,
    activation, 445, 446
    inhibition, 444, 445
  lymphocyte effects, 443, 444
  matrix metalloproteinase gene regulation, 502
  neutrophil effects, 253
  receptor structure and function, 439–442
  side effects, 439
  structures of therapeutic steroids, 439, 440
  transcription factor interactions, 445–447
Gout, neutrophil role, 250, 251
GP-39, features and functions, 272
Graft-versus-host disease (GVHD),
  acute murine graft-versus-host disease, scleroderma model, 302, 303
  autologous bone marrow transplantation, 489
  CD40 blockade effects, 101
  chronic graft-versus-host disease mouse, lupus model, 300, 301
  CTLA4 antibody effects, 100
GVHD, see Graft-versus-host disease

H

HBC, see Hepatitis C virus
HBV, see Hepatitis B virus
Heat shock protein 70, antigen binding in rheumatoid arthritis, 328
Hemochromatosis, linkage disequilibrium, 7
Hepatitis B virus (HBV), arthritis induction and features, 18
Hepatitis C virus (HCV),
  arthritis induction and features, 18, 19
  vasculitis role, 397, 398
Herpes simplex virus 1 (HSV-1), arthritis induction and features, 18

Heterozygosity, analysis, 11, 12
HIV-1, *see* Human immunodeficiency virus 1
HLA, *see* Human leukocyte antigen
HPV, *see* Human papilloma virus
HSV-1, *see* Herpes simplex virus 1
HTLV-1, *see* Human T-cell lymphotropic virus I
Human immunodeficiency virus 1 (HIV-1),
    apoptosis effects, 25, 26
    autoimmune rheumatic disease induction, 20, 21
    complement role, 158
    cytokine profile in infection, 25
    molecular mimicry, 23, 24
    phases of infection, 20
    receptors, 20
Human leukocyte antigen (HLA),
    allele analysis in autoimmune disease, 6
    genetic association data, importance of understanding, 8, 9
    hemochromatosis, 7
    immunotherapy, 495
    polymorphism assessment, 10
    processing alteration in rheumatoid arthritis, 328, 329
    rheumatoid arthritis susceptibility, 327, 328
    systemic lupus erythematosus susceptibility, 311, 312
Human papilloma virus (HPV), apoptosis effects, 25, 26
Human T-cell lymphotropic virus I (HTLV-I),
    apoptosis effects, 26, 27
    arthritis induction and features, 19, 20
    diagnosis of infection, 20
    molecular mimicry, 23, 24
    vasculitis role, 397
Humoral immune response, *see also* B-cell; Immunoglobulin,
    autoimmunity checks, 73
    complement regulation, 152
    overview, 59, 60

I

IBM, *see* Inclusion-body myositis
ICAM-1, *see* Intercellular adhesion molecule-1
ICOS, *see* Inducible costimulator
IL-1, *see* Interleukin-1
IL-2, *see* Interleukin-2
IL-4, *see* Interleukin-4
IL-6, *see* Interleukin-6
IL-10, *see* Interleukin-10
IL-11, *see* Interleukin-11
IL-13, *see* Interleukin-13
Immune complex,
    assays,
        overview, 138, 139
        technical issues, 139, 140
    C1q autoantibodies, 136
    complement modification, 127, 128
    effects on tissue, 136, 137
    history of study, 128, 129
    lipoprotein antigens and heart disease, 138
    pathogenesis role,
        clearance defects, 131–133
        localization, physiochemical composition effects, 133–135
        overview, 127
        rearrangement and persistence, 135, 136
        rheumatoid arthritis, 130, 131
        systemic lupus erythematosus, 129, 132, 133–135, 137, 138, 140
        vasculitis, 129, 130
    precipitin curve, 127, 128
    therapeutic targeting, 137
Immunoglobulin, *see also* Autoantibody; B-cell; Immune complex,
    antigen interactions, 68
    anti-idiotype antibodies, 62
    constant regions, 60
    effector functions, 66
    expression, 64, 66, 67
    gene recombination, 63, 64, 67
    humanization, 62
    isotype switching, 65, 66
    monoclonal antibody production, 61, 62
    RAG genes in rearrangement, 63
    somatic mutation, 65
    structure, 60–62
    variable regions, 61
Inclusion-body myositis (IBM),
    adhesion molecule expression in muscle lesions, 365, 366
    clinical features, 363
    cytokine expression, 365, 366, 370

histopathology, 363, 364, 371
T-cells,
   cytotoxic effector mechanisms, 368, 369
   myoblast interactions,
      CD4+ T-cells, 370, 371),
      CD8+ T-cells, 370
   phenotype and activation state, 366
   receptor repertoire of autoaggressive cells, 366–368
Inducible costimulator (ICOS), structure and function, 94
Infliximab, anti-tumor necrosis factor therapy, 481
Intercellular adhesion molecule-1 (ICAM-1), LFA-1 interactions in T-cell activation, 90, 91
Interleukin-1 (IL-1),
   arthritis role, 234, 235, 262
   inhibition therapy,
      overview, 479, 480
      recombinant receptor antagonist, 480, 481, 509
   osteoporosis role, 416, 417
   receptor antagonist, 234, 235, 335, 336, 480
Interleukin-2 (IL-2),
   receptor, structure and T-cell regulation, 82
   upregulation by T-cell signaling, 82
Interleukin-4 (IL-4), immunotherapy, 479, 484
Interleukin-6 (IL-6),
   arthritis role, 235, 236, 262
   bone cell development and differentiation role, 283, 284
   inhibition therapy,
      monoclonal antibody, 483, 484
      receptor monoclonal antibody, 484
   osteoporosis role, 415, 416
Interleukin-10 (IL-10),
   arthritis role, 238, 336
   immunotherapy, 479, 484
   immunotherapy, 510
   systemic lupus erythematosus dysregulation, 42
   systemic lupus erythematosus role, 318, 319, 484
Interleukin-11 (IL-11), immunotherapy, 484
Interleukin-13 (IL-13), immunotherapy, 510

Ischemia-reperfusion injury, complement role, 157
Isoprostanes,
   activities, 171, 172
   synthesis, 171

L

LAD, see Leukocyte adhesion deficiency
LAT, T-cell receptor signaling, 79, 80
Lck, T-cell receptor signaling, 75, 76, 97
Leukocyte adhesion deficiency (LAD),
   complement role, 155
   neutrophil defects, 255, 256
Leukocyte rolling, adhesion molecules and mechanism, 227, 228
Leukotrienes,
   overview of effects, 161
   receptors, 170
   types and functions, 169, 170
LFA-1, ICAM-1 interactions in T-cell activation, 90, 91
LFA-3, CD2 interactions in T-cell activation, 91
Lining cell, features and functions, 287, 288
Linkage disequilibrium,
   hemochromatosis, 7
   overview, 6, 7, 12
   rheumatoid arthritis, 329
Lipoxins, types and functions, 171
Lipoxygenase,
   catalytic reaction, 169
   5-lipoxygenase features, 169
LJP394, lupus therapy, 494, 495
Lyme arthritis, histopathology, 347

M

MAC, see Membrane attack complex
Macrophage,
   functional overview, 225, 226
   inflammation role, 225–227
   rheumatoid arthritis role,
      angiogenesis role, 228, 229
      foreign substance removal from synovial fluid, 231
      matrix degradation, 231, 232, 235, 334
      origin of cells, 227
      persistence role,

adhesion molecule expression, 349
apoptosis, 353
fibroblast-like synoviocyte
    interaction, 352
products and effects,
    anti-inflammatory molecules,
        335, 336
    chemokines, 334, 335
    colony-stimulating factors, 236
    growth factors, 335
    interleukin-1 receptor antagonist,
        234, 235, 335, 336
    interleukin-10, 238, 336
    matrix metalloproteinases, 334
    overview, 232
    transforming growth factor-β,
        236–238
    tumor necrosis factor-α,
        232–234, 334
Marfan syndrome,
    clinical manifestations, 423, 424
    elastin-associated microfibrils, 424
    FBN1 gene,
        antisense therapy, 427
        mutations, 425
        structure, 424, 425
        transgenic mouse models, 425, 426
    fibrillin-1
        pathogenesis role, 426
        structure, 424
    heredity and gene mutations, 423
    treatment, 426, 427
MASP proteases, complement activation, 147
Matrix metalloproteinases (MMPs), *see also
    specific proteases*,
    cartilage degeneration, 403, 404, 406
    chondrocyte role in osteoarthritis,
        273, 274
    classification and general features,
        500, 501
    inhibitor therapy,
        biosynthesis inhibitors,
            cytokine-modulating drugs, 509, 510
            growth factors, 508
            nitric oxide inhibition, 510
            transcription factors, 508, 509
        chemical inhibitors,
            hydroxamate compounds, 508
            specificity, 506
            table, 507

tetracycline and homologs, 507, 508
design of inhibitors, 504–506
furin as target, 506
tissue inhibitors, 506
osteoarthritis targets, 511, 512
posttranslational regulation,
    activation cascades, 503, 504
    tissue inhibitors, 504
structure, 500
synoviocyte expression in rheumatoid
    arthritis, 334
tissue distribution, 499, 500
transcriptional regulation,
    inhibition, 502, 503
    stimulation, 501, 502
MCP, *see* Membrane cofactor protein
Mediterranean fever, familial genetics, 3
Membrane attack complex (MAC),
    assembly, 148, 468
    disease role, 152
    functions, 151
Membrane cofactor protein (MCP),
    decay-accelerating factor chimera in
        therapy, 472
    inhibition of complement activation, 153
    soluble factor in therapy, 471
Memory T-cell, *see* T-cell
Metalloproteases, *see* Matrix metalloproteinases
Methotrexate (MTX), apoptosis
    induction, 49
    anti-inflammatory effects, 454
    B-cell effects, 454
    complications, 460
    dosing for rheumatic disease, 459, 460
    indications, 460
    neutrophil effects, 253, 254
    structure, 452
    T-cell effects, 453
Microsatellite, genetic marker analysis, 11
Mimicry, *see* Molecular mimicry
Mitogen-activated protein kinase pathways,
    rheumatoid arthritis
    role, 342
MMPs, *see* Matrix metalloproteinases
Molecular mimicry,
    rheumatoid arthritis role, 328
    viral antigens and self proteins, 22–25
Monocyte,
    adhesion molecules and trafficking,
        227–230

chemotaxis, 229, 230
functional overview, 225, 226
products and effects in arthritis,
    interleukin-1, 234, 235
    interleukin-6, 235, 236
    interleukin-10, 238
    oncostatin M, 235
    overview, 232
rheumatoid arthritis persistence role,
    adhesion molecule expression, 349
    T-cell interaction, 349, 350
MRL/lpr/lpr mouse,
    lupus model, 297, 298
    vasculitis model, 301
MTX, *see* Methotrexate
c-Myc, rheumatoid arthritis role, 342, 343
Mycophenolate mofetil, indications, 462
Myoblast,
    CD4+ T-cell interactions, 370, 371
    CD8+ T-cell interactions, 370
    immunological properties in culture, 370
Myositis, animal models, 303

N

Neutrophil,
    abundance, 243
    acquired deficiencies, 256
    adhesion molecules, 245, 246
    antirheumatic drug effects on function,
        colchicine, 254
        glucocorticoids, 253
        methotrexate, 253, 254
        nonsteroidal anti-inflammatory drugs, 253
    congenital disorders,
        Chediak–Higashi syndrome, 255
        chronic granulomatous disease, 254, 255
        leukocyte adhesion deficiency, 255, 256
        neutropenia, 254
    cytokine production, 244
    degranulation, 246, 247
    development, 243, 244
    disease roles,
        gout, 250, 251
        rheumatoid arthritis, 251, 252
        vasculitis, 252, 253
    granules, 243, 244
    microtubules, 245
    phagocytosis, 246
    receptor classes, 249
    signal transduction,
        activation, 249, 250
        chemotaxis, 248, 249
        superoxide production, 247, 248
    tissue injury, 243
    trafficking, 228–230, 244–246
    vasculitis role, 252, 253
New Zealand Black mouse, lupus model, 297
NF-AT, *see* Nuclear factor of activated T-cells
NF-κB, *see* Nuclear factor-κB
Nitric oxide (NO),
    apoptosis induction in cartilage, 274, 275
    cartilage degeneration role in osteoarthritis, 407
    inhibition in osteoarthritis, 510
    scleroderma role, 377
    tissue damage in inflammatory myopathies, 368
Nitrogen mustard, dosing for rheumatic disease, 458
NO, *see* Nitric oxide
Nonsteroidal anti-inflammatory drugs (NSAIDs),
    cyclooxygenase inhibition, 161, 166, 253
    neutrophil effects, 253
NOR90, autoantigen, 122
NSAIDs, *see* Nonsteroidal anti-inflammatory drugs
Nuclear factor of activated T-cells (NF-AT),
    T-cell receptor signaling, 78, 79, 94
    binding sequence, 117
    inflammation role, overview, 113, 114
    nuclear translocation, 118
    regulated functions, 118
    structural motifs, 113, 114
    therapeutic targeting, 123
Nuclear factor-κB (NF-κB),
    autoimmune disease role, 122
    binding sequence, 114
    domains, 115, 116
    glucocorticoid effects, 445–447
    inflammation role, overview, 113, 114
    inhibitor regulation, 116, 117

knockout mice, 122
nuclear translocation, 116
regulated genes, 115
regulated processes, 117
rheumatoid arthritis,
 defects, 48
 role, 340, 341, 345
structural motifs, 113, 114
therapeutic targeting, 123, 479
Nur77
autoimmune disease role, 122
domains, 121
inflammation role, overview, 113, 114

O

OA, *see* Osteoarthritis
Oct-1, autoimmune disease role, 122
Oncostatin M (OSM), arthritis role, 235
Oral tolerance,
 cytokine mediation, 491, 492
 mechanisms, 491, 492
 myelin basic protein in experimental autoimmune encephalomyelitis, 492
 rheumatoid arthritis trials, 493
OSM, *see* Oncostatin M
Osteoarthritis (OA),
 bone changes, 401, 402
 cartilage degeneration,
  collagen expression, 405
  cytokine regulation, 406, 407
  fibrillation, 403
  markers, 408, 409
  matrix metalloproteinases, 403, 404, 406, 499
  nitric oxide role, 407
  ossification, 406
  proteoglycan synthesis, 403–405
  sites, 402, 403
 chondrocyte role,
  cartilage homeostasis imbalance, 272
  extracellular matrix gene expression, 272, 273
  matrix degradation,
   matrix metalloproteinases, 273, 274
   signaling pathways, 274, 275
 clinical presentation, 401
 gene therapy, 510, 511
 synovitis and systemic inflammation, 407

treatment,
 molecular targets, 409, 410, 511
 screening techniques for early damage, 409
Osteoblast,
 alkaline phosphatase production, 286
 apoptosis, 289, 290
 control of development and differentiation,
  adhesion molecules, 285
  cytokines, 283, 284
  growth factors, 282, 283
  overview, 281
  systemic hormones, 284, 285
 lining cell differentiation, 287
 matrix protein secretion, 285, 286
 origin and differentiation, 279–281
Osteoclast,
 apoptosis, 289, 290
 control of development and differentiation,
  adhesion molecules, 285
  cytokines, 283, 284
  growth factors, 282, 283
  overview, 281
  systemic hormones, 284, 285
 histology, 288
 matrix degradation in bone resorption, 288, 289
 origin and differentiation, 279–281
 rheumatoid arthritis role, 346, 347
Osteocyte,
 features and functions, 287
 osteoporosis changes, 417, 418
Osteogenesis imperfecta,
 clinical features, 430, 431
 gene mutations,
  COL1A1, 431–433
  COL1A2, 431–433
  genotype-phenotype correlation, 433–435
 heredity, 423
 types, 430–432
Osteoporosis,
 definition, 413
 etiology and bone loss patterns, 413, 414
 glucocorticoids, pathogenesis of bone loss, 419, 420
 senescence, pathogenesis of bone loss, 418, 419

sex steroid deficiency, pathogenesis of
  bone loss,
    interleukin-1 role, 416, 417
    interleukin-6 role, 415, 416
    osteocyte changes, 417, 418
    protective mechanisms of sex steroids,
      414, 415
    tumor necrosis factor role, 416
  treatment,
    overview of drugs, 420
    parathyroid hormone, 420, 421

P

PAF, see Platelet-activating factor
Palmerston North mouse, lupus model, 299
Parathyroid hormone (PTH),
  bone cell development and differentiation
    role, 284, 285
  osteoporosis treatment, 420, 421
Paroxysmal nocturnal hemoglobinuria
  (PNH), complement
  activation, 153
Parvovirus B19
  apoptosis effects, 26
  arthritis induction and features, 15, 16
PCR, see Polymerase chain reaction
PDGF, see Platelet-derived growth factor
Phagocytosis,
    complement role, 152
    neutrophils, 246
Phospholipase A_2 (PLA$_2$),
    calcium-independent enzymes,
      164, 165
    catalytic reaction, 162
    regulation of expression, 164, 165
    small secreted calcium-dependent
      enzymes, 162, 164
    types, 162, 163
Phospholipase C (PLC), T-cell receptor
  signaling, 77, 78
Phototherapy, apoptosis induction, 49
PKC, see Protein kinase C
PLA$_2$, see Phospholipase A$_2$
Platelet-activating factor (PAF),
  acetylhydrolase, 171
  biosynthesis, 170
  functions, 170, 171
  receptor, 171

Platelet-derived growth factor (PDGF),
  rheumatoid arthritis
  role, 262
PLC, see Phospholipase C
PM, see Polymyositis
PNH, see Paroxysmal nocturnal
  hemoglobinuria
Polyarteritis nodosa, see Vasculitis
Polymerase chain reaction (PCR), diagnosis
  of viral infection, 21
Polymorphonuclear leukocyte, see Neutrophil
Polymyositis (PM),
  adhesion molecule expression in muscle
    lesions, 365, 366
  autoantigens, 367
  clinical features, 363
  cytokine expression, 365, 366, 370
  histopathology, 363, 364, 371
  T-cells,
    cytotoxic effector mechanisms, 368, 369
    myoblast interactions,
      CD4$^+$ T-cells, 370, 371),
      CD8$^+$ T-cells, 370
    phenotype and activation state, 366
    receptor repertoire of autoaggressive
      cells, 366–368
Population stratification, case control study
  problem, 7, 8
Promoter, transcriptional regulation, 111–113
Prostacyclin synthase, features, 167
Prostaglandins,
  history of study, 161
  inflammation role, 168
  receptors,
    clusters, 168, 169
    G protein coupling, 167
    peroxisome-activated receptors, 169
    PGD$_2$, 168
    PGE$_2$, 168
    PGF$_{2\alpha}$, 168
    PGI$_2$, 168
    thromboxane A$_2$, 168
  subclasses, 167
  synthesis, 165–167
Protein kinase C (PKC), T-cell receptor
  signaling, 78, 79, 94
Proteoglycan-induced arthritis, features of
  model, 296
PTH, see Parathyroid hormone

R

RA, *see* Rheumatoid arthritis
RANK, osteoclast differentiation role, 281, 282
Rap1, T-cell anergy role, 101, 103
Ras, T-cell receptor signaling, 79, 103
Rheumatoid arthritis (RA),
    antigen processing alterations, 328, 329
    apoptosis,
        defects in synovial cells, 47
        induction by therapeutics, 48, 49
        signaling in synovial cells, 47, 48
    B-cell role,
        affinity maturation, 331, 332
        autoantibodies, 332
        rheumatoid factor production, 332
    chondrocyte role, 275
    complement role, 156
    cytokine profile, 110
    genetic susceptibility, 327, 328
    immune complexes in pathogenesis, 130, 131
    immunotherapy,
        cytokines, 338, 339
        immunoglobulin removal, 338
        T-cell modulation, 331, 338
    linkage disequilibrium analysis, 329
    macrophage role,
        angiogenesis role, 228, 229
        foreign substance removal from synovial fluid, 231
        matrix degradation, 231, 232, 235, 334
        origin of cells, 227
        products and effects,
            anti-inflammatory molecules, 335, 336
            chemokines, 334, 335
            colony-stimulating factors, 236
            growth factors, 335
            interleukin-1 receptor antagonist, 234, 235, 335, 336
            interleukin-10, 238, 336
            matrix metalloproteinases, 334, 346
            overview, 232
            transforming growth factor-β, 236–238
            tumor necrosis factor-α, 232–234, 334
    membrane changes, 325, 326
    neutrophil role, 251, 252
    osteoclast role, 346, 347
    pannus lesions, 326, 327, 346
    persistence,
        adhesion molecules,
            expression and integrin ligation, 348
            fibroblast-like synoviocytes and synovial lining, 348, 349
            macrophages, 349
            monocytes, 349
    antigen-specific T-cell role, 350–352
    apoptosis in persistence,
        fibroblast-like synoviocyte, 352, 353
        induction as therapeutic approach, 353, 354
        macrophage, 353
        synovial tissue, 352
        T-cell, 353
    cell–cell interactions,
        endothelial cell ligands, 347, 348
        macrophage–fibroblast-like synoviocyte interaction, 352
        T-cell–fibroblast-like synoviocyte interaction, 349
        T-cell–monocyte interaction, 349, 350
    Lyme arthritis comparison, 347
    spread to Old World from Americas, 15
    synoviocyte role,
        adhesion molecule expression, 261
        antigen presentation, 260, 261
        cytokine and growth factor production, 261–263
        fibroblast-like synoviocytes, 336–338
        matrix degradation, 263, 264, 337
        oncogene expression and proliferation, 263
    T-cell role,
        cytokine expression, 329, 330
        receptor repertoire, 330, 331
        T-helper types, 330
    transcriptional regulation,
        AP-1, 342, 345
        C/EBPβ, 341, 342, 345, 346
        Erg-1, 343
        fibroblast-like synoviocytes, 343–346
        mitogen-activated protein kinase pathways, 342
        c-Myc, 342, 343

nuclear factor-κB, 340, 341, 345
overview, 339, 340
STAT, 343
treatment, see specific therapies
viruses in pathogenesis, 21, 22, 47, 328
Rheumatoid factor,
B-cell receptor activity, 220
immune complexes, 130, 131
normal versus pathogenic, 70–72
rheumatoid arthritis pathogenesis, 332
Rheumatoid vasculitis, see Vasculitis
Risk,
probability calculations, 3, 4, 8
relative risk, 5, 6
study design in evaluation, 5–7
RNA polymerase, transcriptional regulation, 111, 113
Rubella, arthritis induction and features, 15, 16, 18

S

Scleroderma,
animal models,
acute murine graft-versus-host disease, 302, 303
tight skin mouse, 302
autoantigens, 375, 376, 378, 379
clinical features and subsets, 375, 377
fibrosis,
cytokine roles, 380, 381
growth factor roles, 381
tissue distribution, 380
myositis, 303
pathogenesis, overview, 376
tolerance loss to self proteins, 379, 380
vasculopathy,
adhesion molecules, 377, 378
endothelial injury, 377, 378
vascular hyperactivity, 377, 378
SHP-1, inhibition of T-cell receptor signaling, 81
Sjögren's syndrome,
molecular mimicry, 23, 24
virus role, 19, 23
SLE, see Systemic lupus erythematosus
SLP-76, T-cell receptor signaling, 79, 80
Soluble complement receptor 1, complement inhibition therapy,

sCR1, 468, 469
sCR1 (desLHR-A), 469, 470
sCR1-SLe^x, 470
SP1, autoantigen, 122
Spondyloarthritis, animal models,
ank/ank mouse, 296
HLA-B27 transgenic rat, 296
STAT,
autoimmune disease role, 122
domains, 121
glucocorticoid effects, 445, 447
inflammation role, overview, 113, 114
kinase interactions, 120, 121
regulated genes, 121
rheumatoid arthritis role, 343
types, 120
Steroid receptors,
amino terminus transactivating domain, 442
DNA-binding domain, 440, 441
ligand-binding domain, 441
regulation of genes, 441, 442
types, 440
Stromelysin, matrix degradation, 263, 264
Sulfasalazine, apoptosis induction, 49
Synovial joint, morphogenesis, 267
Synoviocyte,
fibroblast-like synoviocyte, rheumatoid arthritis persistence role,
adhesion molecule expression, 348, 349
apoptosis, 352, 353
macrophage interaction, 352
T-cell interaction, 349
rheumatoid arthritis role,
adhesion molecule expression, 261
antigen presentation, 260, 261
cytokine and growth factor production, 261–263, 336, 337
fibroblast-like synoviocytes, 336–338
matrix degradation, 263, 264, 337
oncogene expression and proliferation, 263
transcriptional regulation in rheumatoid fibroblast-like synoviocytes, 343–346
types and features,
type A, 259, 260, 325
type B, 259, 260, 325, 336

Systemic lupus erythematosus (SLE),
  animal models,
    induced lupus,
      16/16 idiotype administration, 299, 300
      chronic graft-versus-host disease mouse, 300, 301
    spontaneous lupus,
      BXSB mouse, 298, 299
      MRL/*lpr/lpr* mouse, 297, 298
      New Zealand Black mouse, 297, 318
      Palmerston North mouse, 299
  antigen receptor-mediated signal transduction,
    aberrant T-cell and B-cell receptor signaling, 319, 320
    CD28/CTLA4:CD80/CD86 costimulation, 320, 321
  apoptosis defects,
    acceleration, 41, 42
    Bcl-2 dysregulation, 42–43
    cell residue clearance dysfunction and autoantibody production, 43, 44
    interleukin-10 dysregulation, 42
    overview, 41
    soluble Fas elevation, 44, 45
  autoantibodies, 515
  complement role, 152, 156, 157
  cytokine profile, 25, 110, 317–3319
  DNA autoantibodies, 71, 72, 316, 317
  drug-induced lupus, 315, 316
  estrogen abnormalities, 313, 314
  gene mapping,
    humans, 45, 46, 312
    mouse models, 46
  genetic susceptibility, 311–313, 515, 516
  immune complexes in pathogenesis, 129, 132, 133–135, 137, 138, 140, 322
  molecular mimicry, 23, 24
  silica exposure, 314
  smoking risks, 314
  T-helper cell imbalance,
    subsets, 317
    Th1 cytokines, decreased production, 317, 318
    Th2 cytokines, increased production, 318, 319
  treatment, *see also specific therapies*,
    gene therapy, 516, 521, 522
    overview of approaches, 322
  ultraviolet light triggering, 314
  viruses in pathogenesis, 21, 22, 315
Systemic sclerosis, *see* Scleroderma

T

Takayasu's arteritis, *see* Vasculitis
T-cell,
  activation, *see also* T-cell receptor, signal transduction,
    B7-1/B7-2:CD28/CTLA4 pathway, 92–98
    CD40 interaction with ligand, 91
    ICAM-1:LFA-1 pathway, 90, 91
    LFA-3:CD2 interactions, 91
    nuclear events, 209, 210
    two-signal model, 89–91
  anergy, 87, 90, 98, 101
  antigen-presenting cell interactions, 87–89
  azathioprine effects, 452, 453
  $CD4^+$ T cell inhibition for rheumatoid disease therapy,
    monoclonal antibodies, 478
    rationale, 477
  cyclophosphamide effects, 451, 452
  cyclosporine effects, 453
  cytotoxic T lymphocyte,
    killer cell inhibitory receptor expression, 206
    killing mechanisms,
      cytotoxic granules, 205
      Fas pathway, 205, 206
    subsets, 205
  γδ T-cell, functions, 208, 209
  inflammatory myopathy role,
    cytotoxic effector mechanisms, 368, 369
    myoblast interactions,
      $CD4^+$ T-cells, 370, 371),
      $CD8^+$ T-cells, 370
    phenotype and activation state, 366
    receptor repertoire of autoaggressive cells, 366–368
  memory T-cell,
    functions, 207, 208
    markers, 206
    subsets, 206, 207

methotrexate effects, 453
migration from thymus, 203
receptor diversity in thymus, 203
rheumatoid arthritis role,
   cytokine expression, 329, 330
   immunotherapy, 331
   persistence role,
      antigen-specific T-cells, 350–352
      apoptosis, 353
      fibroblast-like synoviocyte interaction, 349
      monocyte interaction, 349, 350
   receptor repertoire, 330, 331
   T-helper types, 330
subpopulations, 199, 200
T helper cell,
   balance modulation with gene therapy, 517, 518
   subsets and functions, 203, 204
thymocyte development,
   negative selection, 202, 203
   positive selection, 202
   stage I, 201
   stage II, 201
   stage III, 202
   thymus features, 200
tissue distribution, 199
tolerance, 87, 99–101, 103
vasculitis role,
   ANCA-associated vasculitides, 393
   polyarteritis nodosa, 393, 394
   rheumatoid vasculitis, 393, 394
T-cell receptor, signal transduction,
   adapter protein linking of signaling cascades, 79, 80
   apoptosis priming of cells, 82, 83
   B7-1/B7-2:CD28/CTLA4 pathway, 92–98
   calcineurin, 78, 79
   defects and disease, 75
   diacylglycerol, 78
   inhibitors, 80
   phospholipase C, 77, 78
   protein kinase C, 78, 79
   protein tyrosine kinases, 75–77, 79
   Ras, 79
   receptor peptide therapy, 478, 479, 495–497
   structure of receptor, 75
   supramolecular clusters, 90

systemic lupus erythematosus,
   aberrant T-cell and B-cell receptor signaling, 319, 320
   CD28/CTLA4:CD80/CD86 costimulation, 320, 321
T-cell activation role, 89
TDT, see Transmission disequilibruim testing
TGF-β, see Transforming growth factor-β
Thromboxane synthase, features, 167
TNF-α, see Tumor necrosis factor-α
Tolerance,
   B-cell, 66, 67, 221
   central tolerance, 487
   definition, 487
   Fas mutation effects, 40
   induction by interruption of costimulation,
      CD28, 99–101
      CTLA4, 99, 100
   mechanisms, 487, 488
   peripheral tolerance, 487
   T-cell, 87, 99–101, 103
   therapeutic approaches to restoration,
      antigen-directed therapy,
         altered peptide ligands, 493, 494
         B-cell tolerance induction, 494, 495
         oral tolerance, 491–493
         rationale, 490, 491
      autologous bone marrow transplantation, 489, 490
      major histocompatibility-directed therapy, 495
      overview, 488, 489, 497
      T-cell receptor-directed therapy, 495–497
TRAIL, apoptosis induction, 38, 40
Transcription, overview, 110–113
Transcription factors, see specific factors
Transforming growth factor-β (TGF-β),
   arthritis role, 236–238, 262, 263
   bone cell development and differentiation role, 284
   isoforms, 502
   knockout mouse, 303
   matrix metalloproteinase gene regulation, 502
   stimulation of collagen production, 193, 194
Transmission disequilibruim testing (TDT), risk probability analysis, 8

Transplant rejection, complement role, 157
Tumor necrosis factor-α (TNF-α),
   arthritis role, 232–234, 262, 334
   gene regulation, 340
   inhibition therapy,
      etanercept, 482, 483
      monoclonal antibodies,
         cA2, 510
         CDP571, 482
         infliximab, 481
      overview, 479, 480
   osteoporosis role, 416
   receptors, 481, 509, 510
Twin studies,
   autoimmune disease risk, 4, 5
   systemic lupus erythematosus, 515

V

Variable number of tandem repeats (VNTRs), genetic marker analysis, 11
Vasculitis,
   animal models,
      ANCA-associated vasculitis, 301, 302
      mercuric chloride induction in rat, 301
      MRL/*lpr/lpr* mouse, 301
      myeloperoxidase-immunized rat, 301
   anti-neutrophil cytoplasmic antibodies, 391, 392
   extravascular pathology, 386
   FcγRIIa receptor polymorphisms, 392, 393
   histopathology, 386
   immune complex,
      formation and deposition, 130, 390, 391
      pathogenesis role, 129, 130
   interplay of T-cells, macrophages, and arterial resident cells,
      giant cell arteritis, 394–396
      Takayasu's arteritis, 394, 396, 397
   leukocytes,
      adhesion molecules,
         expression, 388
         posttranslational modification, 389, 390
         regulation, 389
      endothelial interactions, 388, 389
   neutrophil role, 252, 253
   syndromes,
      overview of types, 385–387
      preferential vascular involvement, 387
   T-cell mediated immune responses,
      ANCA-associated vasculitides, 393
      polyarteritis nodosa, 393, 394
      rheumatoid vasculitis, 393, 394
   viral infection in pathogenesis, 397, 398
Versican, features and functions, 270
vFLIPs, *see* Viral FLICE-inhibitory proteins
Viral FLICE-inhibitory proteins (vFLIPs), death receptor signal blocking, 27
Vitamin D, bone cell development and differentiation role, 284
VNTRs, *see* Variable number of tandem repeats

Z

ZAP-70, T-cell receptor signaling, 77, 79, 94, 97